Y0-ABS-733

Synthesis and Chemistry of Agrochemicals

ACS SYMPOSIUM SERIES **355**

Synthesis and Chemistry of Agrochemicals

Don R. Baker, EDITOR
ICI Americas Inc.

Joseph G. Fenyes, EDITOR
Buckman Laboratories, Inc.

William K. Moberg, EDITOR
E. I. du Pont de Nemours & Co.

Barrington Cross, EDITOR
American Cyanamid Company

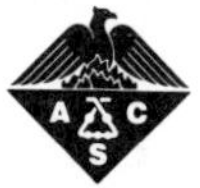

American Chemical Society, Washington, DC 1987

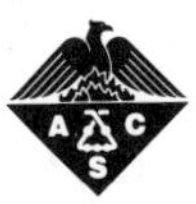

Library of Congress Cataloging-in-Publication Data

Synthesis and chemistry of agrochemicals/Don R. Baker, editor...[et al.].

p. cm.—(ACS symposium series, ISSN 0097-6156; 355)

"Developed from a series of symposia sponsored by the Division of Agrochemicals at the 189th-192nd Meetings of the American Chemical Society."

Bibliography: p.

Includes indexes.

ISBN 0-8412-1434-4

1. Pesticides—Synthesis—Congresses. 2. Pesticides—Testing—Congresses.

I. Baker, Don R., 1933- . II. American Chemical Society. Division of Agrochemicals. III. American Chemical Society. Meeting. IV. Series.

TP248.P47S96 1987
668′.65—dc19 87-22304
ISBN 0-8412-1434-4 CIP

Copyright © 1987

American Chemical Society

All Rights Reserved. The appearance of the code at the bottom of the first page of each chapter in this volume indicates the copyright owner's consent that reprographic copies of the chapter may be made for personal or internal use or for the personal or internal use of specific clients. This consent is given on the condition, however, that the copier pay the stated per copy fee through the Copyright Clearance Center, Inc., 27 Congress Street, Salem, MA 01970, for copying beyond that permitted by Sections 107 or 108 of the U.S. Copyright Law. This consent does not extend to copying or transmission by any means—graphic or electronic—for any other purpose, such as for general distribution, for advertising or promotional purposes, for creating a new collective work, for resale, or for information storage and retrieval systems. The copying fee for each chapter is indicated in the code at the bottom of the first page of the chapter.

The citation of trade names and/or names of manufacturers in this publication is not to be construed as an endorsement or as approval by ACS of the commercial products or services referenced herein; nor should the mere reference herein to any drawing, specification, chemical process, or other data be regarded as a license or as a conveyance of any right or permission, to the holder, reader, or any other person or corporation, to manufacture, reproduce, use, or sell any patented invention or copyrighted work that may in any way be related thereto. Registered names, trademarks, etc., used in this publication, even without specific indication thereof, are not to be considered unprotected by law.

PRINTED IN THE UNITED STATES OF AMERICA

ACS Symposium Series

M. Joan Comstock, *Series Editor*

1987 Advisory Board

Harvey W. Blanch
University of California—Berkeley

Alan Elzerman
Clemson University

John W. Finley
Nabisco Brands, Inc.

Marye Anne Fox
The University of Texas—Austin

Martin L. Gorbaty
Exxon Research and Engineering Co.

Roland F. Hirsch
U.S. Department of Energy

G. Wayne Ivie
USDA, Agricultural Research Service

Rudolph J. Marcus
Consultant, Computers & Chemistry Research

Vincent D. McGinniss
Battelle Columbus Laboratories

W. H. Norton
J. T. Baker Chemical Company

James C. Randall
Exxon Chemical Company

E. Reichmanis
AT&T Bell Laboratories

C. M. Roland
U.S. Naval Research Laboratory

W. D. Shults
Oak Ridge National Laboratory

Geoffrey K. Smith
Rohm & Haas Co.

Douglas B. Walters
National Institute of Environmental Health

AUGUSTANA UNIVERSITY COLLEGE
LIBRARY

Foreword

The ACS SYMPOSIUM SERIES was founded in 1974 to provide a medium for publishing symposia quickly in book form. The format of the Series parallels that of the continuing ADVANCES IN CHEMISTRY SERIES except that, in order to save time, the papers are not typeset but are reproduced as they are submitted by the authors in camera-ready form. Papers are reviewed under the supervision of the Editors with the assistance of the Series Advisory Board and are selected to maintain the integrity of the symposia; however, verbatim reproductions of previously published papers are not accepted. Both reviews and reports of research are acceptable, because symposia may embrace both types of presentation.

Contents

FUNGICIDES

OTHER CONTROL METHODS

Preface

REVOLUTIONARY CHANGES have linked chemistry with agriculture during this century. Agricultural chemicals, properly chosen and applied, offer great benefit to food and fiber producers and consumers alike. The need for new agrochemicals has not abated. Indeed, the growing demand for safe and effective agricultural chemicals has spurred major research effort for new products. The prime goal of researchers is discovering materials that will economically control plant pathogens, insect pests, and weeds and at the same time be of minimal risk to humans and the environment in general.

The challenge for scientists who seek to discover and develop new crop protection chemicals has escalated dramatically. It is becoming increasingly more difficult to satisfy the many safety requirements of the various regulatory agencies. The costs associated with development of a new agrochemical are escalating. Until recently, the challenge has been compounded by the lack of regular scientific interchange among those chemists involved in the discovery process. With the ever-increasing world population, the assistance that these new compounds bring to food production is critical. We hope that the work reported here will be useful to those who accept this challenge.

We have organized a series of symposia at each national meeting of the American Chemical Society, beginning with the St. Louis meeting in 1984. The aim of these symposia has been to provide a forum for presenting the synthesis and chemistry of new agrochemical agents. In addition, chemists have seized their opportunity to discuss the biological properties of the new materials. These symposia are providing a focus for agricultural chemists.

In a similar vein, we hope that this book will provide a view of the current synthetic effort in the agrochemical field. In this volume, a variety of topics has been assembled, ranging from that first symposium to the recent one held in Anaheim in 1986. The chapters in this collection show varied approaches to the discovery process in the agrochemical field, and they represent the current status of these synthetic efforts. The information has been updated to convey the current state of the endeavor.

In the past, publication of new synthetic chemistry and the structures of novel agrochemicals has been largely in the patent literature because most of the major advances come from the agrochemical industry. Many interesting discoveries have not been made accessible because the compounds lacked commercial potential. The agrochemical synthesis symposia have provided at least a parallel avenue for synthesis chemists to make their discoveries public. Furthermore, these symposia provide a unique forum for this assemblage of pesticide chemistry.

Because most of the synthetic effort in the U.S. agrochemical industry is devoted to the development of new herbicides and insecticides, much of the information found in this book is devoted to these two major fields. An effort was also made to give representation to the other important areas of agrochemical synthesis. We particularly appreciate the efforts of those who provided these extraordinary chapters.

We express appreciation to the authors for sharing this large amount of useful chemistry and, most importantly, for sharing their practical insight into the workings of biologically active molecules. We thank the companies and organizations that have cleared much of this work for publication. We hope that by providing an overview of the chemical and biochemical tools available for agrochemical discovery and by sharing viewpoints of many scientists, this volume can contribute to continuing the successful partnership of chemistry and agriculture.

DON R. BAKER
ICI Americas Inc.
Richmond, CA 94804

JOSEPH G. FENYES
Buckman Laboratories, Inc.
Memphis, TN 38108

WILLIAM K. MOBERG
Agricultural Products Department
E. I. du Pont de Nemours & Co.
Wilmington, DE 19898

BARRINGTON CROSS
Agricultural Research Division
American Cyanamid Company
Princeton, NJ 08540

June 9, 1987

Chapter 1

Overview of Agrochemical Development

Don R. Baker [1], Joseph G. Fenyes [2], William K. Moberg[3], and Barrington Cross[4]

[1]ICI Americas Inc., 1200 South 47th Street, Richmond, CA 94804
[2]Buckman Laboratories, 1256 North McLean Boulevard, Memphis, TN 38108
[3]Agricultural Products Department, E. I. du Pont de Nemours & Co., Experimental Station, Building 402, Wilmington, DE 19898
[4]Agricultural Research Division, American Cyanamid Company, P.O. Box 400, Princeton, NJ 08540

Since the earliest of recorded time, man has fought with the environment in tilling his fields. At first largely by hand, then with the hoe, and later the plow. First with the aid of animals, later with machinery. Chemicals too, gradually found a place in providing a suitable environment. The Romans used salt to remove unwanted vegetation, and sulfur was used to control a variety of pests. The dawn of the twentieth century saw many inorganic compounds being used as agrochemicals. Then, the 1940's saw the coming of the first generation of synthetic organic agrochemicals including DDT (1), 2,4-D (2), and parathion (3).

As technology advances, each step brings certain blessings and often unexpected problems. Such was the case with the first generation of organic agrochemicals. The farmer's yields were greater and costs were lower. But the first generation compounds did not solve all of the problems. DDT was too persistent and had an adverse effect on some species of wildlife (4-5). There was accumulation in the food chain, thin eggshells, and genetic effects in some species. Because of these various health and environmental concerns, DDT became embroiled in controversy (6-7). Parathion was too toxic for the average home gardener, indeed, it was too toxic for the average farmer. Even a fine herbicide like 2,4-D had its limitations. It is primarily active on broadleaf plants. This makes it fine for some weeds in small grains and grasses, but useless for broadleaf crops. Here was a need for later generations of herbicides. As 2,4-D controlled the broadleaf weeds, the resistant weeds such as wild oats (*Avena fatua*), Johnsongrass (*Sorghum halepense*), and

0097-6156/87/0355-0001$06.00/0
© 1987 American Chemical Society

foxtails (Setaria sp.) became problems in the United States. In Europe the problem weeds were the cleavers (Galium sp.), chickweed (Stellaria sp.), blackgrass (Alopecurus myosuroides), and wild oats. Wild oats became such a problem in Europe that control of this single weed was incentive enough to develop herbicides solely for its control. Compounds such as diclofop-methyl (8), difenzoquat (9), and flamprop (10) were developed to meet this need.

The metallic fungicides used in the first half of the twentieth century were largely replaced by the protective fungicides such as captan (11-12) and later the new systemics such as benomyl (13).

Gradually the unwanted side effects of these first generation agrochemicals made it apparent that a successful agrochemical must have the proper environmental, toxicological, and cost characteristics in addition to its basic useful action. Each of these general requirements has several criteria that must be satisfied before a particular compound is commercialized (14). Tens of thousands of compounds must be prepared and tested before one is found that has a suitable combination of properties that will warrant commercial development. Since the cost of generating any new product is staggering, only products targeted toward markets which have a high potential for profit are developed. A negative side effect of this process is that chemicals for minor crop markets are often ignored. Therefore, any process that can lessen the number of compounds prepared and tested before a commercial product is found is of major importance.

The question is often asked, "How do you discover a new agrochemical?" The random synthesis and screening method gave us the first generation of agrochemicals. As we have seen, however, these compounds were not without their problems. The next successful approach is exemplified by the organophosphate insecticides. Here the dimethyl or diethyl dithiophosphate group was attached to just about any type of available building block. This approach was later extended to include the phosphonate analogs. Through a comparison of the insecticidal and toxicological data, structure-activity theories were developed which provided a means for the synthesis of safer compounds. A similar approach was used in the 2,4-D area. All manner of substituted phenoxy and benzoic acids and their derivatives were prepared. As a result, much was learned about the structural relationships for the auxin type action. This analog synthesis procedure has often been called "me too chemistry". The patent literature abounds with examples of such a strategy tried on almost everything that has shown a modicum of biological activity. Just as 2,4-D is a mimic of natural auxin, most critical natural products peculiarly associated with plants, insects or microorganisms have been studied with a wide variety of mimics, and analogs. Now it is a common practice for research organizations to do their own "me too chemistry" on their promising compounds. The ·urpose of this approach is to fully understand the structure-activity relationships of those new compounds before the scientific community at large becomes aware of their significance, primarily to solidify and defend primary patent positions.

Another interesting approach is the design of new compounds that interact with a critical enzyme of interest. This strategy has been fruitful in pharmaceutical research, resulting in major compounds such as cimetidine. Some have labeled this strategy as biochemical design. The same strategy is indeed possible in the agrochemical area. As yet we know of no commercial agrochemicals that have come by this route; but, this is none the less a flourishing area for current research (15). A current example is the use of bioisosteres. Agrochemical discovery groups also employ techniques such as quantitative structure-activity relationships (QSAR) as exemplified by the strategy of Corwin Hansch (16). Related to this approach is the use of molecular modeling and computer aided synthetic design (17). These new tools promise to yield interesting new compounds which may someday find commercial use.

To date, the greatest degree of success has come as a consequence of opportunity. Some, for want of a better label, have called it serendipity (18). However, in a real sense it is much more than luck. Usually this takes the form of someone recognizing an unusual result. Many individuals seeing the same event may not have the required insight. The unexpected result may be one compound out of a group of compounds, which for some unknown reason, has unusual properties or characteristics when compared with others in the group. It may be a compound that has chemically or metabolically changed into another compound which is strangely active. It may be an impurity in an otherwise inactive compound. It may be an intermediate on the path to preparation of another material. It may be that a creative new screening test shows activity for a seamingly inactive material. It certainly pays to keep alert. Benjamin Franklin perhaps said it best when he remarked, "The harder I work, the luckier I get!"

Herbicides

The basic idea behind the early herbicides was that you sprayed a group of plants with a compound and the weeds were killed leaving the crop unharmed. This type of compound has come to be known as a post-emergent herbicide. Fairly quickly, it was found that for certain crops such as corn, cotton, and soybeans, it was hard to find compounds that killed the weeds without injury to the crop. The second generation of herbicides included those that required application to the soil before the crop and weeds emerged. In this way many of the troublesome weeds could be eliminated in selective crops. Included were compounds such as the trifluralin, atrazine, and the chloracetamide herbicides. Here the farmer had to be convinced to spray his field before the crop and weeds emerged. For some herbicides, maximum activity required a variation of this pre-emergent surface application method. Trifluralin suffers from light instability and high volatility. It was found that shallow incorporation in the soil greatly aids its herbicidal effect. Incorporation (19) was absolutely essential for the herbicidal action of the thiolcarbamate (20) herbicides because of their volatile nature.

With the advent of these second generation compounds came the finding that many different steps in the plant's biochemistry are susceptible to chemical exploitation (21-28). Those pathways that are different from other forms of life are prime targets for attack in the design of new agrochemicals (30). Toxicologically safer compounds are more likely to be found by this approach.

The first chapter in the herbicide section is devoted to synthetic efforts related to the herbicide Command, currently being developed by FMC Corporation. Here we see detailed the various synthetic and structure-activity relationships of this important group of compounds. These compounds exert their phytotoxic effect by their bleaching action on a wide variety of economic weeds. An important observation was that soybeans were not affected at normal use rates. These compounds act upon the carotene and chlorophyll biosynthesis of the plant. Here are a group of synthetic pathways that are peculiar to plants and a few microorganisms and are susceptible to chemical attack.

This spectacular bleaching effect is discussed in other chapters of this work, such as the N-benzylideneamino heterocycles of the Shell workers, the nicotinamides of Stauffer, the pyridazines of American Cyanamid and the furanones of Chevron. Various aspects of carotenoid biosynthesis inhibition have been presented in other places (27,31), however, we see here some of the exciting new chemistry associated with these powerful compounds.

The discovery process for Dow's Tandem herbicide and the synthesis details associated with the hundreds of new compounds prepared during the discovery process of this interesting new herbicide are described in another chapter. The finding in field tests that Tridiphane and Atrazine were synergistic is an example of opportunity presenting itself and an aware biologist recognizing the significance of the phenomenon.

The workers at American Cyanamid present some of the synthetic and biological characteristics of the sulfur analogs of their imidazoline family of herbicides. This is an example of replacing the carbonyl of the imidazolinone with an isosteric moiety. This is an interesting account of the synthesis and structure-activity relationships in a very active series of herbicides.

Other interesting new chemistry using bioisosteres is presented in the benzylnitramines of American Cyanamid, the vinylogous ureas of Stauffer, the tetrahydrofuranes of Chevron, and triazinones of FMC. The nitramines of this current example seem to function as a bioisostere of a carboxylic acid. The vinylogous ureas are another example of a possible homologous bioisostere at work. And finally, the triazinones appear to behave as imide bioisosteres. These certainly are concepts which merit wider attention.

The studies devoted to the natural herbicide, cyanobacterin, and the rigid peptide reported by the USDA workers show herbicidal effects and give insight into the potential geometry or fit for other active compounds that have the desired spatial and electronic characteristics.

Insecticides

Prior to the advent of DDT and the organophosphates, the natural pyrethrins (32,33) found considerable use but were limited by their instability. The discovery of permethrin by Michael Elliot (34) proved a turning point for the new synthetic pyrethroids. Here were very active compounds that did not suffer from the stability problems of the natural compounds. And even now pyrethroid-like compounds continue to interest synthetic chemists due to their high insecticidal activity and relatively low mammalian toxicity. You would think that by now most of the very active compounds would have been found. But it seems that persistence and originality pay off. Workers at du Pont and FMC detail the structure-activity relationships for two groups of new pyrethroid-like compounds. Chemists at Dow reveal some of the intricacies in the synthesis of the cyclopropane carboxylate end of the molecule.

Carbamates and phosphates continue to be made by chemists the world over. Amazingly, they continue to find very active materials. Chemists at Shell and at Ricerca describe their efforts with this active area. Other interesting types of active compounds such as the oxadiazoles and diazenecarboxamides are also described.

Even compounds related to DDT (35) are of interest. Iowa State workers describe some diphenylchloronitroalkane compounds and their synthesis and biological properties.

These new compounds offer the possibility of less persistance than DDT. Many are quite active. USDA chemists have found that perfluorinated sulfonamides and sulfonates have a delayed action on the fire ant.

Natural products such as the avermectins and milbemycin produce very active insecticides. Chemistry in this area is presented in one chapter. Juvenile hormone activity (36) still is of interest, and current work is described in this field.

Fungicides

Advances in fungicide chemistry were recently reviewed (37). Recent fungicide research points out a factor common to all areas -- the growing problem of pest resistance (38-39). Since bacteria and fungi can go through their life cycle quite rapidly, resistance to a control agent can develop rapidly. This is particularly true if the compound affects only one biochemical target site in the pest. Today we are seeing resistance develop to many of our most useful fungicides, which again points out the pressing need to find new products.

Fungicide research receives less attention by synthesis chemists in the United States than do the herbicide and insecticide disciplines. Overseas chemists find a much greater market for fungicides than do their American counterparts. One of the chapters indicates the interest of the Japanese in fungicides. Two chapters attest to England's contributions to fungicide chemistry. These ergosterol biosynthesis inhibitors continue to attract effort from around the world as evidenced by these workers and the reports from American authors.

Organosilicon compounds seem to have found a niche in fungicides. Interesting chemistry and the biological response to it is described for a new oganosilicon fungicide.

Laetisaric acid, a hydroxylated fatty acid isolated from a soil fungus, is described. Its structure-activity relationships led to the design of even more active and simpler compounds. This example provides another illustration of the value of natural compounds and the valuable information that they provide.

Other Control Methods

This section of the book presents a variety of synthetic experience in a wide assortment of agrochemical applications outside the standard areas. Included are such areas as strigol, pheromones, chemical hybridizing agents, and plant growth regulators (40).

Conclusions

The chapters of this book provide a look at the current synthesis rational employed in the agrochemical industry. We beleive this collection chronicles a significant proportion of the recent advances in the field. Only a very few compounds have those characteristics that encourage commercialization. The considerable body of knowledge reported here hopefully will aid those interested in the design of future active materials.

Literature Cited

1. Muller, P. Helv. Chim. Acta 1946, 29, 1560-80.
2. Zimmerman, P. W.; Hitchcock, A. E. Contrib. Boyce Thompson Inst. 1942, 12, 321.
3. Martin, H.; Shaw H. BIOS, Final Report 1946, No. 1095.
4. Ware, G. W. Residue Reviews 1975, 59, 119-40.
5. Benvenue, A. Residue Reviews 1976, 61, 37-112.
6. Beatty, R. G. The DDT Myth; John Day Co.: New York, 1973.
7. Marco, G. J.; Hollingworth, R. M.; Durham, W., eds. Silent Spring Revisited; American Chemical Society: Washington, DC, 1986.
8. Becker, W.; Langelueddeke, P.; Leditschke, H.; Nahm, H.; Schwerdtle, F. German Patent 2 223 864, 1973.
9. Walworth, B. L.; Klingsberg, E. U. S. Patent 3 882 142, 1975.
10. Jeffcoat, B.; Harries, W. N.; Thomas, D. B. Pesticide Sci. 1977, 8, 1-12.
11. Kittleson, A. R. U. S. Patent 2 553 770, 1951.
12. Kittleson, A. R. Science 1952, 115, 84-6.
13. Delp, C. J.; Klopping, H. L. Plant Dis. Rep. 1968, 52, 95.
14. Ragsdale, N. N.; Kuhr, R. J., eds. Pesticides: Minimizing the Risks; ACS Symposium Series No. 336; American Chemical Society: Washington, DC, 1987.
15. Magee, P. S.; Kohn, G. K.; Menn, J.J., eds. Pesticide Synthesis Through Rational Approaches; ACS Symposium Series No. 255; American Chemical Society: Washington, DC, 1984.
16. Hansch, C.; Leo, A. Substituent Constants for Correlation Analysis in Chemistry and Biology; Wiley: New York, 1979.
17. Olsen, E. C.; Christoffersen, R. E.; eds. Computer Assisted Drug Design; ACS Symposium Series No. 112; American Chemical Society: Washington, DC, 1979.
18. D'Amico, J. J. in Innovation and U. S. Research; Smith, W.N.; Arson, C. F., ed.; ACS Symposium Series No. 129; American Chemical Society: Washington, DC, 1980, pp 143-6.
19. Antoginini, J. J. Am. Sugar Beet Technologists, 1962, no. 2, 94-9.

20. Tilles, H. J. Am. Chem. Soc. 1959, 81, 714-27.
21. Crafts, A. S. in Advances in Pest Control Research, vol. 1, Metcalf, R. L., ed.; Interscience: New York, 1957, pp 39-80.
22. Crafts, A. S. The Chemistry and Mode of Action of Herbicides; Interscience: New York, 1961.
23. Corbett, J. R.; Wright, K.; Baillie, A. C. The Biochemical Mode of Action of Pesticides, 2nd ed.; Academic Press: London, 1984.
24. Audus, L. J., ed. Physiology and Biochemistry of Herbicides; Academic Press: London, 1964.
25. Ashton, F. M.; Crafts, A. S. Mode of Action of Herbicides; Wiley: New York, 1973.
26. Kearney, P. C.; Kaugmann, D. D. Herbicides: Chemistry, Degradation and Mode of Action; 2nd edition, vol. 1-2; Dekker: New York, 1975.
27. Moreland, D. E.; St.John, J. B.; Hess, F. D., eds. Biochemical Responses Induced by Herbicides; ACS Symposium Series No. 181; American Chemical Society: Washington, DC, 1982.
28. Fletcher, W. W.; Kirkwood, R. C. Herbicides and Plant Growth Regulators; Granada: London, 1982.
29. Heitz, J. R.; Downum, K. R., eds. Light-Activated Pesticides; ACS Symposium Series No. 339; American Chemical Society: Washington, DC, 1987.
30. Hedin, P. A., ed. Bioregulators for Pest Control; ACS Symposium Series No. 276; American Chemical Society: Washington, DC, 1985.
31. Britton, G.; Goodwin, T. W., eds. Carotenoid Chemistry and Biochemistry; Pergamon: Oxford, 1982.
32. Cassida, J. E. Pyrethrum: The Natural Insecticide; Academic Press: New York, London, 1973.
33. Jacobsen, M.; Crosby, D. G. Naturally Occurring Insecticides; Marcel Dekker: New York, 1971.
34. Elliott, M., ed. Synthetic Pyrethroids; ACS Symposium Series No. 42; American Chemical Society; Washington, DC, 1977.
35. Coats, J. R., ed. Insecticide Mode of Action; Academic Press: New York, London, 1982.
36. Menn. J. J.; Beroza, M., eds. Insect Juvenile Hormones: Chemistry and Action; Academic Press: New York, 1972.
37. Green, M. B.; Spilker, D. A., eds. Fungicide Chemistry: Advances and Practical Applications; ACS Symposium Series No. 304; American Chemical Society: Washington, DC, 1986.
38. Georghiou, G. P.; Saito, T., eds. Pest Resistance to Pesticides; Plenum Press: New York, London, 1983.
39. Glass, E. H.; et. al. Pesticide Resistance: Strategies and Tactics for Management; National Academic Press: Washington, DC, 1986.
40. Mandava, N. B., ed. Plant Growth Substances; ACS Symposium Series No. 111; American Chemical Society: Washington, DC, 1979.

RECEIVED June 9, 1987

HERBICIDES

Chapter 2

3-Isoxazolidinones and Related Compounds

A New Class of Herbicides

J. H. Chang, M. J. Konz, E. A. Aly, R. E. Sticker, K. R. Wilson, N. E. Krog, and P. R. Dickinson

Agricultural Chemical Group, FMC Corporation, Box 8, Princeton, NJ 08543

Several 2-aryl- and 2-phenylmethyl-3,5-isoxazolidinediones were synthesized and found to be bleaching herbicides with good tolerance by soybeans. The most active member, 2-(2-chlorophenyl)methyl-4,4-dimethyl-3,5-isoxazolidinedione, failed to perform in the field due to its instability in soil. To improve the chemical stability by molecular modifications, a series of 3-isoxazolidinones were prepared and found to be highly active bleaching herbicides with excellent soybean tolerance. Synthesis and structure-activity relationships are discussed. One of the most active compounds, 2-[(2-chlorophenyl)methyl]-4,4-dimethyl-3-isoxazolidinone (FMC 57020), has been developed for commercial use.

In an effort to find new agricultural herbicides a new class of broad spectrum soybean herbicides, the 3-isoxazolidinones, was discovered. The discovery, synthesis, and structure - activity relationships of this new class of herbicides and the related compounds will be discussed.

3,5-Isoxazolidinediones

Isoxazolidinediones have been of interest in the last 20 years for their antiphlogestic, analgesic, and local anesthetic properties (1-4). As no herbicidal activity had been reported and since heterocyclic ring systems have played a large role in the development of new and useful herbicide products, a synthesis program was initiated to investigate the potential of 2-aryl- and 2-phenylmethyl-3,5-isoxazolidinediones (1) as weed control agents. In each case, a similar set of targets were prepared.

0097-6156/87/0355-0010$06.00/0
© 1987 American Chemical Society

Synthesis. Synthesis was accomplished as shown in Schemes 1 and 2. Reduction of the nitrobenzene with zinc/ammonium chloride gave the corresponding hydroxylamine 2. Due to the difficulty in purification, the crude reduction product was used in the reaction with dimethylmalonyl dichloride. This procedure was satisfactory in that yields of 50 to 80% of the dione 3 could be obtained.

Benzaldoximes (4), obtained from the corresponding benzaldehyde and hydroxylamine, were selectively reduced to the hydroxylamine 5 with sodium cyanoborohydride by the procedure of Borch, Bernstein, and Durst (5). Upon scaling-up this reduction, we found it convenient to dissolve the oxime in methanol containing methyl orange as an indicator. Methanol solutions of sodium cyanoborohydride and hydrochloric acid were then added simultaneously with the rate of acid addition adjusted so as to maintain the red-orange transition point of the indicator. Yields were quite satisfactory, in the range of 60-80%. Reaction of the hydroxylamine with the malonyl dichloride gave the desired compounds (6).

Herbicidal Activity. The 2-phenylisoxazolidinediones (3) were tested at 8 kg/ha on lima beans, wild oats and crabgrass. Although no significant kill was observed, the test species were injured as evidenced by their chlorotic condition and stunted appearance.

Similar results were observed from 2-phenymethylisoxazolidinediones (6) with the exception of the compound containing a chlorine in the two position of the aromatic ring, coded FMC 55626 (6, x=2-Cl). In preemergent applications, FMC 55626 completely controlled the test species. In this case, the germinating species emerged bleached, an effect that proved sufficient to cause the death of the plant. This test generated a great deal of interest because the only species that was not bleached were soybeans. In foliar applications, bleaching was also evident but no significant control resulted.

The herbicidal activity of FMC 55626 at 1 kg/ha is summarized in Table I. Crops other than soybeans, e.g., cotton, corn, and wheat, are not tolerant. Velvetleaf and lambsquarters were quite susceptible (85-98%) whereas cocklebur and jimsonweed control ranged from 55-80%. Among the grass species, johnsongrass was the least susceptible (20% control).

Structure-Activity Relationships. With this encouraging data, an extensive synthesis program was undertaken with the objective of improving activity while maintaining tolerance toward soybeans. These results are summarized in Tables II-IV.

The choice of substituents in the aromatic ring is limited to halogen with chlorine being the most effective. The position of this substituent is also important in that it must be on the two-position of the ring. A similar situation exists in multi-substituted analogs. The 2,5-dichloro and 2,4-dichloroisoxazolidinedione were active but neither substitution pattern was as effective as a single chlorine at the two-position.

A number of functionalities at the four-position of the heterocyclic ring were also investigated. Geminal dialkyl substitution was found to be essential for activity. Maximum effectiveness was

3,5-Isoxazolidinediones

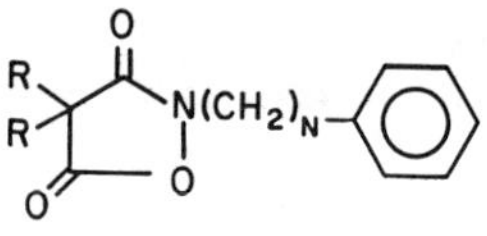
O
R
R
N(CH2)N
O
O

1 N= 0- 1

Structure 1

2-Phenyl-4,4-Dimethyl-3,5-Isoxazolidinediones

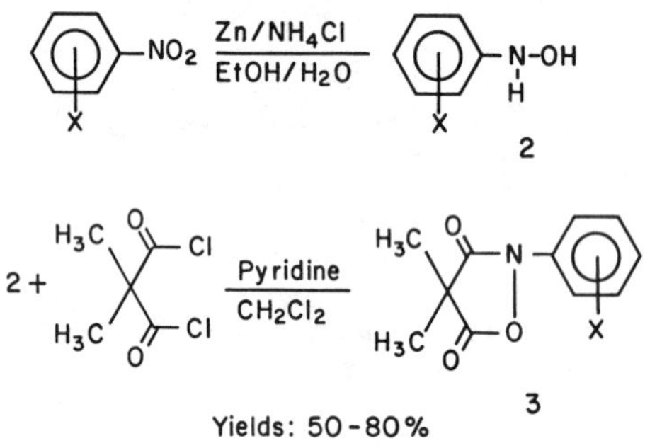
NO2
Zn/NH4Cl
EtOH/H2O
N-OH
H
X
2
2+
H3C
Cl
Pyridine
CH2Cl2
N
O
X
Yields: 50-80%
3

X=H; 2-Cl
4-Cl; 4-CH3

Scheme 1

2-Phenylmethyl-4,4-Dimethyl-3,5-Isoxazolidinediones

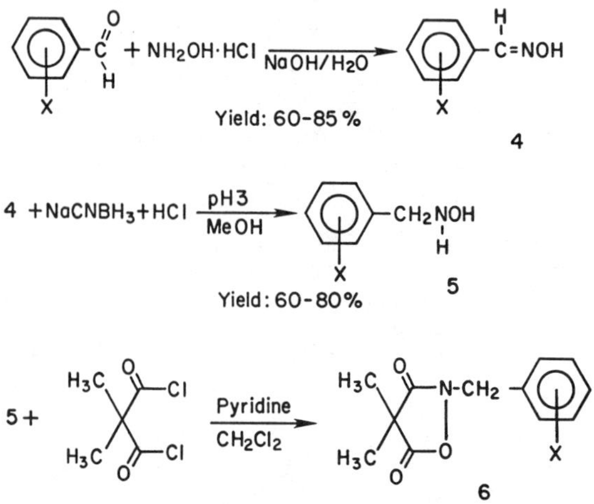
C
H
+ NH2OH·HCl
NaOH/H2O
C=NOH
X
Yield: 60-85 %
4
4 +NaCNBH3+HCl
pH3
MeOH
CH2NOH
H
5
Yield: 60-80%
5+
H3C
Cl
Pyridine
CH2Cl2
N-CH2
O
6

Yield: 50-60% X=H; 2-Cl
4-Cl; 4-CH3

Scheme 2

Table I. Pre-emergent Herbicidal Activity of FMC 55626

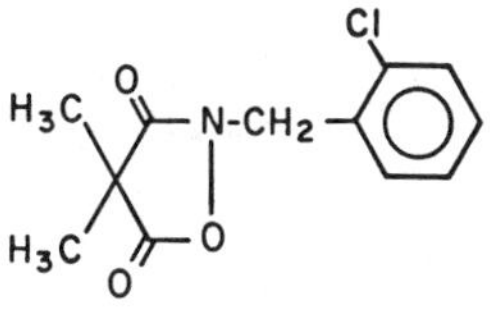

Crops	% Control at 1 kg/ha
Soybean	0
Cotton, Corn, Wheat	90–100
Broadleaf Weeds	
Velvetleaf, Lambsquater	85–98
Cocklebur, Jimsonweed	55–80
Grass Weeds	
Barnyardgrass, Crabgrass	100
Johnsongrass, Greenfoxtail	20–50

Table II. Herbicidal Activity at 8 kg/ha

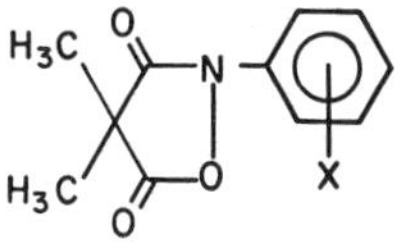

X = H; 2-Cl; 4-Cl; 4-CH_3

Test Species: Lima Beans, Wild Oats, Crabgrass

Results

No Significant Kill (Pre-or Postemergent)

Test Species Chlorotic and Stunted

Table III. Herbicidal Activity at 8 kg/ha

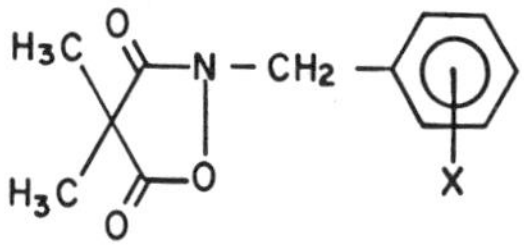

Test Species: Lima Bean, Wild Oats, Crabgrass

X	Preemergent % Control	Postemergent % Control
H	7	24
4-CH	9	10
4-Cl	14	14
2-Cl*	100	23

*FMC 55626

Table IV. Structure–Activity Relationships

Aryl Substituents

H_3C, H_3C; N-CH_2-(phenyl)-X

Monosubstitution
2-Position
Active: Cl > Br > F
Inactive: CH_3; CH_3O; CF_3; NO_2

3-and 4-Position
Inactive: Cl; F; CH_3; CH_3O; CF_3

Multiple Substitution
Active: 2,5-DiCl >2,4-DiCl
Inactive: 2,3-DiCl; 3,4-DiCl; 2,6-DiCl

4-Position of Heterocyclic Ring

R_2, R_2; N-CH_2-(2-Cl-phenyl)

Active
$R_1 = R_2 = CH_3 > R_1 = CH_3, R_2 = CH_3CH_2$

Inactive
$R_1 = R_2 = H; CH_3CH_2; -(CH_2)_2-$
$R_1, R_2 = CH_3, H; CH_3, Cl$

2-Position of Heterocyclic Ring

H_3C, H_3C; N-R

Inactive
R = (2-Cl-phenyl)-CH(CH_3)-; (2-Cl-phenyl)-CH_2CH_2-; (2-Cl-phenyl)-OCH_2-
(2-Cl-phenyl)-C(=O)-; (2-Cl-phenyl)-NH-C(=O)-
(thienyl)-CH_2-; (furyl)-CH_2-

observed when R_1 and R_2 were methyl. Surprisingly, spirosystems such as cyclopropyl were totally inactive.

A similar situation occurred when the (2-chlorophenyl)methyl was replaced with related structures. For example, the 1-(2-chlorophenyl)ethyl and the 2-(2-chlorophenyl)ethyl analogs not only were ineffective in weed control, but the typical bleaching response was also absent.

The principal conclusion was that the structural requirements for activity were quite specific and that FMC 55626 apparently represented the most active compound in this class.

Field Test Results. During the course of this program, FMC 55626 was field tested at rates from 0.5 to 4 kg/ha. As under greenhouse conditions, the germinating seedlings were bleached but the plants rapidly outgrew this injury. The result (Table V) was minimum weed control of even the most sensitive species--velvetleaf (63%), pigweed (40%) and barnyardgrass (33%).

These results appeared to be inconsistent with the general experience in translation of greenhouse application rates to field conditions. One of several possible explanations was that FMC 55626 could be susceptible to microbial degradation. As shown in Table VI, microbial degradation does appear to be a factor. In autoclaved field soil, barnyardgrass and velvetleaf were readily controlled at 0.5 kg/ha whereas, in non-autoclaved soil, there was essentially no control at this rate.

Chemical degradation could also be a factor. As many soils contain nitrogenous bases, such as ammonia and ethanolamine, it was of interest to determine the chemical reactivity of FMC 55626 with amines.

Treatment of FMC 55626 with triethylamine (Scheme 3) resulted in gas evolution, presumably carbon dioxide, and formation of complex reaction products. Although the components of this reaction have not been identified, the NMR spectrum did show a peak that could be assigned to the methine proton of an isobutyric acid. In the case of two primary amines (methylamine and aniline), cleavage of the acyl oxygen bond occurred to give the bis-amides 7. These amides are similar in activity to FMC 55626 and, like FMC 55626, are several times more active in autoclaved soils.

Conclusion. Chemical transformation of FMC 55626 could occur in the soil but which of the two pathways is dominant is unknown. In any event, the end products appear to be herbicidally inactive. In conclusion, isoxazolidinediones were found to be herbicidally active but also appear to be susceptible to microbial and/or chemical degradation.

3-Isoxazolidinones

It is clear that the instability of FMC 55626 greatly reduces its field performance. The search for a solution to this problem became our prime concern. The observed gas evolution under mildly basic conditions suggests that the decarboxylation of FMC 55626 is a facile process. It was, therefore, desirable to remove the "lactone" carbonyl group from the isoxazolidinedione system 6 to

Table V. Pre-emergent Herbicide Field Test

FMC 55626

Species	%Control at 30 Days (4 kg/ha)
Velvetleaf	63
Pigweed	40
Barnyardgrass	33

Table VI. Herbicidal Activity of FMC 55626 in Field Soil Samples

	% Control			
	Autoclaved		Non Autoclaved	
Species	0.5kg/ha	2kg/ha	0.5kg/ha	2kg/ha
Barnyardgrass	80	100	10	10
Velvetleaf	100	100	10	96

Reaction of FMC 55626 with Amines

Et_3N/CH_2Cl_2, 25° → Gas Evol. + Complex Mixture (CO_2?) $[(CH_3)_2CH\text{-}C(=O)\sim]$

RNH_2/CH_2Cl_2, 25° → 7

$R = CH_3$; phenyl

Scheme 3

improve the stability of the heterocyclic ring by releasing some of the ring strain and preventing the decarboxylation reaction. The results of this operation are the 3-isoxazolidinones (8), a new class of compounds that possess a high level of herbicidal activity and excellent soybean tolerance.

Synthesis. The synthesis of these new compounds are shown in Schemes 4-8. Condensation of β-chloropivaloyl chloride with trimethylsilyl chloride-treated benzylhydroxylamine in methylene chloride in the presence of pyridine gave a hydroxamic acid derivative 9 in good yield. It is important to block the hydroxyl group of the hydroxylamine to ensure the desired N-acylation; otherwise, a stable mixture of 40:60 N- and O-acylated products (9, 10) will be obtained. This isomeric mixture is not only difficult to separate but also reduces the efficiency of the synthesis.

Upon treatment with one equivalent of base, chloropivaloyl hydroxamic acid 9 will smoothly cyclize to form 3-isoxazolidinone 8 in good yield. An excess of base in the cyclization, or treatment of the resulting benzyl-3-isoxazolidinone with base will result in a ring expansion product 11 -- a 1,3-oxazine-4-one. This ring expansion process is apparently induced by the base abstraction of the acidic benzyl proton followed by N-O bond cleavage and intramolecular addition of the resulting alkoxide to the newly formed acylimine 12 to form the 1,3-oxazine-4-one ring (6).

An alternate route to the substituted 3-isoxazolidinones is shown in Scheme 6. Condensation of β-chloropivaloyl chloride with hydroxylamine followed by base-induced cyclization of the resulting hydroxamic acid gave 4,4-dimethyl-3-isoxazolidinone (13). Phase-transfer catalytic alkylation of the 3-isoxazolidinone gave both N- and O-alkylated products (14, 15). The ratio of the N- and O-isomers depends on the catalytic conditions. Using KOH/tetrabutylamonium bromide (TBAB)/THF (7), a mixture of 77:23 N/O isomers was obtained. If K_2CO_3/18-Crown-6(18-C-6)/CH_3CN was used, a 95:5 mixture of N/O isomers was obtained. The undesired O-alkylated isomers can be separated by a column chromatography.

When a strong electron-withdrawing group is present in the benzyl halide, e.g. 2-chloro-4-nitro-benzyl bromide (Scheme 7), the normal phase-transfer alkylation will give only ring expansion product (16). However, if the reaction temperature is kept at 0°C, the rearrangement process can be suppressed completely.

A series of 5-alkoxy-3-isoxazolidinones (17) was prepared as shown in Scheme 8. Employing the same method discussed previously, a 5-chloro-3-isoxazolidinone (18) was prepared. This reactive chloride can be easily replaced by nucleophiles such as alcohols to give the desired alkoxy derivatives. Some ring-opening products (19) derived from deprotonation of the acidic benzyl proton were also observed.

Herbicidal Activity. As with FMC 55626, all of the active 3-isoxazolidinones cause bleaching of the emerging weed seedlings. Results observed to date indicate that these compounds affect carotene and chlorophyll biosynthesis (8, 9). Typical greenhouse activity data for preemergence application of FMC 57020 (8, X=2-Cl) on some representative weed species are shown in Table VII. The

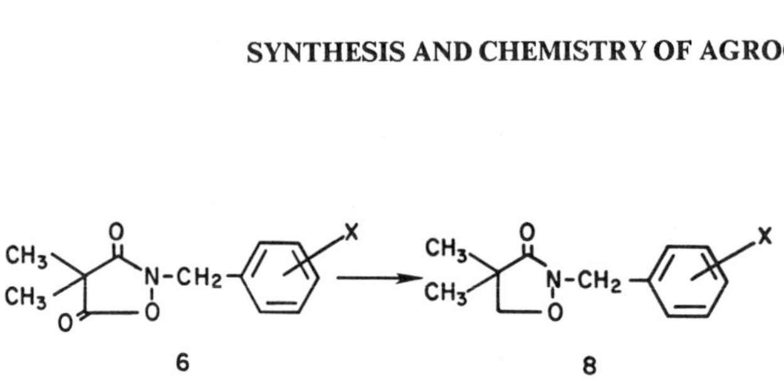

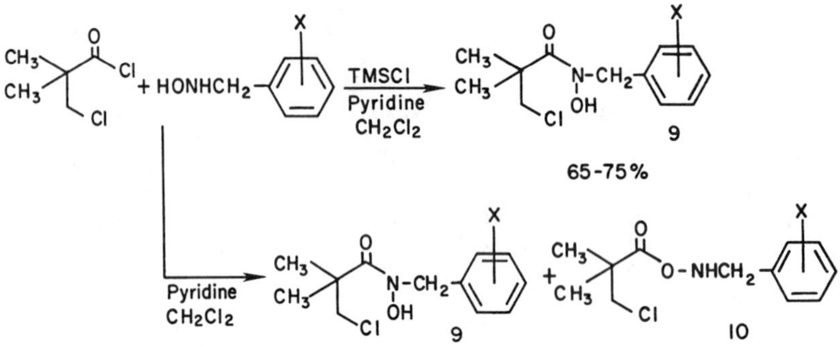

CH3 CH3 O N-CH2 X O O 6 → CH3 CH3 O N-CH2 X O 8

CH3 CH3 O Cl Cl + HONHCH2 X TMSCl Pyridine CH2Cl2 → CH3 CH3 O N-CH2 OH Cl X 9 65-75%

Pyridine CH2Cl2 → CH3 CH3 O N-CH2 OH Cl X 9 + CH3 CH3 O O-NHCH2 Cl X 10

Scheme 4

CH3 CH3 O N-CH2 OH Cl X 9 1eq KOH MeOH CH3 CH3 O N-CH2 O X 8

XS KOH MeOH KOH MeOH

CH3 CH3 O NH O X 11

CH3 CH3 O HB N=CH O⊖ X 12

CH3 CH3 O :B H N-CH O X

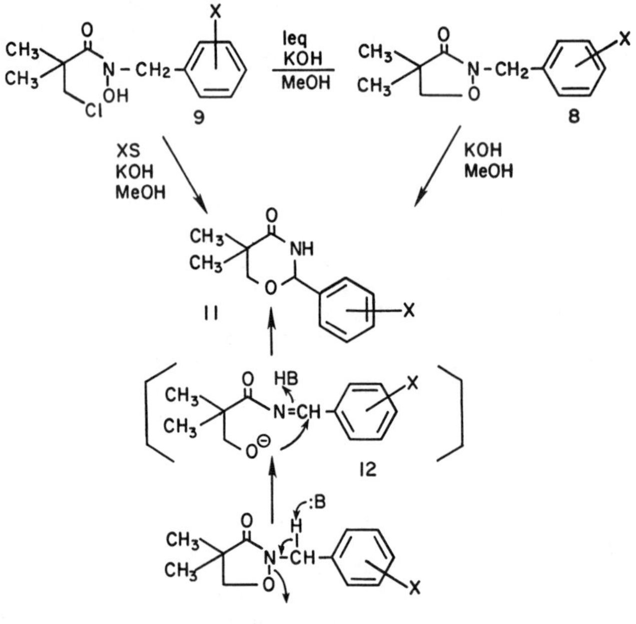

Scheme 5

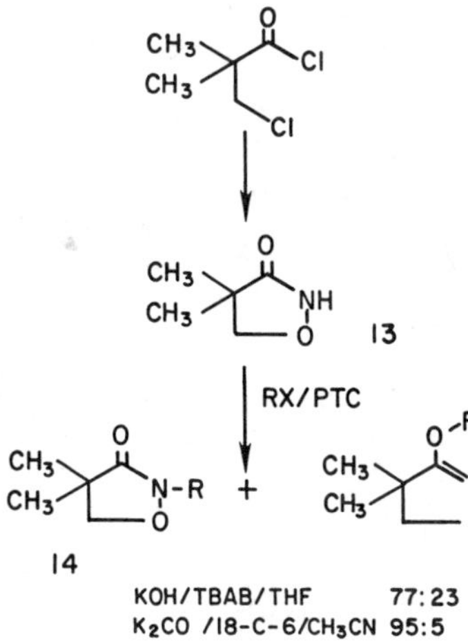
RX/PTC
13
14
15
KOH/TBAB/THF 77:23
K2CO /18-C-6/CH3CN 95:5

Scheme 6

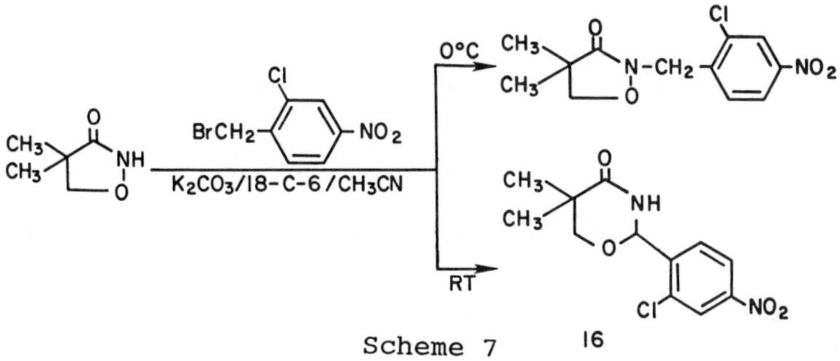
0°C
RT
K2CO3/18-C-6/CH3CN
16

Scheme 7

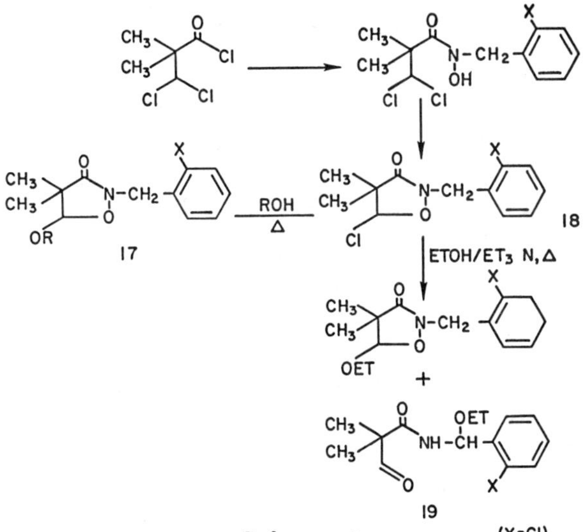
ROH
Δ
ETOH/ET3 N,Δ
17
18
19
(X=Cl)

Scheme 8

activity is expressed in terms of BE_{95} which is defined as the rate (in kg/ha) required to achieve 95% control.

Structure-activity Relationships. It has been found that the position of substitution on the phenyl ring is critical for herbicidal activity. For example, a series of chloro-substituted benzyl-3-isoxazolidinones shown in Table VIII demonstrates activity ranging from inactive to very active. It is clear from this table that the *ortho*-substituent is necessary for activity. In addition to the *ortho*-position, the second substituent must be at the C_4 or C_5 position to be active.

Substituent effects at the *ortho*-position are also observed. Halogen is the only group of substituents which show significant herbicidal activity. Among the four halogens, chlorine gives the most active compound which is followed by bromo, fluoro and iodo derivatives in a descending order. The non-substituted benzyl derivative still shows some bleaching effect at higher rate. Other substituents, such as CH_3, OCH_3, CN, SCH_3, C_6H_5, CF_3 and NH_2 at the *ortho*-position give inactive compounds.

In the case of multiply substituted benzyl analogs, halogen is important for a high level of herbicidal activity. The relative activity for some disubstituted analogs is shown below. The most active member in this series is 2-chloro-4-fluoro analog.

Various groups at the 5-position of the heterocyclic ring, were introduced as discussed in the synthesis section. The herbicidal activity of these compounds ranges from the very active methoxy derivative to the totally inactive methyl and phenyl derivatives (Table IX). The chloro and hydroxy derivatives are fairly active while the methylthio analog is only slightly active. It appears that the oxygen linkage is essential for a high level of herbicidal activity. Again, the observed herbicidal response is a typical bleaching of emerging weed seedlings.

Among the 5-alkoxy derivatives, the relative activity can be ranked in the order shown below. The most active member is 5-methoxy derivative.

An interesting structure-activity observation is that the 3-isoxazolidinones (8) are only slightly more active than their synthetic precursor hydroxamic acids (9) (Table X). For example, the difference in activity between FMC 57020 and its precursor hydroxamic acid toward these 4 species of weeds is very small. They both show a bleaching herbicidal response with excellent soybean tolerance. They also demonstrate a parallel substituent effect, i.e. they both follow the same relative activity order among different substituents such as those shown in Table X.

Finally, the sensitivity of the C_4 position of the heterocyclic ring with respect to the alkyl substituent was examined (Table XI). Results of this investigation have indicated that very small changes in the 4-substituent can cause a significant reduction of activity.

Summary. Synthesis of 3,5-isoxazolidinediones has led to the discovery of a new class of herbicides, the 3-isoxazolidinones. Various structural modifications based on the parent heterocyclic ring were made. A number of very active compounds derived from 2-benzyl analogs and 5-alkoxy derivatives were found. This class of

Table VII. Herbicidal Activity

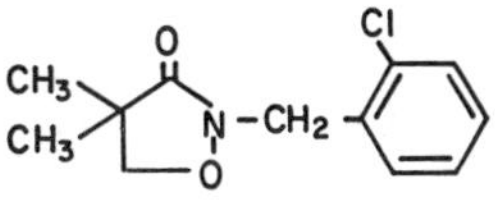

FMC 57020

	BE_{95} (Kg/ha)
Barnyard Grass	.04
Green Foxtail	.25
Velvetleaf	.06
Wild Mustard	.50

• Soybean Tolerance 2 kg/ha

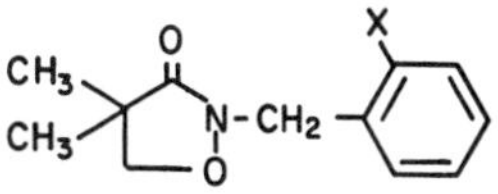

X:
Cl > Br > F > I > H >> CH_3
CH_3, OCH_3, CN, SCH_3,
C_6H_5, CF_3, NH_2------ Inactive

Table VIII. Structure–Activity Relationships

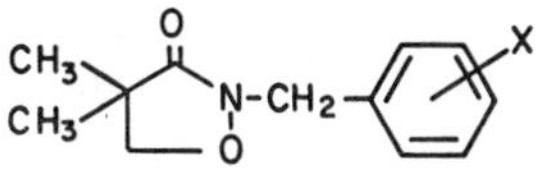

X	Activity
2-Cl	++
2,4-Cl_2	+
2,5-Cl_2	+
2,4,5-Cl_3	+
4-Cl	−
3,4-Cl_2	−
2,6-Cl_2	−
2,3-Cl_2	−

+ + : Very Active
+ : Active
− Inactive

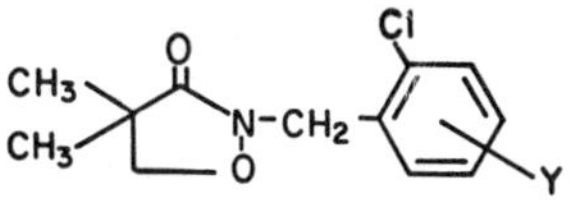

Y:
H ~ 4-F > 5-F > 4-Cl > 5-Cl >> 5-OCH_3 > 5-NO_2

Table IX. Range of Activity

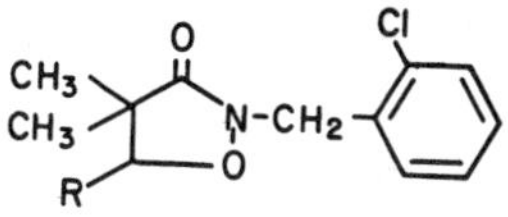

R	Activity
OCH_3	++
Cl	+
OH	+
SCH_3	±
NH_2	−
C_6H_5	−
CH_3	−

++: Very Active
+: Active
±: Slightly Active
−: Inactive

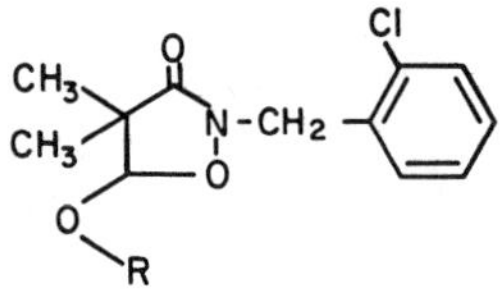

R:
$CH_3 > C_2H_5$, $CH_2CH=CH_2$, $CH_2C\equiv CH$, $CH(CH_3)_2 > COCH_3$

Table X. Comparison of 3-Isoxazolidinones with Hydroxamic Acids

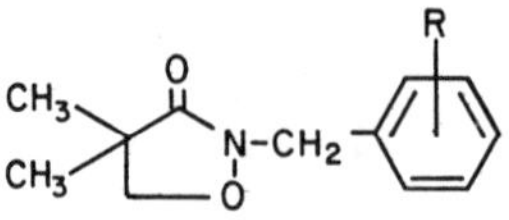

8 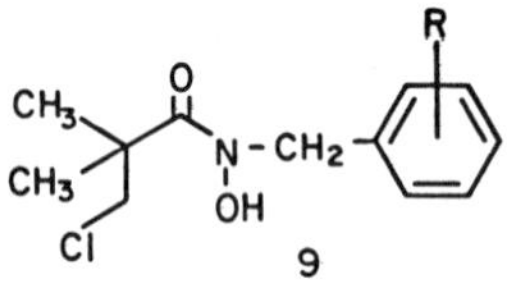 ≳ 9

R = 2-Cl

	BE_{95} (Kg/ha) 8	9
Barnyardgrass	.04	.06
Green Foxtail	.25	.50
Velvetleaf	.06	.06
Wild Mustard	.50	1.00

R: 2-Br, 2-F, 2,4-Cl_2, 2,6-Cl_2, H, 2-CH_3, 2-OCH_3, 3-CF_3, 4-Cl, 3,4-Cl_2

Table XI. Effect of Alkyl Substituent

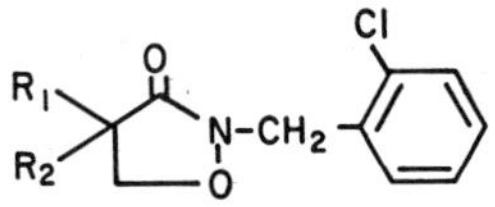

R_1	R_2
C_6H_5	H
H	H
CH_3	CH_2Cl
H	CH_3

Inactive

herbicides generally causes severe bleaching on a broad spectrum of emerging weed seedlings with excellent safety margins toward soybeans. One of the most active compounds, FMC 57020, has been developed for commercial use by FMC Corporation under the FMC registered trademark, Command (10-13).

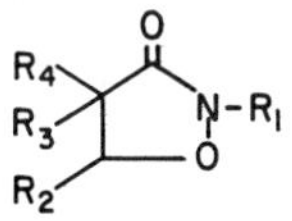

3-Isoxazolidinones

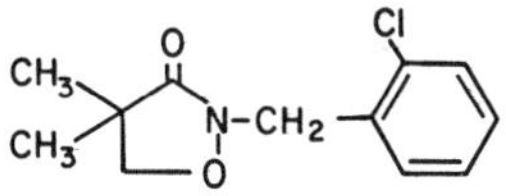

FMC 57020

Literature Cited

1. Matter, M.; Gerber, H. U.S. Patent 3,007,936, 1961.

2. Michel, K.; Gerlach-Gerber, H.; Vogel, Ch.; Matter, M. Helv. Chim. Acta 1965, 48, 1973.

3. Zinner, G.; Moll, R. Arch. Pharm. 1966, 299, 562.

4. Zinner, G.; Ruthe, H.; Boese, D. Pharmazie 1974, 29, 16.

5. Borch, R. F.; Bernstein, M. D.; Durst, H. D. J. Amer. Chem. Soc. 1971, 93, 2897.

6. A similar rearrangement was observed by Uno, H.; Kurokawa, M. Chem. Pharm. Bull. 1978, 26, 549.

7. Takahata, H.; Hashizume, T.; Yamazaki, T. Heterocycles 1979, 12, 1449.

8. Warfield, T. R.; Carlson, D. B.; Parrish, D. S.; Zenk, G. J. NCWCC Proceedings 1983, 38, 4.

9. Sandmann, G.; Boger, P. Z. Naturforsh 1986, 41C, 729.

10. Warfield, T. R.; Halvorson, G. C.; Dobbins, L. D.; Hopper, D. M. NCWCC Proceedings 1985, 40, 80.

11. Warfield, T. R.; Carlson, D. B.; Bellman, S. K.; Guscar, H. L. Weed Sci. Abstr. 1985, 25, 105.

12. Konz, M. J. U.S. Patent 4,302,238, 1981.

13. Chang, J. H. U.S. Patent 4,405,357, 1983.

RECEIVED May 12, 1987

Chapter 3

Synthesis and Herbicidal Activity of Pyridazines Based on 3-Chloro-4-methyl-6-[*m*-(trifluoromethyl)phenyl]pyridazine

Dale L. Shaner, Laurine M. Speltz, and Stephen S. Szucs

Agricultural Research Division, American Cyanamid Company, Princeton, NJ 08540

Greenhouse evaluation in a random herbicide screen showed that 3-chloro-4-methyl-6-[m-(trifluoromethyl)phenyl]pyridazine was sufficiently active to serve as a lead for a synthesis project. Related 3-chloropyridazines were prepared by a sequence based on the addition of acyl anion equivalents of substituted benzaldehydes to the appropriately substituted acrylate esters. Using 3-chloropyridazines as key intermediates, a variety of other 3-substituted-pyridazines were prepared. The effect of altering substitution at each position of the pyridazine and phenyl rings on herbicidal activity was examined.

The first pyridazine for which plant growth regulating activity was patented was maleic hydrazide (1). Since the introduction of MH in the late 1940's, at least four other pyridazines have been developed as herbicides: Pyramin by BASF in 1962, Kusakira by Sankyo in 1970, Zorial by Sandoz A. G. in 1971 and pyridate by Chemie Linz in 1976 (2).

We first became interested in pyridazines as herbicides when a number of pyridazines synthesized in a CNS project at our Lederle division were evaluated in our primary herbicide screen. One of these compounds, AC 228,764, controlled eleven of the twelve weed species at 8 kg/ha in the preemergence test. All of the test species were bleached, emerging white from the soil. In our secondary evaluation at 4 kg/ha, AC 228,764 controlled ten out of eleven annual grass and broadleaf weed species with selectivity in cotton, soybeans and rice. This spectrum of activity and crop

N–N
Cl
CF_3 H CH_3

AC 228,764

0097-6156/87/0355-0024$06.00/0
© 1987 American Chemical Society

selectivity stimulated sufficient interest to designate the sample, 3-chloro-4-methyl-6-[m-(trifluoromethyl)phenyl]pyridazine, as a lead for a synthesis project.

Based on available herbicide data for related Cyanamid pyridazines and patented compounds, the following structural modifications were proposed: 1) substitution of the chlorine at the 3-position; 2) replacement or derivatization of the 4-methyl group; 3) introduction of substituents at the 5-position; 4) alternate substitution in the 6-phenyl ring as well as reduction to the corresponding cyclohexyl derivatives and replacement of the phenyl by heterocycles; and 5) oxidation and quaternization of the nitrogens at positions 1 and 2.

Essentially every analog and derivative prepared in the project was ultimately derived from the corresponding 3-chloro-pyridazine. With the exception of a few 3-chloropyridazines which originated from a Friedel-Crafts acylation of benzene, the large majority of chloropyridazines were prepared by a sequence based on the addition of the masked acyl anion equivalent of a benzaldehyde to the appropriately substituted acrylate ester.

X-C₆H₄-CHO —(a,b; c,d)→ R_6CO–CH(R_5)–CH(R_4)–COOR —(e)→ dihydropyridazinone —(f)→ pyridazinone —(g)→ 3-chloropyridazine (R_6–C₄HN₂–Cl)

a. p-TsOH, morpholine, THF

b. KCN, H_2O

c. $R_5CH{=}CHR_4COOR$, NaOMe, THF

d. 70% HOAc

e. $N_2H_4 \cdot H_2O$, EtOH, H_2O

f. Br_2, gl HOAc

g. $POCl_3$

This procedure has previously been reported by Lederle chemists (3, 4) and was used to prepare our original screening sample. For preparing a series of substituted phenyl analogs, the choice of benzaldehyde fixed the position of the substituent and the choice of an alkyl- or aryl-substituted acrylate fixed the substitution in the 4- and/or 5-position. All intermediates in this sequence were routinely tested in our herbicide screens, but very few of these, including the dihydropyridazinones and the pyridazinones, showed any significant activity.

In addition to being evaluated in their own right for comparison with the lead, the 6-(substituted-phenyl)-3-chloropyridazines (R-Cl) were also used as key intermediates for preparing analogs containing other substituents in the 3-position. Displacement by a variety of alkoxides and amines gave the corresponding 3-alkoxy- and 3-mono- or disubstitutedaminopyridazines. Hydrogenolysis over 10% palladium on carbon in ethanol containing ammonium hydroxide gave the corresponding 3-hydro analog. For those pyridazines containing a phenyl group bearing a halogen or certain ortho-substituents, the 3-chloropyridazine was either hydrogenated over 10% palladium on carbon in glacial acetic acid or was converted to the 3-thiomethyl analog using a sodium mercaptide salt for subsequent Raney nickel desulfurization.

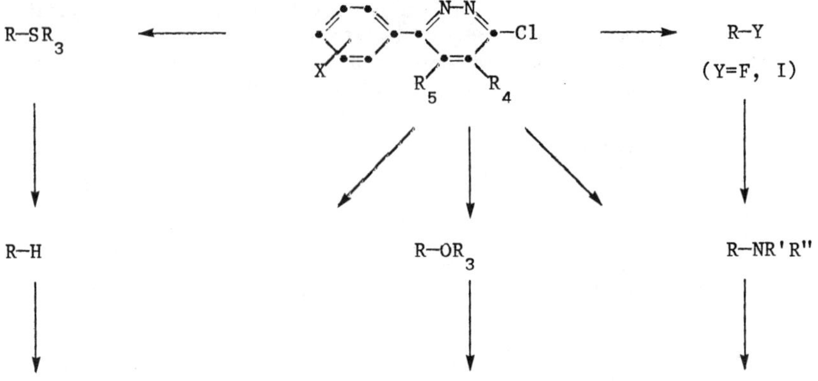

6-CYCLOHEXYLPYRIDAZINES

PYRIDAZINE N-OXIDES

PYRIDAZINIUM SALTS

Similarly when a displacement of a 3-chloropyridazine by ammonia or certain alkyl-substituted amines proceeded very slowly or resulted in very low yields, other 3-halopyridazines were used. The 3-iodopyridazines were prepared by heating the corresponding 3-chloropyridazines with sodium iodide and hydriodic acid in refluxing 2-butanone. The 3-bromopyridazines were prepared from the corresponding 3(2H)-pyridazinones by heating with phosphorous oxybromide. The 3-fluoropyridazines were prepared from the corresponding 3-chloro intermediates by heating with potassium fluoride in sulfolane at 190-200° (5, 6).

A number of pyridazines were selected for further derivatization based on their herbicidal activity. Pyridazines containing methoxy, substituted-amino, chloro, and hydrogen in the 3-position were selectively reduced using platinum oxide in trifluoroacetic acid to yield the corresponding 6-cyclohexyl derivatives (7). Selected analogs were also oxidized in the 1-and/or 2-positions using meta-chloroperbenzoic acid (8) and were quaternized with methyl iodide in refluxing acetonitrile (9) to yield the corresponding pyridazine N-oxides and pyridazinium salts.

For the purpose of comparing the pre- and postemergence data acquired in a variety of tests over a two-year period, the herbicidal activity was expressed as an "averaged rating" over a spectrum of eight annual grass (*Echinochloa crus-galli*, *Digitaria* spp., *Phalaris* spp., *Setaria viridis* and *Avena fatua*) and broadleaf (*Ipomoea* spp., *Brassica kaber*, and *Sida spinosa*) weed species common to most of the tests. This averaged rating was determined for each pyridazine by summing the rating given to each of the selected weed species and dividing by the number of weeds tested, typically eight. The rating scale used in the herbicide evaluation ranged from zero, as observed by no effect relative to the control plant, to nine, indicating the death of the plant.

Figure 1 compares the averaged ratings at 1 kg/ha of the lead pyridazine (R_3=Cl) with other analogs substituted in the 3-position. The 3-hydro analog not only controlled all species preemergence but also had a higher level of postemergence activity. Although the 3-aminopyridazine had no detectable activity at 1 kg/ha, the dimethylamino analog gave preemergence control comparable to that of the 3-hydro analog and significantly increased the level of postemergence activity. The 3-methoxy analog also showed higher levels of both pre- and postemergence activity in comparison with the lead. As a result of these findings, all 3-chloropyridazines containing substitution in the 6-phenyl ring were routinely converted to the 3-hydro, 3-dimethylamino, and 3-methoxy analogs.

One of the most interesting comparisons to evolve in the project in terms of activity and economics was the effect of changing substituents at the 3-position for analogs containing an unsubstituted phenyl group in the 6-position (Figure 2). 3-Chloro-4-methyl-6-phenylpyridazine (R_3=Cl) gave the same level of weed control as the *m*-trifluoromethylphenyl lead. Interestingly, the 3-hydro analog did not produce the marked increase in activity, particularly in the preemergence application as was observed for the *m*-trifluoromethylphenyl analog. However the same significant increase in activity in both pre- and postemergence applications was observed for the unsubstituted-phenyl 3-methoxy and 3-dimethylaminopyridazines. The 3-methylaminopyridazine was nearly as active as the dimethylamino analog but the removal of the methyl substitution (3-NH_2) or homologation (3-NHEt) resulted in a significant reduction in activity.

The most active pyridazine of the group was the 3-methoxy analog, AC 247,909. Like most of the active pyridazine analogs, preemergence application of AC 247,909 caused bleaching. As the most active postemergence pyridazine herbicide, AC 247,909 caused rapid necrosis, suggesting a potential use as a contact-type herbicide. As in the 3-amino series, an extension of the alkyl chain resulted in the loss of activity. Besides methyl, other substituents introduced at the 3-position included alkylsulfonyl, cyano, carboxy, and amido. These pyridazines were inactive at 1 kg/ha and in some cases at 8 kg/ha.

The effect of substitution at the 4- and 5-positions relative to AC 247,909 is summarized in Figure 3. Removal of the 4-methyl

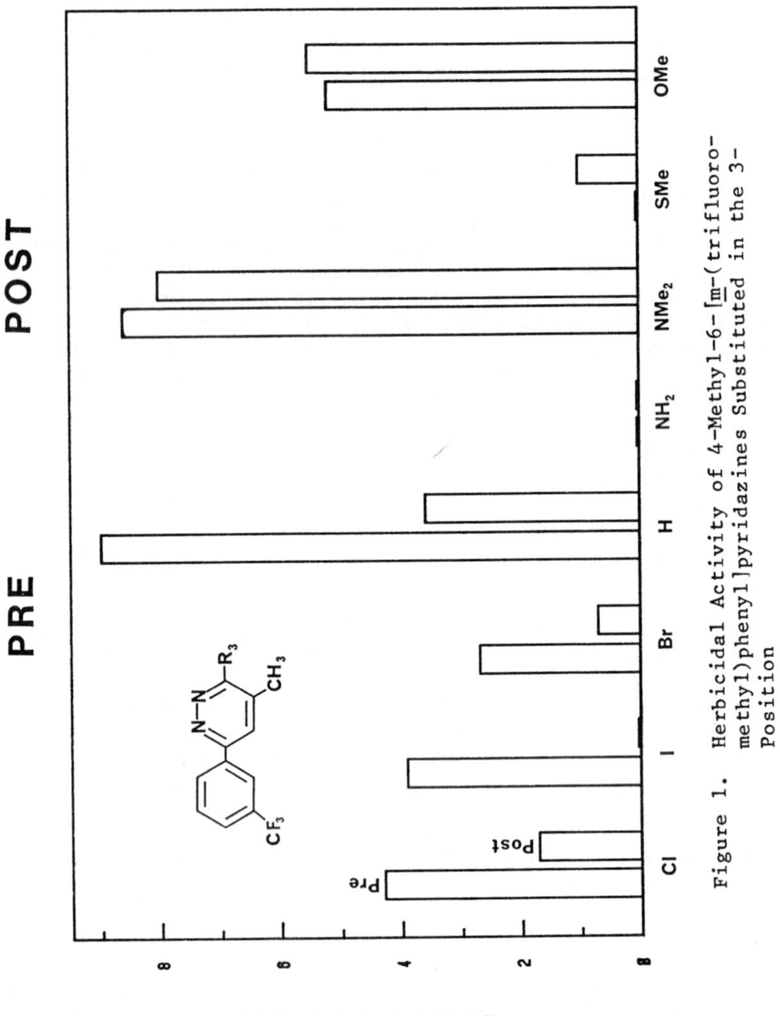

Figure 1. Herbicidal Activity of 4-Methyl-6-[m-(trifluoromethyl)phenyl]pyridazines Substituted in the 3-Position

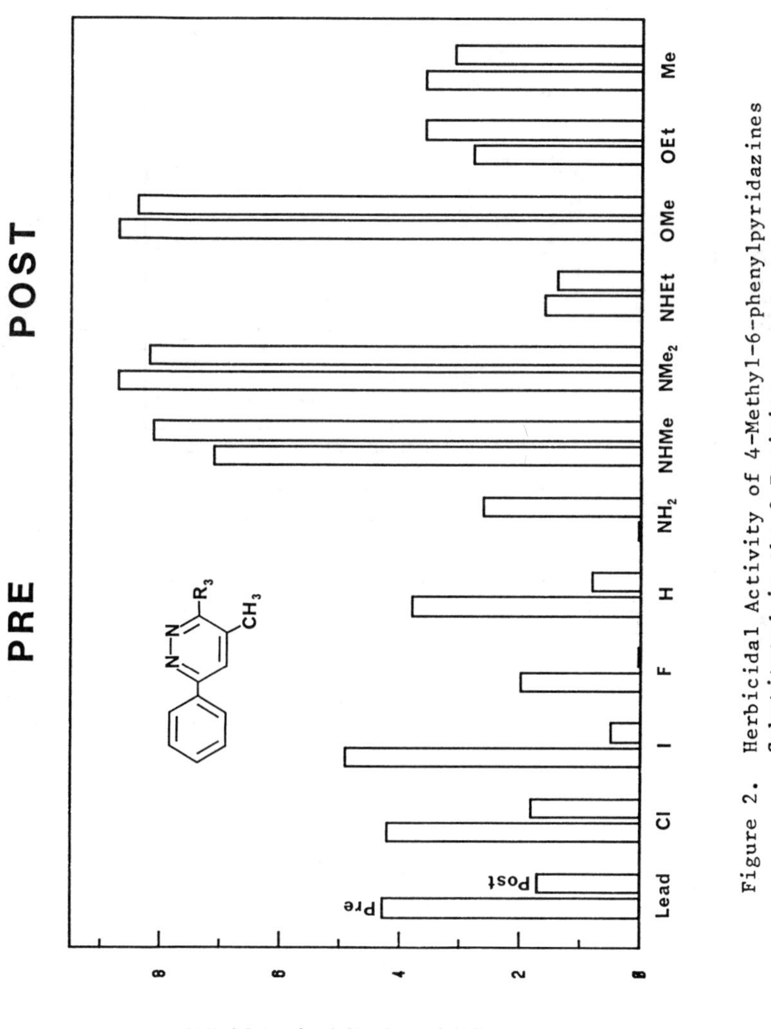

Figure 2. Herbicidal Activity of 4-Methyl-6-phenylpyridazines Substituted in the 3-Position

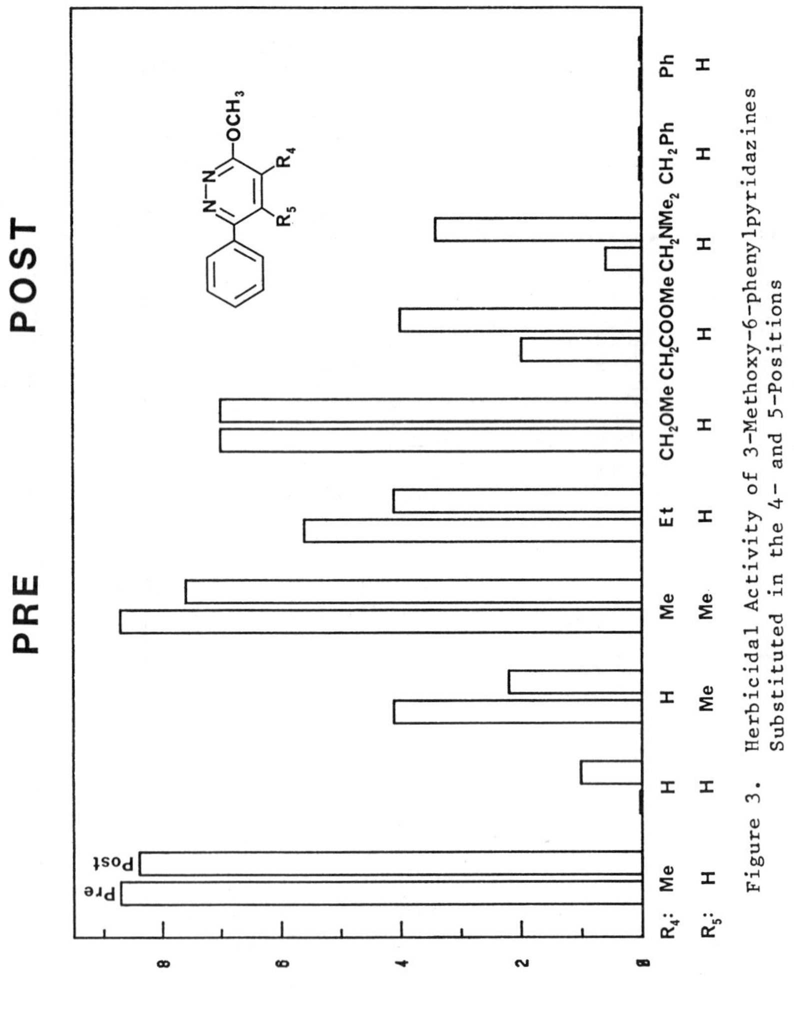

Figure 3. Herbicidal Activity of 3-Methoxy-6-phenylpyridazines Substituted in the 4- and 5-Positions

group resulted in poor herbicidal activity at 2 kg/ha. Movement of the methyl from the 4- to the 5-position resulted in a substantial reduction in activity, but the introduction of a second methyl group at R_5 resulted in a herbicidal response nearly identical to that of AC 247,909. Comparisons at lower rates showed that the 4,5-dimethyl analog was somewhat less active. This slightly diminished activity for the 4,5-dimethyl analog was also observed in the parallel comparison between 3-dimethylaminopyridazines.

Derivatization of the methyl group at R_4 generally resulted in a similar spectrum of weed control, but at lower levels of activity. Some examples include the ethyl, methoxymethyl, carbomethoxymethyl and dimethylaminomethyl. Substitution at R_4 by benzyl, phenyl, or t-butyl resulted in a complete loss of herbicidal activity at 2 kg/ha.

The effect of monosubstitution in the phenyl ring of selected 3-methoxypyridazines is shown in Figure 4. In general substituents in the 6-phenyl ring decreased the level of activity across a spectrum of weeds in the order meta $\geq$ ortho $>$ para.

Both pre- and postemergence data from the monosubstituted phenyl analogs were evaluated using the Hansch 3X regression analysis program. Significant equations were generated for the meta-substituted analogs. A high degree of correlation of both pre- and postemergence activity was obtained for a representative grass and broadleaf weed species as a function of the independent variables π and B_4. Across a spectrum of weed species, none of the two dozen monosubstituted phenyl or the nine disubstituted phenyl analogs exceeded the activity, and certainly the cost efficacy, of the unsubstituted phenyl analog, AC 247,909.

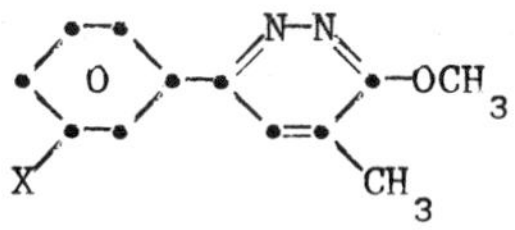

[Structure: 6-(3-X-phenyl)-3-methoxy-4-methylpyridazine; labels: N–N, O, OCH3, CH3, X]

Wild Oats

Preemergence:

$$\log (MW/ED_{85}) = 2.48\ (\pm 0.52) + 0.71\ (\pm 0.40)\ \pi - 0.34\ (\pm 0.22)\ B_4$$

$$n = 11 \qquad R^2 = 0.70$$

Postemergence:

$$\log (MW/ED_{85}) = 2.55\ (\pm 0.47) + 0.71\ (\pm 0.36)\ \pi - 0.30\ (\pm 0.20)\ B_4$$

$$n = 10 \qquad R^2 = 0.76$$

Morningglory

Preemergence

$$\log (MW/ED_{85}) = 2.08\ (\pm 0.40) + 0.59\ (\pm 0.30)\ \pi - 0.18\ (\pm 0.17)\ B_4$$

$$n = 11 \qquad R^2 = 0.72$$

Postemergence:

$$\log (MW/ED_{85}) = 2.88\ (\pm 0.36) + 0.45\ (\pm 0.28)\ \pi - 0.35\ (\pm 0.16)\ B_4$$

$$n = 11 \qquad R^2 = 0.78$$

where ED_{85} was the lowest estimated dose required to obtain a rating of eight.

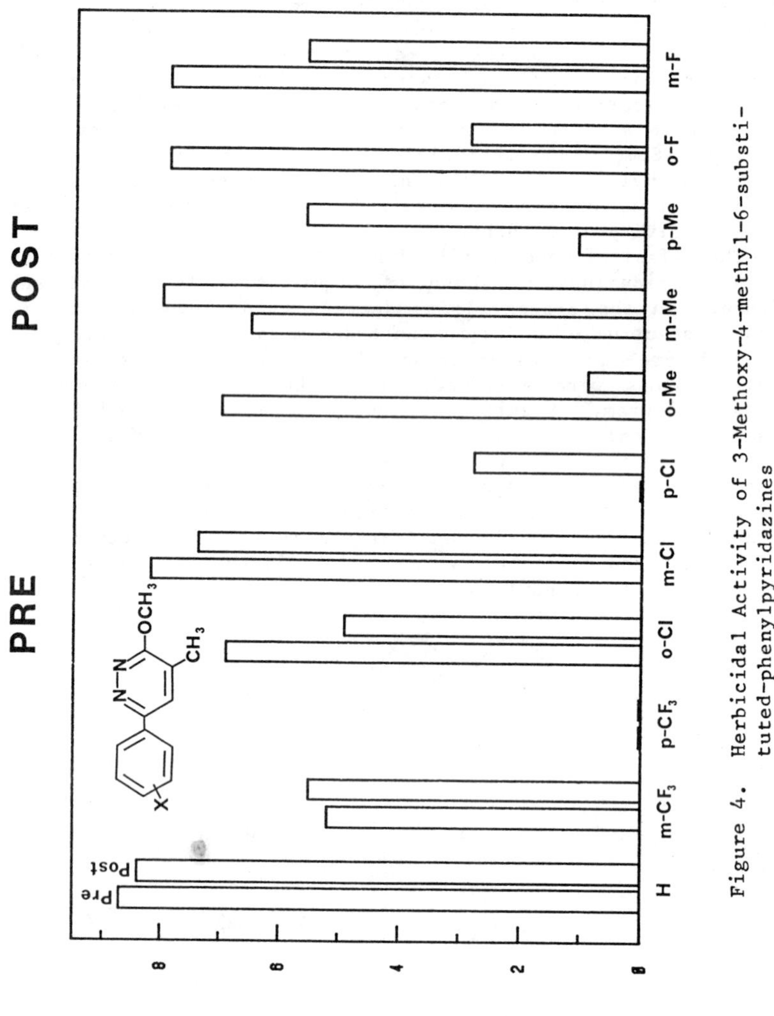

Figure 4. Herbicidal Activity of 3-Methoxy-4-methyl-6-substituted-phenylpyridazines

The structure-activity relationship developed for substituents in the 6-phenyl ring in the 3-methoxy series was paralleled in the 3-chloro and 3-dimethylamino series but not in the 3-hydro series (Figure 5). Conversion of AC 247,909 to its 2-oxide resulted in a reduction of preemergence activity and a complete loss of post activity at 1 kg/ha. Similarly, loss of both pre and post activity was observed for the 2-oxides of both the 3-chloro-and the 3-hydrogen pyridazines relative to their respective parent pyridazines. Although m-trifluoromethyl substitution in the phenyl of the 3-methoxypyridazine resulted in lower activity both pre and post, m-trifluoromethyl substitution in the 3-hydropyridazine resulted in a level of preemergence activity equivalent to that of AC 247,909. This was unusual since very few of the 3-hydropyridazines showed activity at 4 kg/ha with phenyl substituents other than m-trifluoromethyl. Furthermore, instead of reducing activity as was observed for the 3-methoxy- and 3-chloropyridazines, oxidation at the 2-nitrogen resulted in improved preemergence activity over that of AC 247,909. In addition, greenhouse tests indicated that the 2-oxide AC 252,588 was selective preemergence in cotton at 2 kg/ha.

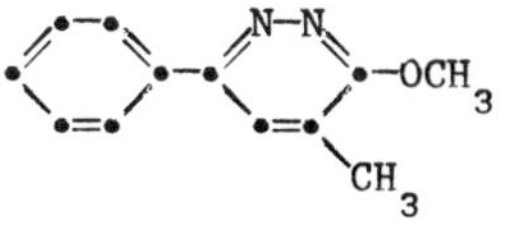

N–N, OCH_3, CH_3

AC 247,909

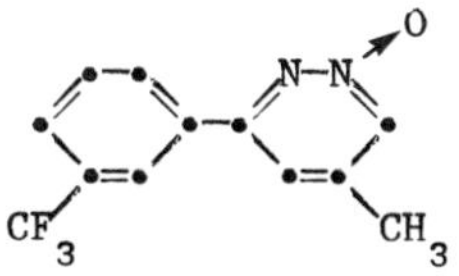

O, N–N, CF_3, CH_3

AC 252,588

Two field candidates emerged from the synthesis project. AC 247,909 had both postemergence non-selective activity and preemergence activity with selectivity in sunflowers. AC 252,588 had preemergence annual grass and broadleaf activity with excellent selectivity in cotton. In the greenhouse, AC 252,588 was found to be more active than Cotoran. In comparison with Zorial, AC 252,588 was two to three times less active across a spectrum of weeds but showed a greater margin of selectivity in cotton at the rate necessary for weed control.

Both compounds were field tested at a number of locations. The level of activity observed in the field trials, however, was not sufficient to warrant continued evaluation. Subsequent greenhouse testing suggested that the failure of AC 247,909 to perform in the field may be due to photodecomposition in postemergence tests and to soil metabolism and volatility in preemergence tests.

Although the synthesis program did not result in any commercial herbicides, two types of pyridazines were discovered which produced unexpected results, both in the level and the type of activity. The first series, which includes the 3-methoxy- and the 3-dimethylaminopyridazines, resulted in a high level of postemergence activity not observed in the lead or in the other 3-substituted-pyridazines. Secondly, based on a comparison with the N-oxides of other pyridazines, the N-oxide of the 3-hydropyridazine resulted in unexpectedly high preemergence activity, yet without phytotoxicity to cotton.

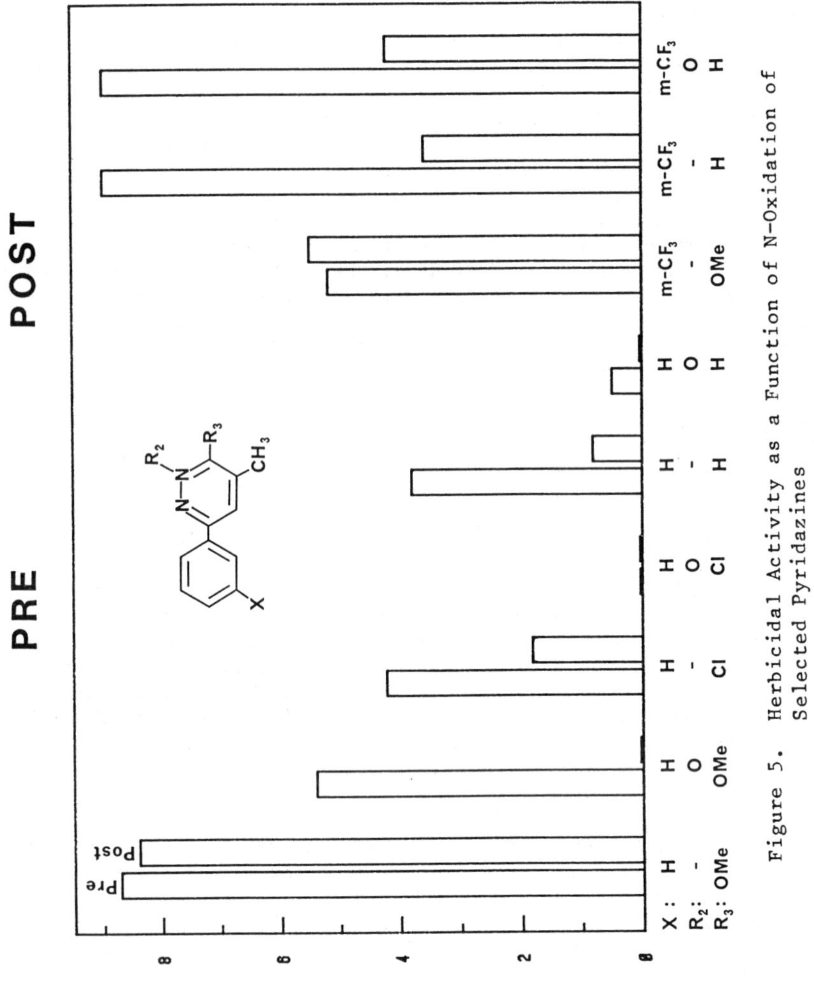

Figure 5. Herbicidal Activity as a Function of N-Oxidation of Selected Pyridazines

Several 3-alkoxy-4-methyl-6-phenylpyridazines, one of which is AC 247,909, have subsequently been disclosed as selective herbicides (10). A patent covering novel pyridazines and pyridazine N-oxides has been assigned to American Cyanamid (11).

Acknowledgments

The authors acknowledge the following individuals who contributed to the synthesis and herbicide evaluations: R. L. Arotin, C. E. Augelli, R. E. Diehl, M. A. Guaciaro, A. W. Lutz, P. A. Odorisio, J. J. Pascavage, H. W. Turpenen, K. Umeda, B. L. Walworth, and D. L. Whitehead.

Literature Cited

1. Worthing, C. R., Ed. The Pesticide Manual; The British Crop Protection Council: Croydon, England, 1983.
2. Fletcher, W. W.; Kirkwood, R. C. Herbicides and Plant Growth Regulators; Granada Publishing Limited: London, 1982; Chapter 1.
3. Albright, J. D.; McEvoy, F. J.; Moran, D. B. J. Heterocyclic Chem. 1978, 15, 881.
4. McEvoy, F. J.; Albright, J. D. J. Org. Chem. 1979, 44, 4597.
5. Finger, G. C.; Starr, L. D.; Dickerson, D. R.; Gutowsky, H. S.; Hamer, J. J. J. Org. Chem. 1963, 28, 1666.
6. Finger, G. C.; Kruse, C. W. J. Amer. Chem. Soc. 1956, 78, 6034.
7. Vierhapper, F. W.; Eliel, E. L. J. Org. Chem. 1975, 40, 2729.
8. Leclerc, G.; Wermuth, C. G. Bull. Soc. Chim. Fr. 1971, 1752.
9. Lund, H.; Lunde, P. Acta Chem. Scand. 1967, 21, 1067.
10. Jpn. Kokai Tokkyo Koho JP 59 01,469 [84 01,469]; Chem. Abstr. 1984, 101, 130699z.
11. Speltz, L. M.; Walworth, B. L. U.S. Patent 4 623 376, 1986.

RECEIVED September 8, 1987

Chapter 4

Synthesis and Herbicidal Properties of *N*-(Benzylideneamino), *N*-(Benzylamino), and *N*-(Phenylazo) Heterocycles

Kurt H. Pilgram, Willy D. Kollmeyer [1]**, Richard D. Skiles, and Larry E. Wittsell**[1]

Biological Sciences Research Center, Shell Agricultural Chemical Company, P.O. Box 4248, Modesto, CA 95352

The search for common structural features within the great variety of organic compounds acting as PS II inhibitors revealed the existence of a vinylogous relationship. By applying hetero-analogy and the principle of vinylogy, a simple model is proposed which unifies the structures of the vast array of PS II inhibitors. In the present work, its predictive value has been tested and confirmed by the preparation of a variety of N-(benzylideneamino) and N-(phenylazo) heterocycles. In these bridged vinylogous ureas, carbamates, and amides, the aromatic and heterocyclic rings are connected via diatomic linkages capable of transmitting substituent conjugative effects. N-(Benzylideneamino) and N-(phenylazo) heterocycles derived from N-aminoimidazolidin-2-one, 4-amino-1,2,4-triazol-3(2H)-one, and 1-aminohydantoin are among the most active members. In general, herbicidal activity is increased with lipophilicity imparted by a meta-substituent on phenyl. meta-CF_3 (and OCF_3) derivatives which showed tolerance on cotton produced severe bleaching, inhibiting carotenoid biosynthesis at the phytoene desaturation stage.

Fundamental problems in a given area of research can often be solved by finding analogies with problems previously solved in other areas of research. This rarely yields the whole solution, but it can provide useful insights and intuitions. For example, the principles of vinylogy and hetero-analogy which are almost as old as organic synthesis itself are familiar to chemists in the solution of certain types of synthetic problems. Since R. C. Fuson's review article (1) in 1935, examples of vinylogous relationships have increased

[1]Current address: E. I. du Pont de Nemours & Co., Wilmington, DE 19898

0097-6156/87/0355-0036$06.00/0
© 1987 American Chemical Society

rapidly in number as well as in variety. Vinylogous relationships have been established in Benary (2), Darzens-Claisen (3), and Vilsmeier-Haack (4,5) reactions as well as in the Pummerer (6,7), Wagner (8), and Wolff (9) rearrangements, to name a few.

However, there are relatively few examples of vinylogous relationships in biological fields. Attention has been drawn to a vinylogous relationship among structures of insecticidal pyrethroids (10,11). 5-Nitro-2-furfurylidene derivatives and their vinylogs figure prominently as antibacterial (12,13) agents, and aryl citronellyl ethers are highly effective as juvenile hormone mimics (14).

Of all commercial herbicides, a great many are inhibitors of photosynthesis (15). Of these, most prevent light-induced reduction of Q_B, the secondary electron acceptor in Photosystem II (PS II) (16). The structures of PS II inhibitors are diverse and cover almost all aspects of organic chemistry. Despite numerous structure-activity studies within classes of PS II inhibitors, little work has been done to correlate activity _across_ class boundaries. Clearly, a system that could accommodate these diverse structures should facilitate the design of new PS II inhibitors. Our work in this field which started in 1967 was based upon the very simple realization that the immense variety of seemingly unrelated PS II inhibitors can be formally derived from the following general structure of type I:

$$-(a{=}b)_l-\overset{|}{N}-(c{=}d)_m-\overset{\overset{X}{\|}}{C}-(e{=}f)_n-R$$

I

wherein a through f = C- or N; X = O or N-;
l, m, n = 0, 1, 2; R = alkyl, cycloalkyl, aryl, O-alkyl, N<

Recognition of the essential structural parts followed by a meaningful reconstruction leads to known PS II inhibitors as exemplified in Chart I.

PS II inhibitors derived from phenols, 4-aminopyridines, 2(and 4)-hydroxypyridines and 1,3-diamino-s-triazines which are capable of assuming tautomeric forms can be described in a similar fashion. Although the generalized vinylogous structure I appears to unify PS II inhibitors of diverse structure, its predictive value remained to be tested.

At this early stage of our work, we decided to explore as many different structures as possible since the number of potentially active PS II inhibitors that can be generated by application of I appeared to be very large, the only limitations being synthetic capacity and feasibility.

Substituents often are required for maximum effect of many herbicides acting as PS II inhibitors. Several herbicides display multiple modes of action. The nature and positions of substituents may cause a shift from one mode of action to another. For example, Diuron [3-(3,4-dichlorophenyl)-1,1-dimethylurea] is a potent PS II inhibitor causing necrosis, whereas the related urea Fluometuron (Chart I) induces albinism in growing plants. Pyrazon [5-amino-4-chloro-2-phenyl-3(2H)-pyridazinone] inhibits the Hill reaction and photosynthetic CO_2 fixation. _meta_-Trifluoromethyl substitution on

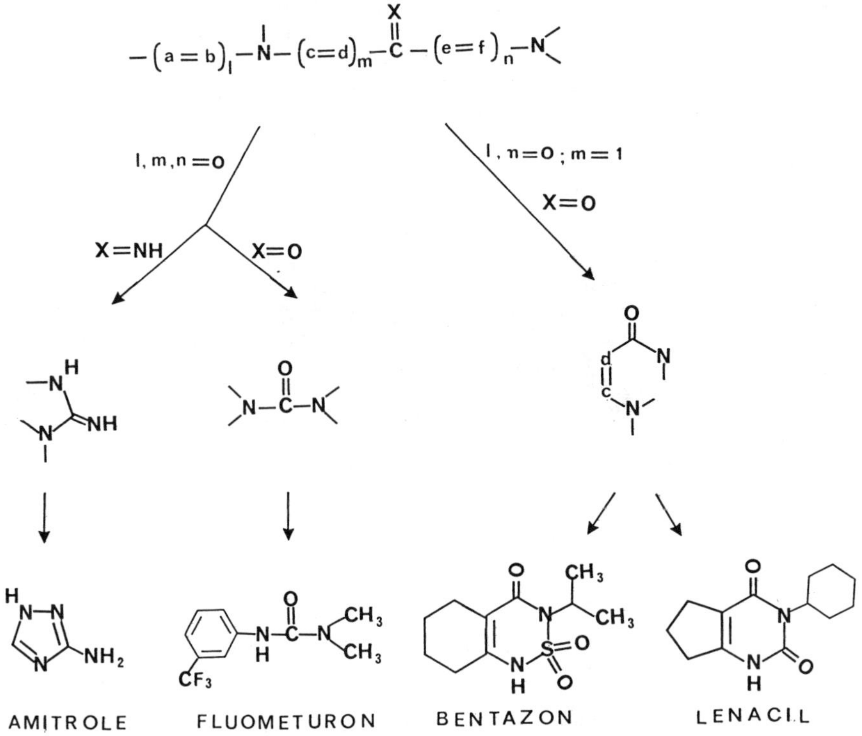

l, m, n = O

X = NH

X = O

l, n = O ; m = 1

X = O

AMITROLE FLUOMETURON BENTAZON LENACIL

Chart I. Application of general structure I to four PS II inhibitors.

the phenyl ring of Pyrazone and mono-methyl substitution of its amino group (to give Norflurazon, Chart II) result in inhibition of carotene biosynthesis. Because of our interest at that time in cotton selective herbicides, it was hypothesized that vinylogous bridged ureas of generalized structural type II should have properties similar to those of Fluometuron (Chart I) and Norflurazon (Chart II).

The present work emphasizes the more generalized structure shown in Table I. The systematic variations with regard to the nature of the heterocyclic ring (a and bridge), the substitution pattern on phenyl (X_n), and the nature of the linkage connecting both rings were selected to arrive at meaningful structure-activity relationships.

Table I. Scope of This Investigation

bridge; a; N; O; linkage; X_n

Linkage:	N=CH	$NH-CH_2$	N=N	CH=N	N=CR	N=CH-CH=N		
Bridge:	$\overset{O}{\overset{\|}{C}}-CH_2$	CH_2-CH_2	N=CH	$CH_2-\overset{O}{\overset{\|}{C}}$	$S-\overset{S}{\overset{\|}{C}}$	$\overset{O}{\overset{\|}{C}}-CHR$		
	$\overset{O}{\overset{\|}{C}}-\overset{O}{\overset{\|}{C}}$	N=CR	$NH-\overset{O}{\overset{\|}{C}}$	$CH_2-CH_2-CH_2$	$O-CH_2-CH_2$			
a:	NH	O	CH_2	NR				
X:	F	Cl	Br	CF_3	OCF_3	SCF_3	NO_2	CHO
	CH_3	OH	OCH_3	O-i-Pr	$OCHF_2$			
n:	0	1	2	3				

Synthesis of N-(Benzylideneamino) Heterocycles

The preparation of the title compounds was approached from two general directions:

(1) Reaction of a substituted benzaldehyde with an N-aminoheterocycle, and

(2) ring closure of an acyclic precursor such as a substituted-benzaldehyde semicarbazone.

The first, path (1), was straightforward since all N-aminoheterocycles used in this work (Table V) were known, and methods for their preparation have been published. The majority of the substituted-benzaldehydes used in this method were prepared according to the Beech (17) method as described (18) for the conversion of 2-bromo-4-toluidine into 2-bromo-4-methylbenzaldehyde. The method is of wide application and gave substituted benzaldehydes in 50-75% yield. The unavailability of certain (polyfluoroalkoxy)anilines precluded synthesis of corresponding aldehydes via this method. These were prepared from anisic acids (Chart III) or reduction of nitrophenols. For example, conversion of meta-anisic acid into 3-(tril,m=O;n=1

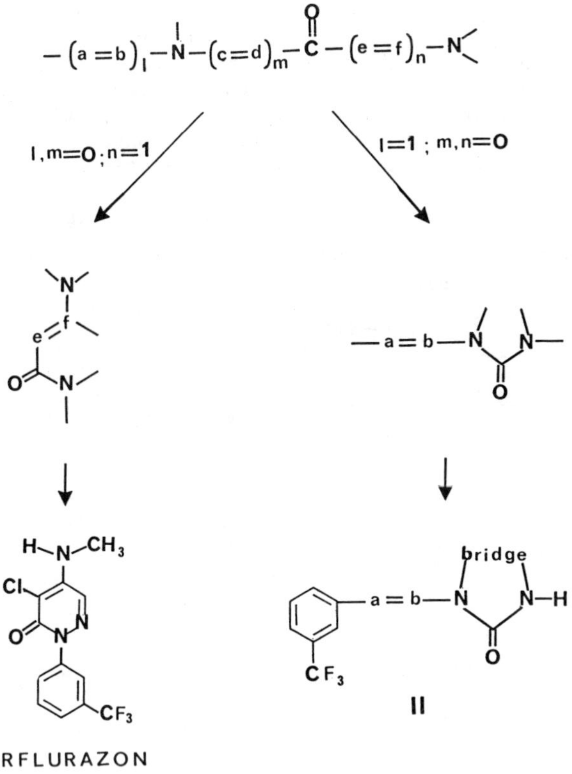

l=1 ; m,n=O

NORFLURAZON

II

Chart II. Formal relationship between norflurazon and title compounds II.

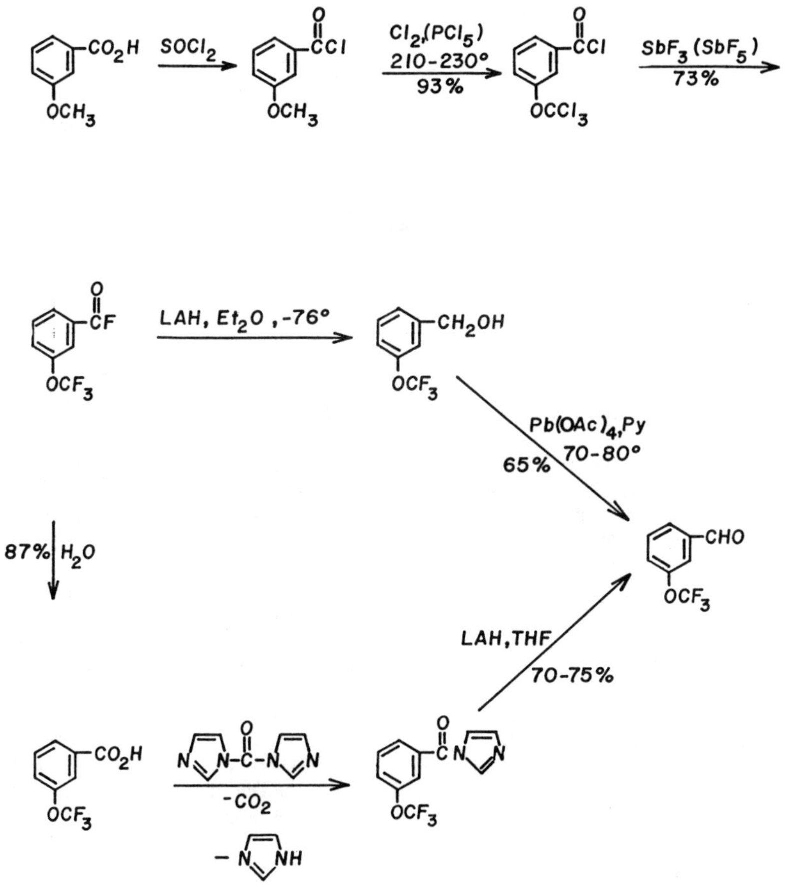

Chart III. Preparation of 3-(trifluoromethoxy)benzaldehyde.

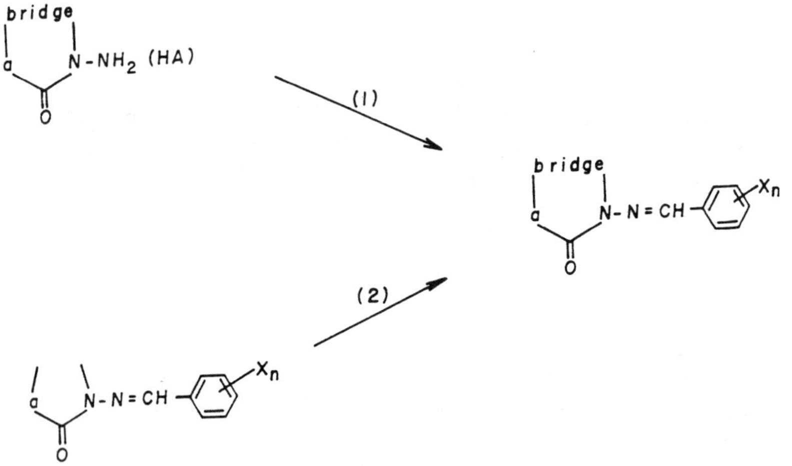

fluoromethoxy)benzoic acid was realized after the method of Yagupolski (19) as detailed for the *para*-isomer. Reaction of 3-(trifluoromethoxy)benzoic acid with N,N'-carbonyldiimidazole followed by reduction with LAH gave 3-(trifluoromethoxy)benzaldehyde in 63% yield. Reduction of the intermediate 3-(trifluoromethoxy)benzoyl fluoride with LAH followed by lead tetraacetate oxidation of the resulting benzyl alcohol gave the aldehyde in 65% yield (20).

Variations of the second strategy can be envisioned depending upon the nature of the "bridge". For example, two pathways, Charts IV and V, leading to 1-(benzylideneamino)hydantoins have been investigated as part of this work. In Chart IV, 3-(trifluoromethyl)benzaldehyde semicarbazone was allowed to react with ethyl chloroacetate in the presence of sodium ethoxide. The anion formed by proton abstraction from the semicarbazone reacted with ethyl chloroacetate to form the first carbon-nitrogen bond. This step is followed by an ester-amide condensation to form a second carbon-nitrogen bond and completing the hydantoin ring. This method has one drawback: Only about 75% of semicarbazone can be utilized. As the concentration of the hydantoin begins to build up, it forms a strongly nucleophilic anion with sodium ethoxide which competes effectively with semicarbazone anion leading to herbicidally uninteresting 3-alkylated-1-(benzylideneamino)hydantoin. Thus, alteration of the ratio of semicarbazone : ethyl chloroacetate : sodium ethoxide to 1.0 : 0.75 : 1.0 allowed for the exclusive formation of desired 1-(benzylideneamino)-hydantoin without alkylation at the 3-position (N-3). However, increasing this ratio to 1 : 1 : 1, or worse, to 1 : 2 : 2, led to formation and isolation of alkylated hydantoin. Thus, about one-fourth of the starting semicarbazone is wasted even under optimum conditions (Chart IV).

The shortcomings of the method in Chart IV have been overcome by an acid-catalyzed ester-amide cyclization step as outlined in Chart V. For example, reaction of ethyl hydrazinoacetate hydrochloride with potassium cyanate proceeded smoothly in aqueous solution to give ethyl 3-aminohydantoate which was converted into the respective 3-(benzylideneamino)hydantoate, by reaction with a substituted ben-

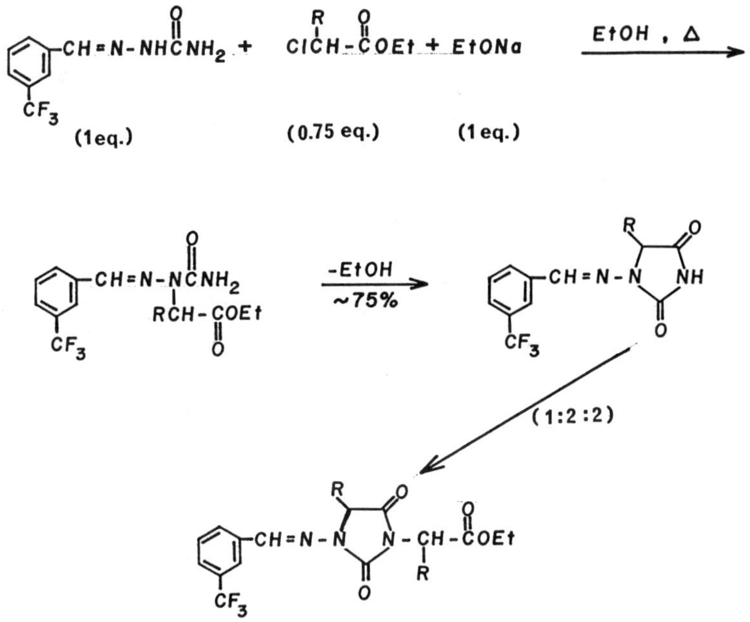

Chart IV. 1-(Benzylideneamino)hydantoins from benzaldehyde semicarbazones.

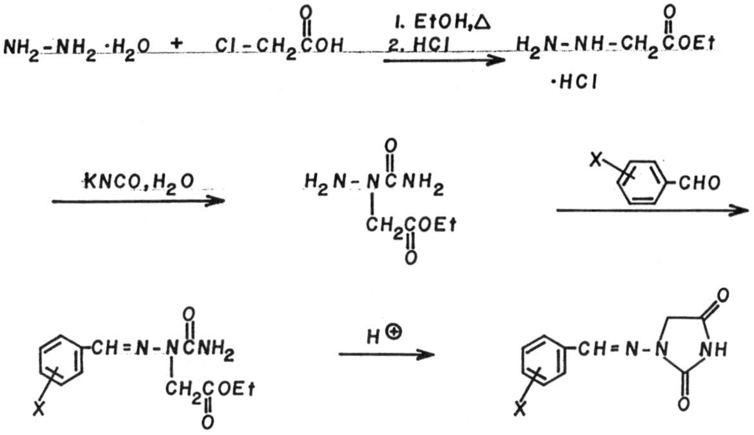

Chart V. 1-(Benzylideneamino)hydantoins from ethyl hydrazinoacetate.

zaldehyde, and then by acid-catalyzed cyclization to the 1-(benzylideneamino)hydantoin. In many instances, chloroacetic acid was treated successively with hydrazine, ethanol, cyanate, aldehyde, and dilute aqueous acid to give the 1-(benzylideneamino)hydantoins in good overall yield without isolation of intermediates (Chart V). This methodology is an adaptation of the process developed for the antibacterial agent nitrofurantoin, 1-[5-(nitrofurfurylidene)amino]-hydantoin (21,22).

Synthesis of Formamidines. N-(Benzylideneamino) heterocycles structurally transform into formamidines by inversion of the azomethine linkage. A series of formamidines related to 1-(benzylideneamino)-imidazolidin-2-ones has been prepared by reaction of substituted formanilides with imidazolidin-2-one (ethylene urea) in thionyl chloride solution. The one-pot method which involves condensation between ethylene urea and an imidoyl chloride, represents a new method for the synthesis of trisubstituted formamidines (Chart VI).

Synthesis of 1-Phenylazo-Imidazolidin-2-ones. Substituent electronic effects are transmitted by the azo link, -N=N-, about 1.5 times more effectively than by a carbon-carbon double bond (23). This difference between azo and ethylenic links may be due to enhanced electronegativity of the nitrogen containing group. For instance, the standard reaction of N-aminoimidazolidin-2-one with aromatic diazonium salts was unsuccessful under a variety of reaction conditions (Table II); none of the desired 1-phenylazo-imidazolidin-2-one could be isolated.

Table II. Attempted Preparation of 1-Phenylazo-imidazolidin-2-ones

$X-C_6H_4-NH_2 \longrightarrow X-C_6H_4-N_2^{\oplus} X^{\ominus}$ + HN N-M (imidazolidin-2-one) ⟶ (0-20°, blocked) $X-C_6H_4-N=N-N$ NH (imidazolidin-2-one)

Diazotization	Solvent	Buffer	M
$NaNO_2$, aq. HCl	H_2O	$NaHCO_3$	H
$NaNO_2$, aq. HBF_4	AcOH	Na_2CO_3	Na
i-C_5H_{11}ONO, AcOH	AcOH-$C_2H_5CO_2H$	NaOH	Li
	THF	NaOC	

However, nitrosobenzenes condensed smoothly with N-aminoimidazolidin-2-one in glacial acetic acid. In many instances, isolation of nitrosobenzenes is cumbersome because of their instability. Higher overall yields (35-56%) were obtained by allowing the crude nitrosobenzene to react with the N-aminoheterocycle, as outlined in Chart VII for the m-CF_3 derivative.

Synthesis of 1-(Benzylamino)imidazolidin-2-ones. Catalytic reduction of 1-(benzylideneamino)imidazolidin-2-ones was only partially sucessful. For example, catalytic reduction over Pd-C with hydrogen in a Parr shaker gave 1-(benzylamino)imidazolidin-2-one in low (32%)

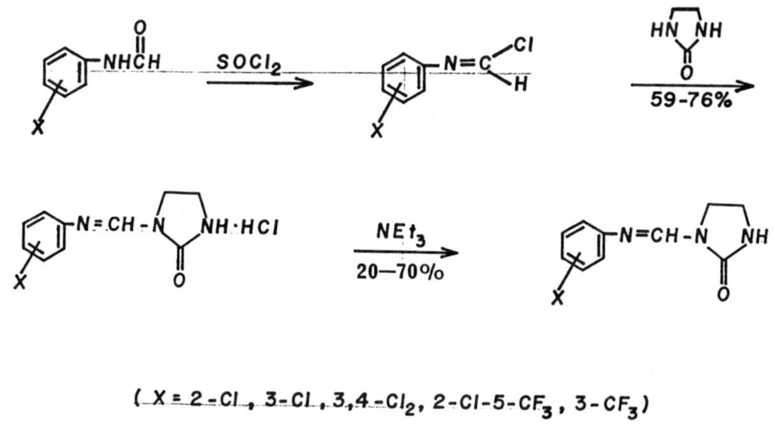

NHCHO SOCl2 N=C(Cl)H; HN NH (C=O) 59-76%

N=CH-N NH·HCl; NEt3 20—70%; N=CH-N NH

(X = 2-Cl, 3-Cl, 3,4-Cl_2, 2-Cl-5-CF_3, 3-CF_3)

Chart VI. Preparation of formamidines.

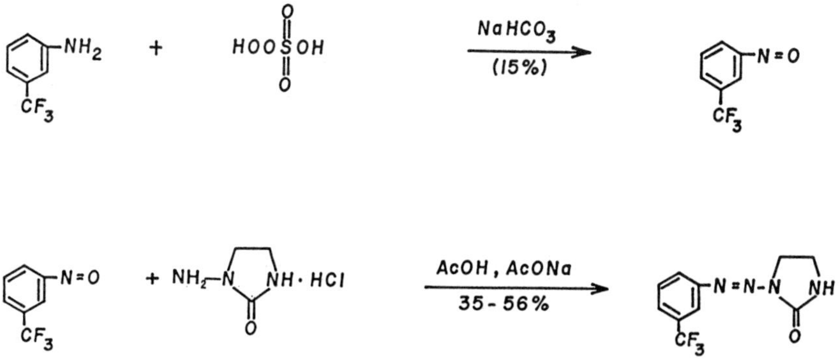

NH_2 + HOOSO2OH; $NaHCO_3$ (15%); N=O; CF_3

N=O + NH_2-N NH·HCl; AcOH, AcONa 35-56%; N=N-N NH; CF_3

Chart VII. Preparation of 1-(3-trifluoromethyl)phenylazo-imidazolidin-2-ones.

yield. However, this method, as well as the Lindlar modification was unsuccessful when the substrate contained a sulfur-containing substituent (X), and when the substituents on phenyl were ortho-Cl, ortho--Br, or ortho-CF_3.

In all instances, reduction of the -CH=N- bond with diborane in tetrahydrofuran proved to be most general. Advantages of this method are:

(1) No cleavage of nitrogen-nitrogen, nitrogen-carbon, or carbon-halogen bonds.

(2) No retardation by sulfur-containing substituents.

(3) No reduction of nitro groups.

In general, the change from unsaturation to saturation of the -CH=N- bond is accompanied by a dramatic increase of the water solubility. In addition, melting points for the reduced products are lower by approximately 100°. The advantages for diborane over catalytic reduction are illustrated in Table III.

Table III. Reduction of 1-(Benzylideneamino)imidazolidin-2-ones

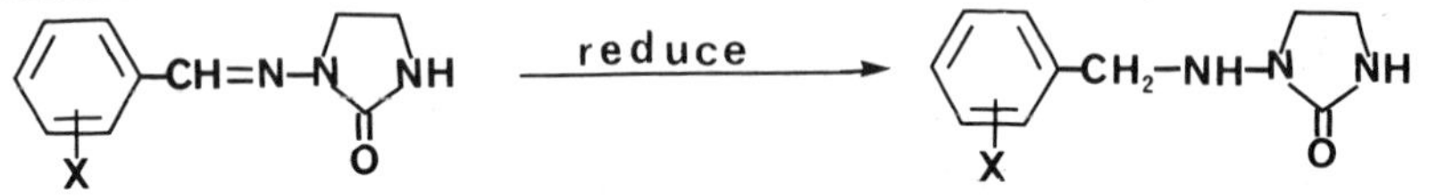

(X-substituted phenyl)-CH=N-N(imidazolidin-2-one)NH —reduce→ (X-substituted phenyl)-CH_2-NH-N(imidazolidin-2-one)NH

X	% Yield B_2H_6	% Yield H_2/Pd-C
H	42	32
2-F	a)	88
2-Cl	68	0.0
2-Br	65	0.0
2-CH_3	87	30
2-CF_3	68	0.0
3-CF_3	82	24
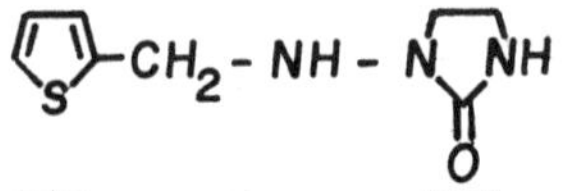 (2-thienyl)-CH_2-NH-N(imidazolidin-2-one)NH	78	0.0
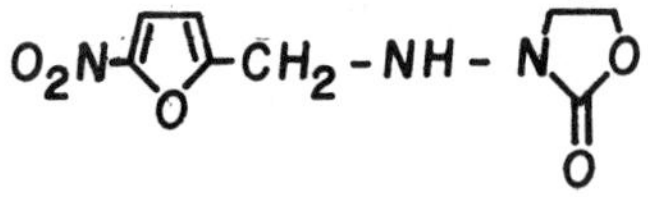 O_2N-(2-furyl)-CH_2-NH-N(oxazolidin-2-one)	42	a)

a) Not done.

Synthesis of 4-(Benzylamino)-Δ^2-1,2,4-triazol-3-ones. These compounds were readily obtained by reduction of the corresponding 4-(benzylideneamino) derivatives with sodium borohydride according to Billman (24).

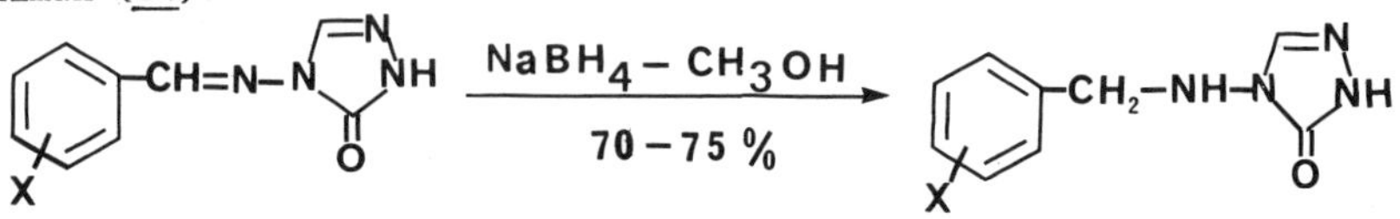

(X-substituted phenyl)-CH=N-N(1,2,4-triazol-3-one)NH —$NaBH_4$ – CH_3OH, 70–75 %→ (X-substituted phenyl)-CH_2-NH-N(1,2,4-triazol-3-one)NH

However, this method was unsuccessful for the reduction of 1-(benzylideneamino)hydantoins.

Herbicidal Activity

Data from the primary herbicide screen of compounds of the following general structure

bridge — a — C(=O) — N — linkage — C_6H_4 — X_n

has provided a reasonably clear picture of the requirements for herbicidal activity.

The Effect of the "Linkage". In considering the structure elements linking the phenyl ring with the heterocycle, we find the azomethine (25,26,27) bridge, -N=CH-, its reduced form, -NH-CH_2-, and the azo (28) grouping, -N=N, very favorable for activity (Table IV). However, substitution of the azomethine unit (R = alkyl, aryl) or chain elongation, -N=CH-CH=CH, resulted in inactive compounds, presumably due to adverse geometry of the resulting structures. In order to account for the high activity of N-(benzylamino) heterocycles containing the -NH-CH_2- bridge, we suggest a process, in soil or plant, leading to unsaturation: -NH-CH_2 $\longrightarrow$ -N=CH-.

Table IV. The Effect of the "Linkage"

Active	Inactive
	-CH=N-
-N=CH-	-NH-C(=O)-
-NH-CH_2-	-N=C(R)-
-N=N-	-N=CH-CH=CH-

Formamidines which contain the -CH=N- link are too susceptible to hydrolysis, in soil and plants, to be effective as herbicides.

Benzamides containing the -NH-C(=O)- bridge are likewise inactive. This may be due to the fact that the amide bond is only about 1/4 to 1/3 as effective as the -N=N- double bond in transmitting conjugation (29,30).

The Effect of a. Changes of the nature of a are of great importance. For example, one of the requirements for activity in this series appears to be a cyclic urea nitrogen atom having pronounced anionic character (NH-acidity). Analogous cyclic carbamates (a = O) are considerably less active, whereas cyclic amides (a = CH_2) are inactive.

Alkylation of the nitrogen atom renders the molecule inactive. N-(Acetoxymethylation) retains preemergent activity while increasing postemergent broadleaf weed activity over that of the parent. Being derivatives of formaldehyde, these hemiaminals hydrolyze readily in soil and plant to the active parent NH-compound.

Thus, herbicidal activity decreases in the following order of a:

$$NH,\ N\text{-}CH_2OAc > O \gg CH_2,\ N\text{-alkyl}$$

The Effect of the "Bridge" (Ring Size). In order to simplify the discussion about the effect of the "bridge" on activity, the structures of the N-aminoheterocycles used in this work rather than the "bridges" alone are presented in Table V. The structures above the dotted line gave herbicidally active *N*-(benzylideneamino) derivatives; whereas, those derived from the structures drawn below the dotted line were herbicidally uninteresting. A number of additional observations can be made.

(1) Herbicidal activity of *N*-(benzylideneamino) derivatives is dependent upon the length of the bridge which determines the ring size. Maximum activity is associated with five-membered ring derivatives. Ring enlargement (5 → 6) is detrimental as evidenced by the inactivity of derivatives containing the tetrahydro-2(1H)-pyrimidinone and tetrahydro-1,4-oxazin-3-one ring systems. Analogous *N*-(benzylideneamino) derivatives containing the imidazolidin-2-one and oxazolidin-2-one ring are active.

(2) Cleavage of the ethylene bridge of herbicidally active N-(benzylideneamino) derivatives containing the imidazolidin-2-one ring results in inactivity as shown by the inability of benzaldehyde 2,4-dimethylsemicarbazones and benzaldehyde hydrazones derived from methyl hydrazinecarboxylate to inhibit plant growth.

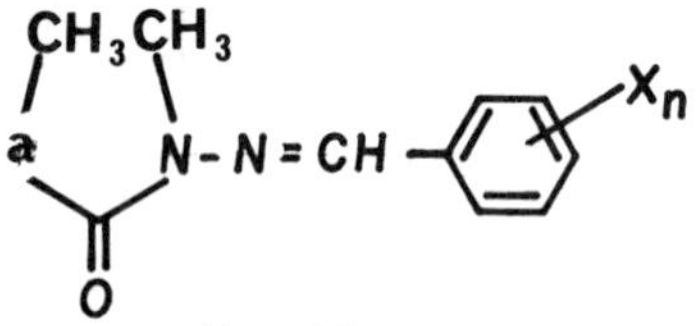

$CH_3\ CH_3$ a N-N=CH-(C$_6$H$_4$)-X_n ; C=O — Inactive

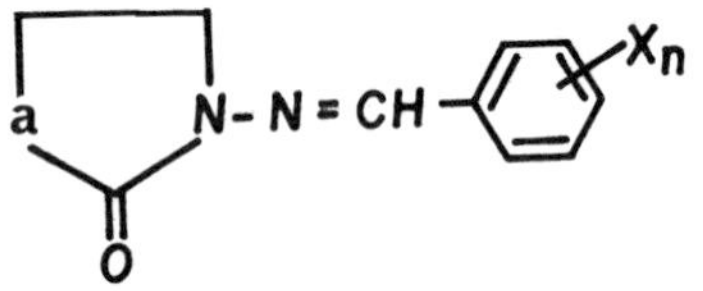

a N-N=CH-(C$_6$H$_4$)-X_n ; C=O (ring) — Active

(a = NH, O)

(3) If the bridge contains one carbonyl group, maximum activity is found in derivatives in which the carbonyl group is adjacent to the NH-group as evidenced by the high activity of N-(benzylideneamino) derivatives prepared from 1-aminohydantoin vs. those prepared from 3-aminohydantoin which are inactive.

(4) Herbicidal activity is retained to a high degree in 1-amino-2-thiohydantoin derivatives.

(5) Derivatives containing the *s*-triazolone ring are among the most active members of this class of compounds showing crop selectivity, whereas the introduction of alkylthio, sulfinyl, and sulfonyl groups cause total loss of activity. Hydroxy derivatives which are tautomers of urazole are likewise inactive.

Table V. N-Amino heterocycles used in this work.

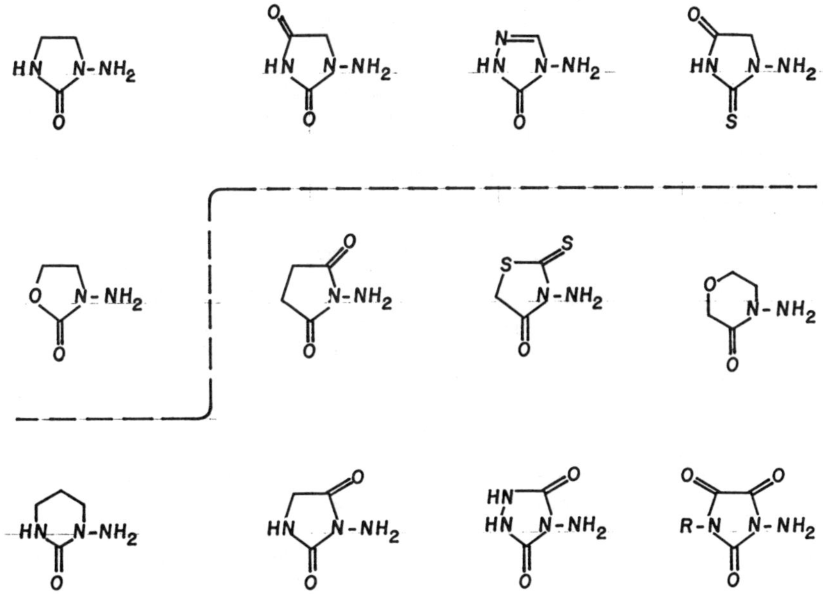

HN N-NH2
O

O
HN N-NH2
O

N
HN N-NH2
O

O
HN N-NH2
S

O N-NH2
O

O
N-NH2
O

S
S
N-NH2
O

O
N-NH2
O

HN N-NH2
O

O
HN N-NH2
O

HN O
HN N-NH2
O

O O
R-N N-NH2
O

(6) The inactivity of derivatives containing the imidazolidin-2,4,5-trione ring is probably due to hydrolytic instability of this ring system in an aqueous environment.

The Effect of Substitution (X_n) on Phenyl. A summary of the effect on phenyl is given in Table VI. The dividing line roughly separates substituents and substitution patterns that give herbicidally active *N*-(benzylideneamino) heterocycles (above the dotted line) from combinations that are herbicidally uninteresting (below the dotted line).

For example, substituents such as OH, OCH_3, and NO_2 in both *ortho*- and *meta*-positions give inactive derivatives. Highest activity is observed with compounds having a strongly electron withdrawing substituent in the *meta*-position on phenyl, followed by substitution in the *ortho*-position. This pattern, i.e.,

meta > *ortho* > *para*

occurs with all substituents. In general, herbicidal activity increases with increasing lipophilicity of X. Although this might explain the activity order of mono-substituted compounds, lipophilicity alone does not account for the differences in the three positional isomers which have approximately the same partition coefficients but vary greatly in their herbicidal activity.

meta-Isomers represent a greater than 10-fold increase in activity over the *para*-isomers. *ortho*-Isomers were only moderately active. *meta*- (Not *ortho*-) isomers produce severe bleaching, inhibiting cartenoid biosynthesis at the phytoene ($C_{40}H_{64}$) desaturation state leading to lycopene ($C_{40}H_{56}$) causing the loss of colored carotenoids and accumulation of colorless phytoene (Flint, D. H., personal communication).

Results

The bleaching properties are especially pronounced in *meta*-CF_3 and *meta*-OCF_3 substituted benzylideneamino derivatives. In this regard, their properties resemble very closely other herbicides containing an aromatic ring bonded to a heterocycle whose bleaching properties are frequently enhanced if there are *meta*-CF_3 (31), *meta*-OCF_3 (26,27), or *meta*-ClO_3 (32) substituents. The particular combination of electron withdrawing properties and lipophilicity undoubtedly combine to give such compounds special properties often associated with effects on membrane permeability.

Compounds which showed appreciable activity in the primary screens were subjected to secondary and tertiary greenhouse tests. Two compounds emerged as the most promising. Both III and IV showed tolerance on cotton, but only III showed a good level of tolerance on soybeans with preemergent control of broadleaf weeds and grasses at 0.2-1.0 lbs/acre in Hanford sandy loam (<1% organic matter content).

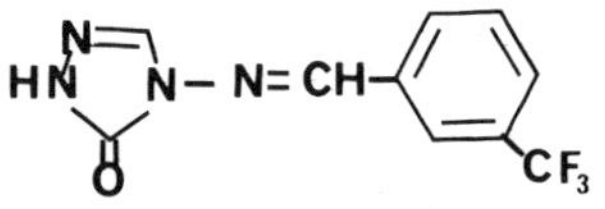

III

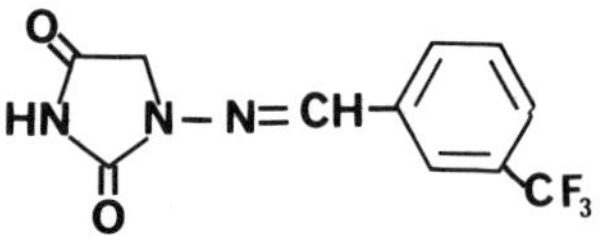

IV

Table VI. The effect of substitution on phenyl.

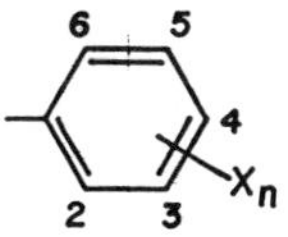

n = 1: 2	n = 1: 3	n = 1: 4	n = 2	n = 3
Cl	CF_3	Cl	2,6-Cl_2	
CF_3	OCF_3	F	2,4-Cl_2	2,3,6-Cl_3
CH_3	SCF_3	Br	2,5-Cl_2	
Br	Cl	CF_3	3,5-Cl_2	
F	Br	CH_3	2-Cl,5-CF_3	
OH	CH_3	OH	3,4-Cl_2	
OCH_3	F		3-Cl, 4-F	
NO_2	OCH_3		2,3-Cl_2	
	OH		3-CF_3, 4-OCH_3	
	NO_2		3-CF_3, 4-OPr^i	
	CHO			
	$OCHF_2$			

Summary and Outlook

This paper illustrates how the principle of vinylogy may serve to direct attention to possible structural similarities in a large number of diverse structures of herbicides with similar activity and mode of action which might otherwise appear unlikely. Structural information such as this on various classes of PS II herbicides in conjunction with intuitive-empirical or computer oriented approaches should facilitate the design of new inhibitors.

Literature Cited

1. Fuson, R. C. Chem. Rev. 1935, 16, 1.
2. Näf, F.; Decorzant, R. Helv. Chim. Acta 1974, 57, 1309.
3. Koppel, G. A. Tetrahedron Lett. 1972, 1507.
4. Jutz, C. Chem. Ber. 1958, 91, 850.
5. Mikhailenko, F. A.; Shevchuk, L. I. Synthesis 1973, 621.
6. Durst, T. In Advances in Organic Chemistry; Taylor, E. C.; Wynberg, H., Eds.; Interscience: New York, 1966; Vol. 6, p 356.
7. Praefke, K.; Weichsel, C. Leibigs Annalen 1979, 784.
8. Wiesner, K.; Ho, P. T.; Ohtani, H. Can. J. Chem. 1974, 52, 640.
9. Smith III, B. A. J. Chem. Soc. Chem. Comm. 1974, 695.
10. Farooq, S. Pestic. Sci. 1980, 11, 242.
11. Elliott, M.; Janes, N. F. Chem. Soc. Rev. 1978, 7, 473.
12. Hayes, K. J. Am. Chem. Soc. 1955, 77, 2333.
13. Kim, H. K.; Bambury, R. E. J. Med. Chem. 1971, 14, 366.
14. McGovern, T. P.; Redfern, R. E. J. Agric. Food Chem. 1979, 27, 82.
15. Wegler, R.; Eue, L. In Chemie der Pflanzenschutz-und Schädlingsbekämpfungsmittel; Wegler, R., Ed.; Springer: Berlin, 1970, Vol. 2, p 165.
16. Moreland, D. E. A. Rev. Pl. Physiol. 1967, 18, 365.
17. Beech, W. F. J. Chem. Soc. 1954, 1297.
18. Jolad, S.D.; Rajagopal, S. Org. Synth, Coll. Vol. 5, 1973, 139.
19. Yagupolskii, L. M.; Troitskaya, V. I. Zh. Obshch. Khim. 1957, 27, 518; Chem. Abstr. 1957, 51, 15517.
20. Stogryn, E. L. J. Med. Chem. 1973, 16, 1399.
21. Uota, H.; Takai, A.; Yokoi, T. J. Pharm. Soc. Japan 1955, 75, 117.
22. Coleman, J. H.; Hayden, Jr., W.; O'Keefe, C. J. U.S. Patent 2 779 786; Chem. Abstr. 1957, 51, 9681.
23. Shawali, A. S.; Altahon, B. M. Tetrahedron, 1977, 33, 1625.
24. Billman, J. H.; Diesing, A. C. J. Org. Chem. 1957, 22, 1068.
25. Kollmeyer, W. D.; Pilgram, K. H. G. U.S. Patent 3 746 704; Chem. Abstr. 1973, 79, 78797.
26. Pilgram, K. H. U.S. Patent 3 830 805; Chem. Abstr. 1974, 81, 152228r.
27. Pilgram, K. H. U.S. Patent 3 884 910; Chem. Abstr. 1975, 83, 79251.
28. Kollmeyer, W. D.; Soloway, S. B. U.S. Patent 3 892 724; Chem. Abstr. 1975, 83, 164179e.
29. Pews, R. G. J. Chem. Soc. Chem. Comm. 1971, 458.
30. Shawali, A. S.; Altahon, B. M. Tetrahedron 1977, 33, 1625.

31. Ridley, S. M. In Carotenoid Chemistry and Biochemistry; Pergamon: Oxford, 1981, p 353.
32. Pilgram, K. H.; Jackson, E. K.; Wittsell, L. E. J. Agric. Food Chem. 1982, 30, 971.

RECEIVED May 12, 1987

Chapter 5

2-Phenoxynicotinamides

A New Class of Bleaching Herbicides

W. J. Michaely and A. D. Gutman

Organic Synthesis Department, ICI Americas Inc., 1200 South 47th Street, Box 4023, Richmond, CA 94804–0023

The 2-phenoxynicotinamides were shown to be excellent bleaching herbicides. The optimum substitution on the 2-phenoxy ring was the meta-CF_3 group. There are significant differences in the optimum substitution patterns for the N-phenyl and N-benzyl nicotinamide series. The aryl analogs (replacing the pyridine ring) were only slightly active.

There are several ways to discover biologically active molecules. Three possible ways seem logical to us. (a) Knowing a three dimensional structure of an enzyme and/or the mechanism of action of the enzyme, appropriate inhibitors can be designed. (b) If one knows several different inhibitors of an enzyme and they inhibit at (or near) the same site, then molecular modeling and QSAR techniques can be used to design new and/or better inhibitors. Sometimes this approach deteriorates to an analogue (me-too) synthesis program. (c) "Randomly" prepare (or buy) compounds about which nothing is known or presumed and apply them to your test systems (insects, plants, fungi, enzymes, etc.). Our colleagues in the pharmaceutical industry have had success in all three approaches, with some excellent success in category (a). Unfortunately, when herbicide chemists attempt to emulate this success, we immolate ourselves because there are very few plant enzymes that are well characterized. Therefore, the two most common approaches are (b) and (c). The nicotinamide class of herbicides was discovered via the "random," (c) synthesis approach. The initial synthesis was prompted by some interesting chemistry described by Villani (1), which showed that the chloro group in 2-chloro-nicotinic acid could be displaced by a phenol (in the presence of a base) to produce the 2-phenoxynicotinic acid. Because the chemistry was interesting and a number of herbicides contain a phenoxy moiety and a benzoic acid group, a few compounds were prepared to determine if there was significant pesticidal activity.

0097–6156/87/0355–0054$06.00/0
© 1987 American Chemical Society

The initial compounds prepared were the 2-(substituted)phenoxynicotinic acids (I, Figure 1). These (substituted)2-phenoxynicotinic acids were devoid of herbicidal activity at our 4 lb/acre screening rate. In order to change the polarity of the products, these nicotinic acids were converted to N-alkyl amides by merely heating them with alkyl isocyanates in the absence of a solvent (II, Figure 1).

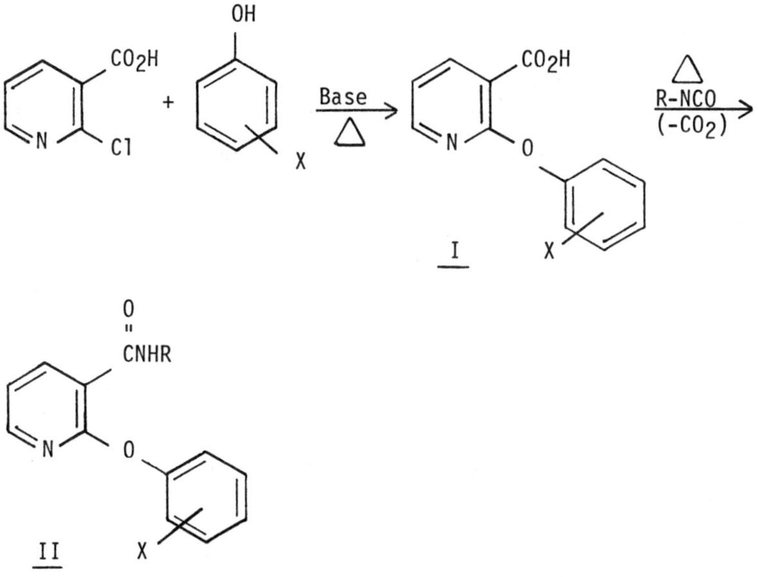

Figure 1. Preparation of N-alkylnicotinamides.

These nicotinic acid intermediates were also converted to their corresponding ethyl esters by reaction with ethyl alcohol in the presence of sulfuric acid. Surprisingly, the alkyl amides had some pre- and postemergent herbicidal activity with bleaching symptomology. The activity was quite weak, less than 50% weed control was observed at 2 lb/acre. The esters, on the other hand, were almost devoid of herbicidal activity.

A research program was initiated to explore the scope of the activity of the 2-phenoxynicotinamides. Holding the amide portion constant, as N-methyl, compounds were prepared from a number of substituted phenols, and after preparing a relatively small number of compounds, it became evident that only the 3-substitution pattern possessed high activity (Figure 2). The results of the study indicated that the 3-trifluoromethyl substitution provided the highest level of activity followed in descending order by: 3-chloro, 3-ethyl and 3-methyl (III, Figure 2). It is interesting to speculate that the herbicidal activity is the result, in part, of a fit on an enzyme site, since CF_3, Cl and CH_3 all have about the same molecular size.

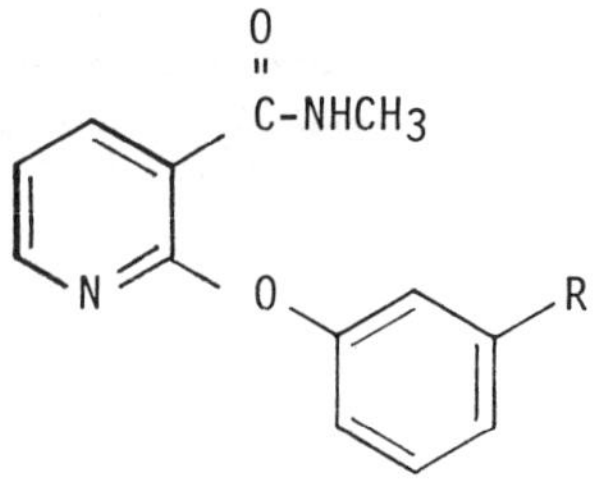

$$\text{III}$$

$3\text{-}CF_3 > 3\text{-}Cl > 3\text{-}C_2H_5 > 3\text{-}CH_3$

Figure 2. Relative Herbicidal Activity vs. the Phenyl Ether Substituent.

Work was next conducted to determine the optimum substitution of the amide group. The substituted phenoxynicotinic acids were reacted with thionyl chloride to produce the acid chlorides, which, in turn, were reacted with a wide variety of primary and secondary amines and anilines to produce the corresponding amides.

The most active compounds were the N-phenyl amides and the N-benzyl amides.

The N-phenyl Nicotinamides (Table I)

In the N-phenyl case all of the secondary aryl amides were very weak or inactive. The biodata on the primary amides is shown in Table I.

When considering a combination of pre- and postemergent herbicidal activity, the 4-chlorophenyl derivative (compound 4, Table I) had clearly superior activity (89% pre- and 74% post-emergent). Considering only the preemergent application method, several compounds showed good levels of activity. The most active compounds contained the 3-chlorophenoxy group and were either unsubstituted or had a 4-chloro or 3-chloro substituent on the N-phenyl group (compounds 15, 7 and 6 in Table I). The comparable 3-trifluoromethylphenoxy compounds were less active (compounds 14, 4 and 3 in Table I), the major difference can be correlated with decreased wild oat control. Despite these clear activity differences, we were unable to obtain a clear Structure Activity Relationship (SAR) for the N-(substituted)nicotinamides. For example, comparing compounds 10, 11, and 13 (all have the N-[4-methylphenyl] group), the order of increasing activity for the phenoxy substituent is $3\text{-}CF_3 < 3\text{-}CH_2H_5 < 3\text{-}Cl$. But, comparing compounds 14, 15 and 16 (all have the unsubstituted N-phenyl group) and compounds 5 and 8 (both have the N-[3,4-dichlorophenyl] group) the orders of activity for the phenoxy substituents are

Table I

N-Phenylnicotinamides

PREEMERGENCE/POSTEMERGENCE ACTIVITY AT 2 LB/ACRE

Compound No.	X	Y	Weed Species: Crab Grass	Wild Oats	Fox Tails	Water Grass	Pig Weed	Mustards	Curly Dock	Average (%)
1	3-CF_3	3-NO_2	90/30	20/30	98/50	20/10	90/90	80/80	75/90	68/54
2	3-CF_3	4-NO_2	0/0	0/0	0/0	0/0	0/0	0/0	0/0	0/0
3	3-CF_3	3-Cl	100/0	20/0	100/20	80/10	100/10	98/10	100/10	85/9
4	3-CF_3	4-Cl	90/80	80/30	100/80	80/50	95/95	95/85	80/100	89/74
5	3-CF_3	3,4-diCl	90/20	10/10	80/20	20/0	90/80	90/80	80/90	66/43
6	3-Cl	3-Cl	100/10	90/10	100/20	95/10	98/10	100/10	95/10	97/11
7	3-Cl	4-Cl	100/10	75/0	100/10	100/10	100/10	100/10	95/10	96/9
8	3-Cl	3,4-diCl	0/0	10/0	10/0	0/0	0/0	0/0	0/0	3/0
9	3-CF_3	3-CH_3	0/0	10/0	0/0	10/0	0/0	30/0	60/0	15/0
10	3-CF_3	4-CH_3	100/10	80/10	100/20	85/0	30/0	10/0	0/0	58/5
11	3-Ethyl	4-CH_3	0/0	10/0	100/20	100/20	100/10	50/0	98/10	65/9
12	3-Ethyl	3-CH_3	0/0	10/0	100/10	75/10	0/0	0/0	80/0	38/3
13	3-Cl	4-CH_3	98/10	50/0	95/10	90/10	80/0	95/10	95/10	86/7
14	3-CF_3	H	100/10	20/0	100/20	100/20	100/20	100/10	100/10	89/13
15	3-Cl	H	100/10	50/0	100/20	100/20	95/20	100/10	95/10	91/13
16	3-Ethyl	H	0/0	10/10	100/100	100/50	90/30	10/0	100/80	59/39
17	3-CH_3	H	0/0	0/0	100/10	20/0	0/0	0/0	80/10	29/3

$3\text{-}C_2H_5 < 3\text{-}CF_3 < 3\text{-}Cl$ and $3\text{-}Cl \ll 3\text{-}CF_3$, respectively. Hence, we found no consistent structural correlations in the N-phenyl series.

After our initial patent applications in this area (2, 3, 4) were filed, a research group at May and Baker Limited filed patents in the same area (5, 6). The information in these patents is covered in a recent publication (7). They came to several conclusions about the SAR of the N-phenyl-2-phenoxynicotinamides. They concluded that the optimum substitution pattern on the 2-phenoxy group was the 3-trifluoromethyl moiety. Their optimum pyridine substituents were the unsubstituted and the 5-methyl nicotinamides. Their optimum N-phenyl substituents were the 4-fluoro and 2,4-difluorophenyl compounds. Combining the greenhouse optimization with field trial results led the May and Baker group to select N-(2,4-difluorophenyl)-2-(3-trifluoromethylphenoxy)-3-pyridine carboxamide (diflufenican) for development as a herbicide for winter wheat and barley.

Sandman et. al. (8) have found the N-phenyl-2-phenoxynicotinamides to be powerful inhibitors of phytoene desaturase. Several bleaching herbicides that inhibit the phytoene to phytofluene transformation have the same 3-trifluoromethylphenyl group (8, 9). This group includes norflurazon, metflurazon, fluridone, fluometuron and fluorochloridone. In the nicotinamide series the same 3-trifluoromethylphenyl group gives optimum herbicide activity.

The N-Benzylnicotinamides

The N-benzylnicotinamides have an interesting herbicidal SAR. There are several important effects of substitution patterns on bioactivity. The variation of herbicidal activity with the nitrogen substituent can be seen in Table II.

From Table II it is clear that the secondary amide (R=H) is the most active. Surprisingly, the highly polar hydroxamic acid (R=OH) is slightly active. This might be explained by *in vivo* reduction to the active parent or possibly polarity in this position is not detrimental to activity. The alkyl amides in Table II appear (with the exception of N-ethyl) to rapidly lose herbicidal activity as the length of the alkyl group increases. For example, when the N-alkyl group contains four or more carbons, all herbicidal activity is lost. The herbicidal activity differences, as a function of application method, are noteworthy. For preemergent application, grass control is usually superior to broadleaf control, but the opposite is true in postemergent application. We do not know the reason for this phenomenon. This result could be due to simple physical differences between grasses and broadleaves. Broadleaves have more exposed horizontal leaf surfaces than grasses, hence, postemergent applications usually produce better leaf coverage on broadleaves.

The substitution pattern for the benzylic carbon is quite simple. Replacing the benzylic hydrogens decreases activity. Polar groups eliminate activity. This can be seen in Table III.

Table II

Herbicide Activity of N-Substituted, N-Benzylnicotinamides

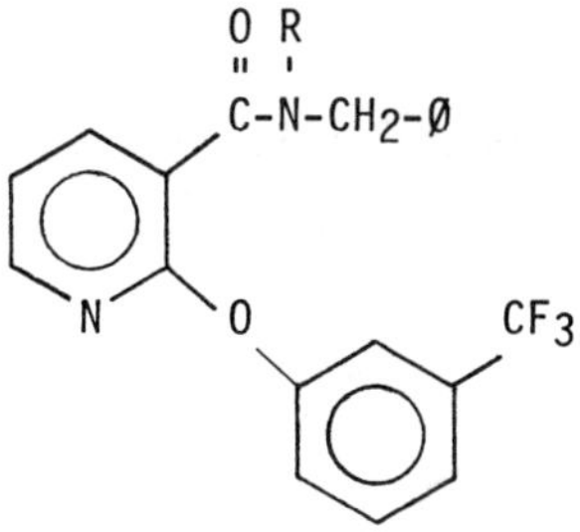

Weed Control (% Grass/% Broadleaf)

R	Preemergent	Postemergent	Rate lb/acre
H	100/90	87/89	4
	100/71	59/84	2
	61/52	32/62	1
	39/17	12/50	1/2
OH	37/20	27/60	4
CH_3	40/16	15/48	4
C_2H_5	65/49	27/85	4
	42/23	13/67	2
	25/8	6/54	1
$\underline{n}C_3H_7$	27/12	12/39	4
$\underline{i}C_3H_7$	7/3	5/11	4
$\underline{n}C_4H_9$	0/0	0/0	4
CH_2CH_2CN	3/0	5/10	4

AUGUSTANA UNIVERSITY COLLEGE
LIBRARY

Table III

Herbicide Activity of Benzylic Substituted Nicotinamides

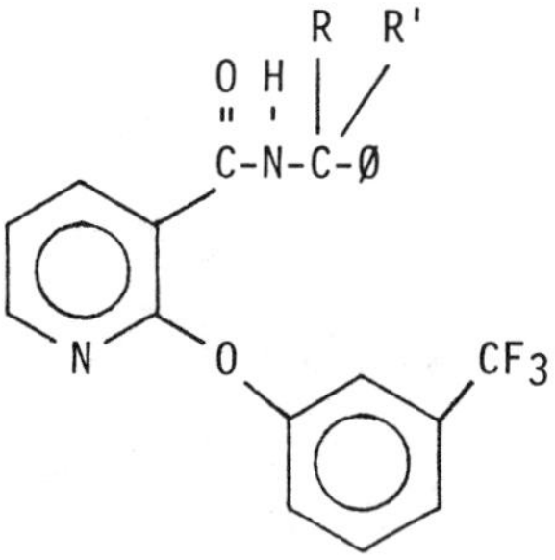

Weed Control (% Grass/% Broadleaf)

R	R'	Preemergent Surface (PES)	Postemergent	Rate lb/acre
H	H	100/90	87/89	4
		100/71	59/84	2
CH_3	H	87/75	68/76	4
		40/14	40/38	2
> C=O		0/0	0/0	4
CN	H	0/3	10/3	4

We have also replaced the benzylic CH_2 by an NH. These (substituted) phenyl hydrazides were inactive.

The optimum substitution pattern on the phenyl group of the ether moiety in the N-benzyl series of compounds is consistent with the pattern seen in N-alkyl and N-phenyl series. In the N-benzyl series, consistently high levels of herbicidal activity are obtained with the 3-trifluoromethylphenyl ethers. Replacing the phenyl ether by a 3-trifluoromethylphenylamine or N-methyl-3-trifluoromethylphenylamine group resulted in total loss of herbicide activity. The substituted benzyl ethers and aliphatic ethers had very low levels of herbicide activity.

The SAR for the N-benzyl phenyl substitution pattern is very different than that for the N-phenyl substitution pattern. In the N-benzyl derivatives, only small groups are tolerated in the para position, even para fluoro is less than half as active as the unsubstituted parent. This phenomenon appears to be a simple size requirement since groups of varying lipophilicities and electronic characteristics such as Cl, Br, CN, CF_3, OCH_3 and CH_3 are all essentially inactive at the 4 lb/acre screening rate.

For substituents in the meta position, size is not as critical as it is for the para position. However, only the meta fluoro compound has herbicidal activity comparable to the unsubstituted parent. All of the other derivatives are substantially less active than these two compounds.

The effect of substituents in the ortho position, on <u>preemergent</u> herbicidal activity, is unclear. The ranking of ortho substituents is $NO_2 > CF_3 > CH_3 > Cl > F > H > Br > OCH_3 > OC_2H_5$. The more active compounds also have a flatter dose response curve. Hence, <u>ortho</u> CF_3 is 93/98 (Gr/Bl) at 4 lb/acre but still 74/92 (Gr/Bl) at 1/2 lb/acre. Surprisingly, most of the ortho substituted compounds are less active, than their corresponding parent, when comparing their <u>postemergent</u> activity.

The Phenyl Analogs of the Pyridine Ring

It has been suggested by Thornber and others (<u>10</u>) that the nitrobenzene ring is equivalent to the pyrdine ring (Figure 3).

This makes some sense based upon electron density and reactivity considerations, but, the nitro group occupies a much larger space than the pyridine nitrogen lone pair of electrons. In order to test this equivalence, we prepared some 3-nitro-2-phenoxybenzamides for comparison to their pyridine analogs. Two of these are shown in Table IV.

As can be seen from Table IV, the nitrophenyl analogs of the nicotinamides are inactive. Interestingly, the 2-(3-trifluoromethylphenyl) benzamides (compound IV minus the nitro group) were moderate herbicides (less than 50% weed control at 1 lb). These compounds are also bleaching herbicides as are the well known 3-phenoxybenzamides. The 3-phenoxybenzamides are also known to be inhibitors of phytoene desaturase (<u>11</u>).

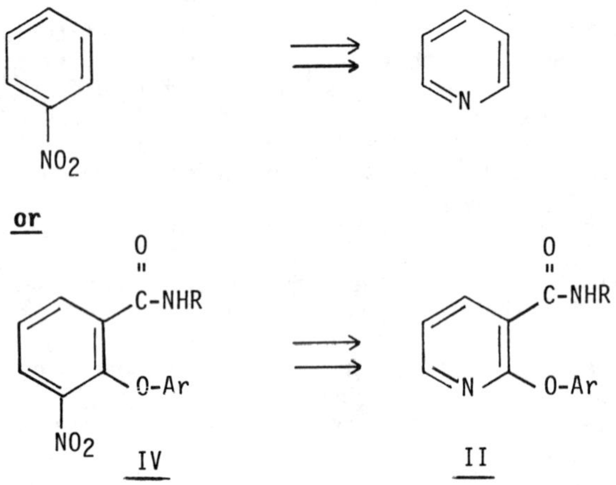

NO_2

or

O
C-NHR
O-Ar
NO_2
IV

O
C-NHR
N
O-Ar
II

Figure 3. Nitrobenzene and Pyridine Structural Equivalence.

Table IV

Comparison of Biological Activities, Some Nicotinamides Versus Their Nitrophenyl Analogs

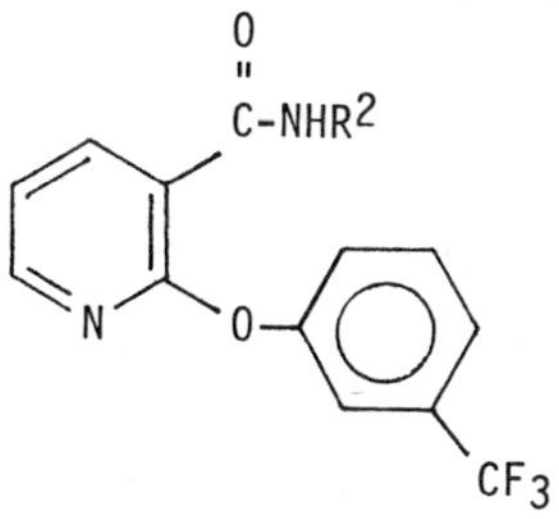

II versus IV

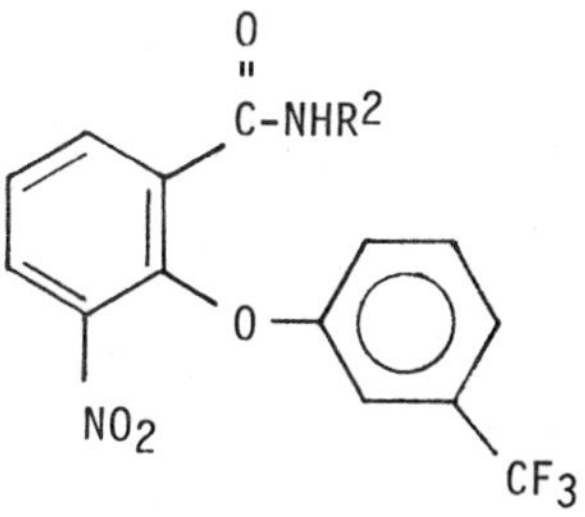

Structure	R^2	PES* Weed Control	Rate (lb/acre)
II	$2\text{-ClC}_6H_4CH_2$-	95%	4
		84%	2
		74%	1
		60%	1/2
		40%	1/4
IV	$2\text{-ClC}_6H_4CH_2$-	0%	4
II	$C_6H_5CH_2$-	88%	4
		89%	2
		57%	1
		29%	1/2
IV	$C_6H_5CH_2$-	0%	4

*PES = preemergent surface

Conclusion

The phenoxynicotinamides represent a novel class of promising preemergence and postemergence herbicides. The results obtained to date indicate that relatively minor variations in structure can have a significant effect on the level of herbicidal activity and spectrum of weeds controlled.

Literature Cited

1. Villani, F. J., et. al., J. Med. Chem. 18, 1-8 (1975).

2. Gutman, A. D. U.S. Patent 4,251,263 (Filed, Sept. 4, 1979; issued, Feb. 17, 1981).

3. Gutman, A. D. U.S. Patent 4,270,946 (Filed, Oct. 1, 1979; issued, June 2, 1981).

4. Gutman, A. D. U.S. Patent 4,327,218 (Filed, Nov. 28, 1980; issued, April 27, 1982).

5. Cramp, M. C.; Gilmour, J.; Parnell, E. W. U.K. Patent App. 2,087,887A (Filed, Nov. 19, 1981).

6. Cramp, M. C.; Gilmour, J.; Parnell, E. W. U.S. Patent 4,618,366 (Filed, June 15, 1984; issued, Oct. 21, 1986).

7. Cramp, M. C.; Gilmour, J.; Hatton, L. R.; Hewett, R. H; Nolan, C. J.; Parnell, E. W. Pestic. Sci. 18, 15-28 (1987).

8. Sandman, G.; Clarke, I. E.; Bramley, P. M.; Boger, P. Z. Naturforsch., C: Biosci, 39C, 443-9 (1984).

9. Dodge, A. D. Progress in Pesticide Biochemistry and Toxicology; Hutson, D. H. and Roberts, T. R., Ed.; John Wiley and Sons Ltd.: New York, 1983; pp 163-197.

10. Thornber, C. W. Chem. Soc. Rev. 8, 563-580 (1979) and references cited therein.

11. Clarke, I. E.; Sandman, G.; Bramley, P. M.; Boger, P. Pest. Biochem. and Phys., 23, 335-340 (1985).

RECEIVED May 12, 1987

Chapter 6

5-Aminofuran-3(2*H*)-ones

A New Development in Bleaching Herbicides

Carl E. Ward, William C. Lo, Patricia B. Pomidor, F. E. Tisdell, Andrew W. W. Ho, Chu-Ling Chiu, David M. Tuck, Carmelita R. Bernardo, Patricia J. Fong, Ahmad Omid, and Katherine A. Buteau

Chevron Chemical Company, Ortho Research Center, Richmond, CA 94804

A novel series of 5-amino-4-phenylfuran-3(2H)-ones was synthesized and found to possess potent bleaching herbicidal activity. The compounds incorporate a vinylogous amide substructure, a feature which is common to a number of other bleaching herbicides that are known to block desaturation of 15- cis phytoene, a step in carotenoid biosynthesis. Synthesis of the furanones was accomplished by three routes the most notable of which utilized a newly discovered transformation of diaryl cyanoketones to 5-amino-2,4-diarylfuran-3(2H)-ones. Herbicidal activity was generally highest for compounds having a meta CF_3 group on the 4-phenyl ring, small alkyl groups on the 5-amino function and a small alkyl or a phenyl substituent at the furan C-2 ring position. Results are interpreted in terms of a hypothetical binding site which could accommodate the 3-furanones as well as certain other known inhibitors of phytoene desaturation.

A great diversity in molecular structure is observed among herbicides which inhibit carotene biosynthesis as is exemplified by the structures of norflurazon, fluridone and difunone (shown below). Nonetheless, many of these compounds, which comprise a subset of the larger group known as bleaching herbicides, appear to inhibit the same step in the biosynthetic pathway to the carotenoids (1). The inhibited step is the desaturation of 15-cis phytoene to 15- cis phytofluene (Figure 1) and the build-up of phytoene in plants and in cell-free systems which have been treated with these herbicides is well documented (2-4).

Although it may not be obvious from first inspection of the structures as they are often drawn, these molecules each possess a nitrogen atom in conjugation with a carbonyl and/or cyano group through one or two double bonds as indicated by the bold lines in the structural formulas. In a modification of the ideas of Sandmann et. al. (2), we hypothesized that it is this vinylogous amide-like configuration of atoms that is one key to the apparently common mode of action of these

0097-6156/87/0355-0065$06.00/0
© 1987 American Chemical Society

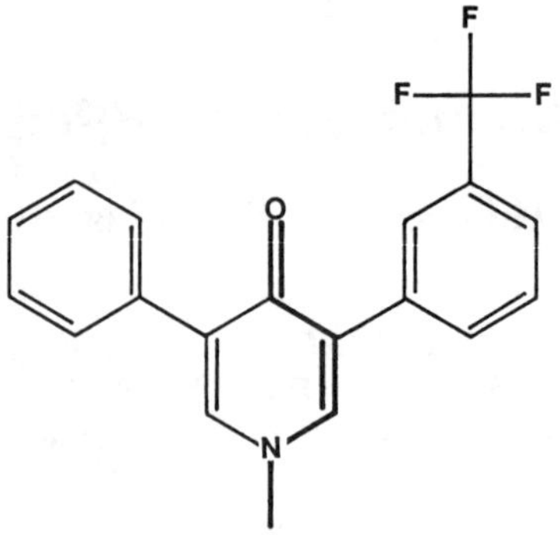

F
F F
O
N

Fluridone

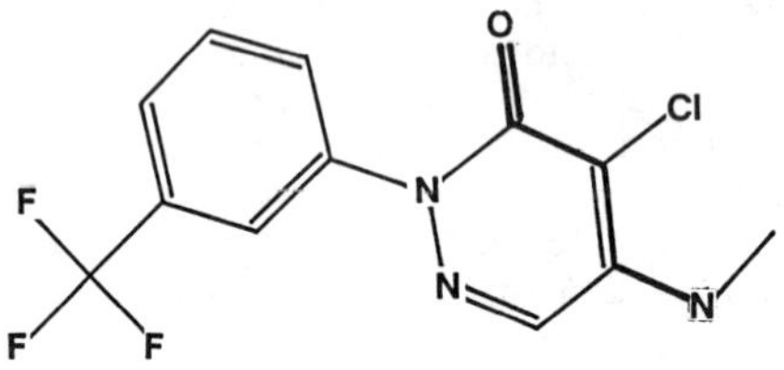

O
Cl
N
F
N
N
F F

Norflurazon

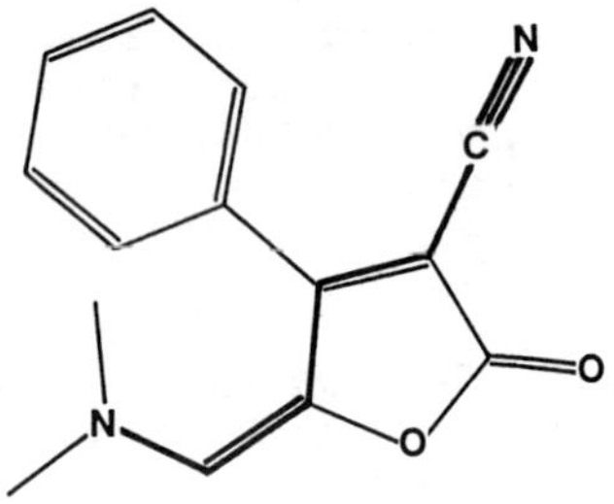

N
C
N
O
O

Difunone

X
O
R^3
O
R^1—N
R^2

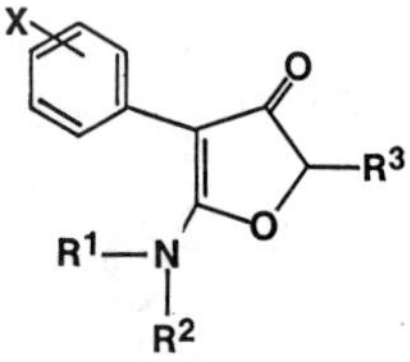

1

herbicides. We now report that we have discovered a new chemical family of bleaching herbicides which incorporates the vinylogous amide substructure. The family of 5-amino-4-phenylfuran-3(2H)-ones represented by structure **1**, is the subject of the present paper (5).

Results and Discussion

Chemistry. Only a few examples of the subject furanones were known prior to our disclosure of this work and none of the reported compounds had been tested for herbicidal activity (6-9). Synthesis of the 3-furanones is accomplished primarily by means of three routes the choice among which depends upon the nature of the substituents R and X. Thus, when R^3 is alkyl or alkenyl, routes 1 and 2 depicted in Scheme I are employed as exemplified for compound **6**, although the synthesis of compounds wherein R^3 is aryl, e.g., phenyl or substituted phenyl, may also be accomplished by means of route 2. In fact, if X is an electron donating group, or if R^3 is an aryl substituent containing a strongly electron donating group, route 2 is preferred. However, the synthesis of many of the 2-aryl compounds was greatly facilitated by our discovery that diaryl cyanoketones undergo a smooth conversion to 5-amino-2,4-diarylfuran-3(2H)-ones upon treatment with bromine in acetic acid as exemplified for compound **7** in Scheme II. Thus, **7** afforded the furanone **12** in 50% yield and treatment of **12** with dimethyl sulfate and aqueous sodium hydroxide in methylene chloride under phase transfer conditions gave **13** in 53% yield after recrystallization. The cyclization can also be conducted in methylene chloride and appears to require the presence of water.

Although the complete mechanism of the reaction is uncertain at this time, we established the intermediacy of **8** by isolating it from a reaction which was worked up immediately after bromine addition. We showed that resubjecting **8** to acetic acid fails to afford any furanone product unless HBr is also reintroduced. This observation is consistent with the proposed rearrangement of **8** to **9** which should be catalyzed by strong acid and which produces an intermediate with a more stable enolic form. Nevertheless, the proposed subsequent series of intermediates represents only one of several possible sequences which could lead to the observed product.

The aminofuranones are weakly basic and exist as the hydrobromide salts (e.g., **11**) in the bromination reaction mixtures. The salts may be isolated or they may be readily converted to the free bases by treatment with aqueous sodium bicarbonate. In general, salt formation with weak organic acids such as acetic acid does not occur but occurs readily with the stronger mineral or sulfonic acids. This weak basicity is due to the extensive delocalization of the nitrogen lone pair into the carbonyl group and is reflected in the infrared spectra of these compounds which each exhibit a weak carbonyl stretching band at approximately 1660 cm^{-1}.

Biology. Test Methods. Compounds were evaluated as preemergence and postemergence herbicides. The test plants (weeds) were lambsquarters (*Chenopodium album*), mustard (*Brassica spp.*), pigweed (*Amaranthus retroflexus*), barnyardgrass (*Echinochloa crusgalli*), crabgrass (*Digitaria sanguinalis*), and wild oats (*Avena fatua*); crops were soybean and rice. In the preemergence tests, seeds of the test vegetation were planted in a pot of sandy clay loam soil and the test solution was sprayed uniformly onto

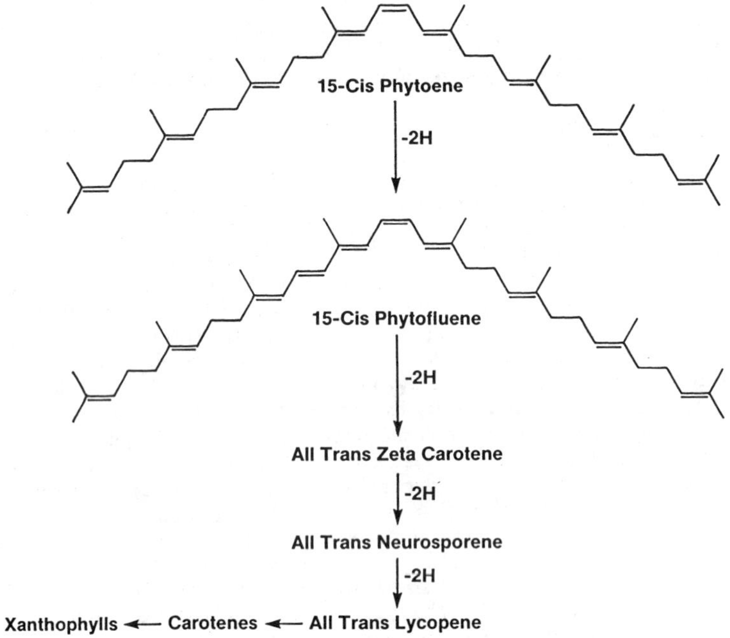

15-Cis Phytoene

-2H

15-Cis Phytofluene

-2H

All Trans Zeta Carotene

-2H

All Trans Neurosporene

-2H

Xanthophylls ← Carotenes ← All Trans Lycopene

Figure 1. Synthesis of Carotenes from Phytoene. (Reproduced with permission from Reference 1. Copyright 1982 Pergamon Press.)

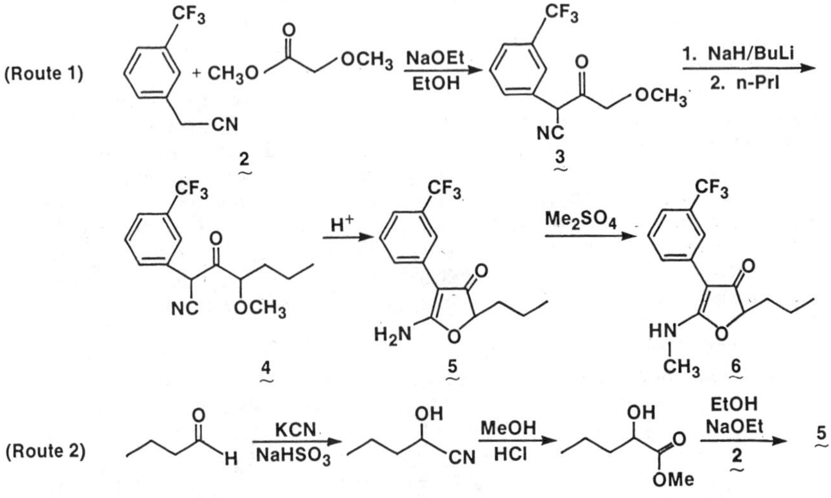

(Route 1) CF_3 ... CN (2) + CH_3O–CO–CH_2–OCH_3 → NaOEt / EtOH → 3 → 1. NaH/BuLi 2. n-PrI → 4 → H^+ → 5 → Me_2SO_4 → 6

(Route 2) butanal (O, H) → KCN / $NaHSO_3$ → (OH, CN) → MeOH / HCl → (OH, O, OMe) → EtOH / NaOEt / 2 → 5

SCHEME I

the soil surface. The solution was prepared by dissolving the test compound in acetone containing a non-ionic surfactant followed by appropriate dilution with an aqueous solution of the same surfactant. The pot was watered intermittently and observed for seedling emergence, health of emerging seedlings etc. for a three week period. At the end of this time, the herbicidal activity of the compound was determined by visual observation of the treated plants in comparison with untreated controls. In the postemergence tests, the developing plants were sprayed when the plants were two to four inches tall. No attempt was made to prevent the spray from reaching the soil. After the plants dried, they were placed in a greenhouse and were periodically subirrigated at their bases as needed. After three weeks, the herbicidal activity was determined as described for the preemergence tests.

Herbicidal Activity. The subject furanones are primarily active as preemergence and preplant incorporated (PRE/PPI) materials and are moderately active when applied postemergence. The structure-activity relationships discussed below pertain to the preemergence activity.

For a given set of substituents, as in this example where R^1 = H, R^2 = CH_3 and X = CF_3, activity is generally highest when R^3 = phenyl or ortho-substituted phenyl (Figure 2). Substitution of the 2-phenyl moiety is preferred in the ortho position and we observe a progressive decrease in activity as the substituent is moved to the meta and para positions (Figure 3). When R^3 = lower alkyl (C1-C3), the level of activity approaches that of the phenyl cases. However, activity falls off rapidly with further increases in chain length or when R^3 = H and essentially vanishes if the 2-position is disubstituted (Figure 2). Branching at the attached carbon in R^3 also tends to lower activity. Turning to the 4-phenyl moiety (Figure 4), we observe that regardless of other factors, activity is always enhanced when X is something other than hydrogen and is attached at the meta position. Almost any such substitution produces measurable herbicidal activity, however, in general, activity is greatest when X = CF_3. Substitutions at the para position of the ring fail to produce activity in all cases if meta substituents are absent. In considering the 5-amino group (Figure 5), we observe that disubstitution always decreases activity thus, one of R^1 or R^2 should be hydrogen in order to maximize activity. In addition, small alkyl groups such as methyl or ethyl substantially increase activity while larger alkyl groups, or especially branching at the carbon attached to nitrogen, substantially lowers activity.

Although they were made solely on intact plants, the above observations suggest a hypothetical binding site, perhaps within the phytoene desaturase complex, that might appear in cross section as shown in Figure 6. Recognition by the complex of the vinylogous amide substructural unit of **13** could occur through interaction with that part of the desaturase which normally recognizes the conjugated region of phytoene. Such a binding site would possess a pocket which accommodates the 4-phenyl substituent and which contains a lipophilic or hydrogen bonding region that recognizes the meta-substituent, particularly the trifluoromethyl group. In addition, the site would incorporate a roughly cone-shaped region which interacts with R^3 and which has a depth approximately equal to the distance across a phenyl ring. This would account for the preference for ortho or no substituents and the progressively negative effect of meta or para substitution when

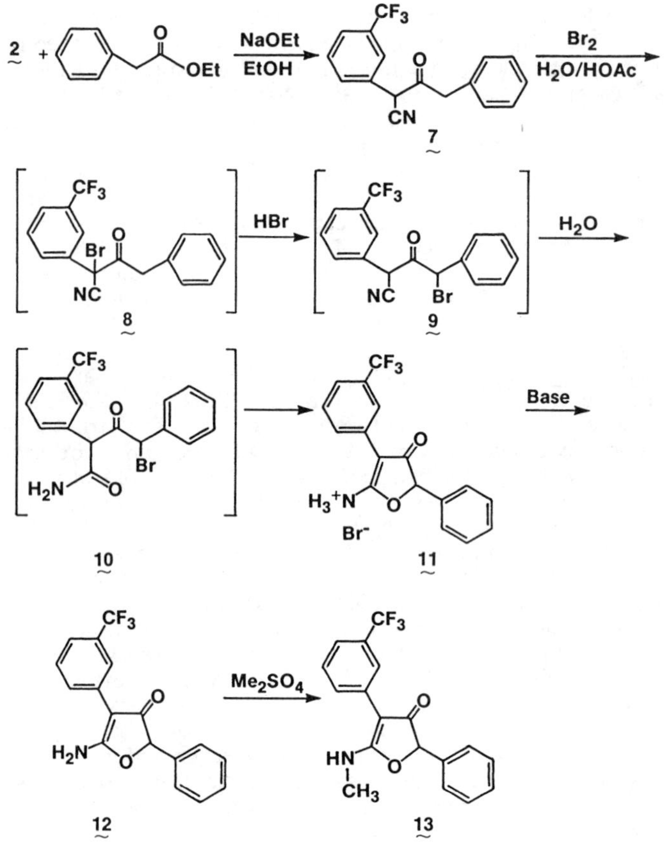

2 + [ethyl phenylacetate] → NaOEt / EtOH → 7 → Br_2 / H_2O/HOAc → [8] → HBr → [9] → H_2O → [10] → 11 → Base → 12 → Me_2SO_4 → 13

SCHEME II

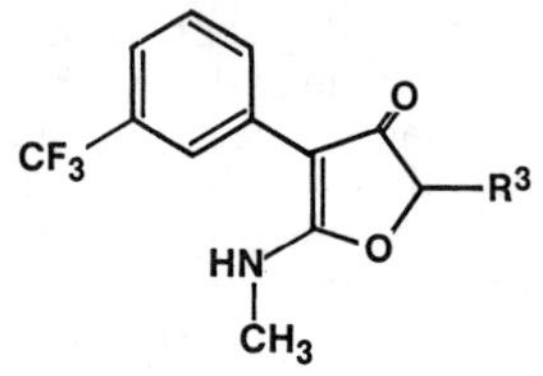

$R^3 = C_6H_5 > n\text{-}C_3H_7 > i\text{-}C_3H_7 > n\text{-}C_4H_9 > H >> (CH_3)_2$

Figure 2. Effect of R^3 on Relative Preemergence Activity.

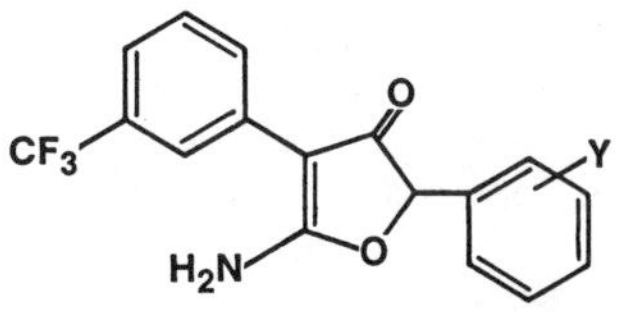

Y = o-Cl > m-Cl >> p-Cl

Figure 3. Effect of Y on Relative Preemergence Activity.

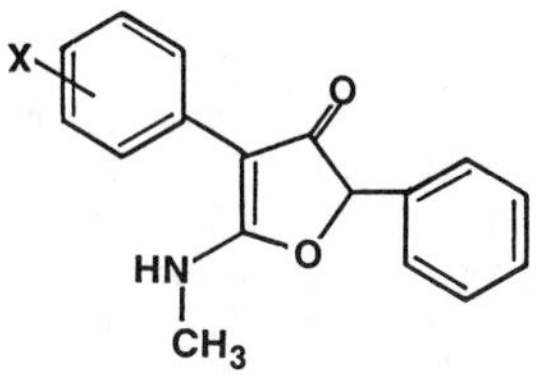

X = m-CF_3 > m-Cl > m-OCH_3 >> H ~ p-Cl

Figure 4. Effect of X on Relative Preemergence Activity.

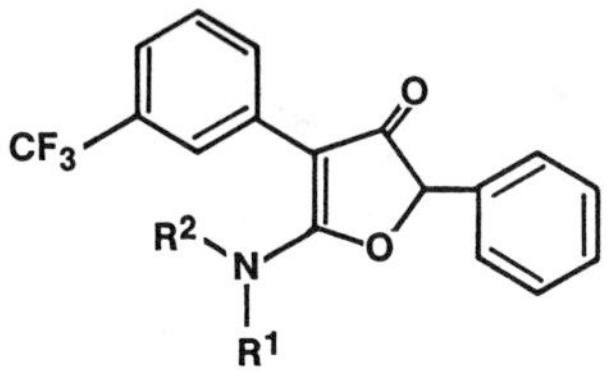

R^1,R^2 = CH_3, H > C_2H_5, H > nC_3H_7, H ~ CH_3, CH_3 > H, H >> iC_3H_7, H

Figure 5. Effect of R^1 and R^2 on Relative Preemergence Activity.

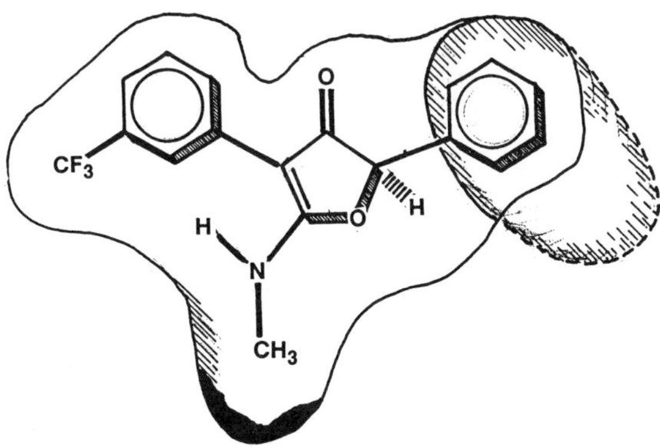

Figure 6. Hypothetical Binding Site.

R^3 is a phenyl ring as well as for the reduced activity observed when alkyl chains are longer than three carbons. The apparent need for a proton on the carbon bearing R^3 may reflect a steric requirement in this region or it may indicate a preference for binding the furanones in their enolic form. The portion of the site which interacts with the exocyclic N-alkyl substituents would include a small lipophilic pocket which would account for the enhanced activity of N-methylated or N-ethylated compounds and for the negative effect of branched or longer N-alkyl substituents.

If our hypothesis is correct, this hypothetical binding site should also accommodate fluridone, norflurazon and difunone and some possible binding orientations of these molecules are compared with furanone **13** in Figures 7-9. Note that we have attempted to depict the molecules in such a way that key structural features, e.g., the CF_3-phenyl and vinylogous amide subunits, occupy the same positions as nearly as possible. Finally, it should be emphasized that considerable further work is required to demonstrate that the furanones actually inhibit phytoene desaturase and to further probe the possibility of a common binding site for the proven inhibitors including those such as fluorochloridone (10) and the m-phenoxybenzamides (4), which do not incorporate the vinylogous amide substructure.

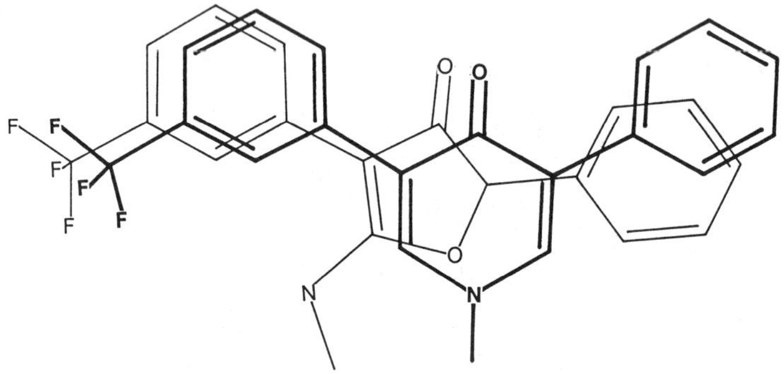

Figure 7. Furanone-Fluridone Comparison.

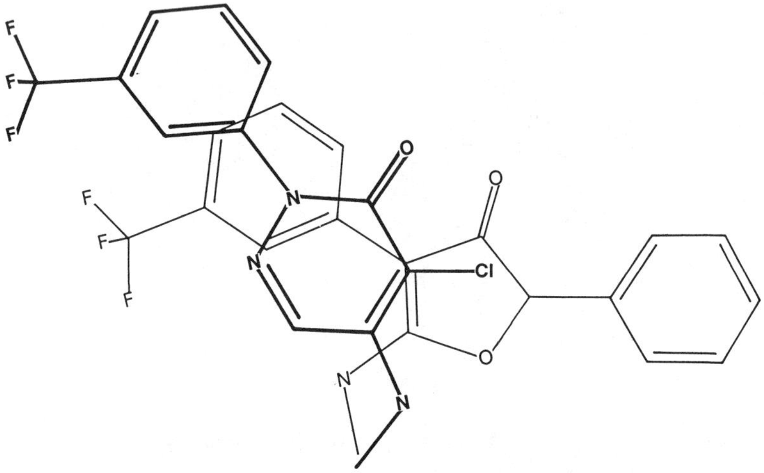

Figure 8. Furanone-Norflurazon Comparison.

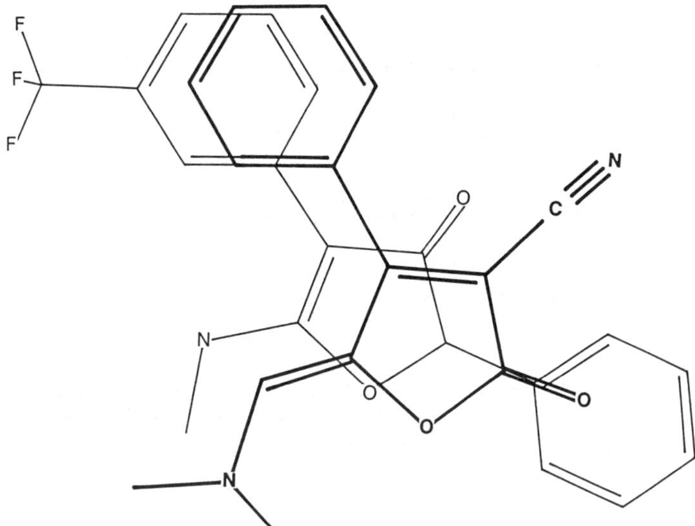

Figure 9. Furanone-Difunone Comparison.

Literature Cited

1. Ridley, S. M. Proc. 6th Int. Symp. on Carotenoids (IUPAC), Liverpool. UK. Britton, G.; Goodwin, T. W., Eds.; Pergamon Press, 1982; p355.
2. Sandmann, G.; Clarke, I. E.; Bramley, P. M.; Boger, P. Z. Naturforsch. 1984, 39c, 443.
3. Clarke, I. E.; Bramley, P. M.; Sandmann, G.; Boger, P. In Biochemistry and Metabolism of Plant Lipids; Wintermans, J. F. G. M; Kuiper, P. J. C., Eds.; Elsevier, Amsterdam, 1982; p549.
4. Clarke, I. E.; Sandmann, G.; Bramley, P. M.; Boger, P. Pestic. Biochem. Physiol. 1985, 23, 335.
5. Ward, C. E. U.S. Patent 4 568 376, 1986.
6. Umio, S.; Kariyone, K.; Kunihiko, T. Japanese Patent 13710, 1969; Chem. Abstr. 1969, 71, 61195e
7. Meier, V. H.; Binder, A. Chem. Zeit. 1980, 104, 302.
8. Capraro, v. H.-G.; Winkler, T.; Martin, P. Helv. Chim. Act. 1983, 66, 362.
9. Speziale, A. J.; Smith, L. R. J. Org. Chem. 1962, 27, 4361.
10. Lay, M. M.; Niland, A. M. Pestic. Biochem. Physiol. 1983, 19, 337.

RECEIVED May 12, 1987

Chapter 7

α-Trichloroethylstyrene Oxides

A New Class of Grass Herbicides

L. D. Markley [1], E. J. Norton[1], L. L. Smith, Jr.[1], and P. S. Zorner [2]

[1]Dow Chemical Company, Midland, MI 48674
[2]Dow Chemical Company, Walnut Creek, CA 94598

Tridiphane, the active ingredient in Dow's new herbicide, TANDEM , is being developed for postemergent grass and broadleaf control in corn. When used in combination with triazine herbicides such as atrazine, it enhances their weed activity by decreasing the rate of glutathione conjugation. Tridiphane is a member of a unique class of α-trichloroethylstyrene oxides discovered by The Dow Chemical Company. The synthesis and herbicidal activity of this group of compounds will be reviewed.

Tridiphane, 2-(3,5-dichlorophenyl)-2-(2,2,2-trichloroethyl)oxirane, 1, is the active ingredient in Dow's new herbicide, TANDEM, which is being developed for postemergent weed control in corn. The material is the outgrowth of many years of research in The Dow Chemical Company in the

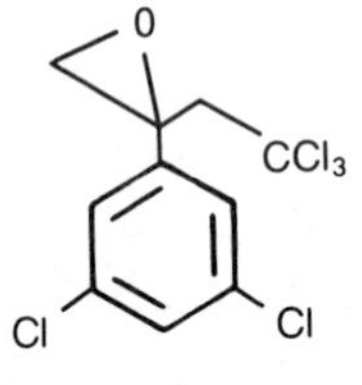

0

CCl_3

Cl Cl

Tridiphane
1

area of α-trichloroethylstyrenes and their epoxides as potential herbicides. The project had its beginning in Dow in the early sixties when by random

0097–6156/87/0355–0074$06.00/0
© 1987 American Chemical Society

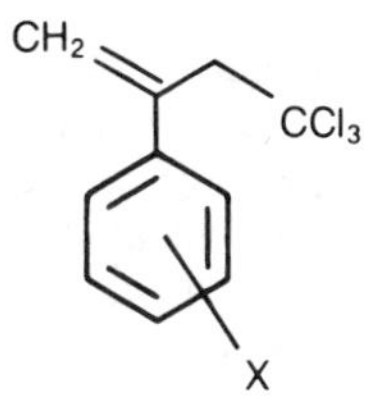

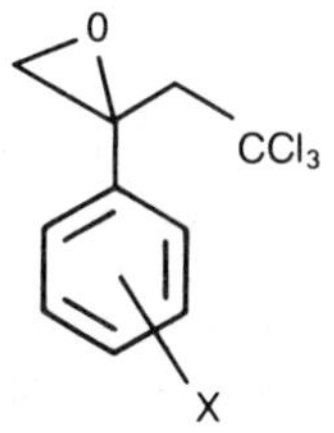

screening, α-(2,2,2-trichloroethyl)styrene, 2, was shown to possess good levels of preemergent herbicidal activity, most effective on grass weeds(1).

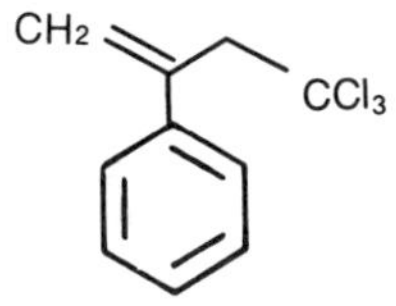

2

It is of historical interest to note that M.S. Kharasch and co-workers (2) had previously reported preparing 2 in their pioneering studies of the addition of halogenated hydrocarbons to olefins. In this case (Scheme I), Kharasch added bromotrichloromethane to α-methylstyrene with either light or acetyl peroxide as the free-radical initiator, and under the reaction conditions elimination of hydrogen bromide occurred, resulting in the formation of α-(2,2,2-trichloroethyl) styrene 2. The light or peroxide-initiated

SCHEME 1

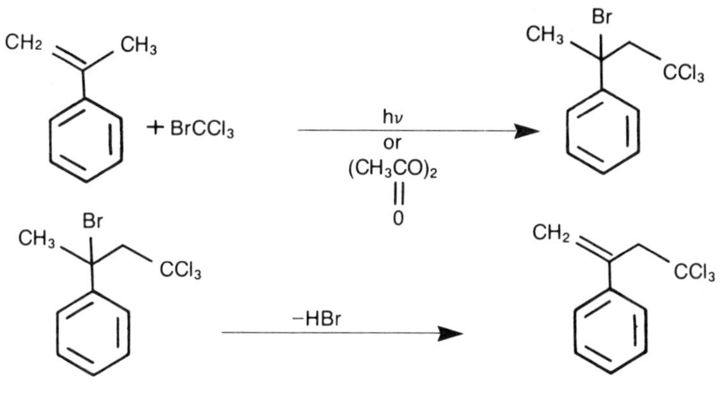

$+ BrCCl_3$ → $h\nu$ or $(CH_3CO)_2$ → $-HBr$ → 2

additions were often limited in that poor yields of one-to-one adducts were obtained and cheaper raw materials such as carbon tetrachloride gave considerably lower yields than the corresponding brominated materials.

In the early sixties, a redox catalyst system for the addition of halogenated hydrocarbons to olefins was discovered at Dow (3). The addition was carried out in the presence of a mixture of cuprous chloride and an amine such as piperidine or cyclohexylamine (Scheme II). Essentially quantitative yields of the one-to-one adducts could be obtained and the new catalyst system worked as well with carbon tetrachloride as bromotrichloromethane. Independently, M. Asscher and D. Vofsi (4) found a similar catalyst system.

Scheme II

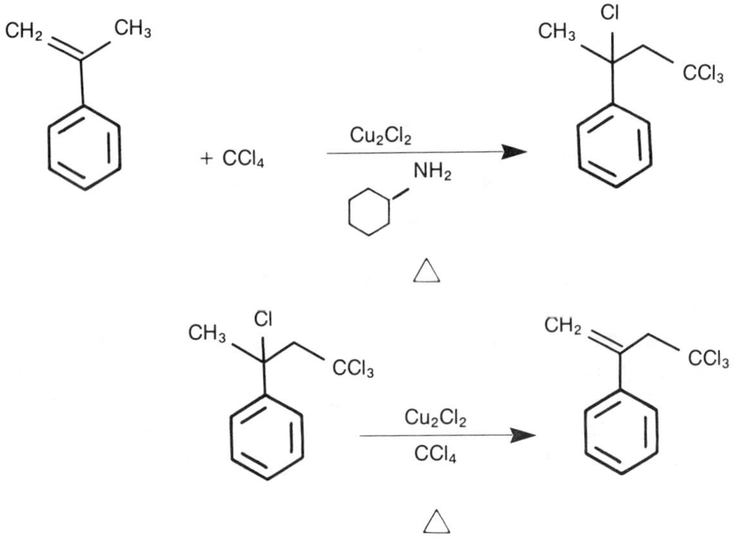

2

With the discovery in Dow that 2 possessed good herbicidal activity, a series of aromatic-substituted analogs were prepared and tested. In general one could conclude from this work that the meta-substituted analogs were the most active, while the corresponding ortho-substituted derivatives were essentially inactive and the para-substituted ones were intermediary. Three of the best compounds included the m-nitro 3, m-trifluoromethyl 4 and m-chloro 5 derivatives.

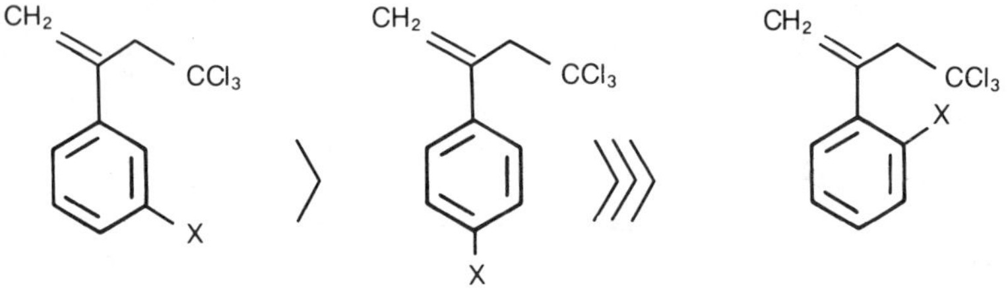

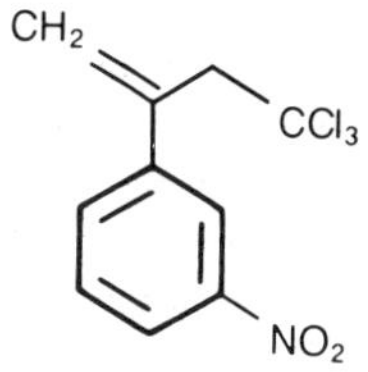

3 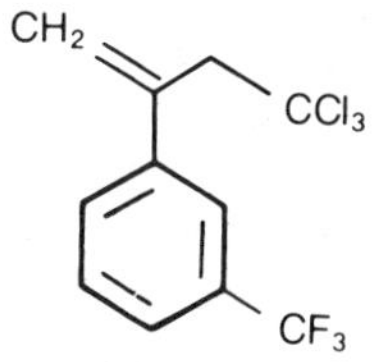 4 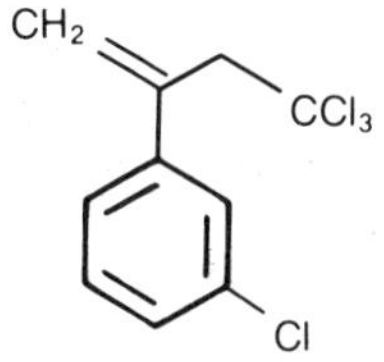 5

A greenhouse comparison of preemergent grass weed activity of these compounds is given in Table I. In addition, their effect on corn and soybeans at somewhat higher rates is included as a measure of crop selectivity.

TABLE I
Preemergent Herbicidal Activity

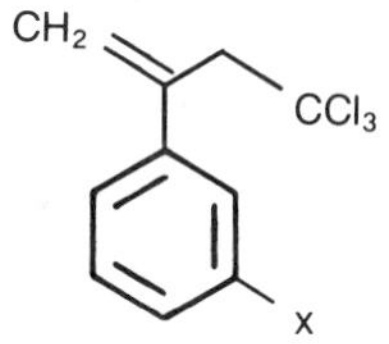

	% Weed Control*											
	Barnyard Grass		Crabgrass		Yellow Foxtail		Johnson Grass		Corn		Soybean	
X/lbs/Acre	1.0	0.50	1.0	0.50	1.0	0.50	1.0	0.50	2	1	2	1
H	50	40	80	40	80	70	80	80	90	85	0	0
NO_2	99	95	100	100	0	0	0	0	0	0	0	0
CF_3	0	0	95	90	95	90	100	100	50	0	0	0
Cl	90	90	95	95	100	95	90	90	95	85	50	30

*Ratings were made two weeks after application

One can see from these results that the original lead, 2, is considerably less active than the three substituted analogs with the exception of its highly injurious effect on corn. The m-nitro-α-(2,2,2-trichloroethyl) styrene 3 was quite safe on corn, however, its spectrum of weed activity was quite narrow. m-Chloro-α(2,2,2-trichloroethyl) styrene 5 has been field tested and shown to provide good annual grass control and upon incorporation in the soil also inhibits yellow nutsedge by destroying the growing points of this difficult-to-control perennial weed (5).

Over the years a general laboratory procedure as outlined in SCHEME III has been developed for the preparation of the desired α-(2,2,2-trichloroethyl) styrenes. As shown, the needed α-methylstyrenes can be prepared by classical routes involving Grignard chemistry and dehydration of the 3⁰ carbinol is accomplished with catalytic amounts of strong acids such as p-toluenesulfonic acid. The addition of carbon tetrachloride or bromotrichloromethane to the subsitited α-methylstyrene has remained essentially the same as first discovered. The final step involves elimination of hydrogen chloride or bromide and in many cases can be accomplished using catalytic amounts of cuprous chloride and heat. Lewis acids such as antimony pentachloride have also been used.(6).

SCHEME III

General Procedure for Synthesis of (α-2,2,2-trichloroethyl) styrenes

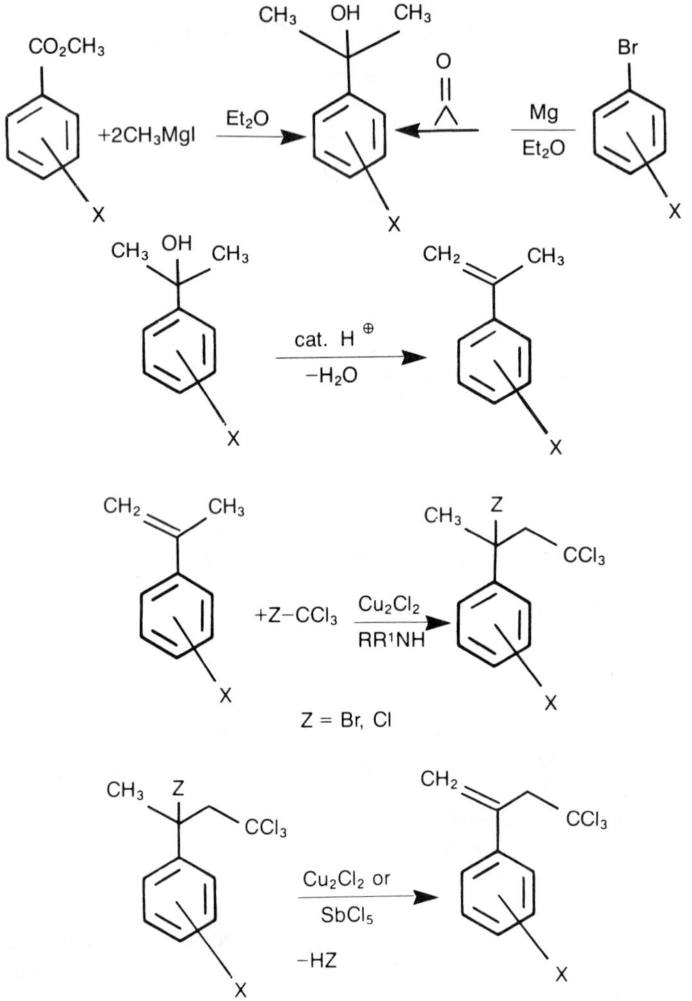

CO_2CH_3 (X-substituted benzene) $+2CH_3MgI$ $\xrightarrow{Et_2O}$ CH_3 OH CH_3 (X-substituted phenyl carbinol) ← acetone ← $\frac{Mg}{Et_2O}$ Br (X-substituted benzene)

CH_3 OH CH_3 (X-substituted phenyl carbinol) $\xrightarrow[-H_2O]{cat.\ H^{\oplus}}$ CH_2 CH_3 (X-substituted α-methylstyrene)

CH_2 CH_3 (X-substituted α-methylstyrene) $+Z{-}CCl_3$ $\xrightarrow[RR^1NH]{Cu_2Cl_2}$ CH_3 Z CCl_3 (X-substituted phenyl)

Z = Br, Cl

CH_3 Z CCl_3 (X-substituted phenyl) $\xrightarrow[SbCl_5]{Cu_2Cl_2\ or}$ $-HZ$ CH_2 CCl_3 (X-substituted styrene)

Discussions between Dow chemists and biologists concerning the mode of action of this unique class of herbicides led to the synthesis and screening of 2-phenyl-2-(2,2,2-trichloroethyl)oxirane, 6. The epoxide was found to be twice as active as the olefin, 2, when applied preemergently and the type of activity of the two materials were similar (7). A series of

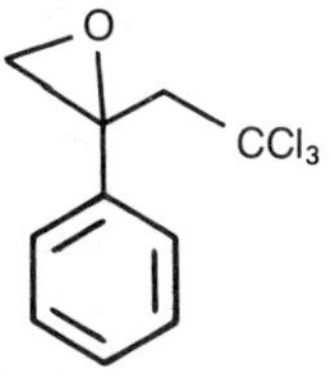

6

aromatic substituted -phenyl epoxides were prepared and again the meta-substituted derivatives were the most active herbicides while the ortho-substituted analogs had little activity. The para-substituted compounds were of intermediary activity (8). It was later shown that the olefins are oxidized in plant tissue to the epoxides. Greenhouse comparisons of the most active epoxides 7-9 as well as 6 are given in TABLE II. As shown the epoxides

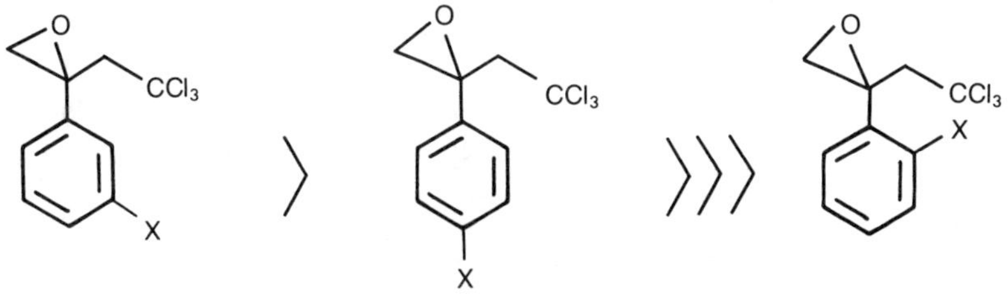

have greater herbicidal activity than their corresponding olefins in TABLE I, however, more crop damage, especially to corn, is also exhibited by the oxiranes. Under field conditions, the m-trifluoromethyl 8 and m-chloro 9 epoxides were shown to effectively control grass weeds at application rates where soybeans were quite tolerant.

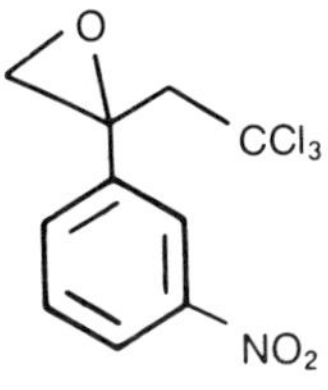

7 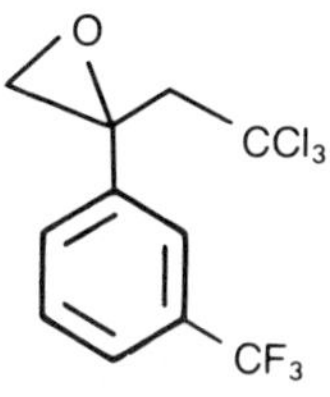 8 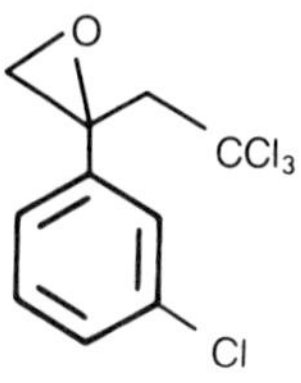 9

TABLE II
Preemergent Herbicidal Activity

	% Weed Control*											
	Barnyard Grass		Crabgrass		Yellow Foxtail		Johnson Grass		Corn		Soybean	
X/lbs/Acre	0.50	0.25	0.50	0.25	0.50	0.25	0.50	0.25	2	1	2	1
H	98	90	90	20	95	60	25	15	98	97	20	10
NO_2	40	0	95	30	0	0	50	0	50	40	0	0
CF_3	95	95	100	95	95	95	95	95	100	95	50	40
Cl	95	95	100	95	85	75	90	90	90	85	60	40

*Ratings were made two weeks after application

The epoxides were prepared from the corresponding olefins either by oxidation with various peracids such as peracetic acid or m-chloroperbenzoic acid or in a two-step procedure via the halohydrin (SCHEME IV). The direct epoxidation procedure is preferred due to the generally low yields of halohydrins obtained in the second method. The halohydrins are active herbicides and will be discussed in a future publication (9).

SCHEME IV

Preparation of Epoxides

CH_2 CCl_3 R $+R^1CO_3H$ O CCl_3 R

OH X CCl3 R X_2 H_2O Base

$X_2=Br_2,Cl_2$

Since the meta-substituted epoxides were the most active herbicides, we next chose to look at the 3,5-disubstituted compounds. The first compound prepared was the 3,5-dichloro derivative, tridiphane, 1. Its precursor, α-(2,2,2-trichloroethy 1)-3,5-dichlorostyrene, showed very little preemergent

O
CCl_3
X X

activity while tridiphane possessed excellent levels of activity and much to our surprise was safe on both corn and soybeans. As can be seen in TABLE III, tridiphane performs at rates in the greenhouse comparable to standards such as alachlor and trifluralin.

TABLE III
Preemergent Herbicidal Activity

	% Weed Control*											
	Barnyard Grass		Crabgrass		Yellow Foxtail		Johnson Grass		Corn		Soybean	
Herb/lbs/A	.125	.0625	.125	.0625	.125	.0625	.125	.0625	2	1	2	1
Tridiphane	98	85	100	70	100	100	100	98	0	0	0	0
Alachlor	70	60	80	20	100	95	70	30	0	0	0	0
Trifluralin	75	60	98	35	98	25	80	20	50	35	0	0

*Ratings were made two weeks after application

With the discovery that the 3,5-dichloro analog was very active (10), a variety of 3,5-disubstituted compounds were prepared and tested. The 3,5-dimethyl epoxide 10 exhibited good activity in the greenhouse but under field conditions did not give season-long weed control while the 3-chloro-5-fluoro derivative 11 was somewhat more active than tridiphane.

0
CCl_3
CH_3 CH_3

10

O
CCl_3
Cl F

11

Tridiphane was field tested for several years as a preemergent grass herbicide for corn and soybeans. Even though it performed well in comparison to standards such as alachlor, it was decided that in order to compete in the mature corn herbicide market we would have to offer the grower a truly unique product. The discovery that tridiphane could synergize triazine herbicides postemergently came at a most opportune time and was made initially in the field as opposed to the greenhouse. In the field test, tridiphane and atrazine were applied separately to 3-4 leaf grass weeds and to corn and the two materials were also applied in combination (TABLE IV). From greenhouse testing it was known that tridiphane inhibited the growth of weeds when applied postemergently, however, in time the weeds would regrow. It was also not surprising to find atrazine ineffectual on grass weeds in as much as it is used for broadleaf weed control. It was surprising to see the dramatic synergistic effect when the two materials were applied in combination.

TABLE IV
Postemergent Field Test

Treatment/lbs/Acre		% Weed Control* Barnyard Grass	Johnson Grass	Corn
Tridiphane	0.50	0	7	0
	1.0	39	20	0
	2.0	44	65	7
Atrazine	1.0	0	0	0
	2.0	47	33	0
Tridiphane and Atrazine	0.5 + 1.0	76	32	0
	1.0 + 1.0	90	93	0
	2.0 + 1.0	98	95	3

*Ratings were made 4 weeks after application

With this discovery, intensive work was carried out in both the greenhouse and field to better define the breadth of the synergism. It was found that the tridiphane-triazine combination was effective in controlling not only grassy weeds but broadleaf weeds as well — including velvetleaf, a broadleaf weed atrazine alone does not control effectively. Laboratory studies have shown that tridiphane slows down the rate of glutathione conjugation of atrazine in giant foxtail, the major route of detoxification of triazine herbicides in foliar tissue (11) as shown in TABLE V (12,13).

Cl
N N
+GSH
EtNH N NH
Atrazine

GST →

SG
N N
EtNH N NH
Glutathione Conjugate

TABLE V

Detoxification of Atrazine in Giant Foxtail

% Atrazine Remaining in Leaf After Application

Time (Hrs)	Atrazine	Tridiphane + Atrazine
6	80	86
24	50	72
72	28	73

The major route of detoxification of tridiphane in corn has also been shown to be glutathione conjugation.

O
CCl_3
Cl Cl
1

+GSH

GST →

OH
GS CCl_3
Cl Cl
Glutathione Conjugate

GSH = γ–Glu–Cys–Gly
GST = Glutathione–S–transferase Enzyme

We have synthesized the glutathione conjugate of tridiphane and shown it to be inactive as a herbicide; however, G. L. Lamoureux and D. G. Rusness (14,15) have found it to be an effective inhibitor of atrazine glutathione conjugation *in vitro*.

Tridiphane is a unique molecule in many ways. It is certainly not a typical epoxide in its chemical reactivity. As shown in SCHEME V, it can be heated in glacial acetic acid at 100°C for eight hours with little or no change.

SCHEME V
Reactions of Tridiphane

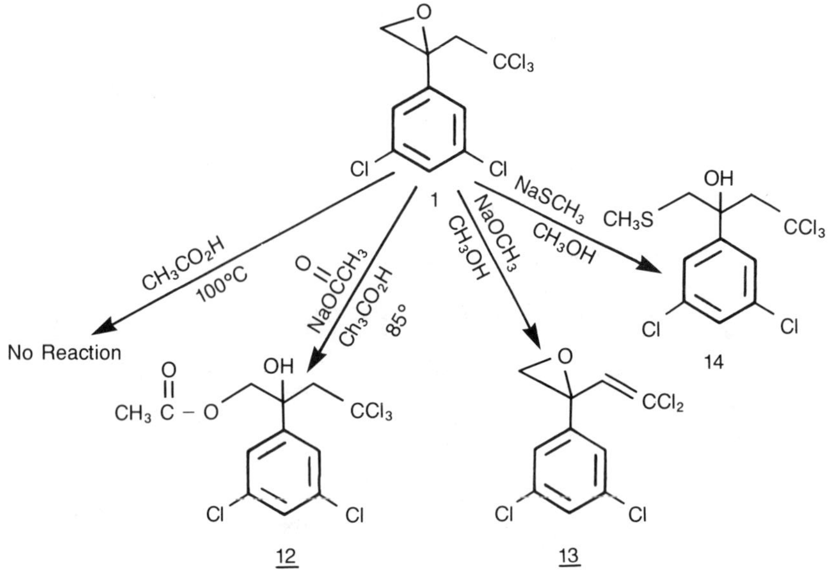

1

CH_3CO_2H, 100°C → No Reaction

$NaOCCH_3$ (O=), Ch_3CO_2H, 85° → 12

$NaOCH_3$, CH_3OH → 13

$NaSCH_3$, CH_3OH → 14

12

13

14

One can open the epoxide, however, by treating it with sodium acetate in acetic acid at 85°C for 48 hours and obtain the gylcol acetate, 12, in quantitative yield. Treatment of tridiphane with one equivalent of sodium methoxide in methanol at room temperature causes hydrogen chloride elimination and formation of the vinyl epoxide, 13, which has little herbicidal activity. In contrast to sodium methoxide, sodium methylthiolate readily opens the epoxide ring giving the β-thioalcohol, 14 in quantitative yield.

Many related compounds have been synthesized and tested at Dow both as herbicides and triazine synergists. Replacement of one of the chlorines in the trichloromethyl group with other substituents as shown below

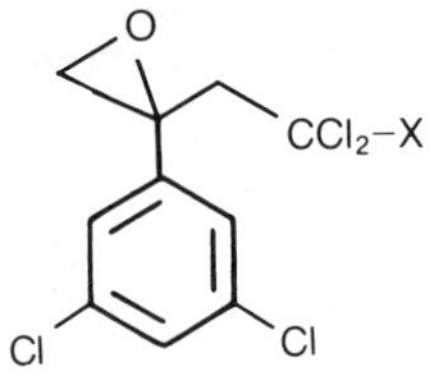

$CCl_2{-}X$

X = H, CH_3, CN, $CONH_2$, CO_2Et, $COCH_3$, CF_3, etc.

resulted in compounds with varying levels of herbicidal activity. It was disappointing, however, to find that none of the compounds were as effective as tridiphane in synergizing atrazine. Replacement of one of the hydrogens on the unsubstituted carbon in the epoxide ring as in 15 or on the carbon adjacent to the trichloromethyl group as in 16 with either a chlorine or a methyl group resulted in compounds devoid of herbicidal

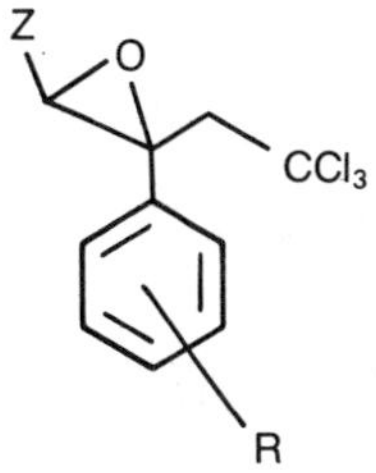

15

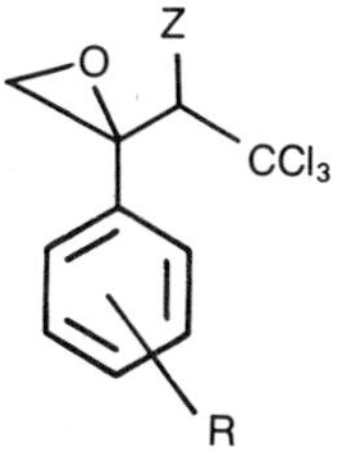

16

Z = Cl, CH_3

activity. Some of the most active herbicidal analogs of tridiphane made were heterocyclic derivatives as shown below.

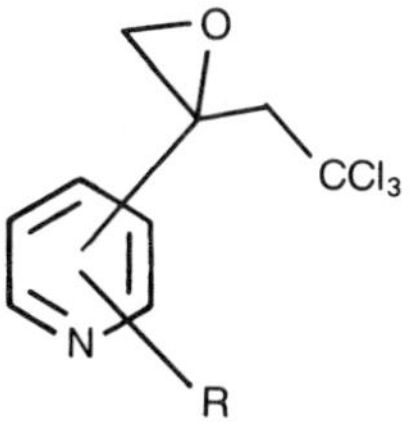

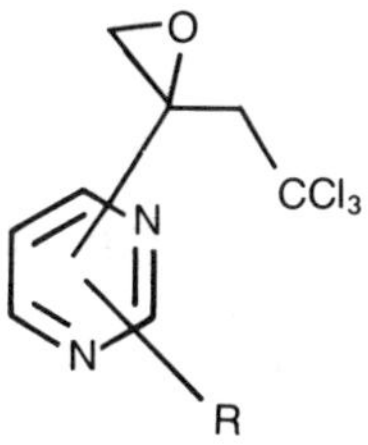

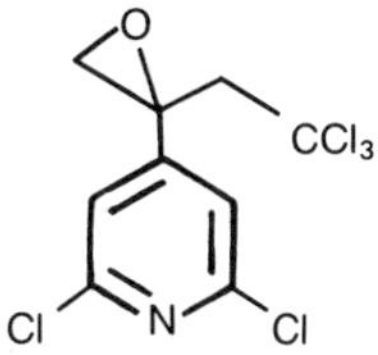

17

Many pyridine compounds as well as primidines were synthesized and screened. The most active material is the direct pyridine analog, 17, which possessed activity equivalent to tridiphane. (16).

The success of the project is due in part to the extraordinary efforts of many Dow scientists. Synthetic chemists who have made many of the compounds include K. E. Arndt, D. L. Decker, L. D. Markley, S. D. McGregor, L. R. Morris, E. J. Norton, T. M. Ozretich, R. G. Pews, J. M. Renga, R. B. Rogers and J. M. Soper. Early-stage greenhouse biologists including B. C. Gerwick, T. W. Holmsen, P. G. Ray, L. L. Smith, Jr. and P. S. Zorner have evaluated the materials as herbicides as well as determined the basis for the tridiphane-triazine synergism.

In summary, with the discovery in Dow that α-(2,2,2-trichloroethyl) styrene possessed unique preemergent herbicidal activity and the synthesis and evaluation of close to one thousand related materials, a new product, tridiphane, the active ingredient in TANDEM* will enter the marketplace in 1986. Tridiphane will be the first postemergent grass herbicide for use in corn and will be used in combination with triazine herbicides such as atrazine and cyanazine.

Literature Cited

1. Mussell, D.R., U.S. Patent 3 373 011, 1968.
2. Kharasch, M.S.; Simon E.; Nudenberg, W. J. Org. Chem., 1953, *18*, 328.
3. Decker, D.L.; Moore, C.; Tousignant, W.F. U.S. Patent 3 454 657, 1969.
4. Asscher, M.; Vofsi, D. J. Chem. Soc, 1963, 1887.
5. Barrons, K.C.; Smith L.L.; Holmsen, T.W. U.S. Patent 4 086 081, 1978.
6. Markley, L.D. U.S. Patent 4 188 436, 1980.
7. Ozretich, T.M. U.S. Patent 3 719 465, 1973.
8. Ozretich, T.M. U.S. Patent 4 018 801, 1977.
9. Markley, L.D. U.S. Patent 3 972 913, 1976.
10. Markley, L.D.; Norton, E.J. U.S. Patent 4 211 549, 1980.
11. Frear, D. S.; Still, G.G. Phytochemistry 1970, 9, 2123.
12. Zorner, P.S.; Olson, G.L. Proc. North Central Weed Control Conference, December 8, 1981, p. 15.
13. Zorner, P.S. Proc. Southern Weed Science Society, 38th Annual Meeting, 1985, p. 484.
14. Lamoureux, G.L.; Rusness, D.G. Proc. 188th National ACS Meeting, 1984.
15. Lamoureux, G.L.; Rusness, D.G. Pestic. Biochem. Physiol., 1986, 26, 323.
16. Markley, L.D.; Soper J.M. U.S. Patent 4 474 602, 1984.

RECEIVED July 20, 1987

Chapter 8

o-(5-Thiono-2-imidazolin-2-yl)aryl Carboxylates

Synthesis and Herbicidal Activity

Michael A. Guaciaro, Marinus Los, Ronald K. Russell, Peter J. Wepplo, Barbara L. Lences, Peter C. Lauro, Philip L. Orwick, Kai Umeda, and Pierre A. Marc

Agricultural Research Division, American Cyanamid Company, P.O. Box 400, Princeton, NJ 08540

The synthesis and herbicidal activities of various imidazolinthiones, in particular the thiono isosteres of imazapyr, imazethapyr and imazamethabenz are discussed. In the synthesis area it is shown that the imidazolinthione ring functions as an *ortho*-directing group in aromatic lithiations. In the biological activity area it is shown that replacement of the imidazolinone carbonyl with a thiocarbonyl results in changes in weed toxicity and crop selectivity.

The imidazolinones are a new class of herbicides discovered and being developed by American Cyanamid Company. Previous papers in the imidazolinone area (1-12) have discussed the preparation and biological activity of various aryl substituted imidazolinones, in particular imazapyr 1 (AC 243,997, registered by American Cyanamid under the trademarks ARSENAL, ASSAULT and CHOPPER), imazethapyr 2 (AC 263,499, discovered and being developed by American Cyanamid under the trademark PURSUIT) and imazamethabenz 3/4 (AC 222,293, discovered and being developed by American Cyanamid under the trademark ASSERT).

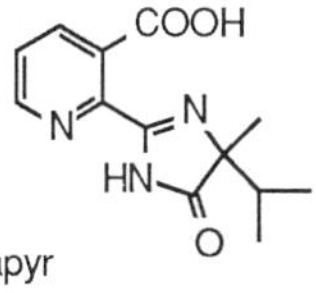

1 Imazapyr

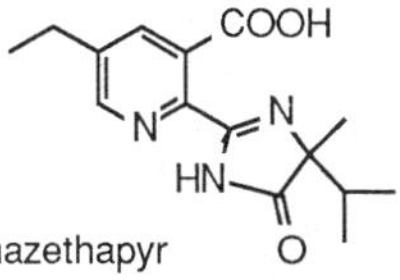

2 Imazethapyr

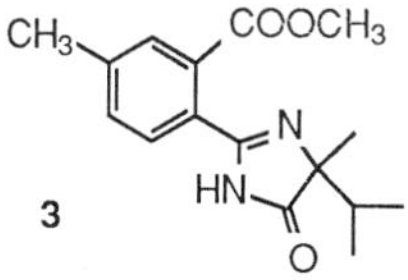

3 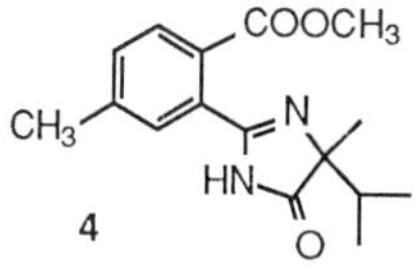 + 4

Imazamethabenz

0097-6156/87/0355-0087$06.00/0
© 1987 American Chemical Society

Prior investigations have dealt with the effects on herbicidal activity produced by changes in the aryl rings, the aryl ring substituents, the nature of the carbonyl function and the alkyl groups on the imidazolinone ring. These changes have all resulted in significant alterations in herbicidal activity and crop selectivity.

Another site where molecular modification might produce changes in herbicidal activity and crop selectivity is the imidazolinone carbonyl. We reasoned that replacing the imidazolinone carbonyl with an isosteric moiety, such as a thiocarbonyl, would affect such properties as imidazolinone ring size and bond angles, electronic distribution, partition coefficients, pKa, chemical reactivity and hydrogen bonding capacity and thus might have some effect on the absorption, translocation and metabolism of the compounds in question, the biochemical responses elicited by the compounds and the resulting plant structural changes.

This paper will discuss the synthesis and herbicidal activity of the imidazolinthione counterparts of the herbicides shown above.

Synthesis

Synthesis of the Thiono Counterpart of Imazapyr. In our synthesis of imidazolinthiones the most efficient point for introduction of the thiocarbonyl group proved to be at the initial stages of the synthesis. Thus treatment of amino amide 5 with phosphorus pentasulfide (13, 14) afforded thioamide 6, which was most efficiently purified by precipitation of its hydrochloride salt.

H_2N—C(iPr)(Me)—C(=O)—NH_2 + P_2S_5 → (1. Dioxane, 90°C; 2. HCl(g); 3. Et_3N) → H_2N—C(iPr)(Me)—C(=S)—NH_2

5 6 80-90%

The thiono counterpart of imazapyr was prepared by treating 2,3-pyridinedicarboxylic anhydride 7 with thioamide 6 (THF, 60°C), affording both possible addition products 8 and 9 as a 60:40 mixture. These regioisomers were separated by fractional crystallization. Treatment of each intermediate with excess sodium hydroxide followed by acidification afforded thioimidazolinyl acids 10 or 11. Since picolinic acid 11 was not active in the herbicide screen below 500 g/ha preemergence and 250 g/ha postemergence and had no apparent crop selectivity, it will not be discussed further.

7 → (6, THF, 60°C) → 8 (COOH, CONH—C(iPr)(Me)—$CSNH_2$) + 9 (CONH—C(iPr)(Me)—$CSNH_2$, COOH)

60 : 40

Treatment of acid 10 with diazomethane (15, 16) afforded methyl ester 12.

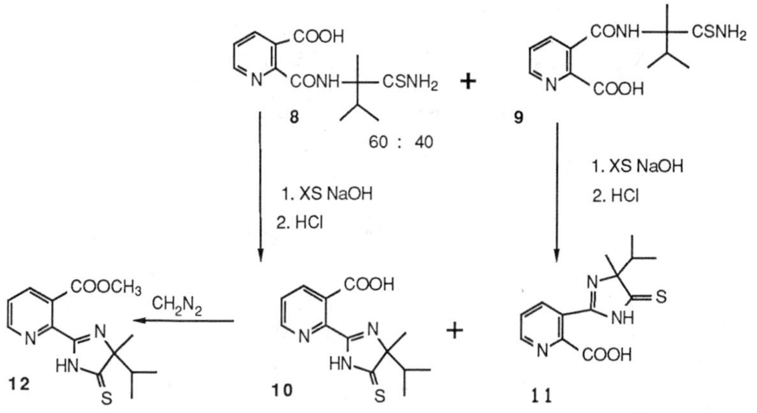

Synthesis of the Thiono Isostere of Imazethapyr. The thiono isostere of imazethapyr was prepared in the same fashion from 5-ethyl-pyridine-2,3-dicarboxylic anhydride 13. The resulting mixture of regioisomers 14 and 15 was treated with aqueous sodium hydroxide to afford acid 16 after acidification and fractional crystallization.

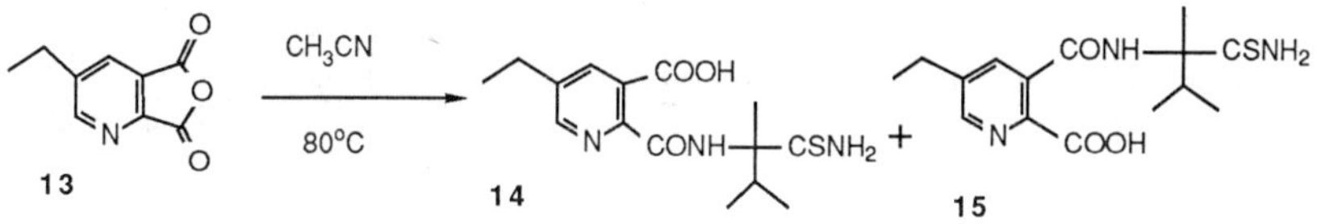

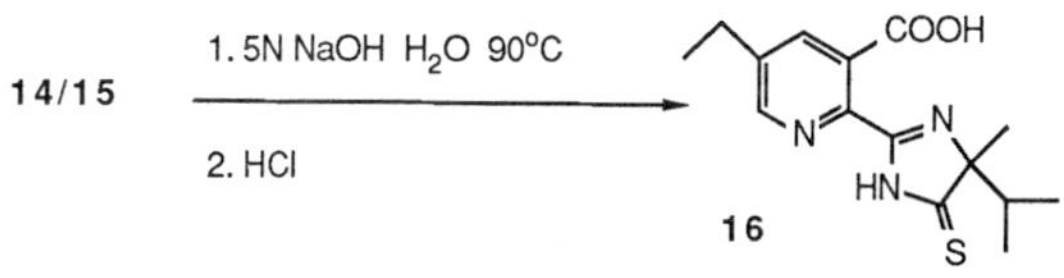

Treatment of acid 16 with dicyclohexylcarbodiimide (DCC) resulted in ring closure to the tricycle 17. Under these cyclization conditions none of the other possible tricycle 18 is detected.

COOH 16 DCC CH_2Cl_2 RT 17

18

Ring opening of tricycle 17 with sodium methoxide afforded the methyl ester 19 in quantitative yield. The use of these tricyclic intermediates allows preparation of a variety of esters simply by varying the alcohol employed (17).

17 cat NaH MeOH RT 100% $COOCH_3$ 19

Synthesis of the Thiono Counterpart of Imazamethabenz. The thiono counterpart of imazamethabenz was prepared by treating 4-methylphthalic anhydride (20) with thioamide 6, affording both possible thiocarbamoyl methylphthalamic acids 21 and 22 in 90% yield as a 55:45 mixture.

CH_3 20 6 CH_3CN RT 90%

COOH CH_3 CONH—CSNH$_2$ 21

+

CH_3 COOH CONH—CSNH$_2$ 22

This mixture underwent cyclization in sodium hydroxide to imidazolinthiones 23 and 24 in 99% yield. The mixture of acids 23 and 24

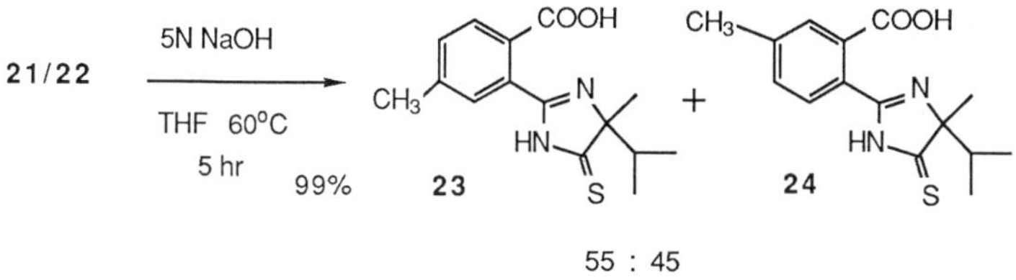

21/22 → (5N NaOH, THF 60°C, 5 hr, 99%) 23 + 24 (55 : 45)

was treated with DCC to afford tricycles 25 and 26, which were easily converted without purification to esters 27 and 28 via treatment with sodium methoxide.

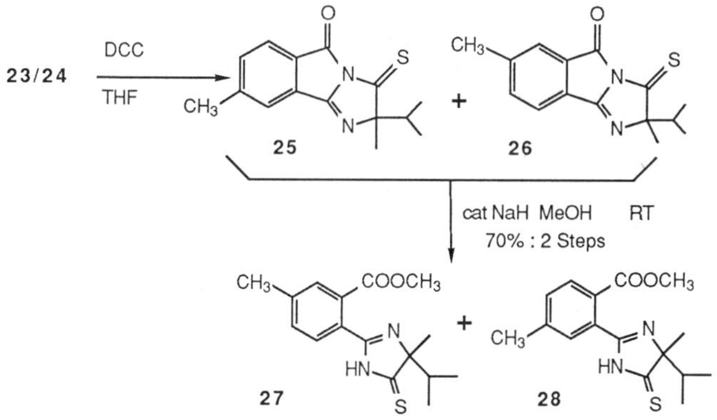

23/24 → (DCC, THF) 25 + 26 → (cat NaH MeOH RT, 70% : 2 Steps) 27 + 28

<u>The Regiospecific Synthesis of 23, 24, 27 and 28.</u> We were interested in testing each of the previously mentioned regioisomers 23, 24, 27 and 28 individually in our greenhouse screens. Since chromatographic separation or fractional crystallization of these regioisomers proved to be tedious and inefficient and we wished to determine if the imidazolinthione ring, like the imidazolinone ring, was an <u>ortho</u>-directing group in aromatic lithiations (<u>18</u>, <u>19</u>), we embarked on the regiospecific synthesis of the above isomers.

Treatment of <u>meta</u>- or <u>para</u>-toluyl chloride (29 or 30) with thioamide 6 in the presence of excess triethylamine at -60°C afforded the thiocarbamoyl toluamides 31 or 32 which, when treated with excess sodium hydroxide, cyclized to the imidazolinthiones 33 or 34.

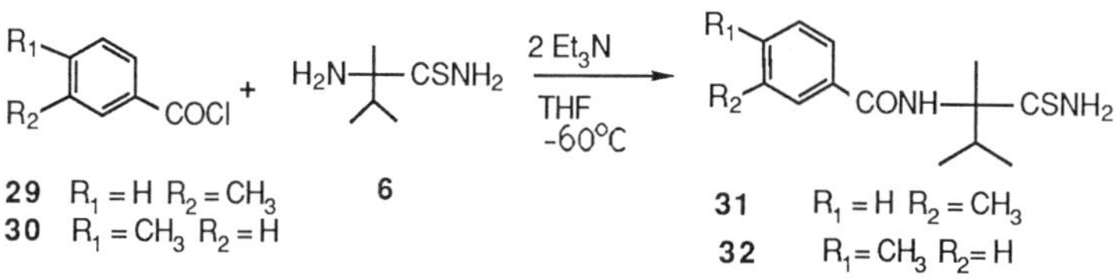

29/30 (COCl) + 6 (H_2N–C–$CSNH_2$) → (2 Et_3N, THF, -60°C) 31/32 (CONH–C–$CSNH_2$)

29 $R_1 = H$ $R_2 = CH_3$
30 $R_1 = CH_3$ $R_2 = H$

31 $R_1 = H$ $R_2 = CH_3$
32 $R_1 = CH_3$ $R_2 = H$

31 OR 32 → 5 equiv 10% NaOH, THF 68°C

33 $R_1 = H$ $R_2 = CH_3$ 47% from 29

34 $R_1 = CH_3$ $R_2 = H$ 50% from 30

Treatment of 33 with two equivalents of <u>sec</u>-butyllithium in the presence of tetramethylethylenediamine (TMEDA) at -70°C with gradual warming to -45°C, followed by a carbon dioxide quench at -70°C and acidification afforded the acid 23 in 62% yield.

33 → 1. 2 sec-BuLi 2 TMEDA, THF -70°C to -45°C; 2. CO_2; 3. H_3O^+ → 62% 23 + trace 35

While it is possible for lithiation of 33 to occur between the methyl group and the imidazolinthione ring, only trace amounts of the resulting sterically crowded acid 35 could be seen in the NMR spectrum of the unpurified product. Similarly, substrate 34 provided the acid 24 in 39% yield after recrystallization.

34 → 1. 2 sec-BuLi 2 TMEDA, THF -70°C to -45°C; 2. CO_2; 3. H_3O^+ → 39% 24

Acids 23 and 24 were carried on, via the tricycles 25 and 26, to the methyl esters 27 and 28 respectively. The yield of ester 28 was low since it was prepared from impure acid 24.

DCC NaOMe

23 $R_1 = H$ $R_2 = CH_3$
24 $R_1 = CH_3$ $R_2 = H$

25 $R_1 = H$ $R_2 = CH_3$
26 $R_1 = CH_3$ $R_2 = H$

27 $R_1 = H$ $R_2 = CH_3$ 39% from **23**
28 $R_1 = CH_3$ $R_2 = H$ 18% from **24**

Biological Activity

The imidazolinthiones were tested in the greenhouse pre- and postemergence on a number of weeds and crops. The grasses were barnyard grass, green foxtail, purple nutsedge, wild oats and quackgrass. The broadleaves were field bindweed, morning glory, wild mustard, velvetleaf, ragweed and matricaria. The crops were spring barley, sugar beets, corn, cotton, rice, sunflower, spring wheat and soybeans. The phenyl analogs were tested on all five grasses while the pyridyl compounds were tested on all but green foxtail. The benzoates were tested on all of the broadleaves except ragweed and matricaria. The nicotinates were tested on all the broadleaves except wild mustard. In all instances weed control is defined as $\geq$90% toxicity and safety towards crops as $\leq$10% toxicity.

Figures 1 to 8 compare the imidazolinthiones to the imidazolinones at various rates of application pre- and postemergence. Figure 1 compares thione 10 to imazapyr (1) at 32 g/ha postemergence while Figure 2 compares the preemergence data for the methyl ester (36) of imazapyr to its thione counterpart 12 at 32 g/ha. In the imazaethapyr area Figure 3 compares the preemergence data for imazethapyr (2) to the data for imidazolinthione 16 at 63 g/ha. In the imazamethabenz area Figure 4 compares the postemergence data at 500 g/ha for the acid mixtures 23/24 and 37/38 while Figure 5 compares the postemergence data for 23/24 and 37/38 at 500 g/ha. Figure 6 compares the preemergence data for the mixture of methyl esters 27/28 and imazamethabenz 3/4 at 500 g/ha. Figure 7 presents a comparison of the biological data for imidazolinone 37 and its imidazolinthione counterpart 23 on specific weeds and cereals postemergence at 250 g/ha. In Figure 8 the preemergence data at 500 g/ha for imidazolinthione 27, imidazolinone 4 and imazamethabenz 3/4 is compared.

Structure-Activity

The Imazapyr Area. When imazapyr (1) is compared to its imidazolinthione counterpart 10 both pre- and postemergence, imazapyr proves to be a more effective total vegetation control agent. As Figure 1 shows, while 10 is comparable to imazapyr at 32 g/ha postemergence in controlling grasses and injuring crops, it is less effective in controlling broadleaves. Thione 10 is much less active than imazapyr preemergence at 32 g/ha in all three categories.

Comparison of the effectiveness of the methyl ester (36) of imazapyr as a total vegetation control agent to thione 12 (Figure 2) shows that introduction of a thiocarbonyl does not improve weed toxicity, providing a compound (12) which is comparable to 36 in terms of overall total vegetation control at 32 g/ha preemergence. At 32 g/ha postemergence thione 12 is much less effective than 36 in controlling weeds.

The Imazethapyr Area. As Figure 3 shows, thione 16 is less effective overall than imazethapyr (2) in preemergence weed control on soybeans, particularly in the broadleaves, where 16 is inactive on morning glory and ragweed. Imidazolinthione 16 is also more injurious to soybeans than imazethapyr and shows no other crop selectivity. Thione 16, postemergence at the same rate, is essentially inactive compared to imazethapyr. The methyl ester (19) of thione 16 is essentially inactive both pre- and postemergence at 63 g/ha.

Structure-Activity in the Imazamethabenz Area. In this category, the mixture of imidazolinones 37/38 is more effective in controlling grasses and broadleaves than the thione mixture 23/24. Preemergence at 500 g/ha (Figure 4) both 23/24 and 37/38 are quite injurious to crops. However, at 500 g/ha postemergence, as Figure 5 shows, thione mixture 23/24 is less injurious to crops than 37/38, showing safety on corn, wheat and rice. The mixture 23/24 is less effective than 37/38 in controlling broadleaves and only controls wild oats in the grass category. In this instance introduction of the thiocarbonyl group imparts some crop selectivity to 23/24.

The thione counterparts of imazamethabenz 3/4 only show herbicidal activity and crop selectivity in the cereals area but are less effective than imazamethabenz in controlling selected weeds on cereals preemergence, as Figure 6 shows. The introduction of a thiocarbonyl group allows green foxtail to completely detoxify the mixture 27/28. In postemergence tests, 27/28 also does not outperform imazamethabenz in terms of weed control in cereals.

In individual tests the *meta*- and *para*-toluic acids 37 and 38 were shown to be injurious to crops both pre- and postemergence. However, imidazolinthione 23 is selectively detoxified by cereals and is more effective in controlling selected weeds on cereals, especially postemergence (Figure 7). Unfortunately, 23 fails to control green foxtail and thus fails to provide a useful new range of activity on cereals.

Of the two regioisomers 27 and 28 only *para*-toluate 27 shows any significant preemergence activity and its selectivity is confined to cereals. As Figure 8 shows, thione 27, imidazolinone 4 and imazamethabenz (3/4) show little difference in overall preemergence weed control with 27 and imazamethabenz being safe on cereals. Again, introduction of a thiocarbonyl group does not improve the herbicidal effect on green foxtail. In postemergence tests 27 is slightly less effective than imazamethabenz in controlling selected weeds on cereals.

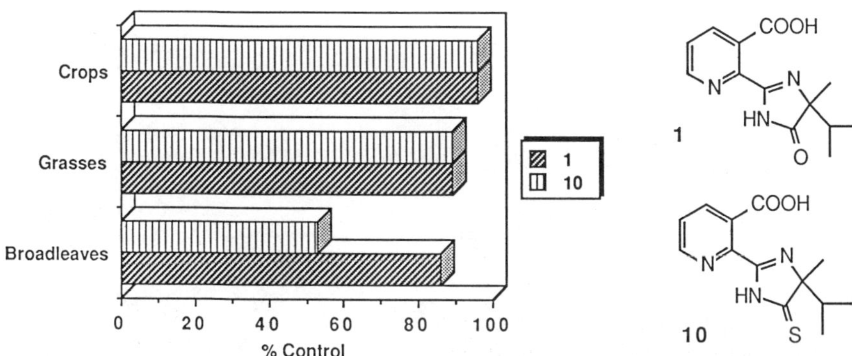

Figure 1. Comparison of 1 to 10 at 32 g/ha postemergence.

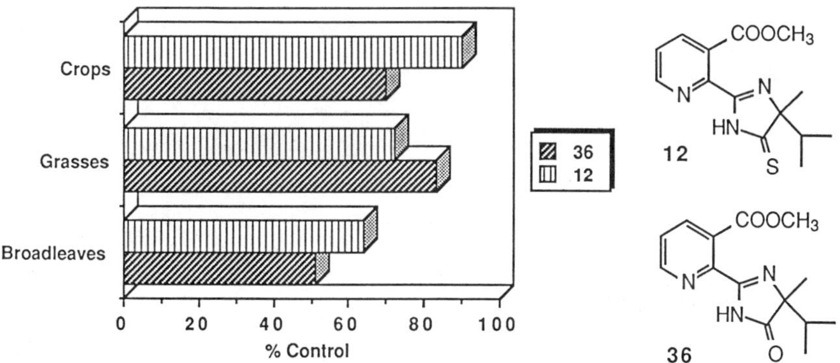

Figure 2. Comparison of 12 to 36 at 32 g/ha preemergence.

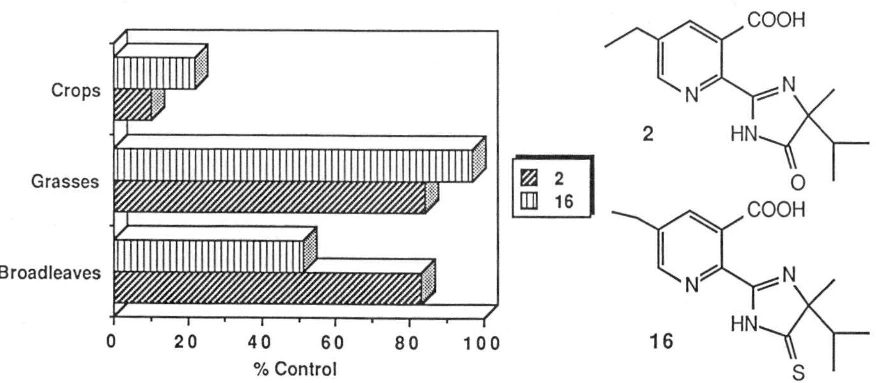

Figure 3. Comparison of 2 to 16 at 63 g/ha preemergence.

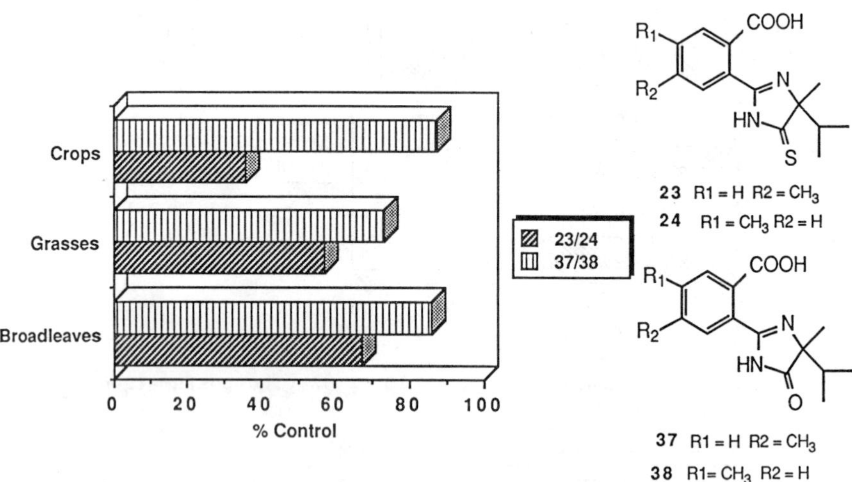

Figure 4. Comparison of 23/24 to 37/38 at 500 g/ha pre-emergence.

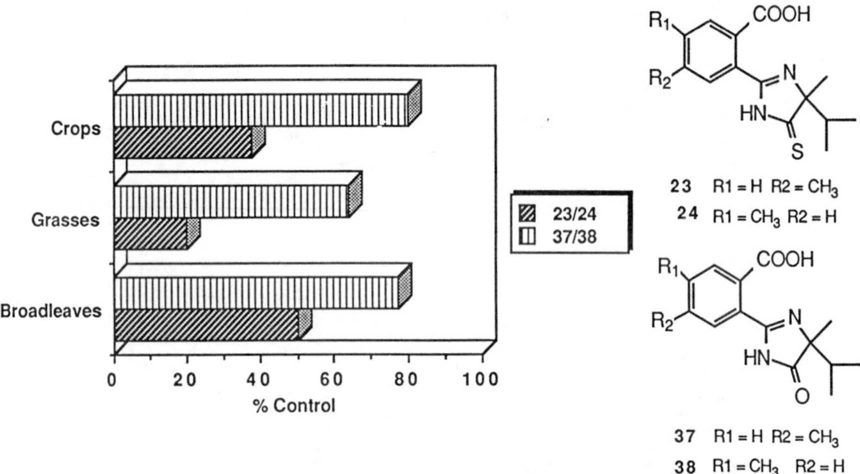

Figure 5. Comparison of 23/24 to 37/38 at 500 g/ha post-emergence.

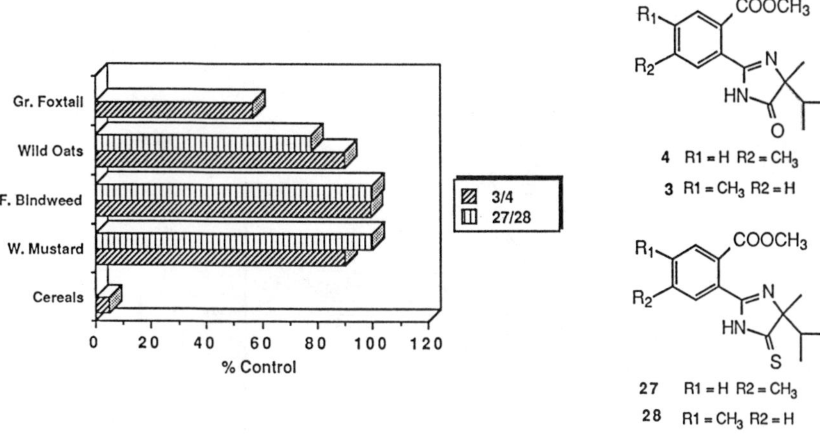

Figure 6. Comparison of 3/4 to 27/28 at 500 g/ha pre-emergence.

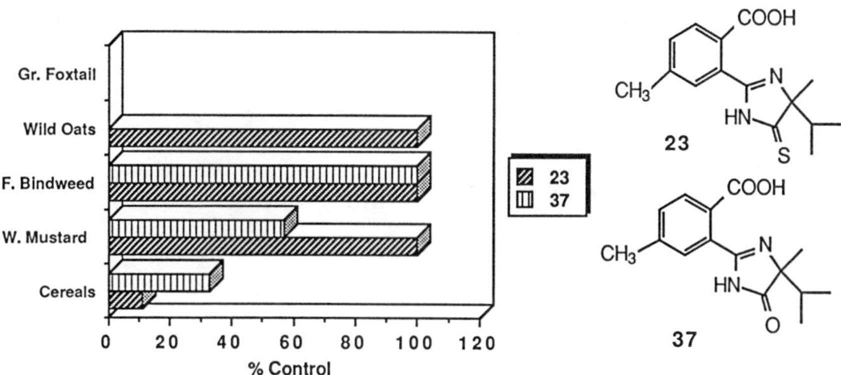

Figure 7. Comparison of 23 to 37 at 250 g/ha postemergence.

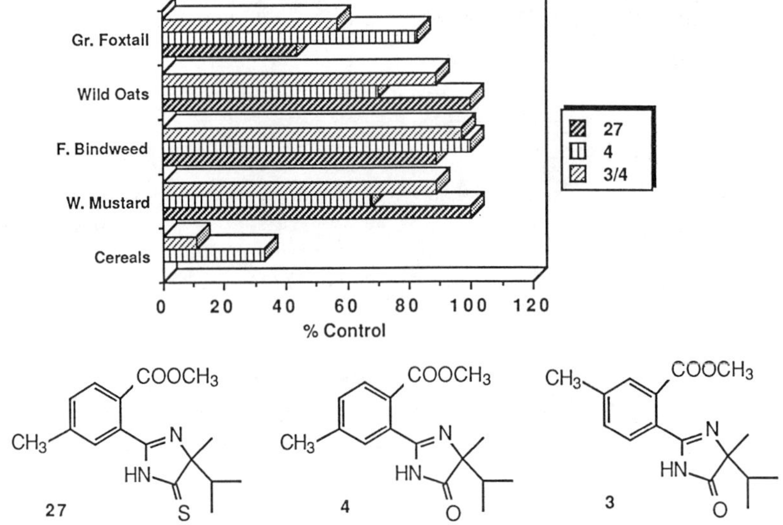

Figure 8. Comparison of 27 and 4 to 3/4 at 500 g/ha pre-emergence.

Literature Cited

1. Los, M.; Ciarlante, D. R.; Ettinghouse, E. M.; Wepplo, P. J., 184th National Meeting, American Chemical Society, 1982; PEST 21.
2. Los, M.; Orwick, P. L.; Russell, R. K.; Wepplo, P. J., 185th National Meeting, American Chemical Society, 1983; PEST 87.
3. Los, M., 186th National Meeting, American Chemical Society, 1983; PEST 65.
4. Los, M., American Chemical Society Symposium Series 1984, 255, 29-44.
5. Los, M.; Wepplo, P. J.; Russell, R. K.; Lences, B. L.; Orwick, P. L., 188th National Meeting, American Chemical Society, Philadelphia, PA, 1984.
6. Los, M.; Wepplo, P. J.; Parker, E. M.; Hand, J. J.; Russell, R. K.; Barton, J. M.; Withers, G,; Long, D. W., 10th International Congress of Heterocyclic Chemistry, University of Waterloo, Ontario, Canada, August 11, 1985.
7. Los, M. U.S. Patent 4 188 487, 1980.
8. Los, M. U.S. Patent 4 297 128, 1981.
9. Los, M. Eur. Patent 41 623, 1981.
10. Los, M. Eur. Patent 133 310, 1985.
11. Los, M. Eur. Patent 133 311, 1985.
12. Los, M. Eur. Patent 166 907, 1986.
13. Reid, E. E. Organic Chemistry of Bivalent Sulfur; Chemical Publishing Company: New York, 1962; Vol IV.
14. Walter, W.; Voss, J. The Chemistry of Amides; Wiley: New York, 1970; pp 383-475.
15. de Boer, Th. J.; Backer, H. J. Org. Syn. Coll Vol. 4, 1963, 943.
16. de Boer, Th. J.; Backer, H. J. Rec. trav. chim. des Pay-Bas, 1954, 73, 229.
17. Los, M. U.S. Patent 4 544 754, 1985.
18. Los, M.; Russell, R. K.; Lauro, P. C.; Lences, B. L.; Hadden, S. K.; Brady, T. E.; Wepplo, P. J., 10th International Congress of Heterocyclic Chemistry, University of Waterloo, Ontario, Canada, August 11, 1985.
19. Los, M.; Russell, R. K.; Lauro, P. C.; Lences, B. L.; Lies, T. A.; Parker, E. M.; Wepplo, P. J., ibid, August 12, 1985.

RECEIVED August 31, 1987

Chapter 9

Benzylnitramines as Herbicides

Synthesis, Resolution, and Effect of Configuration on Activity

D. W. Ladner, S. J. Rodaway, and Barrington Cross

Agricultural Research Division, American Cyanamid Company, Princeton, NJ 08540

A series of benzylnitramines were prepared by either nitration of the carbamates or N-alkylation of nitrourethane, followed by ammonolysis. These represent one-phenylnitramines, known broadleaf herbicides. Nastic responses and growth inhibition observed for this class suggested similarity to the auxin type herbicides. To determine if the preference for the (*R*) -configuration extended to nitramines, 1-(2',6'-dichlorophenethyl)nitramine was resolved and the absolute configuration determined by asymmetric synthesis. A comparison of the (+) and (-) isomers in herbicidal and in vitro assays was performed and the results are discussed.

The phenylnitramines, **1**, a class of plant growth regulators affecting root geotropism and shoot phototropism, was reported in 1954 by ICI (1). Twenty years later American Cyanamid(2) received patent for herbicidal phenylnitramines generically represented by structure **2** . Efficacy was dependent

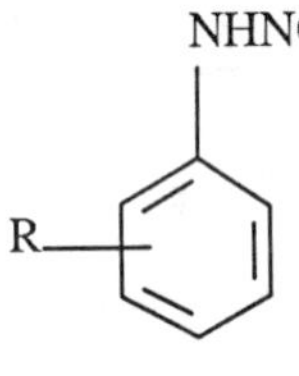

1

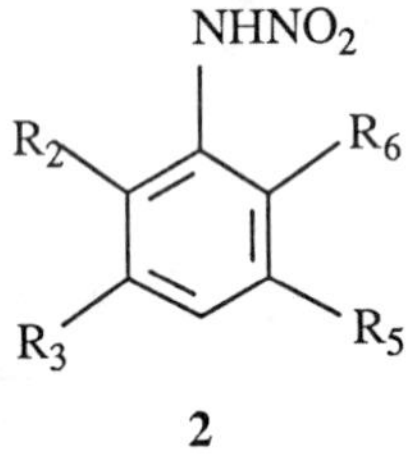

2

on substituents and their position and differed from the ICI compounds such as AC 78,167, since 4-substituents were detrimental for herbicidal activity. The 2,3,5,6 tetrachloro-*N*-nitroaniline, AC 78,299, was the most active in this series. The substituents at the 2,6-positions not only improved activity, but increased the stability of the compounds. Rearrangement can occur with certain nitro-substituted or electron rich *N*-nitoanilines, and the decomposition can be explosive. AC 78,299, on the other hand, is stable up to its melting point of 143°.

Nastic or leaf curling effects, and stem elongation caused by AC 78,299 and its close analogs contrasted with the growth inhibitory response of AC 78,167 type compounds. This structure-activity behaviour, namely the effect of a

0097–6156/87/0355–0100$06.00/0
© 1987 American Chemical Society

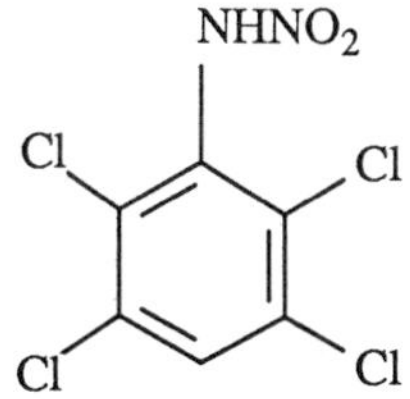

$NHNO_2$ Cl Cl Cl Cl

AC 78,299

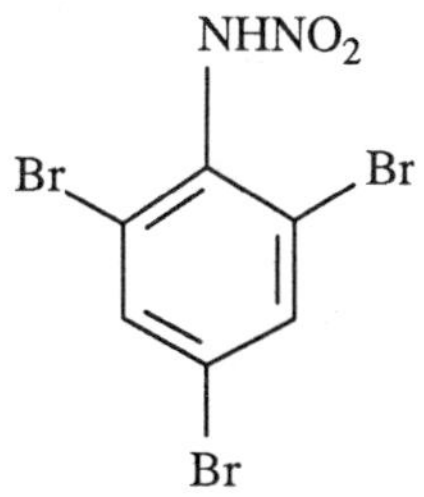

$NHNO_2$ Br Br Br

AC 78,167

4-substitutent, reminded us of the activity of benzoic acids. This series of herbicides are known to be auxins, but have been shown to be auxin-antagonists when 4-substituted. This particular structural feature has figured prominantly in the development of an auxin receptor model(3). We therefore hypothesized that phenylnitramines interact at the auxin receptor because of three observations: the physiological effects, the structure-activity relationships and the chemical similarity of a nitramino group to a carboxylic acid.

The biological resemblence of nitramino groups to carboxylic acids has been examined in other systems (4). Both groups are strong organic acids, a property frequently associated with uptake and translocation (5), however, the pKa's of nitramines reported in the literature are consistently 0.50-0.55 units higher than the corresponding benzoic acids(6). Additionally, in order to ionize, nitramines, require an α-proton. This latter property makes phenylnitamines more closely isosteric with phenylacetic acids (also auxins) rather than benzoic acids, however.

If the nitramino group is also acting as a physiological replacement for either COOH or CH2COOH, the logical task would be to prepare and test the benzyl analogs which could be similar to the CH2COOH group, as in the herbicide **fenac**. Benzyl nitramines are reported to be more thermally stable than the phenyl counterparts(7-8). Improving the known alkylation reaction with halides and nitrourethane seemed plausible(9). Preparation of nitrourethane however, was not a particulary high-yield process(10). Direct nitration with 90% nitric acid succeeded, but a modification using cupric nitrate and acetic anhydride gave a somewhat higher yield. N-nitrourethane was isolated and used as its ammonium salt. The stable salt was reacted in DMF with various benzyl halides at 80° to give initial products which were not isolated, but treated with ammonia and acidified to give the desired products (Table 1). A phase-transfer variation also succeeded, but only for unhindered cases. This DMF reaction was quite satisfactory for most of the nitramines prepared from either the halide or mesylate. A summary of herbicidal activity appears in Charts 1 and 2. Activity was primarily limited to pre-emergence application for most of the series, with the trichloro-analog being the most active. This differs from the phenyl series, in which the tetrachloro was the most active, but compares favorably with the **fenac** structure. We suspect this is just a reflection of a required ideal lipophilicity for activity. The non-chlorinated analogs were much less active.

A more unusual compound was AC 233,866, which showed some beneficial growth-regulating effects as well as being a mildly active herbicide.

TABLE 1. SYNTHESIS OF BENZYLNITRAMINES

$$\underset{\displaystyle R}{\mathrm{Ar-\overset{}{C}H-X}} \xrightarrow[\text{DMF}\ 80°\text{-}90°]{(EtO_2C-\bar{N}-NO_2)NH_3} \xrightarrow[2.\ HCl]{1.\ NH_3} \underset{\displaystyle R}{\mathrm{Ar-CH-NHNO_2}}$$

Ar	R	X	Yield
Ph	H	Br	71
4-Cl-Ph	H	Cl	30
2,4-diCl-Ph	H	Cl	55
2,6-diCl-Ph	H	Br	73
2,6-diCH_3-Ph	H	OMs	53
2,3,6-triCl-Ph	H	Br	64
2,4,6-triBr-Ph	H	OMs	69
2,3,5-tri-I-Ph	H	OMs	45
2-Cl-4,5-methylenedioxy-Ph	H	Cl	20
2,3,5,6-tetra-Cl-Ph	H	OMs	45
2,6-diCl-Ph	CH_3	OMs	18
1-naphthyl	H	Cl	50
1-(2-Me)napthyl	H	Cl	70

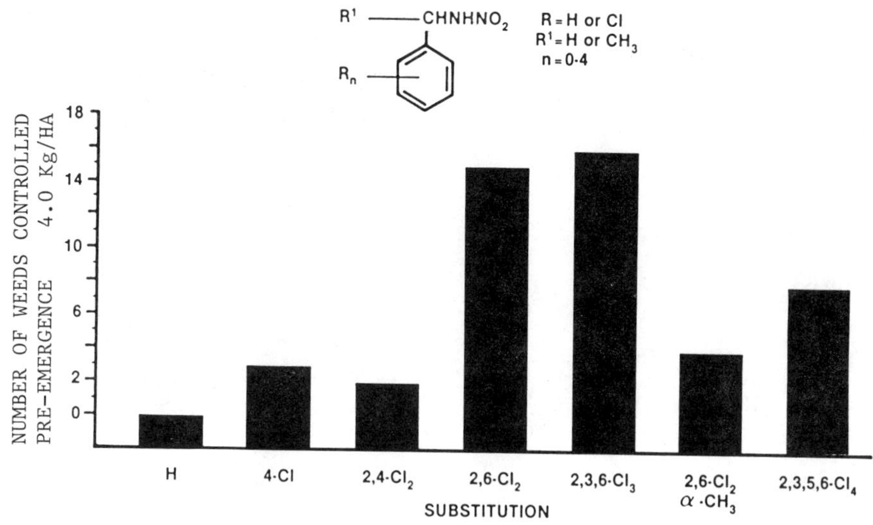

CHART 1. HERBICIDAL ACTIVITY OF CHLOROBENZYLNITRAMINES

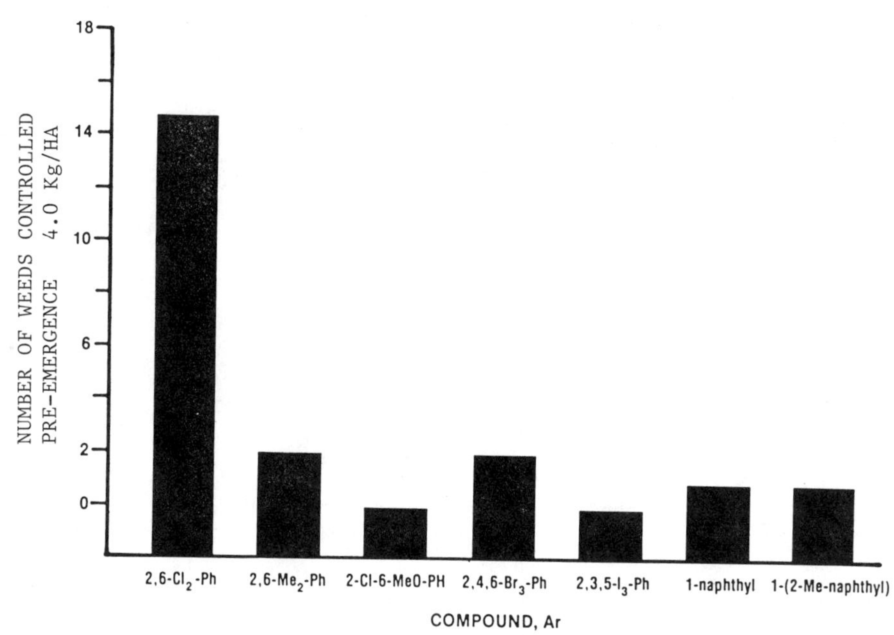

CHART 2. ACTIVITY OF MISCELLANEOUS ARYLMETHYLNITRAMINES.

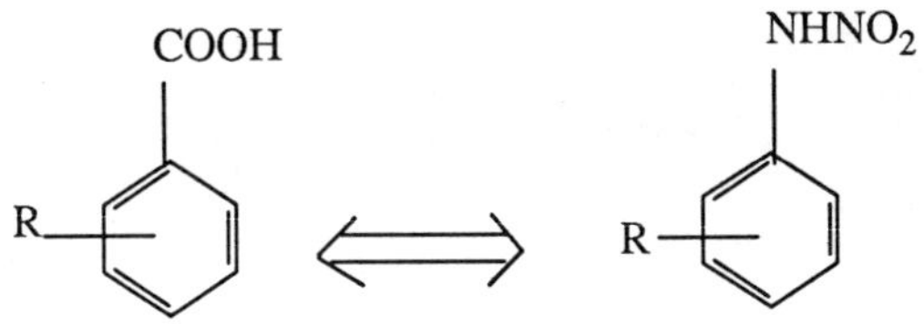

COOH

R

NHNO$_2$

R

benzoic acid analogy

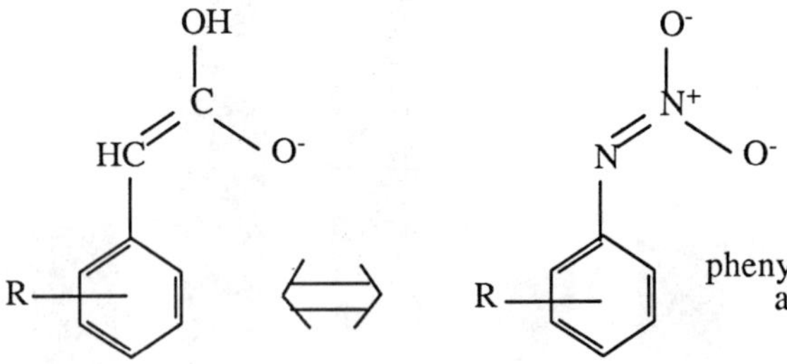

OH

C

HC

O$^-$

R

O$^-$

N+

N

O$^-$

R

phenylacetic acid analogy

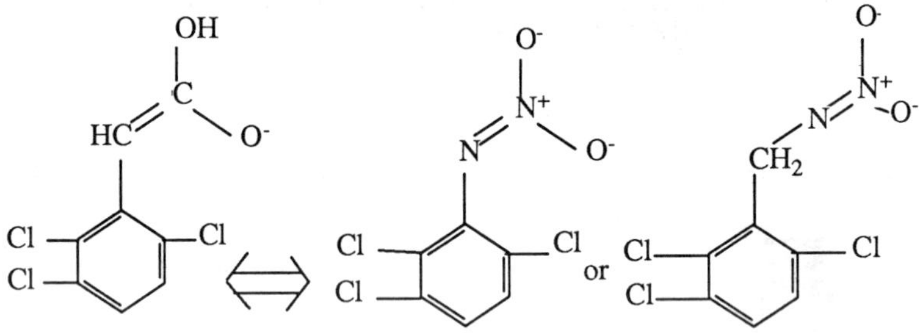

OH

C

HC

O$^-$

Cl

Cl

Cl

fenac

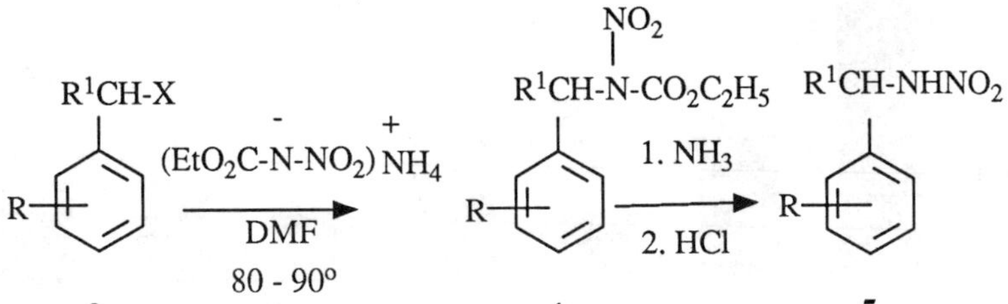

O$^-$

N+

N

O$^-$

Cl

Cl

Cl

or

O$^-$

N+

N

O$^-$

CH$_2$

Cl

Cl

Cl

R^{1}CH-X

R

3

X = Cl,Br, OSO$_2$CH$_3$

$(EtO_2C\text{-}\overset{-}{N}\text{-}NO_2)\overset{+}{N}H_4$

DMF

80 - 90°

NO$_2$

R^{1}CH-N-CO$_2$C$_2$H$_5$

R

4

1. NH$_3$

2. HCl

R^{1}CH-NHNO$_2$

R

5

We noted that it possessed the added structural feature of an asymmetric carbon atom, similar in that respect to the 2-phenylpropionic type of herbicides. Our intention was to resolve this material, if sufficient quantity could be prepared. Since steric effects presumably limited yields obtained by standard methods, alternatives were investigated as shown. These involved preparation and

A. **6** (H_3C, O; Cl, Cl) $\xrightarrow{NH_2OH}$ **7** (H_3C, NOH; Cl, Cl) $\xrightarrow{NOCl}$ **8** (H_3C, $NHNO_2$; Cl, Cl) $\xrightarrow[HOAc]{NaBH_4}$ **AC 233,866** (H_3C, $NHNO_2$; Cl, Cl)

B. **9** (H_3C, NH_2; Cl, Cl) $\xrightarrow{ClCO_2Et}$ **10** (H_3C, $NHCO_2Et$; Cl, Cl) $\xrightarrow{HNO_3}$ $\xrightarrow[2.\ HCl]{1.\ NH_3}$ **AC 233,866**

C. **AC 233,498** (CH_2NHNO_2; Cl, Cl) $\xrightarrow{2\ BuLi}$ [**11** ($HC{=}N{-}NO_2^{-2}$; Cl, Cl)] $\xrightarrow{CH_3I}$ (not observed) **AC 233,866**

$$R\text{-}CH_2\text{-}CH_2\text{-}NO_2 \xrightarrow{2\ BuLi} R\text{-}CH{=}CH\text{-}NO_2^{-2}$$ (Ref. 11)

reduction of a nitrimine, preparation of the carbamate and subsequent nitration, and an attempt to methylate the dianion, **11** , in a procedure analogous to that of Seebach(11). The first two were moderately successful in some runs, but still not particulary advantageous over the original route. The latter gave benzaldehyde as the only isolable product. The best route was a variation of the original which was an extension of the conditions introduced by Mitsunobu(12), as shown. This very direct approach avoids possible elimination reactions reduces the number of steps. A reaction entirely analogous to this for alkylation of β-nitroesters has subsequently appeared(13) and the mechanisms must be very similar. The reaction was complete in an hour and the yield was 41%. Having sufficient quantity permitted not only more definitive biological testing of the compound, but also a traditional resolution into optical isomers. The preparation of the (+) - and (-) - α-phenethylamine salts was straightfoward and after three recrystallizations and hydrolysis, a 10% recovery of each chiral isomer was obtained.

$$\text{1-(2,6-dichlorophenyl)ethanol} \xrightarrow[\text{Ph}_3\text{P, EtO}_2\text{CNHNO}_2,\ 25^\circ,\ 30\text{ min}]{\text{EtO}_2\text{CN=NCO}_2\text{Et}} \xrightarrow[\text{2. HCl}]{\text{1. NH}_3} \text{2,6-Cl}_2\text{C}_6\text{H}_3\text{CH(CH}_3\text{)NHNO}_2$$

$$RCH_2OH \xrightarrow[\text{Ph}_3\text{P, EtO}_2\text{CCH}_2\text{NO}_2]{\text{EtO}_2\text{CN=NCO}_2\text{Et}} RCH_2CH(NO_2)CO_2Et$$

In the method used for the preparation of AC 233,866, there was the likelihood that the reaction proceeded with stereospecific inversion. Since other Mitsunobu-type reactions are known to do so, an asymmetric synthesis establishing absolute configuration was possible. In order to accomplish this, a resolution of the starting alcohol was carried out as shown via the acid phthalates. The optical purity of (+) - **12a** was found to be 94 ±5% by NMR analysis using the optically active shift reagent Eu(tfc)$_3$, or NMR of the diastereomeric *O*-methylmandelates. Conversion of the (+)-alcohol **12a** to the product gave the nitramine with a rotation of -242°. That inversion had taken place was demonstrated by performing the Mitsunobu reaction on the unsubstituted (*S*)- (-)-1-phenylethanol **13** which gave the (+) product, **14a**. In contrast, direct nitration of (*S*) - (-) **15** under conditions expected to give retention led to the (-) product , **14b**. The absolute configuration of **12a** was established by reductive removal of the chlorine to obtain the alcohol of (*S*) configuration, and retention was presumed. The optical isomers were then compared to the racemate in the standard pre-emergence herbicide test described previously. Although the (*S*) -(-) isomer was generally more active than the (*R*)-(-) isomer, the differences were not as striking in all species. (Chart 3)

An in vitro bioassay was then performed to measure the auxin-like properties of these compounds, based on a procedure from Cleon Ross(14)(Fig. I). This assay is based in principle on the growth response to auxins of stem segments of *Pisum sativum*. Measurement of segment weight and transectional area was compared to the untreated control.In this manner, a response curve was obtained for each compound. Indoleacetic acid (IAA) gave a typical response curve, as shown; AC 78,299 gave an auxin-like response while AC 78,167 was inactive(Fig. 2).

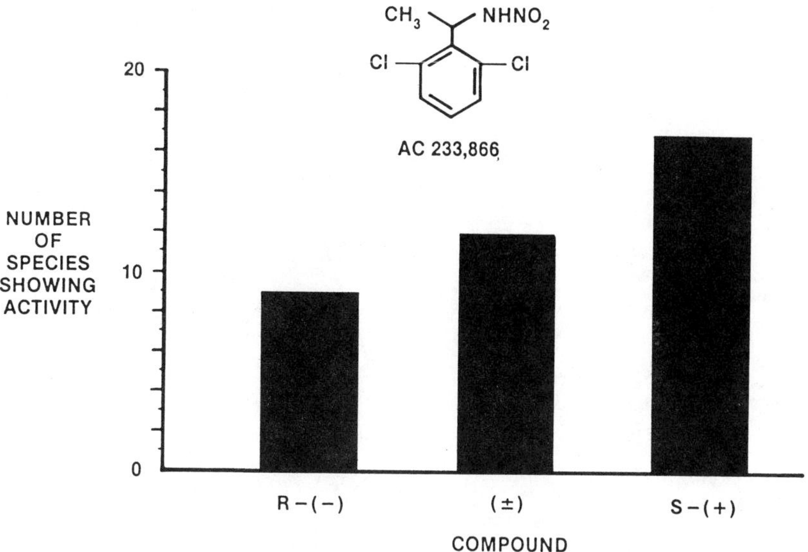

CHART 3. PRE-EMERGENCE ACTIVITY RANGE OF RACEMIC AND CHIRAL AC 233,866

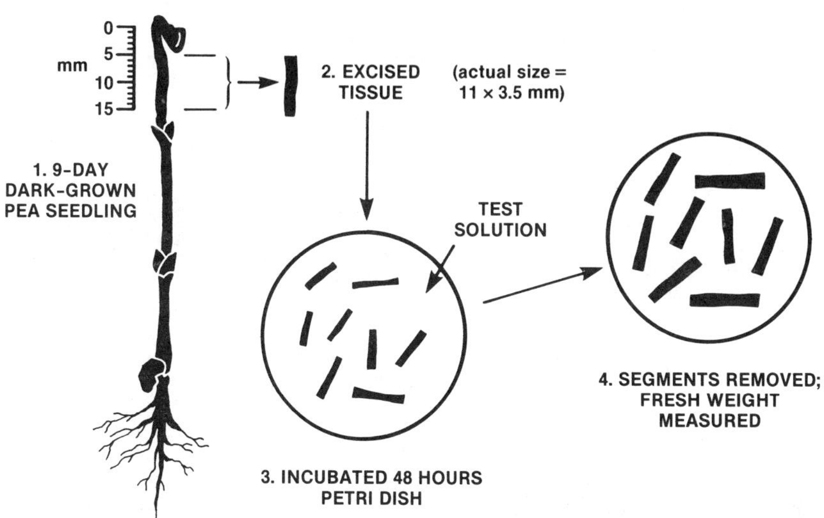

FIGURE 1. PEA EPICOTYL GROWTH BIOASSAY FOR AUXINS

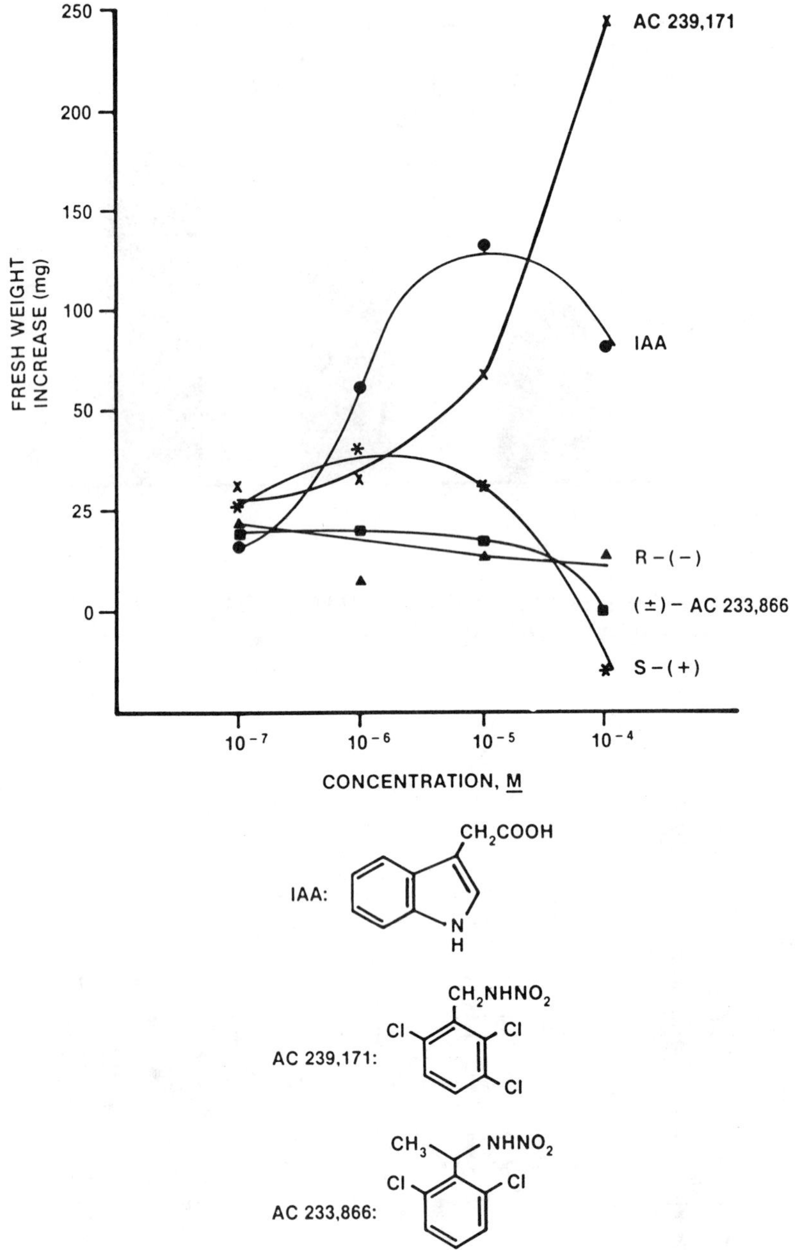

FIGURE 2. PEA EPICOTYL BIOASSAY OF BENZYLNITRAMINES

CH_3 OH Cl Cl → CH_3 O-phth≠ Cl Cl

CH_3 | (-)-$PhCHNH_2$ → (±)Salts ⇄ (+)Salt

HCl

CH_3 OH Cl Cl ← NaOH (+)-phthalate

(+)

50 mole % $Eu(tfc)_3$

$\Delta\delta = 6.45$

94.5% o.p.

$[\alpha]_D = 5.89°$

OCH_3 | (-)PhCHCOCl ←

H_3CO CH_3 O_2C H Cl Cl

(+),(-)

δ 3.43 (3.41)

≠phth = CO_2H C(O)-

AC 239,171 was also auxin-like(Fig. 3), and although less responsive than IAA, its activity continued to increase at the higher rate. AC 233,866, the racemic compound, showed only a slight inhibitory effect; the (*R*)-(-) isomer was inactive. The (*S*)-(+) isomer, on the other hand showed a stronger growth inhibitory response. The slight enhancement at lower concentrations is not necessarily significant. A simple test for auxin antagonism on this compound was negative: lower doses of the compound had no effect on IAA activity, and at the higher rate, no amount of IAA could reverse the inhibitory response.

We concluded from these tests that some of these nitramines are indeed behaving like auxins, but that neither the racemic nor individual antipodes of the α-methylbenzyl compound can be so classified. Underscoring the difference in behavior was the greater activity shown by the (*S*) isomer rather than the expected (*R*), as in the case of phenylpropionic and phenoxypropionic acids(15). While the most herbicidally active nitramines seem to be auxins, others which are interesting growth regulants (e.g. AC 78,167 and AC 233,866) are apparently neither auxins nor auxin antagonists. We conclude that our initial hypothesis concerning the interchangeability of carboxyl and nitramino may be correct, but the mode of action of nitramines is not confined to the auxin/anti-auxin class.

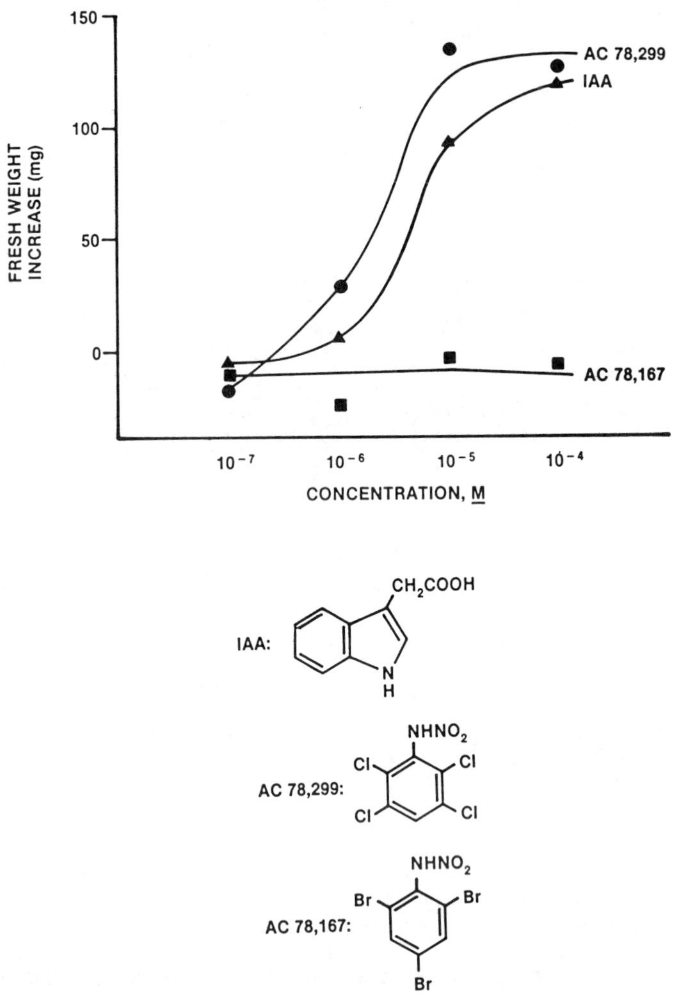

FIGURE 3. PEA EPICOPYL BIOASSAY OF PHENYLNITRAMINES

CH_3 OH Cl Cl (*S*)-(+) **12a** $\xrightarrow{a}$ $\xrightarrow{b,c}$ CH_3 $NHNO_2$ Cl Cl (*R*)-(-) *inversion*

12a ↓ d

CH_3 OH (*S*)-(-) *retention* **13** $\xrightarrow{a}$ $\xrightarrow{b,c}$ CH_3 $NHNO_2$ (*R*)-(+) *inversion* **14a**

CH_3 $NHCO_2Et$ (*S*)-(-) **15** $\xrightarrow{e}$ $\xrightarrow{b,c}$ CH_3 $NHNO_2$ (*S*)-(-) *retention* **14b**

a. PhP, $EtO_2CN{=}NCO_2Et$, EtO_2CNHNO_2

b. NH_3

c. HCl

d. H_2, NaOMe, 10% Pd-C, MeOH, 1 atm

e. HNO_3, Ac_2O

Patents covering these compounds and their use as growth regulants have issued(16).

Acknowledgment

The authors acknowledge the following individuals who contributed to the preparation of compounds and the biological evaluations: B. Walworth, R. Herrick, P. Bhalla, T. D. O'Neal, M. Blair, R. Depew, J. Cadet, D. Whitehead and L. Larue.

Literature Cited

1. Jones, R.L.; Metcalfe, T.P.; Sexton, W.A.; J. Sci. Food Agric., 1954, 5, 38.
2. Cross, B; Gastrock, W.; 1974, US 3 844 762.
3. Katekar, G.F.; Geissler, A.E.; Phytochemistry, 1983, 21, 27 and references therein.
4. Alston, T. A.; Porter, D. J. T.; Bright, H. J.; Acc. Chem. Res., 1983, 16, 418.
5. Crisp, C.E.; Larson, J.E.; 5th Inter. Symp. of Pest. Chem.(IUPAC), Kyoto, 1982.
6. Salymon, G.S.; Grachev, I.V.; Porai-Koshits, B.A.; Sbornik Staiei Obshei Khem., 1935, 2, 1315.
7. Lamberton, A.H.; Quarterly Rev., 1951, 5, 75.
8. Soll, H.; in Houben-Weyl, 1958, 11, pt.2, 99.
9. Gillibrand, M.I.; Lamberton, A.H.; J. Chem. Soc., 1949, 1883.
10. Brian, R. C.; Lamberton, A.H.; J. Chem. Soc., 1949, 1663.
11. Henning, R.; Lehr, F.; Seebach, D.; Helv. Chem. Acta,, 1976, 59, 2213.
12. Mitsunobu, O.; Wasa, M.; Sano, T.; J. Amer. Chem. Soc., 1972, 94, 679.
13. Mitsunobu, O.; Yoshida, N.; Tetrahedron Lett., 1981, 22, 2295.
14. Ross, C.; Plant Physiology Lab Manual; Wadsworth Publishing Co.: Belmont, CA , 1974; p. 124.
15. Aubert, B. et al.; Swed. J. Agric. Research, 1979, 9, 57.
16. Neal, T.D.; Bhalla, P.R.; Cross, B.; 1983, US 4 367 339.

RECEIVED May 29, 1987

Chapter 10

α-Cyano Vinylogous Ureas

A New Class of Herbicides

W. J. Michaely, H. M. Chin, J. K. Curtis, and C. G. Knudsen

**Organic Synthesis Department, ICI Americas Inc.,
1200 South 47th Street, P.O. Box 4023, Richmond, CA 94804–0023**

A novel class of N,N'-diphenyl vinylogous urea herbicides was shown to have several strict structural requirements. All of the following are important for optimum herbicide activity: an alpha-cyano group; a beta-(vinyl)hydrogen; an N-methyl group on the enamine nitrogen and the volume of the substituent in the ortho position on the amide phenyl should not exceed 71 cubic Angstroms. Other substituents on the enamine phenyl and the amide phenyl groups usually diminish activity.

Several of the older and more common herbicides have been shown to interfere with one or more steps of photosynthesis. A number of these are powerful inhibitors at or near photosystem II (PS II) (1). Beginning in 1981, J. N. Phillips and J. L. Huppatz and their group at CSIRO (Australia) have shown that a series of cyanoacrylate (vinylogous carbamate) herbicides are potent inhibitors of PS II (2-6).

Although the CSIRO group elucidated the probable mechanism of action, the initial discoveries in this area were reported in three patents, claiming herbicide activity, to BASF (1969-1970) (7-9). In determining their mode of action, Huppatz and Phillips demonstrated that several structural variations could significantly enhance the PS II inhibition of the vinylogous carbamates (2-6). This enhanced activity, encouraged us to work in the area. It seemed reasonable to us that since both the carbamates and vinylogous carbamates are herbicides and the ureas are herbicides, the vinylogous ureas should be herbicides (see Figure 1). Furthermore, the carbamates (*e.g.*, X=Cl; Furloe), the vinylogous carbamates (*e.g.*, R'=CH_3, R=alkyl) and the ureas (*e.g.*, X=Cl; Diuron) are *all* PS II inhibitors at the thylakoid membrane (Hill reaction inhibition) (1-6).

It is possible that these vinylogous compounds are simply bioisosteres (10) of their parents. There are some subtle structural differences between the classes which are disturbing. The

0097–6156/87/0355–0113$06.00/0
© 1987 American Chemical Society

N-phenyl vinylogous carbamates require the N-alkyl group for herbicidal activity and the commercial ureas and/or the carbamates do not have this requirement. In the N-aliphatic case, primary amino compounds are equally as active as their secondary amino derivatives. The optimum activity occurs when the number of aliphatic carbons in the ester and the amine group together equal twelve, and the polar vinylogous carbamate moiety is within two carbons of one end of this C_{12} unit. For example, the ethyl ester with the N-*n*-decyl vinylogous carbamate is about equal in activity to the *n*-decyl ester with the N-ethyl. An oxygen within the ester further enhances activity and allows the ester to be longer. In the N-decyl case the ethoxyethyl ester (C_2H_5-OC_2H_5-) is about 200 times more active than its simple ethyl ester (11). Most of the biological data of Huppatz and Phillips were done using a Hill reaction assay (isolated chloroplasts) and included very little greenhouse or field data. From inhibition studies with diuron and metribuzin, they concluded that there is binding to the thylakoid membrane at the quinone B site. The general conclusions were: there is a lipophilic pocket and there is hydrogen bonding to the carbonyl oxygen and to the oxygen of the alkoxyester (2-6, 11).

Preparation of Vinylogous Ureas

The BASF procedure (Figure 2) required the use of the highly toxic phosgene (7, 8). The CSIRO procedure was more advantageous since it allowed us to easily vary the substituted amine group (Figure 3). The cyanoacetamides were prepared from cyanoacetic acid and diisopropyl carbodiimide (Figure 4). The diisopropyl urea was easily removed via water washes to give the cyanoacetamides in high yield (82-94%). We also obtained the desired cyanoacetamides from the unstable cyanoacetyl chloride in lower yields (35-62%). The cyanoacetamide was then converted into the desired vinylogous urea via either a two step procedure or a convenient one-pot procedure. Both procedures yielded desired product in good yield (69-89%) (Figure 4).

As work progressed, we desired an acid intermediate that would allow us a broader spectrum of structural variants on the amide nitrogen. We found that the desired vinylogous carbamic acid could be prepared directly from cyanoacetic acid (Figure 5). When R equals (substituted)benzyl, an approximate 1:1 ratio of desired products and decarboxylated products was obtained. When R equals (substituted)phenyl, only the desired carboxylic acid intermediates were obtained. The impure vinylogous carbamic acids could easily be purified by base extraction. These acids were converted to vinylogous ureas via their stable acid chlorides.

These procedures were not useful for the preparation of compounds containing an electron withdrawing group on the enamine nitrogen. For these compounds we used the procedure illustrated in Figure 6. Although either (or both) hydrogen(s) attached to

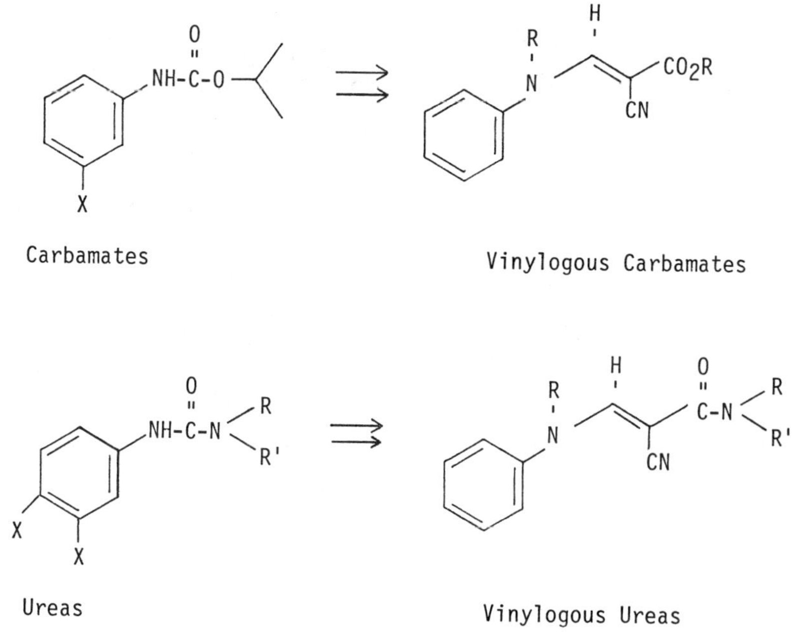

Carbamates

Vinylogous Carbamates

Ureas

Vinylogous Ureas

Figure 1. Structural Similarities

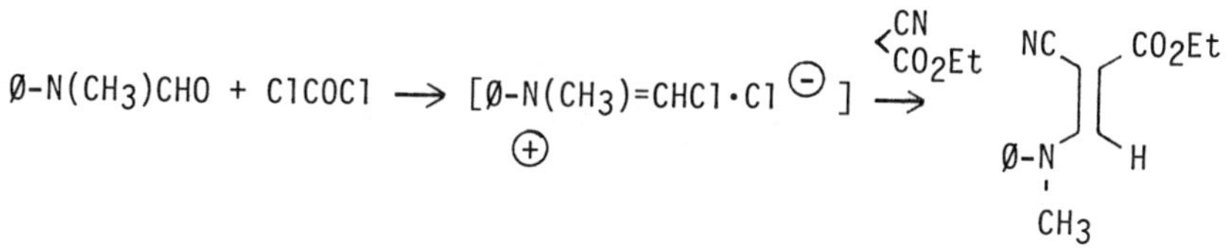

Ø-N(CH_3)CHO + ClCOCl ⟶ [Ø-N(CH_3)=CHCl·Cl$^{\ominus}$] ⟶

Figure 2. Procedure Described in BASF Patent

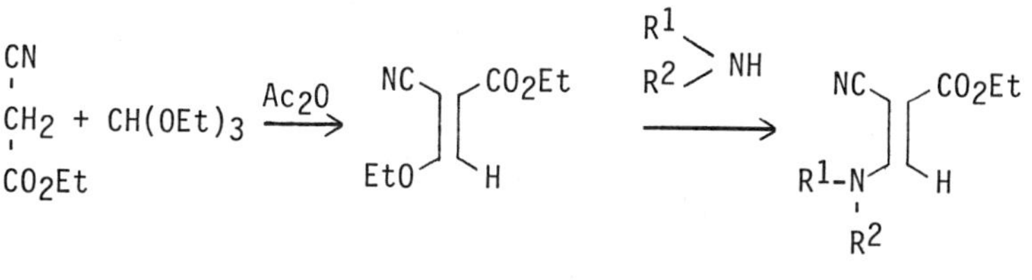

Figure 3. Phillips and Huppatz Procedure

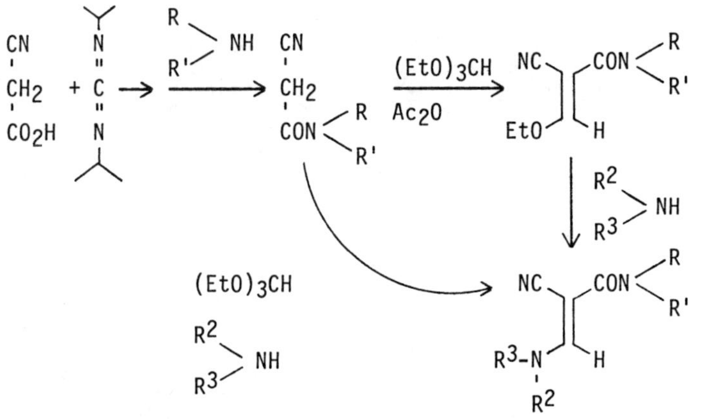

Figure 4. General Method of Vinylogous Urea Preparation

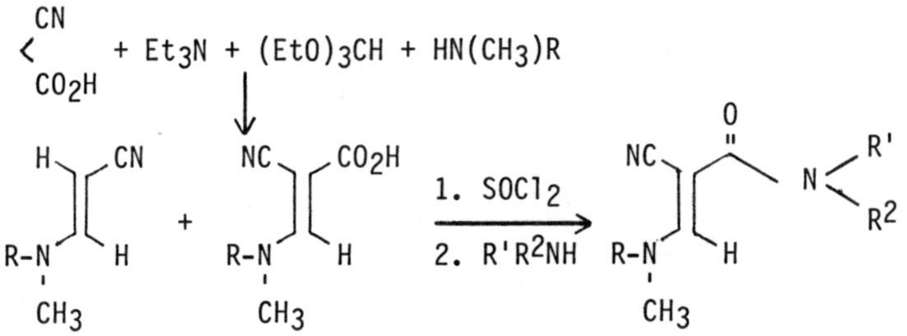

Figure 5. Preparation of Vinylogous Ureas Via Vinylogous Carbamic Acid

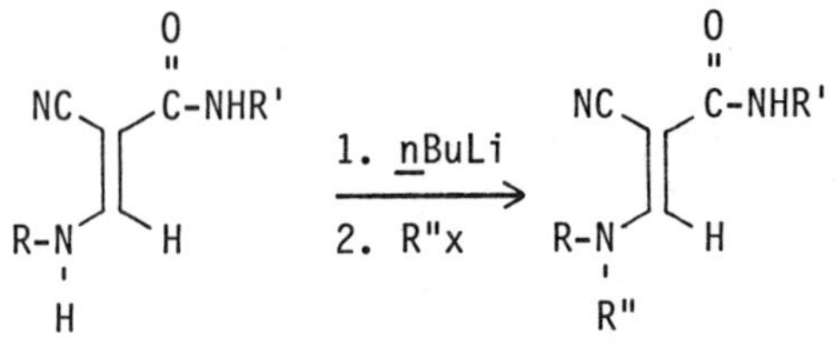

R"=R'''CO, R'''SO2, Aliphatic, etc.
X=Cl, Br

Figure 6. Method for Substituent Variation On The Enamine Nitrogen

the two nitrogens could be abstracted, only the enamine nitrogen was alkylated or acylated. Several explanations seem possible. The enamine nitrogen is cross conjugated to the cyano group and would be expected to be slightly more acidic as a vinylogous cyanamide. The enamine NH compounds were found to have a Z-configuration and the disubstituted enamines had an E-configuration. Hydrogen bonding between the enamine hydrogen and the amide carbonyl could easily be detected spectroscopically. If the enamine hydrogen were abstracted first, the lithium would be expected to coordinate to the amide carbonyl. After alkylation or acylation the final products had the E-configuration, indicating that double bond isomerization had occurred either under the reaction conditions or during the workup.

Structural Requirements for Herbicide Activity

The four substituents on the double bond of the vinylogous urea can be considered distinct areas for substituent variation (Figure 7). For two of these areas the substituent requirements are quite simple. Substituting anything for the vinyl hydrogen tremendously reduces or eliminates herbicidal activity. This includes simple alkyls, alkyl ethers, alkylthio ethers, halogens, etc. For example, replacing the vinyl hydrogen by a methyl group gives a compound that is 1/2 to 1/8 the herbicidal activity of its hydrogen analog.

The other group that has even stricter requirements is the cyano group. We have replaced the cyano group by hydrogen and by electron withdrawing groups such as acetyls, aryls, aryl or alkyl sulfonyls, esters and amides. In all cases the herbicidal activity disappeared.

The substituent requirements on the enamine nitrogen were more flexible. In general, the NH enamines were inactive. But, the N,N-dialkyl enamines were moderately active. The N-CH_3 with N-phenyl or N-benzyl compounds had excellent activity (Figure 8). The benzyl series was slightly less active than the phenyl series and substituents on the benzylic carbon also decreased activity. In both series, aryl substituents were usually less active than the unsubstituted parent (Figure 8). When n=2 (phenethyl) or larger, all herbicidal activity is lost. All polar groups, attached to the enamine nitrogen, eliminated activity.

The amide nitrogen substituent pattern was quite different (Figure 9). When R is aliphatic and R' is H or aliphatic, there are good levels of both pre- and postemergent herbicide activity with control of both broadleaves and grasses. This level of activity was usually greater than 1/4 lb/acre. When R' was (substituted) phenyl, R could not be larger than methyl without substantial decrease of activity. The N-aryl amides frequently had excellent postemergent broadleaf weed control (>95%) at doses of 1/10 lb/acre or less. The one major criteria for levels of herbicidal activity was the nature of the ortho substituent (Table I). The volume of the ortho substituent should be less than 71 cubic Angstroms,

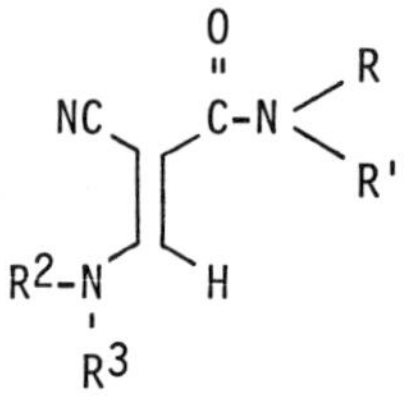

Figure 7. Generic Structure For The Vinylogous Ureas

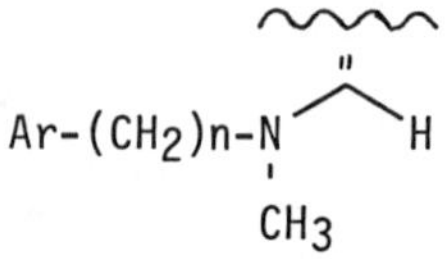

n=1 (Benzyl)
Ar=(Substituted) aromatic

- 4-Substituents: H>>F>>all other substituents
- 3-Substituents: H>F>Cl>>CH_3>>OCH_3
- 2-Substituents: H$\geq$F>CH_3>Cl>OCH_3

n=0 (Phenyl)
Ar=(Substituted) aromatic

- 4-Substituents: H only
- 3-Substituents: H>F>CH_3~Cl>>OCH_3
- 2-Substituents: H>F>>all others

Figure 8. The Aryl Enamine Substituent Requirements

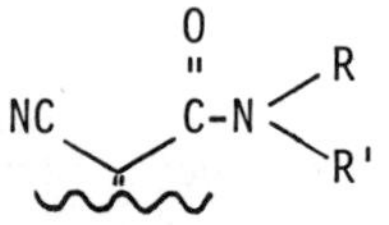

R=H,$CH_3$$\geq$$C_2H_5$$\geq$other aliphatics
R'=(Substituted)aryl, aliphatics

Figure 9. The Amide Substituent Requirements

Table I. Ortho Substituted Alpha-Cyano Vinylogous Ureas: $C_6H_5N(CH_3)CH{=}C(CN)CONH(ortho\text{-}X)Aryl$

#	X	Act(1,2)	Log P(3)	MR(4)	Vol(5)
1	H	A	0.00	1.03	6.47
2	F	E	0.14	0.92	15.17
3	OH	P	-0.67	2.85	15.69
4	NH_2	A	-0.23	5.42	31.16
5	CN	E	-0.57	6.33	34.01
6	CL	E	0.71	6.03	35.83
7	CH_3	E	0.56	5.65	39.22
8	OCH_3	A-E	-0.02	7.87	45.14
9	BR	E	0.86	8.88	45.76
10	I	E	1.12	13.94	61.43
11	CHO	A	-0.65	6.88	61.77
12	NO_2	E	-0.28	7.36	64.34
13	CF_3	A-E	0.88	5.02	70.61
14	CO_2H	P	-0.32	6.93	86.91
15	$N(CH_3)_2$	P-A	0.18	15.55	86.94
16	$COCH_3$	P-A	-0.55	11.18	109.50
17	SO_2NH_2	P-A	-1.82	12.28	113.10
18	CH_2CH_3	A	1.02	10.30	113.90
19	$CONH_2$	P	-1.49	9.81	120.20
20	$CH(CH_3)_2$	P	1.53	14.96	128.92
21	SO_2CH_3	P	-1.63	13.49	136.20
22	$S(O)CH_3$	P	-1.58	13.70	142.90
23	SCH_3	A-E	0.61	13.82	143.50
24	CO_2CH_3	P	-0.01	12.87	172.02
25	OCH_2CH_3	P	0.38	12.47	174.50
26	$SO_2N(CH_3)_2$	P	-0.78	21.88	206.80
27	$CO_2CH_2CH_3$	P	0.51	17.47	344.60

1. Postemergent broadleaf activity (mustard, sesbania, sicklepod, velvetleaf and annual morningglory) -- active means it exceeds 75% average control at the indicated dose
2. Codes: P=Inactive at 4 lb/acre
   A=Active at 4 lb - 1/4 lb/acre
   E=Active at 1/4 lb - 1/40 lb/acre
3. Log P (N-octanol/water) - calculated
4. Molar Refractivity
5. Volume=(L1)X(B4)(squared)X(3.14)(12)

but larger than hydrogen, for best activity. The compounds in Table I are arranged according to the increasing volume of the ortho substituent, using Verlops parameters (12) to calculate the volume. There are two exceptions to the size criteria. First, small, highly polar groups (e.g., OH and NH_2; compounds 3 and 4 in Table I) that can strongly hydrogen bond, are less active than their size would indicate. Second, some large nonpolar groups (e.g., C_2H_5 and SCH_3; compounds 18 and 23 in Table I) are more active than their size would indicate. Other phenyl substituents, including the 2,6-disubstituted phenyl, are less active than the simple ortho-monosubstituted phenyl compounds.

Mode of Action

Since the ureas, carbamates and vinylogous carbamates are all PS II inhibitors (Figure 1), it is not surprising that these compounds are also powerful PS II inhibitors. The more active compounds (Table I) were considerably more active than atrazine (Table II) in the Hill reaction assay. The Hill reaction assay frequently does not correlate with whole plant (greenhouse) activity (1 and 2 and references cited therein). However, vinylogous ureas do correlate fairly well (Table III). Other assays including the carotinoid biosynthesis and acetolactate synthesis (ALS) assays showed little or no activity for these compounds.

Due to solubility difficulties and the use of highly polar solvents such as dimethyl formamide (DMF) or dimethyl sulfoxide (DMSO) we had some difficulty in obtaining reproducible results. For all biological tests great care had to be taken to ensure that homogeneous testing solutions were used. As an extra precaution, we usually tested the reference compounds and standards using the same solvents and surfactants.

Table II. Calculated Concentration for 50% Inhibition (IP 50) of Photosynthesis in Thylakoid Membranes From Pea Via the Hill Reaction

Compound Number	Substituent X	IP 50 (ppm)
Atrazine	-	0.48
5	CN	0.23
6	Cl	0.14
8	OCH_3	0.63
9	Br	0.08
10	I	0.16
12	NO_2	0.23
13	CF_3	1.12
23	SCH_3	0.25

Table III. Postemergent Broadleaf Control in Greenhouse Tests

Compound Number	% Broadleaf Control (1)	Rate (lb/acre)
5	67	0.10
	88	0.25
6	84	0.10
	88	0.25
8	75	0.25
9	81	0.25
10	97	0.05
	99	0.10
	99	0.25
12	90	0.25
13	76	0.25
23	77	0.25

1. Broadleaf weeds: mustard, sesbania, sicklepod, velvetleaf and annual morningglory.

Acknowledgments

We would like to thank several members of Stauffer's Biochemical Design group: David Diaz and M. M. (Alex) Lay for the Hill reaction assays and Desiree Bartlett for the ALS and carotinoid biosynthesis assays.

Literature Cited

1. Moreland, D. E. Ann. Rev. Plant Physiol. 1980, 31, 597-638.
2. Huppatz, J. L.; Phillips, J. N. Z. Naturforsch., C 1984, 39 C, 617-22.
3. Huppatz, J. L.; Phillips, J. N. Z. Naturforsch., C 1984, 48, 55-58.
4. Huppatz, J. L.; Phillips, J. N. Agric. Biol. Chem. 1984, 48, 55-58.
5. Huppatz, J. L.; Phillips, J. N. Agric. Biol. Chem. 1984, 48, 51-54.
6. Huppatz, J. L.; Phillips, J. N.; Rattigan, B. M. Agric. Biol. Chem. 1981, 45, 2769-73.
7. Scheurmann, H.; Fisher, A. S. African Patent 6 805 817, 1969; Chem. Abstr. 1970, 72, 20790x.
8. French Patent 1 579 902, 1969; Chem. Abstr. 1970, 72, 121209v.
9. Fischer, A. German Patent 1 950 601, 1971; Chem. Abstr. 1971; 75, 47729h.
10. Thornber, C. W. Chem. Soc. Rev. 1979, 8, 563-579.
11. Phillips, J. N.; Huppatz, J. L. IUPAC Fifth Int. Cong. of Pest. Chem. Aug. 29, 1982, in Kyota, Japan; Paper #IVb-13.
12. Verloop, A.; Hoogenstraaten, W.; Tipker, J.; in Drug Design; Ariens, E. J., Ed.; Academic: New York, 1976; Vol. 7, p 165.

RECEIVED July 8, 1987

Chapter 11

2-Aryl-1,2,4-triazin-3-ones and 2-Aryl-1,2,4-triazepin-3-ones

Synthesis and Herbicidal Activity

M. J. Konz, S. J. Cuccia, and S. Sehgel

Agricultural Chemical Group, FMC Corporation, P.O. Box 8, Princeton, NJ 08543

New 2-aryl-1,2,4-triazin-3-ones and 2-aryl-1,2,4-triazepin-3-ones were prepared in a three step reaction sequence from readily available aryl isocyanates and aminoacetals or ketals. The key step in the reaction scheme was the formation of 2-arylsemicarbazides by the treatment of arylureas with the aminating reagent 0-(4-nitrophenyl)hydroxylamine. 2-Aryl-1,2,4-triazin-3-ones were herbicidally active in preemergent tests at rates from 0.50 to 0.06 kg/ha. Tolerance towards such crops as cotton and soybean, however, was marginal.

The synthesis and testing of heterocyclic compounds for herbicidal activity has been of continuous interest in our laboratories. As one phase of this program, a search of the literature indicated only a relatively few 2-aryl-1,2,4-triazin-3-ones (1, n=0) and 2-aryl-1,2,4-triazepin-3-ones (2) had been reported, and of those, none appeared to have been examined for herbicidal properties. A synthesis program was therefore initiated in order to access their potential as weed control agents.

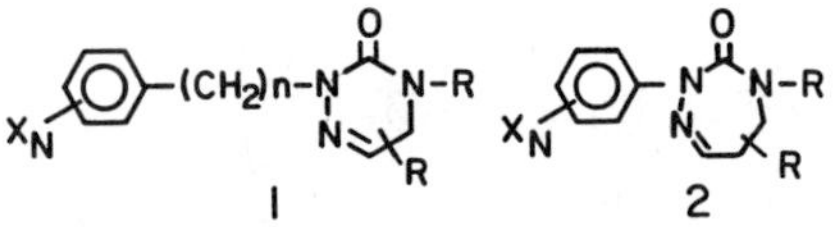

1 n=0.1

2

0097–6156/87/0355–0122$06.00/0
© 1987 American Chemical Society

Synthesis

Treatment of 2-arylsemicarbazides with dicarbonyl or alpha-substituted carbonyl compounds is a common method for the formation of 2-aryl-1,2,4-triazin-3-ones (Scheme 1) (2). Reduction and then alkylation in the case of 3 or alkylation in the case of 4 would provide access to compounds with substituents at the 4-, 5- and 6-positions of the heterocyclic ring. Neither approach, however, has been reported to give triazin-3-ones where the heterocyclic ring is unsubstituted at the 5- and 6-positions.

As 2-aryl-4-alkyl-1,2,4-triazin-3-ones were the first compounds of interest, a reaction scheme was proposed that could provide these compounds (Scheme 2). The first step in the sequence is the reaction of aryl isocyanates and aminoacetals to form the corresponding urea. Treatment of the urea with an aminating reagent would provide a semicarbazide containing the functionalities for the formation of the triazine ring through acidic hydrolysis of the protected carbonyl and then ring closure. By the appropriate choice of aminoacetals or ketals, one could not only selectively introduce substituents at each position of the triazine ring but extend this reaction sequence to include the synthesis of triazepin-3-ones (2).

The results of this reaction sequence are summarized in Scheme 3. Reaction of phenyl isocyanates with methylaminoacetaldehyde dimethyl acetal gave the corresponding ureas (5) in 90-95% yields. The urea was then treated with sodium hydride, and after the reaction mixture had cooled to 5°C, the aminating reagent was added all at once. Of three aminating reagents-O-(mesitylenesulfonyl) hydroxylamine (2), O-(2,4-dinitrophenyl)hydroxylamine (3) and O-(4-nitrophenyl)hydroxylamine (3), the latter was preferred as it is a stable, recrystallizable solid. The crude product from this reaction mixture consisted of the semicarbazide and the urea which are conveniently separated by flash chromatography (silica gel). The conversion of urea to semicarbazide ranged from 25-65% and the yields, based on the recovered urea, were from 50-90%. The lower conversion and yields were consistently obtained where a chlorine atom was at the 2-position of the aromatic ring. The semicarbazide was then heated in aqueous hydrochloric acid (1-2 hours, 80-90°C) to give the triazin-3-ones(1) in recrystallized yields of 50-90%.

2-Aryl-1,2,4-triazepin-3-ones (2) were also prepared from the appropriate aryl isocyanate and 3-(methylamino)propionaldehyde diethyl acetal (Scheme 4). The yields in each reaction step were comparable to those for the synthesis of the triazin-3-ones.

The synthesis of 2-benzyl-1,2,4-triazin-3-ones (1, n=1) was approached from another direction (Scheme 5) as 2-benzylsemicarbazides could not be obtained through amination of the corresponding ureas. Benzophenone hydrazone was first treated with phenyl chloroformate and then with methylaminoacetaldehyde dimethyl acetal to give the semicarbazone 7. From this point, the desired triazin-3-ones could be obtained either by formation of the triazine ring and then alkylation (Path A) or by alkylation and then formation of the heterocyclic ring (Path B). Of these, Path A is the lower yielding method due to the difficulty in recovering the highly water soluble 4-methyl-1,2,4-triazin-3-one (8) and the predominant side-product formation in the alkylation step.

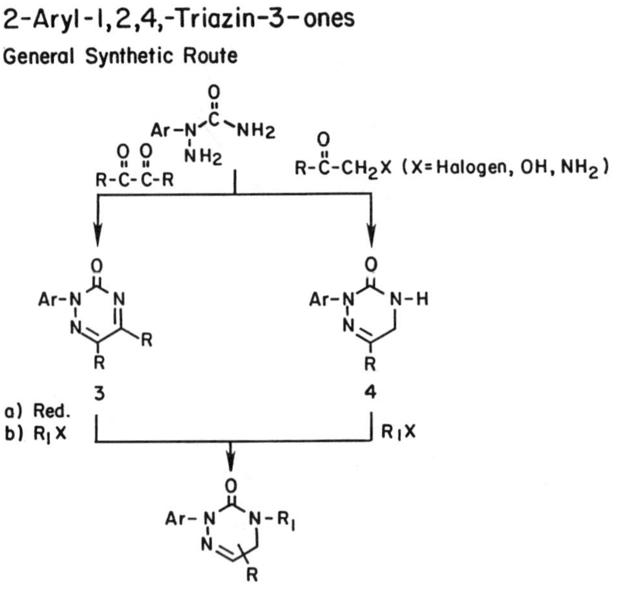

2-Aryl-1,2,4,-Triazin-3-ones

General Synthetic Route

Ar-N(NH2)-C(=O)-NH2

R-C(=O)-C(=O)-R

R-C(=O)-CH2X (X=Halogen, OH, NH2)

3

4

a) Red.

b) R1X

R1X

Scheme 1

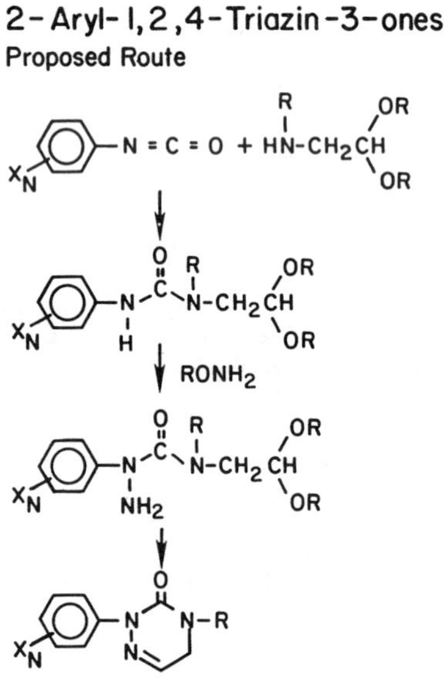

2-Aryl-1,2,4-Triazin-3-ones

Proposed Route

N=C=O + HN(R)-CH2CH(OR)2

RONH2

Scheme 2

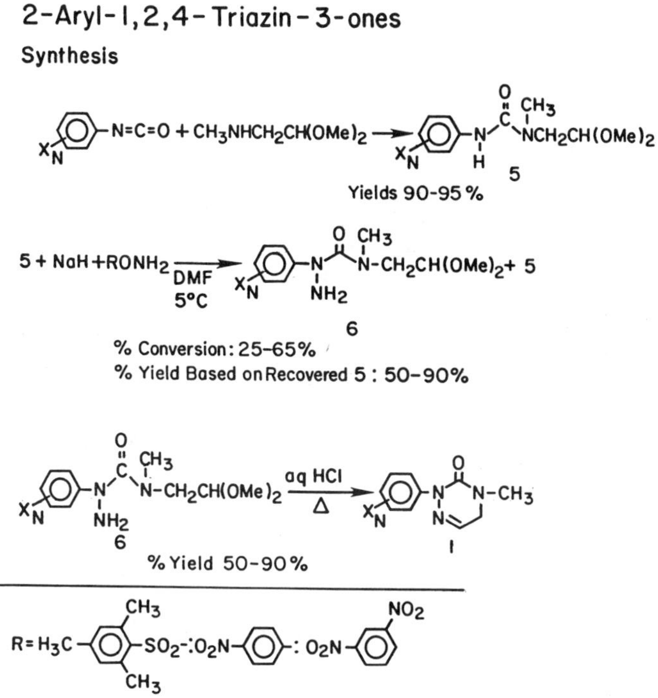
2-Aryl-1,2,4-Triazin-3-ones
Synthesis
N=C=O + CH3NHCH2CH(OMe)2
NCH2CH(OMe)2
5
Yields 90-95 %
5 + NaH + RONH2
DMF
5°C
N-CH2CH(OMe)2 + 5
NH2
6
% Conversion: 25-65%
% Yield Based on Recovered 5 : 50-90%
aq HCl
Δ
N-CH3
1
% Yield 50-90%
R = H3C
SO2- : O2N- : O2N-
NO2

Scheme 3

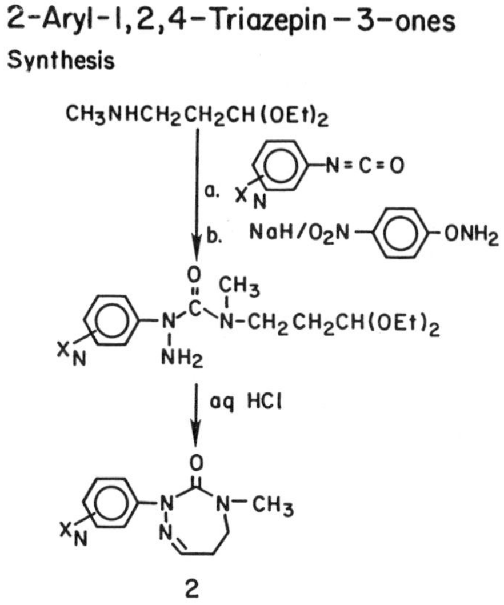
2-Aryl-1,2,4-Triazepin-3-ones
Synthesis
CH3NHCH2CH2CH(OEt)2
a.
N=C=O
b. NaH/O2N-
ONH2
N-CH2CH2CH(OEt)2
NH2
aq HCl
N-CH3
2

Scheme 4

Herbicidal Activity

The first triazin-3-ones and triazepin-3-ones that were examined for potential weed control were substituted by chlorine in the 4-position of the aromatic ring (Table I). In preemergent applications, the 2-(4-chlorophenyl)-1,2,4-triazin-3-one was the only effective compound, providing ≧80% weed control at 1 kg/ha. This compound also inhibited the Hill reaction but it was less effective than diuron (pI_{50} of 5.9 vs. 7.4). The 2-(4-chlorophenyl)-1,2,4-triazepin-3-one, despite a pI_{50} of 5.1, was ineffective in controlling the test species even at 8 kg/ha. Apparently, this compound is not reaching the primary site of herbicidal activity.

Since the triazin-3-ones appear to be Hill reaction inhibitors and may be considered as a class of cyclic ureas, disubstitution of the aromatic ring would be expected to increase activity. The 2-(3,4-dichlorophenyl)-1,2,4-triazin-3-one, however, was found to require >4 kg/ha for acceptable weed control, despite a respectable pI_{50} of 6.9 (Table II). This difference in weed control between the two compounds suggests the aromatic substitution pattern in this class is quite different from that of a "urea" like compound. This, apparently, is the case (Table III). 2,4-Disubstitution as well as the choice of halogen is important for activity. The most effective combination appears to be a fluorine at the 2-position of the aromatic ring with either a chlorine or bromine at the 4-position. However, it is only with the fluorine/bromine combination that some degree of crop tolerance is observed, and then only at the lowest acceptable weed control rate.

Further improvements in herbicidal activity were obtained by introducing an alkoxy function at the 5-position of the aromatic ring (Table IV) (4). The triazin-3-one with propynyloxy at this position was the most effective, providing ≧80% weed control at 0.031-0.062 kg/ha. Soybeans were the most tolerant crop but the difference in weed control rates and the lowest rate for minimum soybean injury may be marginal.

Substitution of the heterocyclic ring was examined and the results are summarized in Table V. For R_1 at the 4-position of the ring, a methyl group was the most effective. At the 5-position of the ring, substitution of a methyl group for a proton offered no improvement in activity and the R and S enantioners were equally effective. At the 6-position of the ring, a methyl group decreased activity by approximately four-fold.

Conclusions

A new synthesis of 2-aryl-1,2,4-triazin-3-ones and 2-aryl-1,2,4-triazepin-3-ones from convenient starting materials has been demonstrated. Of these compounds, the triazin-3-ones were found to have herbicidal properties and with appropriate aromatic substituents, weed control can be obtained at low application rates. However, the weed control/crop tolerance ratio may limit the commercial application of the more active triazinones.

2-Aralkyl-1,2,4-Triazin-3-ones

Synthesis

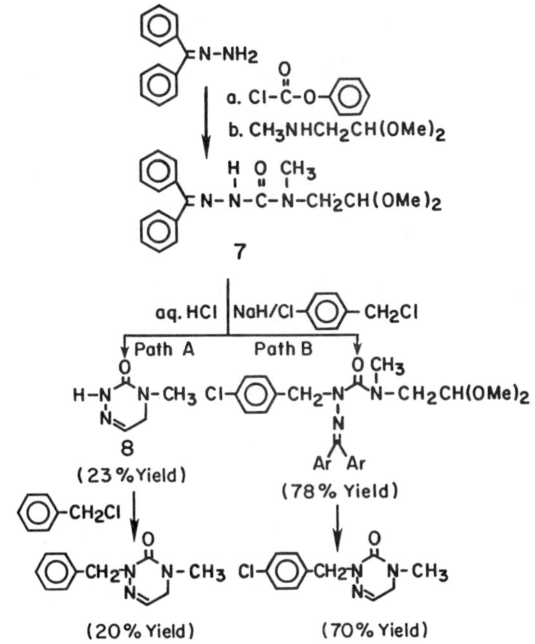

a. $Cl-C(=O)-O-C_6H_5$

b. $CH_3NHCH_2CH(OMe)_2$

7

aq. HCl | NaH/Cl-C_6H_4-CH_2Cl

Path A — **8** (23% Yield); $C_6H_5CH_2Cl$ → (20% Yield)

Path B — (78% Yield) → (70% Yield)

Scheme 5

Table I. Preemergent Herbicidal Activity and Inhibition of Hill Reaction (pI_{50})

	Rate (kg/ha) for ≧ 80% Control	pI50
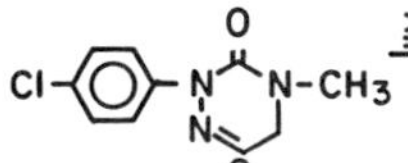 Cl-⟨⟩-N(triazinone)N-CH_3	1	5.9
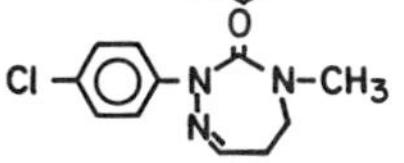 Cl-⟨⟩-N(triazepinone)N-CH_3	>8	5.1
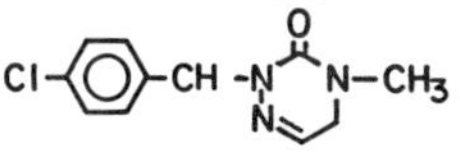 Cl-⟨⟩-CH-N(triazinone)N-CH_3	>8	(<3.5)
Diuron		7.4

Test Species Barnyardgrass, Greenfoxtail
Morningglory, Velvetleaf

Table II. Preemergent Herbicidal Activity and Inhibition of Hill Reaction (pI_{50})

	Rate (kg/ha) for ≧80% Control	pI50
Cl-C6H4-N(N=CH-CH2-N(CH3)-C=O) [4-chlorophenyl]	1	5.9
Cl,Cl-C6H3-N(N=CH-CH2-N(CH3)-C=O) [dichlorophenyl]	>4	6.9
Diuron		7.4

Test Species: Barnyardgrass, Greenfoxtail Morningglory, Velvetleaf

Table III. Preemergent Herbicidal Activity

X_N	Rate (kg/ha) for ≧ 80% Control	Rate (kg/ha) for ≦20% Crop Injury
2,4-DiCl	4	–
2,5-DiCl	>4	–
2-F,4-Cl	0.25	0.125
2-F,4-Br	0.25	0.25

Test Species: Barnyardgrass, Greenfoxtail Morningglory, Velvetleaf Cotton, Soybean

Table IV. Preemergent Herbicidal Activity

R	X	Rate (kg/ha) for ≧ 80% Control: Grasses	Broadleafs	Rate (kg/ha) for ≦ 20% Soybean Injury
$(CH_3)_2CH$	Br	0.125	0.25	>0.25
$HC{\equiv}CCH_2$	Br	0.062	0.25	0.125
$(CH_3)_2CH$	Cl	0.062	0.25	0.125
$HC{\equiv}CCH_2$	Cl	0.031	0.062	0.125
CH_3	Cl	0.125	1.0	0.125

Table V. Structure-Activity Relationships
Heterocyclic Ring

[Structure: Cl, F, $(CH_3)_2CHO$ substituted phenyl attached to N of triazinone ring bearing N–R_1 and R_2]

R_1
4-Position of Ring
$CH_3 > CH_3CH_2 > CH_3O \gg H$

R_2
5-Position of Ring
$H = CH_3$
(Stereochemistry has no effect)

6-Position of Ring
$H > CH_3$

Acknowledgments

We are indebted to Dr. Blaik P. Halling for the determination of pI_{50} values, to Dr. Fredrick W. Hotzman for the whole plant testing data, and to Drs. Kenneth R. Wilson and John W. Lyga for their comments pertaining to the synthetic aspects.

Literature Cited

1. Neunhoeffer, H.; Wiley, P. E., "Chemistry of 1,2,3-Triazines and 1,2,4-Triazines, Tetrazines and Pentazines," in A. Weissberger (ed.), The Chemistry of Heterocyclic Compounds, Vol. 33, Interscience, New York, 1978.
2. Tamura, Y.; Minamikawa, J.; Sumoto, K.; Fujii, S.; Iheda, M. J. Org. Chem. 1973, 38, 1239.
3. Sheradsky, T.; Salemnick, G.; Nir, Z. Tetrahedron 1972, 28, 3833.
4. Mitsuru, S. K.; Hitoshi, T. K.; Katsumasa, K. O.; Tatsuo, M. H. U.S. Patent 4 318 731, 1982.

RECEIVED May 15, 1987

Chapter 12

Chiral 3-Benzyloxytetrahydrofuran Grass Herbicides Derived from D-Glucose

William Loh

Chevron Chemical Company, Ortho Research Center, Richmond, CA 94804

A novel series of chiral grass herbicides based on the benzyloxy substituted tetrahydrofuran ring system has been prepared. These compounds are readily accessible synthetically from diacetone-D-glucose which serves as a chiral template possessing the appropriate stereochemistry for elaboration to the active herbicides. The degree of herbicidal activity is related to the molecular shape of these compounds and especially to the orientation of the substituents around the tetrahydrofuran ring. The chemistry and empirical structure-activity relationships of these compounds will be discussed.

Sugar herbicide RE 39571, 5,6-dideoxy-1,2-O-(1-methylethylidene)-3-O-(2-methylphenylmethyl)-α-D-xylo-hexofuranose (Figure 1), a representative of a novel series of chiral grass herbicides, has been demonstrated in our laboratories to possess a high level of preemergence herbicidal activity against grassy weeds with safety on soybeans, cotton, peanuts, and several other broadleaf crops. This herbicide has also been demonstrated to possess some broadleaf weed activity.

Herbicide RE 39571 and its analogues represent new herbicide chemistry (1) and are chemically based on the common sugar D-glucose. This makes these compounds environmentally attractive products. These compounds are readily accessible synthetically from diacetone-D-glucose which serves as a chiral template possessing the appropriate stereochemistry for elaboration to the active herbicides.

Empirical Structure-Activity Relationships

In view of the structural novelty of this series of chiral herbicides, it was imperative to determine to what extent herbicidal activity is specifically linked to its molecular structure, and to define its structure-activity relationship requirements as a preliminary step toward designing even more potent representatives for this new series of herbicides. The

0097–6156/87/0355–0130$06.00/0
© 1987 American Chemical Society

original lead compound for this research was derived from our random screening program.

In our attempts to optimize the herbicidal activity of this novel series of chiral compounds, a systematic study of the structure-activity relationships was undertaken. Practically all parts of the basic tetrahydrofuran ring were subjected to structural variations. The key structural modifications around the tetrahydrofuran ring can be classified as follows:

1. modifying and varying the shape and size of the substituent at the C-4 ring carbon position (using the carbohydrate nomenclature),
2. varying the aromatic substitution pattern around the benzyl group, as well as replacing the phenyl ring entirely by other aromatic or heterocyclic ring systems,
3. modifying the substituents on the dioxolane acetal ring to exploit the stability as well as the steric and lipophilic characters of this ring,
4. changing the ring size of the rings (one or both), and
5. changing the stereochemistry around the tetrahydrofuran ring.

A great variety of different substituents were investigated at the C-4 ring carbon position (Figure 2). Of particular interest are compounds substituted with an alkyl or 1-hydroxyalkyl group (but not hydroxymethyl) (2), as these substituents resulted in compounds possessing the highest level of biological activity. Variation from the optimum alkyl chain length of two carbons decreased the activity (Figure 3). The ketone derivatives were also active but the aldehyde was not.

We then examined the aromatic substitution pattern around the benzene ring. The substitution pattern as well as the type of substitution on the phenyl ring played an important role in the potency of these compounds. It was apparent from our findings that the highest biological activity was obtained when the phenyl ring was substituted at the ortho position by a F, CH_3, or Cl atom. However, the ranking of these three atoms could vary depending on what the substitution pattern was around the tetrahydrofuran ring, but they were consistently the most active herbicides (Figure 4). In contrast, moving these substituent groups from the ortho to the para position led to a reduction in activity relative to the parent compound. Moreover, moving these substituents to the meta position led to an even further reduction in activity relative to the parent compound.

Meta substitution with either electron withdrawing or electron donating groups consistently led to compounds with diminished activity indicating that the meta position cannot tolerate any substitution. As an added example, a trifluoromethyl analogue at the ortho position was active whereas the meta substituted one was inactive. However, not all ortho substitution was favorable. An ortho cyano or an ortho methoxy group led to very weak activity and compounds with an ortho carboxymethyl or carboxyethyl group were devoid of activity. Bulky substituents around the ring led to inactive compounds suggesting some steric effects around these positions.

Turning our attention to disubstituted benzyloxy compounds, we found that they in general were weaker except for the 2,6-Cl_2 and 2,6-F_2 compounds. The activity-lowering effects of the meta or para substituents are seen in the 2,4- and 3,4-disubstituted compounds.

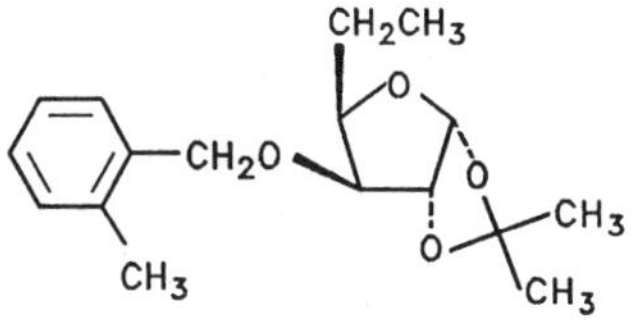

Figure 1. RE 39571.

Alkyl	CH_3, C_2H_5, $n-C_3H_7$, $n-C_4H_9$, $i-C_4H_9$
Alkenyl	$CH=CH_2$, $CH_2CH=CH_2$
Hydroxyalkyl	CH_2OH, $CH(OH)CH_3$, $CH(OH)C_2H_5$
Aldehyde	CHO
Ketone	$COCH_3$, COC_2H_5, COC_3H_7

R, R where R = $OCH_2C_6H_5$, $OCOCH_3$, Cl, OH

O R^1, O R^2 where R^1 = H; R^2 = OC_2H_5, C_6H_5

R^1 = R^2 = H, CH_3, C_2H_5

Figure 2. Range of substituents investigated at the C-4 ring carbon position.

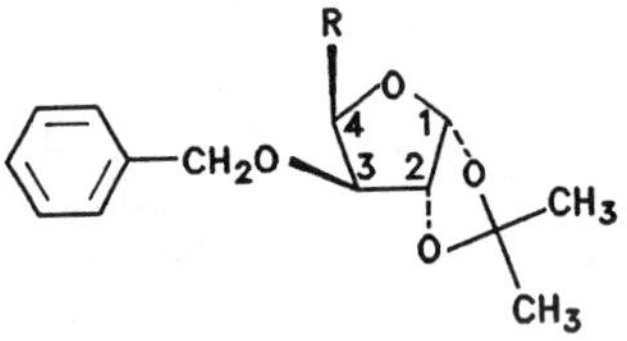

R = C_2H_5 > $n-C_3H_7$ > CH_3 >> $CH=CH_2$ > CH_2Cl > CH_2OCH_3 >> $n-C_4H_9$ > $i-C_4H_9$

R = $CH(OH)CH_3$, $CH(OH)C_2H_5$ >> $CH(OH)C_3H_7$

Figure 3. Effect of C-4 substitution on relative herbicidal activity.

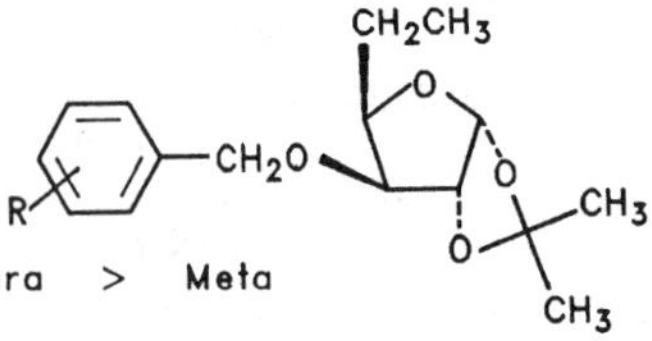

Ortho > Para > Meta

Ortho Set

F > CH_3 > Cl > H > 2,6-Cl_2 >> OCH_3 > CN > CO_2CH_3

Figure 4. Effect of aromatic substitution on relative herbicidal activity.

Interestingly, when the benzene ring was replaced by other heterocycles such as pyridine or thiophene, herbicidal activity was retained (3).

The relative herbicidal activity of the compounds that resulted from the modifications of the dioxolane ring are shown in Figure 5. The size and length of the R^1 and R^2 substituents had a marked effect on herbicidal potency. The highest biological activity was obtained when the ketal substituents were small alkyl groups such as methyl or ethyl. Increasing the size of these groups led to a reduction in herbicidal activity. The only halogenated alkyl group that resulted in high potency was fluoromethyl. The chloromethyl group in contrast resulted in decreased activity.

The following furo-dioxane series was also investigated where the 5-membered acetal ring has been replaced by a 6-membered ring (4). In this case, the acetal functional group has been changed to an ether-type function. The trend in the aromatic substitution pattern was found to be similar to the RE 39571 series (Figure 6), but they were slightly weaker.

At this point, several other pertinent questions needed to be resolved. Since RE 39571 is chiral and is the D-isomer, the question that can be raised is whether the L-isomer, its enantiomer is herbicidal. Does the biological activity reside in both enantiomers or in just one enantiomer? This question was answered when the desmethyl enantiomer of RE 39571 was synthesized and tested (Figure 7). Interestingly, this enantiomer was inactive (tested at 2.8 kg/ha) demonstrating that all the herbicidal activity resides in the D-isomer.

Another question that needed to be raised was whether the configuration at the C-3 carbon position where the benzyloxy group is attached to plays an important role in activity. The 3-epimer was synthesized and tested in our screens and was found to be essentially devoid of herbicidal activity. This result clearly demonstrated that a cis relationship between the ethyl group and the benzyloxy group is required for activity.

Removal of the acetal group or the benzyl group led to inactivity. Interestingly, the hydroxymethyl derivative was not active whereas the 1-hydroxyethyl and 1-hydroxypropyl groups at the C-4 carbon position led to good herbicides.

The criteria required for optimum herbicidal activity for these sugar compounds can now be summarized as follows:

1. a C-4 ring substituent that is preferably an ethyl group,
2. an ortho substituent on the phenyl ring, preferably a methyl, fluorine, or chlorine group,
3. an acetal with two substituents of appropriate size such as methyl or ethyl, and
4. a D-threo configuration about the C-3 and C-4 carbons with a cis relationship of their substituents.

Related Herbicides with Similar Characteristic Structural Features

It became increasingly apparent as research progressed that we needed to know if any other known herbicides possibly possessed or shared these same characteristic structural features. A literature survey revealed several herbicides that need to be mentioned here which possess or incorporate the same characteristic structural features. These are the

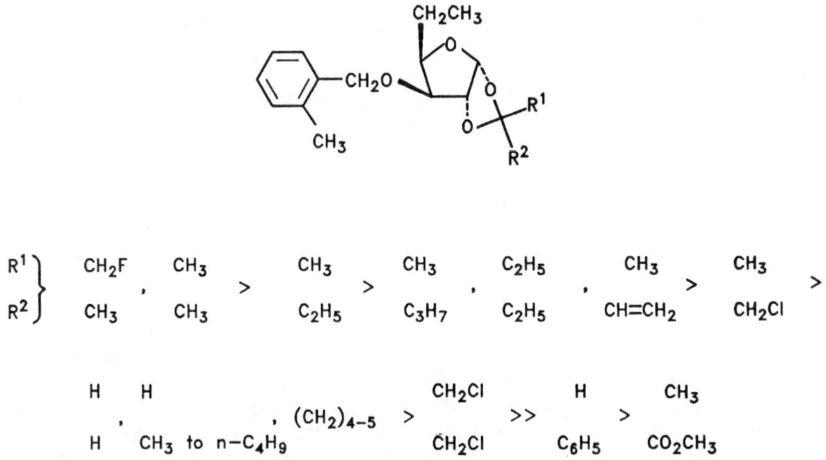
CH2CH3
CH2O
CH3
R1
R2
R1, R2: CH2F/CH3 , CH3/CH3 > CH3/C2H5 > CH3/C3H7 , C2H5/C2H5 , CH3/CH=CH2 > CH3/CH2Cl >
H/H , H/CH3 to n-C4H9 , (CH2)4-5 > CH2Cl/CH2Cl >> H/C6H5 > CH3/CO2CH3

Figure 5. Effect of ketal substituents on relative herbicidal activity.

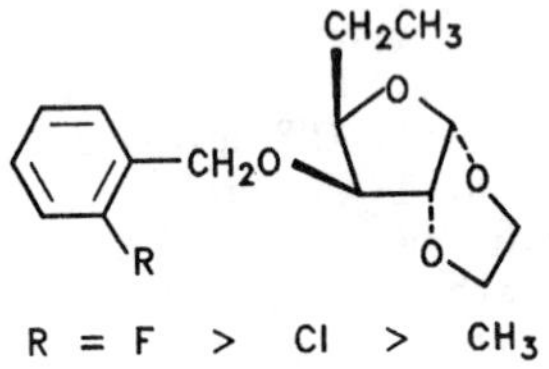
CH2CH3
CH2O
R
R = F > Cl > CH3

Figure 6. Relative herbicidal activity.

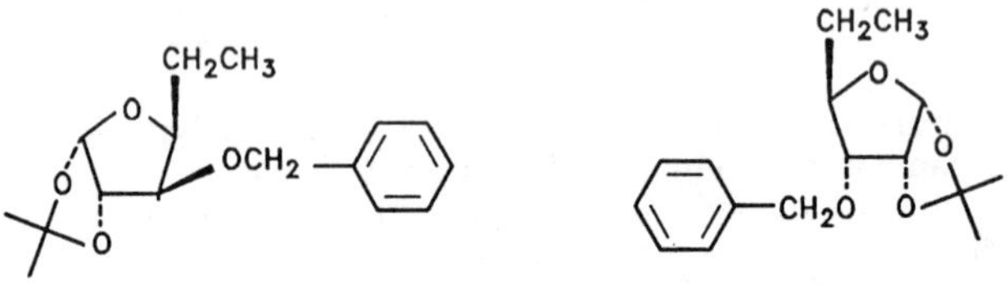
CH2CH3
OCH2
CH2CH3
CH2O

RE 39571 enantiomer 3-epimer

Figure 7. Comparison compounds.

cineole Shell Cinch (5), dioxolane Shell WL 29226 (6,7), and dioxane FMC 39871 (8) (Figure 8).

Relationships that immediately become apparent between RE 39571 and the other compounds are:

1. the presence of a short alkyl chain, i.e., methyl or ethyl vicinal to the benzyloxy group,
2. a benzyl group preferentially substituted at the ortho position,
3. a cis relationship between the above two groups, and
4. a common glycol or glycerol fragment.

Additionally, computer and Dreiding modelling immediately demonstrated that all four of these structures can be overlapped or superimposed on top of each other (Figure 8), the alkyl groups overlapping over each other, as well as the benzyl groups and the glycol oxygen atoms.

Hypothetical Biological Binding Site for Sugar Herbicide

It is now apparent that the degree of herbicidal activity is related to the molecular shape of the sugar molecule and especially to the orientation of the benzyloxy and alkyl groups. These observations therefore suggest a hypothetical biological binding site that might appear in partial cross section as shown (Figure 9) in this representation. This representation of the binding site consists of a cleft capable of accommodating the benzyl portion of the molecule and a pocket or cavity that accepts the alkyl group. The herbicide fits the binding site in a lock-and-key or complementary relationship and can bind only to those compounds that can share a common denominator of structure and that is, the backbone that contains the benzyloxy group and the alkyl group oriented as shown. The binding site clearly demonstrates complete stereospecificity as it can distinguish between stereoisomeric forms. This offers an explanation as to why the enantiomer of RE 39571 is not herbicidal. It cannot fit the binding site and therefore cannot elicit the biological response.

Even though there is great diversity in molecular structure of these related herbicides such as RE 39571, Cinch, WL 29226, and FMC 39871, the similar spectrum of biological activity possessed by all of these herbicides therefore lead us to postulate that they all appear to fit the same binding site and share a common mode of action.

Metabolite Studies

The metabolic fate of the desmethyl analogue of RE 39571 has been evaluated in barnyard grass shoots. The major metabolite was identified as the debenzylated sugar derivative which was devoid of any herbicidal activity.

Synthesis

The first step in the 5-step synthesis sequence of RE 39571 involved benzylation of the commercially available diacetone-D-glucose with α-chloro-o-xylene employing either NaH or NaOH as base. The use of differently substituted benzyl halides afforded the corresponding substituted products. Selective deisopropylidenation at the 5,6-position with aqueous acetic acid then gave the terminal diol (Scheme 1). The terminally unsaturated sugar can be generated from the 5,6-diol via a

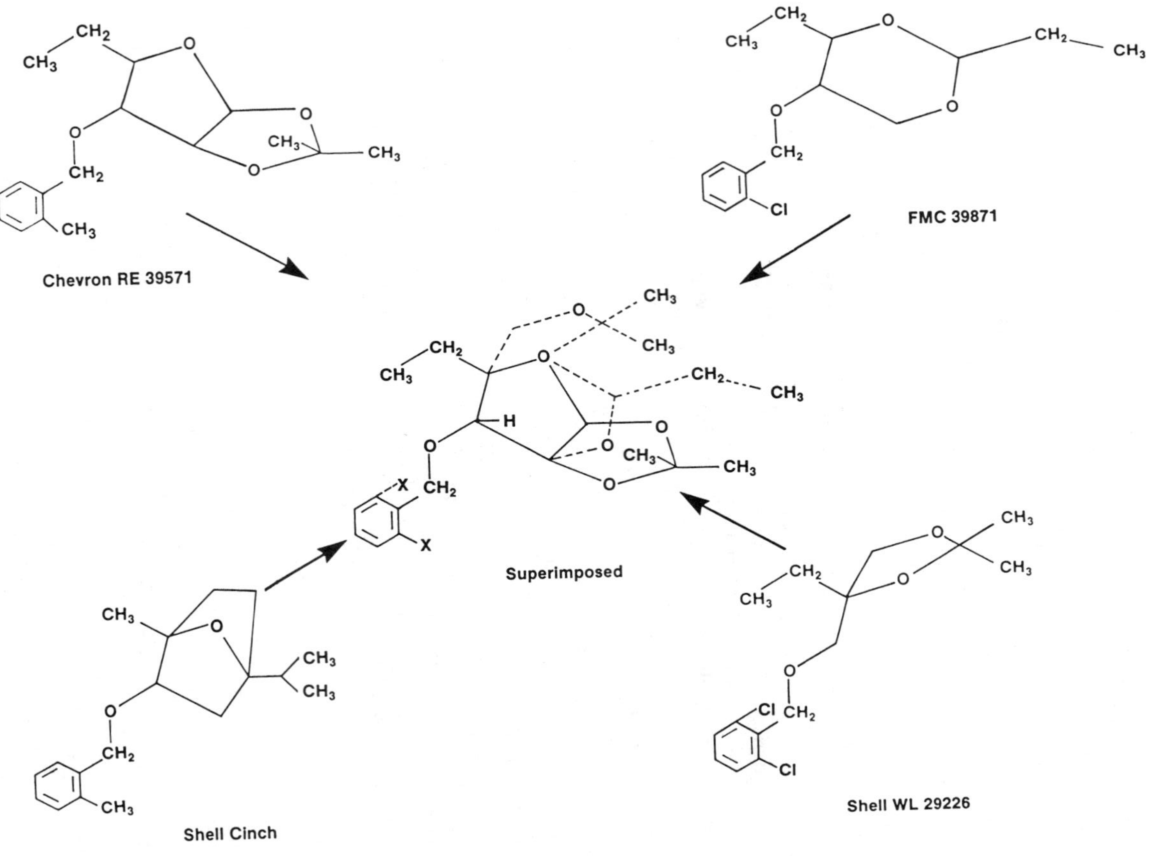

Figure 8. Structural overlap of herbicides related to RE 39571.

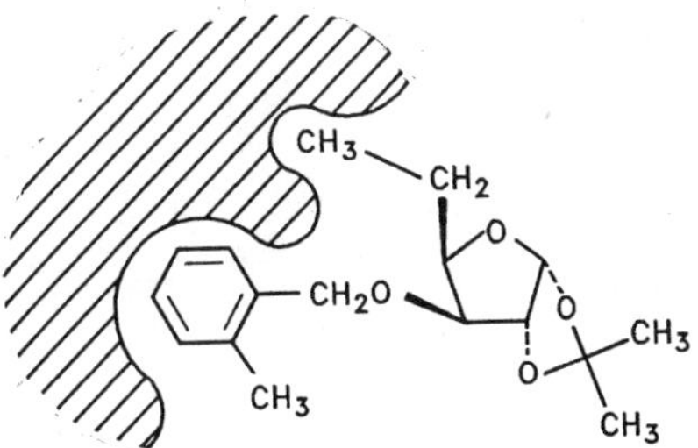

Figure 9. Hypothetical biological binding site.

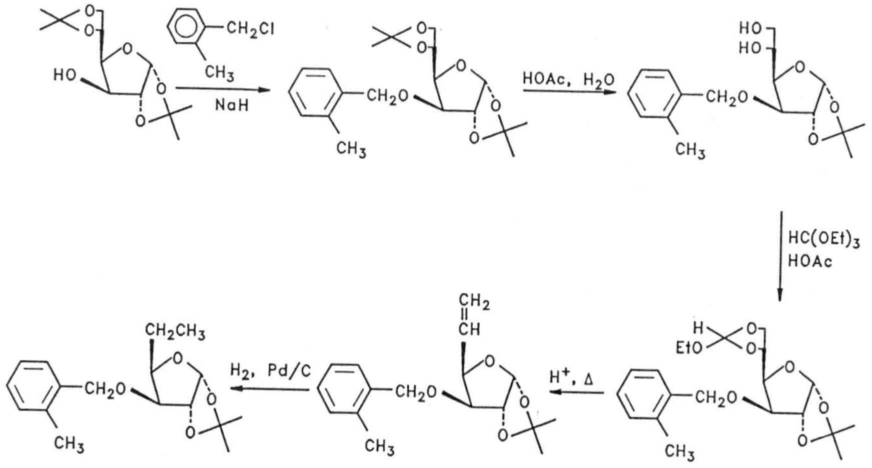

Scheme 1. Synthesis of RE 39571 via D-glucose.

cyclic thionocarbonate, followed by treatment with trimethyl phosphite (9). However, the acid catalyzed decomposition of the cyclic ethyl orthoformic ester provided a simpler, higher yielding route generating only innocuous side-products and was the method of choice. This method also offered consistent results with different aromatic substituents. Subsequent reduction by catalytic hydrogenation with Pd/C then afforded cleanly the saturated sugar derivative in high yield with no debenzylation being observed. If debenzylation is desirable, this is accomplished cleanly by hydrogenolysis under catalytic transfer hydrogenation conditions (10) employing 20% $Pd(OH)_2/C$ and cyclohexene as hydrogen donor.

An alternate approach to the synthesis of these sugar derivatives employed the commercially available diacetone-D-xylose as starting material (Scheme 2). Deprotection of the 3,5-isopropylidene group followed by selective tosylation of the primary hydroxyl group gave the known 5-O-tosyl-α-D-xylofuranose derivative (11). Coupling of the tosylate with a Grignard reagent in the presence of dilithium tetrachlorocuprate as catalyst (12) produced the ethyl substituted tetrahydrofuran derivative which was then benzylated with the appropriately substituted benzyl halide. This procedure was satisfactory for the synthesis of a variety of different aryl derivatives and also allowed entry into different C-4 substituted derivatives.

The enantiomer of the desmethyl analogue of RE 39571 was prepared in a similar manner employing L-xylose instead of D-xylose.

Modification of the ketal substituents involved deketalization of RE 39571 with aqueous trifluoroacetic acid followed by reaction with the appropriately substituted ketone or aldehyde and anhydrous copper sulfate as the dehydrating agent (Scheme 3). If the glycoside-ether is the desired product, this can readily be obtained by glycosidation with methanol in the presence of hydrogen chloride followed by alkylation of the 2-hydroxyl group with the appropriate halide.

The 3-epimer sugar derivative was synthesized in a similar manner as the parent compound except that the hydroxyl group at the C-3 position in diacetone-D-glucose was initially epimerized (13) by oxidation with methyl sulfoxide and acetic anhydride followed by reduction with sodium borohydride.

The furo-dioxanes can also be synthesized from RE 39571 by conversion to the glucoside with methanol and hydrogen chloride, followed by alkylation of the hydroxyl group at the C-2 position with ethyl bromoacetate. The product was then reduced with lithium aluminum hydride to the alcohol and cyclized by acid catalysis (Scheme 4).

Summary

In summary, these compounds represent a novel series of chiral grass herbicides that provide yet another example where chirality is very important for herbicidal activity. Additionally, the use of the sugar D-glucose as a chiral and enantiomerically pure starting material also offers the advantage of having the correct stereochemistry established inherently in the molecule.

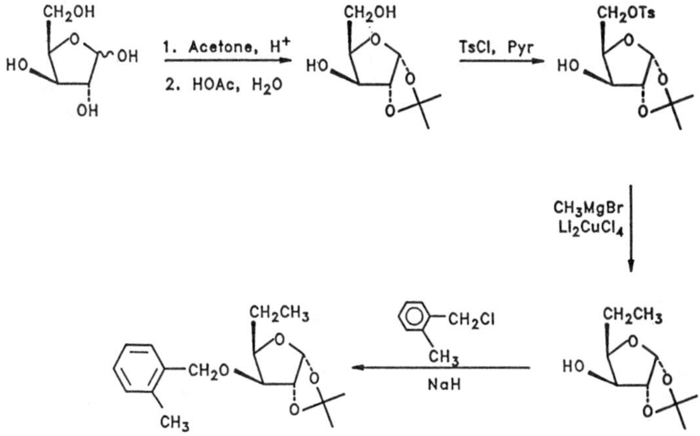

1. Acetone, H^+
2. HOAc, H_2O
TsCl, Pyr
CH_3MgBr
Li_2CuCl_4
NaH

Scheme 2. Alternate synthesis route via D-xylose.

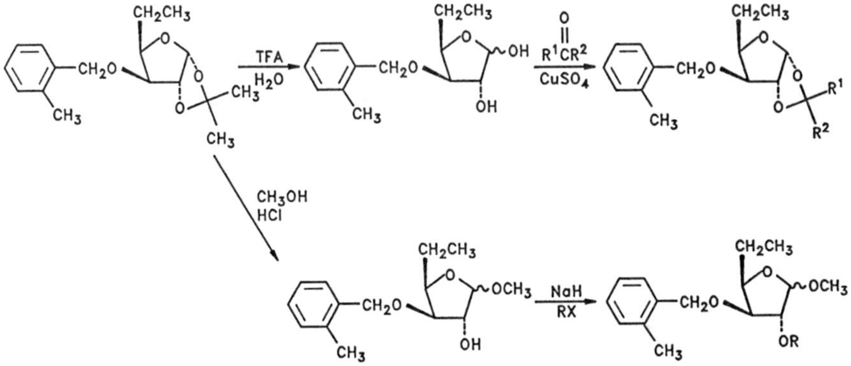

TFA
H_2O
$CuSO_4$
CH_3OH
HCl
NaH
RX

Scheme 3. Ketal and glycoside synthesis.

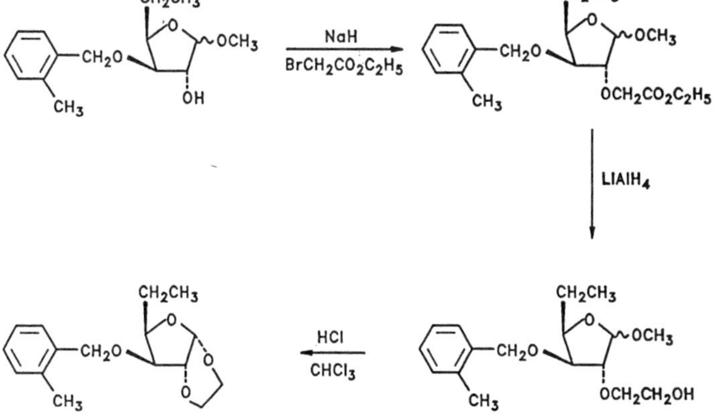

NaH
$BrCH_2CO_2C_2H_5$
$LiAlH_4$
HCl
$CHCl_3$

Scheme 4. Furo-dioxane synthesis.

Acknowledgments

I wish to thank A. Omid for his contribution to the biological testing and Y. S. Chen for the metabolism studies. I am also grateful to M. S. Singer for his computer-assisted modelling studies and to D. C. Aven for her technical assistance.

Literature Cited

1. Loh, W. U.S. Patent 4 429 119, 1984.
2. Loh, W. U.S. Patent 4 521 240, 1985.
3. Loh, W. U.S. Patent 4 515 618, 1985.
4. Loh, W. U.S. Patent 4 534 785, 1985.
5. Payne, G. B.; Soloway, S. B.; Powell, J. E.; Roman, S. A.; Kollmeyer, W. D. U.S. Patent 4 542 244, 1985.
6. Kirby, P.; Turner, R. G. Proc. 12th Br. Weed Control Conf. 1974, 2, 817.
7. Barker, M. D.; Isaac, E. R.; Kirby, P.; Smith, G. C. U.S. Patent 3 919 252, 1975.
8. Konz, M. J. U.S. Patent 4 207 088, 1980.
9. Horton, D.; Thomson, J. K.; Tindall, C. G., Jr. Methods Carbohydrate Chem. 1972, 6, 297.
10. Hanessian, S.; Liak, T. J.; Vanasse, B. Synthesis 1981, 396.
11. Tipson, R. S. Methods Carbohydrate Chem. 1963, 2, 247.
12. Fouquet, G.; Schlosser, M. Angew. Chem. Internat. Edit. 1974, 13, 82.
13. Stevens, J. D. Methods Carbohydrate Chem. 1972, 6, 123.

RECEIVED May 12, 1987

Chapter 13

Synthesis and Activity of Analogs of the Natural Herbicide Cyanobacterin

Janet L. Carlson [1], **Timothy A. Leaf** [2], **and Florence K. Gleason** [2]

[1]Department of Chemistry, Macalester College, St. Paul, MN 55105
[2]Gray Freshwater Biological Institute, University of Minnesota, Navarre, MN 55392

The natural product cyanobacterin has been found to inhibit photosynthetic electron transport in other organisms. A series of analogs of cyanobacterin were prepared as potential herbicides. Several of the analogs also inhibit the growth of the test photosynthetic organisms. The synthesis and structure-activity relationships of these analogs are discussed.

Cyanobacterin, a natural product isolated from the freshwater cyanobacterium (blue-green alga) Scytonema hofmanni UTEX 2349, has been shown to be highly toxic toward other cyanobacteria and green algae (1). It interrupts photosynthetic electron transport at a site in Photosystem II, but not at the same site as classical PS II inhibitors such as DCMU (3-(3,4-dichlorophenyl)-1,1-dimethylurea) act(2). Cyanobacterin, whose structure is shown in Figure 1, is the first example of a halogenated metabolite to be isolated from a freshwater alga. A related compound, the α,β-unsaturated lactone resulting from dehydration of cyanobacterin, was also isolated from Scytonema hofmanni but is not algicidal (3).

The total synthesis and x-ray structure determination of racemic cyanobacterin was recently reported by Williard and coworkers (4). An x-ray structure determination of the natural product has also been published (5).

We have prepared a series of analogs (in racemic form) by a modification of the reported synthesis and tested them for inhibition of PS II.

Biological Activity of the Analogs

The relative potency of the analogs was determined by the concentration required to inhibit PS II (6). In this assay, the concentration of analog which caused complete inhibition of the evolution of oxygen by thylakoid membranes isolated from Synechococcus sp ATCC 27146 was determined using $K_3Fe(CN)_6$ as the electron acceptor.

0097-6156/87/0355-0141$06.00/0
© 1987 American Chemical Society

The data shown in Tables I-III indicates that the presence of a halogenated ring is necessary but not sufficient for an analog to inhibit oxygen evolution by the thylakoid membranes. Substitution of the chlorine by bromine yielded an analog whose inhibitory activity is similar to the natural product. However, substitution by hydrogen resulted in an inactive analog. Similarly, a closely related analog having a methyl group in the position occupied by the chlorine in cyanobacterin and methoxyls instead of the methylenedioxy group is also inactive.

As shown in Table II, removal of the methylenedioxy group produces an analog with greatly reduced inhibitory activity. However, replacement of the methylenedioxy group by an additional chlorine in the para position partially restores inhibitory activity. The presence of chlorine in the para position alone is not sufficient to cause inhibition.

The analog lacking the methoxyl also showed some activity. (See Table III.) Moving the chlorine from one aromatic ring to the other destroyed inhibitory activity. Not surprisingly, the completely unsubstituted analog did not inhibit oxygen evolution.

Analog Synthesis

The analogs were prepared by a modification of the published synthesis. In the key step, the α-anion of a dihydrocinnamic acid ester was coupled with an acetylenic ketone. (See Scheme A.) After separation of the resulting diastereomers by medium pressure liquid chromatography, the slower moving isomer having the priority antireflective (PARF) (7) configuration shown was allowed to react with silver nitrate in aqueous dimethoxyethane to yield the analog. When the published procedure using methanol was employed, the NMR spectra of the product indicated that additional methoxyls were sometimes added.

A representative synthesis of the dihydrocinnamic acid ester (shown in Scheme B) begins with the bromination of vanillin (8). The catechol obtained upon demethylation (9) is not purified as it is air sensitive. Instead, the crude product is alkylated with dibromomethane (4) to yield the methylenedioxy compound which can be recrystallized with ease.

A Horner-Wittig reaction with triethylphosphonoacetate produces a cinnamate in high yield (4). The yield varied from 58% to >99% for other analogs. The alkene is then reduced with sodium borohydride and nickel chloride in methanol and dimethoxyethane (10). (Catalytic hydrogenation on noble metal catalysts is known to cause extensive dehalogenation of aromatic bromides (11). We observed 10-50% debromination using $NaBH_4/NiCl_2 \cdot 6H_2O$ depending on the reaction time.) For other analogs the yield ranged from 44% to >99%.

In some cases, the requisite cinnamic acid was commercially available and could be reduced after esterification. Partial reduction was seen when the carboxylic acid was used as the substrate. After hydrolysis and silylation, the desired intermediate ester was obtained.

The synthesis of the acetylenic ketone, shown in Scheme C, began with the appropriately substituted ketone or aldehyde. In the

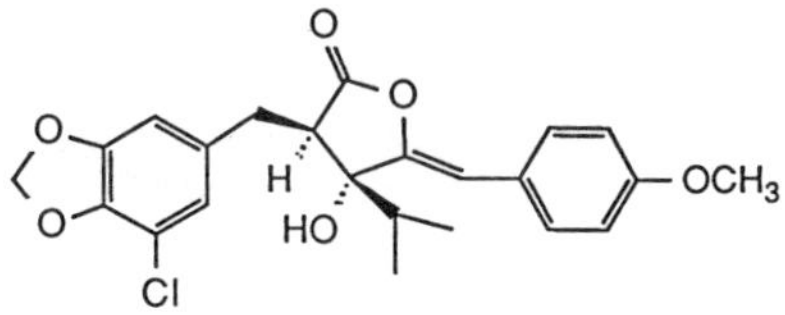

Figure 1. Cyanobacterin.

Table I. Analogs of Cyanobacterin Having One Modified Aromatic Ring

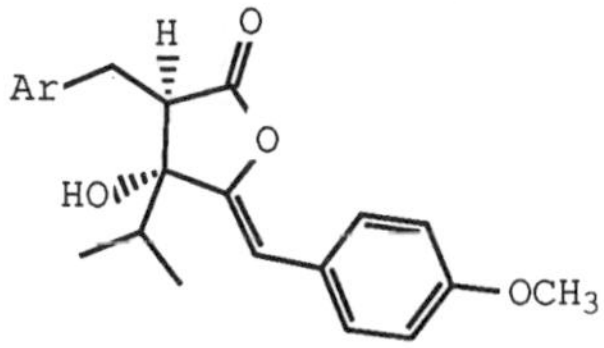

Ar =	Complete Inhibition of the Hill Reaction with $K_3Fe_3(CN)_6$
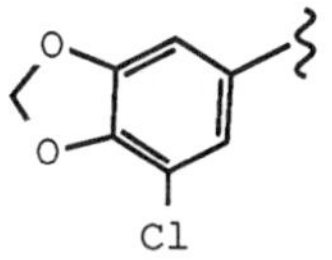 O, O, Cl	25 nM (natural product)
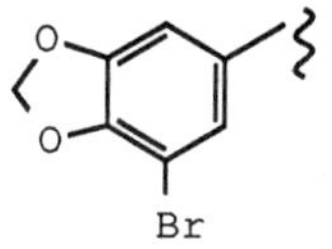 O, O, Br	60 nM
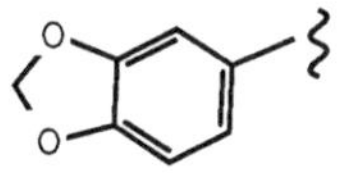 O, O	Not Active
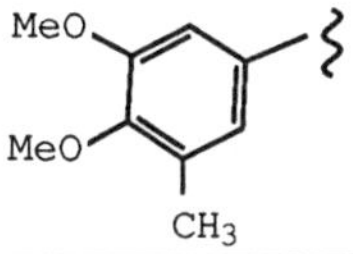 MeO, MeO, CH_3	Not Active

Table II. Analogs of Cyanobacterin Having One Modified Aromatic Ring

Ar =	Complete Inhibition of the Hill Reaction with $K_3Fe_3(CN)_6$
3-chlorophenyl (Cl)	1.5 μM
4-chlorophenyl (Cl)	Not Active
3,4-dichlorophenyl (Cl, Cl)	136 nM
phenyl	Not Active

Table III. Analogs of Cyanobacterin

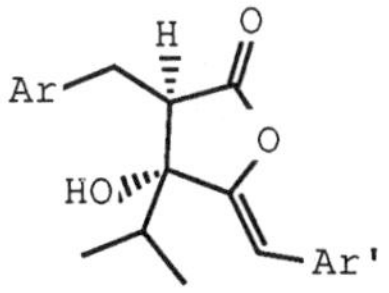

H O
Ar
O
HO
Ar'

Ar =	Ar' =	Complete Inhibition of the Hill Reaction with $K_3Fe_3(CN)_6$
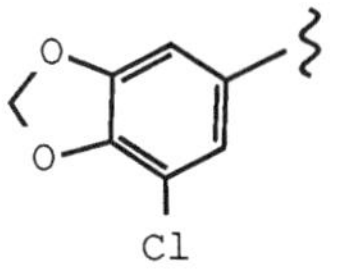 O O Cl	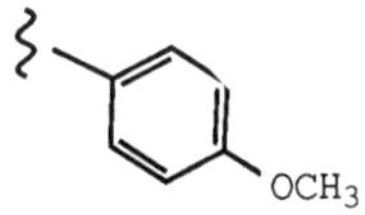 OCH_3	25 nM (natural product)
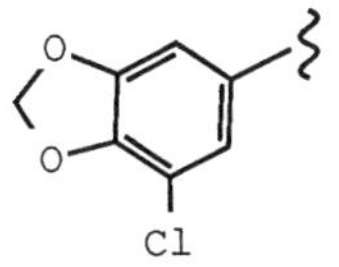 O O Cl	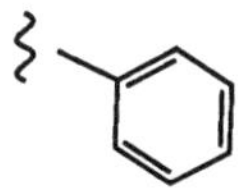	143 nM
O O	Cl	Not Active
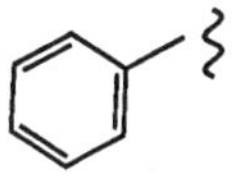	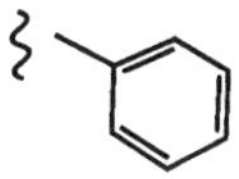	Not Active

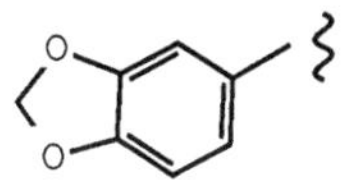

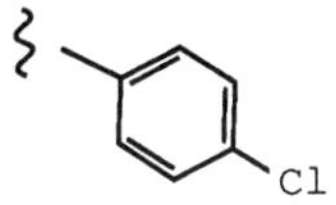

OTMS
A
+
B
OCH3
Br
LDA
OH
+ diastereomer
OH
Br
OCH3
AgNO3
OCH3
OH
Br

Scheme A. Synthesis of Cyanobacterin Analogs.

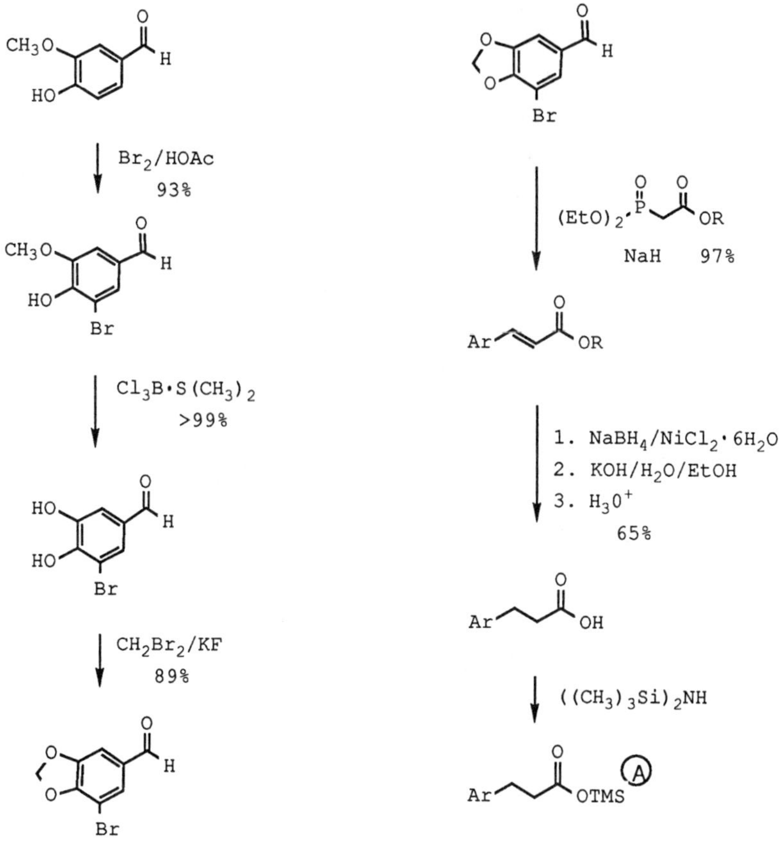

Br_2/HOAc 93%

$Cl_3B \cdot S(CH_3)_2$ >99%

CH_2Br_2/KF 89%

$(EtO)_2P(O)CH_2C(O)OR$ NaH 97%

1. $NaBH_4/NiCl_2 \cdot 6H_2O$
2. $KOH/H_2O/EtOH$
3. H_3O^+
65%

$((CH_3)_3Si)_2NH$

Ar–CH₂CH₂–C(O)OTMS (A)

Scheme B. Preparation of a Dihydrocinnamic Acid Ester.

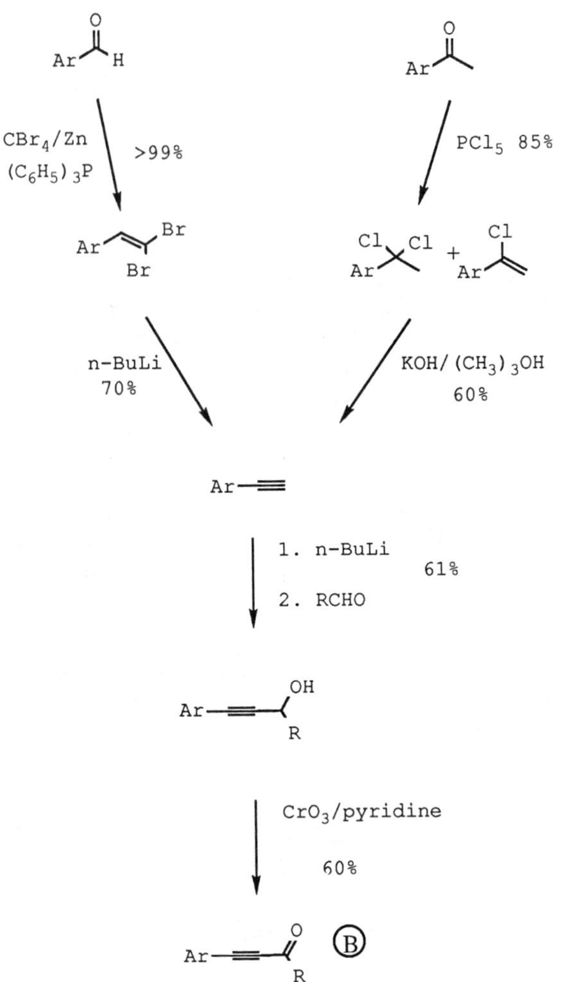

Scheme C. Preparation of an Acetylenic Ketone.

case of the p-anisaldehyde, Normant's (12) procedure was used. A Wittig-type reaction yielded the dibromide in excellent yield. The yield of the reaction depends on the degree to which the product can be washed from the sticky triphenylphosphine oxide/zinc bromide mass. Elimination and transmetallation followed by protonation gave the acetylene.

Alternatively, conversion to the acetylene from the ketone was accomplished using a modification of standard procedures (from Organic Reactions). We found that in the case of the p-chloro compound, the dehydrohalogenation step proceeded much more cleanly when t-butanol was employed instead of ethanol which is more commonly used. (The by-product in the reaction was determined to be 1-ethoxy-2-(4'-chlorophenyl)ethylene.)

Alkylation of the acetylenic anion with isobutyraldehyde gave the propargylic alcohol which was then oxidized using Collin's reagent to yield the requisite ketone.

Conclusion

We have prepared several analogs of cyanobacterin which inhibit PS II. The results of the assays of these analogs indicate that analogs that act at the same site as cyanobacterin must have a halogen present in the ring in which chlorine is found in the natural product.

Acknowledgments

We wish to thank Andrew Buirge, Christopher Fotsch and Myra Kueker (students at Macalester College) for preparing some of the intermediates in the analog syntheses. Prof. Thomas R. Hoye generously provided laboratory facilities for J.L.C. during her sabbatical leave at the University of Minnesota. Rita King (graduate student at the U. of M.) obtained high resolution (300 MHz) NMR spectra of the analogs. We are grateful to Prof. Paul G. Williard for helpful discussions. Finally we wish to acknowledge the support of the Minnesota Sea Grant and the Faculty Development Program (sponsored by the Bush Foundation) at Macalester.

Literature cited

1. Mason, C.P., Edwards, K.R., Carlson, R.E., Gleason, F.K., Wood, J.M., Science, 1982, 215, 400.
2. Gleason, F.K., Case, D.E., Plant Physiol., 1986, 80, 834.
3. Gleason, F.K., Paulson, J.L., Arch. Microbiol., 1984, 138, 273.
4. Jong, T-T., Williard, P.G., Porwoll, J.P., J. Org. Chem., 1984, 49, 735.
5. Gleason, F.K., Porwoll, J., Flippen-Anderson, J., George, C., J. Org. Chem., 1986, 51, 1615.
6. Gleason, F.K., Case, D.E., Sipprell, K.D., Magnuson, T., Plant Sci., 1986, 46, 5.
7. Carey, F.A., Kuehne, M.E., J. Org. Chem., 1982, 47, 3811.
8. Hann, R.M., Spencer, G.C., J. Amer. Chem. Soc., 1927, 49, 535.
9. Williard, P.G., Fryle, C.B., Tetrahedron Letters, 1980, 3731.

10. Satoh, T., Nanba, K., Suzuki, S., Chem. Pharm. Bull., 1971, 19, 817.
11. "Sodium Borohydride," Thiokol/Ventron Div., Danvers, Mass.
12. Villieras, J., Perriot, P., Normant, J.F., Synthesis, 1975, 458.

RECEIVED May 12, 1987

Chapter 14

Conformationally Rigid Peptides as Models for Selective Herbicides

J. V. Edwards[1], H. G. Cutler[2], P. S. Zorner[3], and C. B. Coffman[4]

[1]Southern Regional Research Center, Agricultural Research Service, U.S. Department of Agriculture, New Orleans, LA 70179
[2]Richard B. Russel Research Center, U.S. Department of Agriculture, Athens, GA 30163
[3]Agricultural Research Center, BASF Chemicals Division, Research Triangle Park, NC 27709–3528
[4]Northeastern Region Beltsville Agricultural Research Center, U.S. Department of Agriculture, Beltsville, MD 20705

Synthetic peptide analogs derived from the phytotoxin tentoxin, have been examined for their phytotoxicity and herbicidal potential to a variety of plants and agronomically significant weeds. Structurally modified analogs included both cyclic and acyclic derivatives. Acyclic tripeptides were modified from the synthetic intermediate tert-butyloxycarbonyl-Leucyl-N(methyl) dehydrophenylalanyl-glycine methyl ester. Modifications at the leucine side chain and dehydrophenylalanine nitrogen were introduced by substituting different alkyl groups. Selective alkylation at the amide bond nitrogen of dehydrophenylalanine provided analogs which showed herbicidal potential. The cyclic peptides induced chlorosis in both barnyardgrass and morningglory. The tripeptide analog tert-butyloxycarbonyl-Valyl-N(ethyl) dehydrophenylalanyl-glycine methyl ester exhibited root growth inhibition in barnyardgrass and inhibited bolting in mustard seed. Similar analogs containing an N-ethylated amide nitrogen and dehydrophenylalanine exhibited some growth regulating activity in wheat coleoptiles. The effects of stereochemical and rigid conformation on biological activity are discussed.

The use of biologically derived chemicals as herbicides has met with limited success. Despite this, biotechnology offers potential for the exploration of naturally occurring compounds as herbicides, which may serve as impetus for new synthetic and structure/function approaches in herbicide developement (1). In this regard we have implemented a program to study biologically active peptides from plants and fungi. Specifically, we focused on phytotoxic cyclic

0097–6156/87/0355–0151$06.00/0
© 1987 American Chemical Society

tetrapeptides secreted by fungi. Cyclic peptides having a diverse range of biological activities in plants have been isolated and structurally characterized (Figure 1) (2-6). These activities vary in both the induced pathological and plant growth regulating response as well as selectivity. For example AM toxin, a host selective toxin secreted by A. mali, induces necrosis on only certain apple leaf cultivars (2), whereas tentoxin (5) (Figure 2), a non-selective toxin, induces chlorosis (a yellowing of plant tissue) in some plants such as lettuce and mung bean but not in others such as corn (7,8). Tentoxin induced chlorosis results from interference with chloroplast development (9-11).

Interestingly, these compounds (Figure 1) share similar structural features, notably the 12-atom peptide rings, which are rich in alkyl amino acid side chains. Some of the peptides contain unusual amino acid side chains possessing olefinic (AM toxin, tentoxin) and epoxide functionalities (HC toxin). In view of these biological and structural characteristics it is timely to explore the role of conformation, side chains, and peptide backbone modifications in the phytotoxic profiles of these peptides. We selected tentoxin as a model for examining some aspects of structure versus function. The conformational rigidity resulting from the 12-atom peptide ring has allowed previous workers to determine bond angles by using NMR techniques to identify preferred conformers associated with biological activity (12 and 13). Our previous analog studies have explored the role of the 12-atom ring in biological activity and compared biochemical profiles for the mode of action of the two conformationally similar analogs tentoxin and [Pro^1] tentoxin (24). Of practical interest is tentoxin's potential as a selective herbicide since it is active in sorghum species similar to johnsongrass but not in corn (7,8).

Recently we reported the total synthesis of tentoxin and a conformationally similar peptide [Pro^1] tentoxin (24). Synthesis of tentoxin requires synthetic steps both common to and different from normal solution phase peptide syntheses due to the presence of unusual modifications including N-methylated amide bonds and a dehydrophenylalanyl residue. An advantage in performing the total synthesis of a peptide such as tentoxin is the convenient approach affording piecemeal assessment of unique functional groups for their role in biological activity. In order to assess the contribution of these unusual modifications to chlorosis induction, synthetic intermediates from the synthesis were assayed for chlorosis induction in lettuce seedlings. Although only one peptide demonstrated induction of significantly low chlorophyll levels in lettuce it was found that this analog also inhibited root growth. Further investigations into sequence requirements for the root inhibition revealed that the tripeptide derivative Boc-Leu-N(CH3)Δ^ZPhe-Gly-OMe (**3**) was sufficient for full biological response (root growth inhibition). The structure of analog **3** (R_1 is isobutyl and R_2 is methyl) which demonstrates root growth inhibiting effects is shown in Figure 3.

Though this peptide has considerably increased conformational flexibility over the cyclic peptide tentoxin, it contains two backbone and side chain modifications which confer increased conformational rigidity to the molecule when compared with backbone non-modified oligopeptides. It is helpful to recall that the conformation of a peptide is determined by its overall three-dimensional structure (14). If the bond angles and bond

Peptide	Biological Activity
Tentoxin cyclo[-N(CH_3)-Ala-Leu-N(CH_3)Δ^ZPhe-Gly-]	Induces chlorosis in some plants (lettuce, mung bean) but not others (corn, tomato) (5,7,8).
HC-toxin cyclo[-Aoe-D-Pro-Ala-D-Ala-]	Inhibits growth of susceptible corn roots (3).
Cyl-2 cyclo-[Aoe-D-O-methylTyr-Ile-Pip-]	Inhibits lettuce root growth elongation and rice seedling growth (6).
cyclo[-Pro-Val-Pro-Val-]	Retards stem growth of rice seedlings.
(D-Val isomer)	Promotes stem growth (4).
Malformin cyclo[D-Cys-D-Cys-Val-D-Leu-Ile]	Induces malformations in corn roots (16-18).
AM-toxin cyclo[-Ala-Hmb-Amp-ΔAla-]	Causes veinal necrosis on apple leaf cultivars (2).

Figure 1. Abbreviated structures and biological activities of phyto-active, cyclic peptides. Abbreviations according to IUPAC-IUB Commission (1972) Biochemistry 11,1726-1732 are used. Δ^Z denotes a dehydroamino acid of the Z configuration.

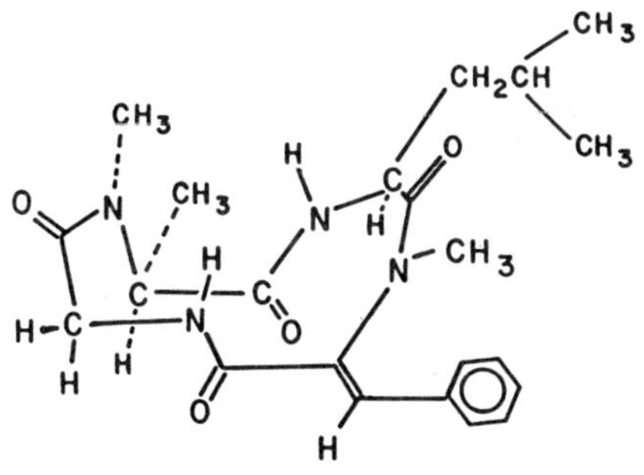

Figure 2. Structure and preferred conformation of tentoxin (5,12).

lengths are held constant the conformation is describable. Important dihedral angles for defining conformation in peptides are the Ψ, ϕ and ω angles (Figure 3). Because of the considerable conformational freedom present in peptides it is desirable to fix and rigidify the conformation in order to probe the relation of conformation to biological activity (15). In the field of mammalian hormone and neurotransmitter peptides this approach has been investigated over the last 10-15 years. For this reason we decided to study the biological effects of structural features which would predictably rigidify and/or change conformation in the tripeptide sequence found to have root growth inhibiting properties. Some structural changes incorporated in this study which either reduce conformational flexibility (15) or change the spatial orientation of the amino acid side chain include: N-alkylation (substitution of a methyl, ethyl, or propyl for a hydrogen at the nitrogen of an amide bond), conversion of an sp^3 center at an α-carbon to a sp^2 center, substitution of a D amino acid for an L amino acid and substitution of a hydrogen at the α carbon with a methyl group. Previously conformational studies by Vitoux et al. (25) on dipeptides containing N-methylation have shown the conformational specificity induced by N-methylation. Conformations of tripeptides containing dehydrophenylalanine have been recently discussed by Chauhan et al. (26).

In initial structure activity relationship studies we have held constant the olefinic moiety at position 2 and varied alkyl groups at the 2 position amide bond. This was made possible through selective N-alkylation. The selective N-alkylation step shown in Figure 4 is pivotal to the synthesis of analogs described here, and preliminary profiles of the structure activity relation for the root growth inhibitors revealed that alkylation at the 2 position of the synthetic intermediate was necessary for biological activity at the 100-500 micromolar level. Utilizing this reaction we have thus far been successful in N-alkylating at dehydrophenylalanine with methyl, ethyl, and propyl groups in good yield.

We focus here on an approach in which synthetic fragments of a naturally occurring cyclic peptide such as tentoxin can be studied as a model for conformationally rigid peptide phytotoxins and for their potential by selective herbicidal activity. Our initial studies include the following steps: 1) Screen synthetic intermediates for phytotoxicity in plants sensitive to tentoxin. 2) Appropriately derivatize synthetic intermediates showing activity at 100 micromolar or less. 3) Test these analogs in a plant assay sensitive to a broad range of biologically active compounds. 4) Test analogs in crop plants and agronomically important weeds both in excised and intact plant tissue. This report constitutes the results of four different plant assays. The modified peptides were initially screened in lettuce and cress seedlings and subsequently tested on agronomically important weeds.

Synthesis

Cyclic peptides of this study were prepared utilizing synthetic routes previously reported. The full details of the synthesis of tentoxin and [Pro^1] tentoxin have been reported elsewhere (24).

Tripeptides utilized in this study were synthesized employing synthetic steps identical to those in the cyclic peptide syntheses. Variations of the N-terminal amino acid and in the alkyl group at the nitrogen of the 2-position dehydrophenylalanine were accomplished through substitution of the appropriate tert-butyloxycarbonyl amino acid and alkyl iodide at the appropriate synthetic step, respectively. The details and physical constants of these synthetic tripeptide analogs will be reported elsewhere (Edwards J. V. and Cutler H. G., unpublished results).

Root growth bioassay of germinating lettuce and curly cress seedlings

Aliquots of oligopeptide compounds to be tested were dissolved in ethyl acetate. One milliliter aliquots of the samples were pipetted onto filter paper and 15 lettuce or cress seeds were uniformly distributed on the the filter paper surface and allowed to imbibe in the dark at 20 to 25°C for 24h. The samples were subsequently placed in a growth chamber in continuous light at 28°C for 72h, and the root lengths were measured.

Wheat coleoptile assay

An assay previously utilized for detecting growth inhibition and promotion and cited for its validity in screening for phytotoxicity was employed. The techniques utilized were those of Cutler et. al. (18).

Petri dish assay for herbicidal activity.

Compounds were applied to sterile filter paper in a petri dish at a concentration of 500 micromolar in a solution of 5% acetone and 95% water. Surface sterilized seeds of lettuce, barnyardgrass, morningglory, and mustard seed were placed on filter paper. A visual assessment of chlorosis was made. Radical and coleoptile lengths were measured seven days after seed germination. Two replications per compound were performed.

Discussion of structure function relationships

The peptides discussed in this structure/activity relation study were initially tested in the lettuce and cress seedling bioassay where the root growth inhibition activity was originally discovered. The results of this study are shown in Table I. It is interesting that replacement of the methyl group at the amide nitrogen of dehydrophenylalanine in **3** with an ethyl group, resulting in **1** gives a shift from inhibition to growth promotion. On the other hand when the stereogenic center at leucine in the N-ethylated analog is converted from the R to S configuration a shift from growth inhibition to growth promotion is observed. Further derivatization in the form of various combinations of R_1 and R_2 group subsitutions gave the root growth responses seen in Table I. Compound **8** is the most rigid of the analogs. A gem dimethyl functionality at the α carbon of the 1 position amino acid in combination with R_2 as a methyl group and a dehydrophenylalanine residue in compound **8** resulted in promoted growth of both lettuce and cress seedlings.

Previously an extended structure function relation analysis was performed to assess the role of varying degrees of conformational rigidity present in the tripeptide sequence (H-Leu-Phe-Gly-OH) on

Table. I Results of _in vitro_ lettuce and cress root growth assay for seven _tripeptide_ analogs.

Compound	Lettuce/Cress Seedling Assays Promotion	*%Root Growth at 10^{-6}M Inhibition
1 Boc-Leu-N(C_2H_5)Δ^ZPhe-Gly-OMe	40-50%(L),19%(C)	
2 Boc-D-Leu-N(C_2H_5)ΔPhe-Gly-OMe		50%(L),80%(C)
3 Boc-Leu-N(CH_3)Δ^ZPhe-Gly-OMe		60%(L),50%(C)
4 Boc-D-Ala-Δ^ZPhe-Gly-OMe		40%(L),20%(C)
5 Boc-Val-N(C_2H_5)Δ^ZPhe-Gly-OMe	40%(C)	
6 Boc-Val-N(CH_3)Δ^ZPhe-Gly-OMe		85%(C)
8 Boc-Aib-N(CH_3)Δ^ZPhe-Gly-OMe	40%(L),90%(C)	

plant growth (Edwards J. V. and Cutler G. G., unpublished results). This approach was the subject of a study done in a wheat coleoptile assay. The wheat coleoptile assay is a primary plant bioassay sensitive to a broad range of biologically active compounds (18). The synthetic tentoxin fragments had activities comparable to other phytotoxic compounds in this assay. These studies showed trends of increased activity as the peptide backbone was modified both structurally and conformationally. For example the order of growth inhibition with wheat coleoptiles was Boc-Leu-Phe-Gly-OMe < Boc-Leu-Δ^ZPhe-Gly-OMe < Boc-Leu-N(CH3)Δ^ZPhe-Gly-OMe. This parallels an increase in backbone rigidity in the tripeptide sequence Leucyl-phenylalanyl-glycine. Interestingly the growth promotion observed from analogs in this assay structurally paralleled analogs found to promote growth in the lettuce seedling assay. The results of a wheat coleoptile study are shown for analogs **1, 3** and **5.** Peptides which were N-ethylated at the two position nitrogen gave significant promotion when compared with the N-methylated sequence (Figure 5).

Promising activites observed against barnyardgrass, morningglory, and mustard seed were found in the herbicidal assays. The highest levels of root growth inhibition were observed in treatments with analogs **1, 2,** and **5** (Figure 5). The same compounds inhibited bolting of mustard seed. It should be noted that these assays (lettuce/cress, wheat coleoptile, and weed) were done in different laboratories under double blind conditions. It is interesting that those analogs which gave promotion in the lettuce and wheat coleoptile assays were the same ones demonstrating promising herbicidal activity in the _in vitro_ weed assays. Compound **5** showed the most herbicidal _promise_ of any compound tested. In the whole plant assays phytotoxic responses observed seemed to be tolerated by the plant. Only in the case of analog **2**

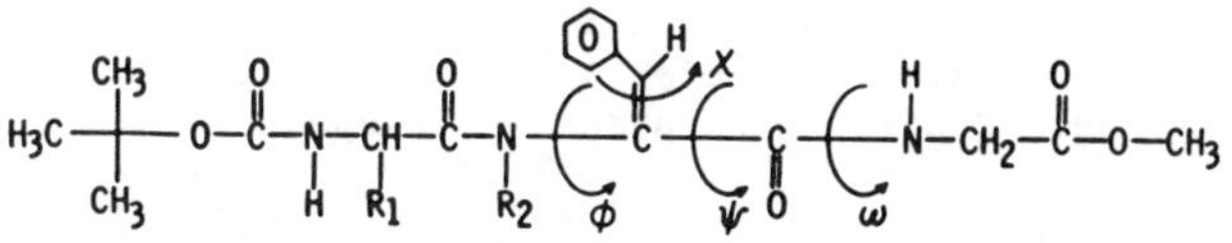

Figure 3. General formula for tripeptides of this study. Arrows with accompanying Greek letters indicate dihedral bond angles.

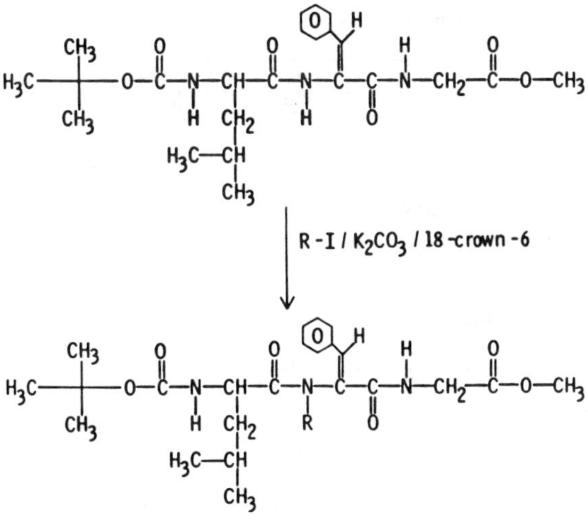

Figure 4. Selective alkylation reaction employed in the preparation of 2-position alkylated tripeptides. R is methyl, ethyl, or propyl.

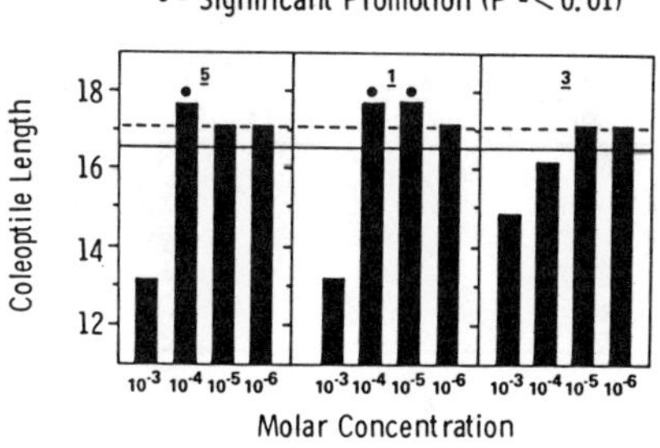

Figure 5. Results of wheat coleoptile assay for three tripeptides (**1**, **3**, and **5**).

have we observed any significant level of phototoxicity (pigweed) in whole plant assays (23) (Edwards and Coffman, unpublished results). These results were observed independent of the present study.

The cyclic peptides tested in this study included tentoxin (Figure 2) and [Pro[1]] tentoxin. [Pro[1]] tentoxin contains a substitution of proline for N-methyl alanine, and is conformationally similar to tentoxin. Previous biochemical studies comparing these analogs have shown both similarities and

Table. II. Results of *in vitro* herbicide assay for seven tripeptide analogs

Compound	Growth (%)* for Barnyard grass. Shoot	Growth (%)* for Barnyard grass. Root	Growth (%)* for mustard seed Total length
1 Boc-Leu-N(Et)Δ^ZPhe-Gly-OMe	79	59	54
2 Boc-D-Leu-N(Et)Δ^ZPhe-Gly-OMe	85	60	110
3 Boc-Leu-N(Me)Δ^ZPhe-Gly-OMe	93	87	98
4 Boc-D-Ala-Δ^ZPhe-Gly-OMe	96	88	86
5 Boc-Val-N(Et)Δ^ZPhe-Gly-OMe	101	10	13
6 Boc-Val-N(Me)Δ^ZPhe-Gly-OMe	83	67	63
7 Boc-Val-N(Pr)Δ^ZPhe-Gly-OMe	107	72	81

*Expressed as shoot ($\pm$0.09%). Abbreviations are explained in Figure 1. Boc denotes *tert*-butyloxycarbonyl.

differences (24). The results of the *in vitro* herbicide assays (Table III) for these analogs demonstrate good chlorosis inducing activity at 100 μM in barnyard grass and morningglory similar to that found in leaf lettuce for both cyclic peptides.

Table. III. Results of *in vitro* herbicide assay for two cyclic peptides (100μM)

Compound	Visual assessment* of Chlorophyll in weeds: Barnyard grass	Pitted moningglory	Lettuce
Tentoxin	XXX	XXX	XXX
[Pro[1]] Tentoxin	XXX	XX	XXX
Control check	X	X	X

XXX = bright yellow, chlorotic.*
XX = dull yellow, spotty dull green.
X = deep green

Conclusions

This study has outlined an approach to exploring the herbicide potential of synthetic intermediates taken from a naturally occurring peptide phytotoxin (tentoxin) while examining the effects of conformationally rigid linear synthetic peptides and the cyclic analogs [Pro^1] tentoxin and tentoxin in selective herbicidal activity. We have examined the comparative responses of various plants and agronomically significant weeds to both linear and cyclic analogs of tentoxin. In this regard it is noteworthy that the linear tripeptide analogs gave rise to an altogether different phytotoxic response than the cyclic analogs. The meristematic root growth inhibition (Table II) observed with linear analogs was not evident with the cyclic analogs, and the chlorosis induction (Table III) observed with tentoxin and [Pro^1] tentoxin was not apparent with the derivatized synthetic fragments of tentoxin.

Previously, reports of di- and tripeptides containing P-terminal 9-aminofluorene-9-ylphosphine oxides have noted herbicidal activity for glycine and threonine, containing adducts (19). A synthetic dipeptide alcohol (Cbz-Prolyl-valinol) which is a derivatized sequence fragment found in the cyclic tetrapeptide HC toxin has been shown to increase corn yields (20). The lack of herbicidal activity in the whole plant herbicide assays in this study and the demonstration of seedling activity with analogs **1**, **2**, and **5** leads one to ask: Can native plant activity of these peptides be induced by altered transport, solubility, or increased resistance to proteolytic enzymes? These areas have been the subject of numerous productive investigations in the field of mammalian neurotransmitter peptides. One possible solution to this question is to examine more than one of these processes via incorporation of amide bond isosteres (21). The use of attached transport agents such as the dipeptide glutamyl-leucine or a β-glucan fragment (giving a glycopeptide) deserve further attention as rational approachs toward herbicide design. Future studies in this area might also benefit from investigating repetitive amino acid and peptide sequences found in plant cell wall proteins such as extensin (22). Finally, possible approaches for the developement of peptide and peptidomimetic herbicides are numerous. It seems likely that investigations into potential applications of peptides to crop plants will receive increased acceptance in the future, as biotechnological approaches to herbicide development increase. As more is learned about the selective phytotoxic properties of naturally occurring peptide phytotoxins and their synthetic analogs, the potential for their application in the rational design of herbicides and plant growth regulators will become apparent.

Literature Cited

1. Alder, E. F., Wright, W. L, and Brown, I. F. In Agricultural Chemicals Of The Future; Hilton, J. L., Ed.; BARC Symposium 8; Rowman & Allanheld. Totowa, 1985 pp 147-155.
2. Ueno, T., Nakashima, T., Hayashi, Y., and Fukami, H. Agric. Biol. Chem. 1975, 39, 1115.
3. Walton, J. D., Earle, E. D., and Gibson, B. W. Biochem. Biophys. Res. Comm., 1982, 107, 185.
4. Ueda, T., Sada, I., Kato. T., and Izumiya, N. Int. J. Peptide Protein Res. 1985, 25, 475

5. Meyer, W. L., Kuyper, L. F., Lewis R. B., Templeton, G. E. and Woodhead, S. H. Biochem. Biophys. Res. Comm. 1974, 56, 234.
6. Hirota, A., Suzuki, A., Suzuki, H. and Tamura, S. Agric. Biol. Chem. 1973, 37, 643.
7. Fulton, K. N. D., Bollenbacher K., and Templeton, G. E., Phytopathol. 1965, 55, 49.
8. Templeton, G. E., Grable, C. I., Fulton, N. D. and Bollenbaher, K. Phytopathol. 1967, 57, 516.
9. Vaughn, K. C. and Duke, S. O. Physiol. Plant. 1984, 60, 257.
10. Steele, J. A., Uchytl, T. F., Durbin, R. D., Bhatnagar, P. and Rich, D. H. Proc. Natl. Acad. Sci. USA. 1967, 73, 2245.
11. Lax, A. R, Vaughn, K. C., Gisson V. A. and Templeton G. E., Photosynthesis Research, 1985, 6, 113.
12. Rich, D. H., and Bhatnagar, P. K. J. J. Am. Chem. Soc., 1978, 100, 2218.
13. Rich, D. H., Jasensky, R. D., and Singh, J., In Neurohypophysical Hormones and Other Biologically Active Peptides; Schlesinger, D. H., Ed.; Dev. Endocrinol. 13; Elsevier North Holland, Inc. 49.
14. Zimmerman, S. S., In The Peptides: Analysis, Synthesis, Biology; Udenfriend, S. and Meienhoffer, J., Eds.; Academic Press: New York 1985; Vol 7, p165.
15. Hruby, V. J. Life Sciences, 1982, 31, 189.
16. Bodansky, M. and Stahl, G. L. Proc. Natl. Acad. Sci. USA, 1974 71, 2791.
17. Curtis, R. W., Plant Physiol., 1976, 57, 365.
18. Cutler, H. G. In Bioregulators: Chemistry and Uses; Ory, R. L. and Rittig, F. R., Ed.; ACS Symposium Series No. 257; American Chemical Society: Washington, D. C. 1984; pp 153-169.
19. Pawel, K., Lejczak, B., Gancarz, R., Jaskulska, E., Mastalerz, P; Wieczorek, J. S., and Zbyryt, I. Pestic. Sci., 1985, 16, 239.
20. Lin, W. and Kauer, J. C. Plant Physiol. 1985, 77, 403.
21. Spatola, A. F., In Chemistry and Biochemistry of Amino Acids, Peptides and Proteins; Weinstein, B., Ed.; Marcel Dekker, New York, 1984, Vol 7, p267.
22. Smith, J. J., Muldoon, E. P. Willard J. J. and Lamport D. T. A. Phytochemistry, 1986, 25, 1021.
23. Genter, W. A. and Danielson, L. L. Weed Science, 1970, 18, 551.
24. Edwards, J. V., Lax, A. R., Lillehoj, E. B. and Boudreaux, G. J.; Int. J. Peptide Protein Res., 1986, 28, 603.
25. Vitoux, B., Aubry, A., Chung, M. T. and Marraud, M. Int. J. Peptide Protein Res. 1986, 27, 617.
26. Chauhan, V. S., Sharma, A. K., Uma, K., Paul, P.K.C. and Balaram, P. Int. J. Peptide Protein Res. 1987, 29, 126.

RECEIVED July 30, 1987

INSECTICIDES

Chapter 15

Synthesis and Insecticidal Activity of Pyrethroids from Substituted Pyrazole Methanol Precursors

Thomas P. Selby

Agricultural Products Department, E. I. du Pont de Nemours & Co., Experimental Station, Building 402, Wilmington, DE 19898

The insecticidal activity and structure-activity relationships of novel pyrethroids prepared by reacting methyl phenyl substituted pyrazole methanols with dichloro chrysanthemic acid chloride are reported. These pyrethroids are active on tobacco budworm, fall armyworm, southern corn rootworm, and aster leafhopper, generally in the concentration range of 1000-250 ppm. Although less active than the pyrethroid standard bifenthrin, the overall structure-activity of these pyrazole pyrethroids with regard to substitution patterns is similar to that previously observed with bifenthrin analogs.

Pyrethroids, due to their high insecticidal activity and low mammalian toxicity (1), have been the subject of much synthetic effort (1-3). Most of the commercially available synthetic pyrethroids are generally related in that they contain the same meta-phenoxybenzyl alcohol, or some close derivative thereof in the molecule, two examples being permethrin and fenvalerate.

More recently, the pyrethroid bifenthrin 1, which was derived from 3-phenyl-2-methylbenzyl alcohol rather than a meta-phenoxybenzyl alcohol was shown to have very high broad spectrum insecticidal activity (4, 5). The methyl group being ortho to the phenyl ring was important for high activity, presumably to keep the two phenyl rings twisted out of plane. Bifenthrin also incorporated a unique trifluoromethyl chloro substituted chrysanthemic acid portion which gave some boost to the overall insecticidal activity over the more traditional dichloro chrysanthemate analog (4).

Reported here is the synthesis and insecticidal activity of some related pyrethroids represented by general formula 2 prepared by condensing methyl phenyl substituted pyrazole methanols with the more readily available dichloro chrysanthemic acid chloride (DV-acid Chloride). All of the pyrethroid samples were also prepared and tested as approximately a 4:3 trans/cis mixture of isomers.

0097-6156/87/0355-0162$06.00/0
© 1987 American Chemical Society

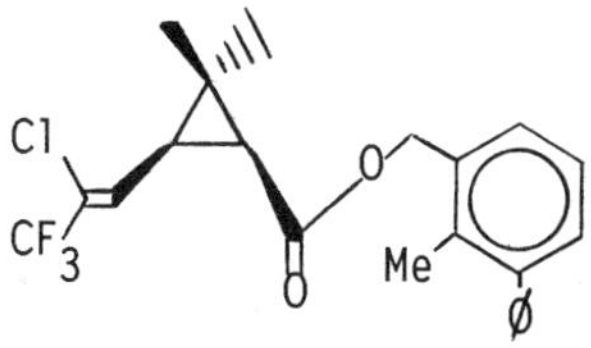

Chemistry

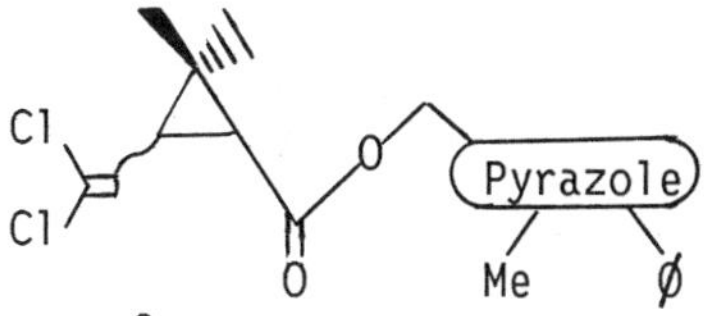

Schemes I-IV illustrate the syntheses of the pyrazole pyrethroids reported here. In scheme-I, condensation of ethyl ethoxymethyleneacetoacetate (3) (6) and ethyl ethoxymethylenetrifluoroacetoacetate (4) (7) with phenylhydrazine in glacial acetic acid initially at room temperature followed by heating at reflux gave the pyrazolecarboxylates 5 (8) and 6 in yields of 43% and 70%, respectively. Reduction with lithium aluminum hydride gave the alcohols 7 and 8 which were then allowed to react with the DV-acid chloride in Et_3N/THF to give the pyrethroid isomer mixtures 9 (9) and 10 (4:3 trans/cis) in 80-85% yield from the carboxylates. Pyrethroid 10 was prepared to determine how the increased lipophilicity over 9 affected insecticidal activity.

In scheme-II, following the procedure of Finar (10) et al., condensation of ethyl 2,4-dioxovalerate (11) with phenylhydrazine was carried out in glacial acetic acid whereby the addition was carried out at ambient temperature followed by heating at reflux. This gave a 55% yield of about a 2:1 mixture of the pyrazolecarboxylates 12 and 13 which were separated by silica gel column chromatography. By the procedure of Tensmeyer (11) et al., condensation of ethyl benzoylpyruvate (14) (12) with methylhydrazine in ethanol initially at ambient temperature followed by heating at reflux gave a 73% yield of a 2:3 mixture of the pyrazole carboxylates 15 and 16 which were also separated by silica gel column chromatography. Reduction of the carboxylates 12, 13, 15 and 16 with lithium aluminum hydride cleanly gave the alcohols which on reaction with the DV-acid chloride gave the pyrethroids isomer mixtures 17, 18, 19, and 20, all in good yield (>80%).

In scheme-III, reaction of 2-methylphenylhydrazine with the bis-dimethylacetal of malonaldehyde in aqueous acidic THF gave 2-methylphenylpyrazole 21 in 70% yield. Formylation at the 4-position of the pyrazole followed by reduction to the alcohol and reaction with DV-acid chloride in Et_3N/THF gave in 70% overall yield from 21 the pyrazole pyrethroid 22 which had an ortho methyl group on the phenyl ring rather than the pyrazole ring. It was felt that the ortho methyl group might still keep the phenyl ring twisted out of plane with the pyrazole ring and thus give rise to an insecticidally active compound.

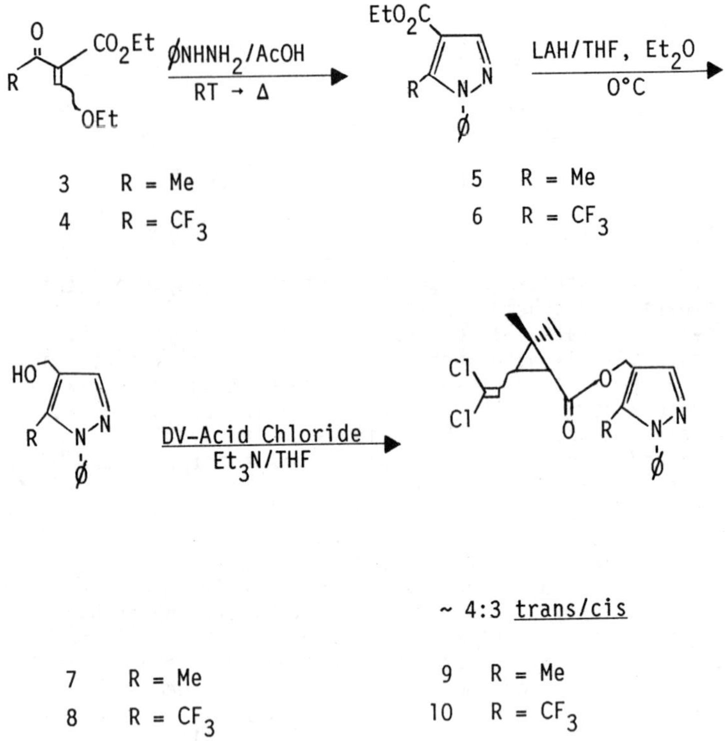

$\phi NHNH_2/AcOH$, RT → Δ

EtO_2C

LAH/THF, Et_2O, 0°C

3 R = Me
4 R = CF_3

5 R = Me
6 R = CF_3

HO

DV-Acid Chloride, Et_3N/THF

Cl Cl

~ 4:3 trans/cis

7 R = Me
8 R = CF_3

9 R = Me
10 R = CF_3

Scheme I. Synthesis of Pyrethroids 9 and 10.

$RCOCH_2COCO_2Et$

$R'NHNH_2$
AcOH or EtOH
RT → Δ

11 R = Me
14 R = Ø

EtO_2C … N–N(R') … R + EtO_2C … R'–N–N … R

	R	R'
12	Me	Ø
15	Ø	Me

	R	R'
13	Me	Ø
16	Ø	Me

1) LAH/THF, ET_2O 0°C
2) DV-Acid Chloride Et_3N/THF

1) LAH/THF, ET_2O 0°C
2) DV-Acid Chloride Et_3N/THF

~ 4:3 <u>trans</u>/<u>cis</u>

	R	R'
17	Me	Ø
19	Ø	Me

~ 4:3 <u>trans</u>/<u>cis</u>

	R	R'
18	Me	Ø
20	Ø	Me

Scheme II. Synthesis of Pyrethroids 17, 18, 19, and 20.

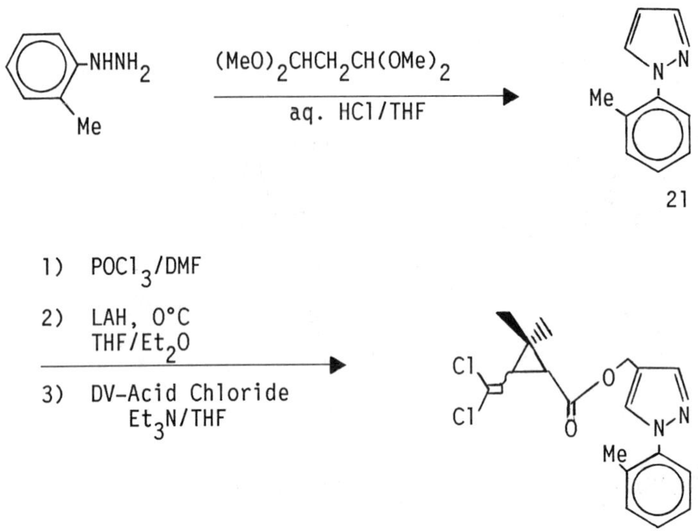

NHNH$_2$ / Me

$(MeO)_2CHCH_2CH(OMe)_2$

aq. HCl/THF

Me, N, N

21

1) $POCl_3$/DMF

2) LAH, 0°C THF/Et_2O

3) DV-Acid Chloride Et_3N/THF

Cl, Cl, O, O, N, N, Me

~ 4:3 trans/cis

22

Scheme III. Synthesis of Pyrethroid 22.

The preparation of various pyrazole-N-methanol containing pyrethroids are shown in scheme-IV. Reaction of 3-phenyl-4-methylpyrazole (23) (13) with aqueous 37% formaldehyde in methanol gave a 83% yield of approximately a 5:1 mixture of the pyrazole-N-methanol isomers 24 and 25. Although not evident by NMR, it was assumed that the minor isomer 25 had the methanol substitution adjacent to the more sterically hindered phenyl group, alkylation thus being favored at the less hindered pyrazole nitrogen. These isomers were not separable either through recrystalization or silica gel chromatography and were reacted together with DV-acid chloride in Et_3N/THF to give the pyrethroid mixtures 26 and 27 which were separated by silica gel column chromatography. Reaction of 3-phenyl-5-methylpyrazole (28) (14) with aqueous 37% formaldehyde gave mainly all 29 contaminated with only a small amount of the isomer 30. Again, it was assumed that alkylation occurred at the less hindered pyrazole nitrogen adjacent to the methyl rather than the ring nitrogen adjacent to the phenyl ring. Recrystalization from acetonitrile gave reasonably pure 29 which on reaction with DV-acid chloride gave the pyrethroid mixture 31. Also, reactions of 3,5-dimethyl-4-phenylpyrazole (32) (15) and 3,5-dimethyl-4- bromopyrazole (33) (16) with aqueous formaldehyde gave the pyrazole-N-methanols 34 and 35 in which isomer formation did not occur since alkylation at either ring nitrogen gave the same product. These alcohols were then converted to the pyrethroid mixtures 36 and 37. Conversion of these pyrazoles to the pyrazole-N-methanols were in the 75-85% yield range and the transformations of these alcohols to pyrethroids were all in the 80-85% range.

	R	R'	R^2
23	H	Me	Ø
28	Me	H	Ø
32	Me	Ø	Me
33	Me	Br	Me

	R	R'	R^2
24	H	Me	Ø
25	Ø	Me	H
29	Me	H	Ø
30	Ø	H	Me
34	Me	Ø	Me
35	Me	Br	Me

~ 4:3 trans/cis

	R	R'	R^2
26	H	Me	Ø
27	Ø	Me	H
31	Me	H	Ø
36	Me	Ø	Me
37	Me	Br	Me

Scheme IV. Synthesis of Pyrazole-N-Methanol Pyrethroids.

Biological Test Results

The insecticidal data, recorded as percent mortality, for these pyrethroids on the third-instar larvae of fall armyworm (*Spodoptera frugiperda*), tobacco budworm (*Heliothis virescens*), corn rootworm (*Diabrotica umdecimpunctata howardi*) and adult leafhopper (*Mascrosteles fascifrons*) are shown in Table-I. The concentration at which they were tested ranged from the initial spray concentration of 1000 ppm to in some cases 50 ppm.

The pyrethroids 9, 17, 19, 26, and 36 which all had the phenyl ring *meta* to the methanol bridge and a methyl group *ortho* to the phenyl generally demonstrated the highest level of insecticidal activity for these compound types. They all demonstrated comparable activity generally in the 1000-250 ppm range.

In the case of pyrethroids 18 and 27 in which the phenyl was adjacent to the alcohol moiety and pyrethroid 20 in which the phenyl was *meta* to the alcohol moiety but no methyl group *ortho* to the phenyl, significant activity was not observed at 1000 ppm. The pyrazole-N-methanol pyrethroid 31, which showed some activity at 1000-250 ppm without a methyl group being *ortho* to the *meta* phenyl, was still less active overall than the pyrazole-N-methanol pyrethroid 36, in which there was a methyl group (actually two methyl groups) *ortho* to the phenyl. Interesting, the 4-bromo-3,5-dimethylpyrazole-N-methanol pyrethroid 37 also demonstrated some insecticidal activity without a phenyl group being on the pyrazole ring. Pyrethroid 22, in which the methyl was substituted at the *ortho* position of the phenyl substituent, was not active at 1000 ppm. The more lipophilic trifluoromethyl substituted pyrazole pyrethroid 10 did have insecticidal activity but was not more active than the other derivatives. Increasing the lipophilicity of the molecule in this case did not improve on the activity although introduction of the trifluoromethyl group would have also resulted in some steric changes as well.

Table I. Insecticidal Data (% Mortality)

Compound	Conc PPM	TBW	FAW	SCRW	ALH
9	1000	100	100	93	98
	250	17	100	26	86
	100	-	23	13	53
10	1000	60	90	100	100
	250	20	40	100	49
	100	40	17	47	-
17	1000	87	100	100	100
	250	0	77	100	39
	100	-	53	80	-
19	1000	43	100	100	100
	250	17	50	26	100
	100	-	-	-	95
26	1000	60	73	100	100
	250	-	0	87	84
	100	-	-	40	68
31	1000	40	60	100	100
	250	-	-	100	64
	100	-	-	27	-
36	1000	100	100	100	100
	250	70	87	100	52
	100	-	0	67	-
37	1000	7	100	100	100
	250	-	17	93	90
	100	-	-	80	71

TBW = Tobacco Budworm
FAW = Fall Armyworm
SCRW = Southern Corn Rootworm
ALH = Aster Leafhopper

Conclusion

In summary, a number of novel pyrethroids as well as alcohol intermediates were prepared. In most cases, the pyrethroids which demonstrated insecticidal activity generally in the concentration range of 1000-250 ppm required the phenyl group meta to the alcohol bridge and preferably a methyl group ortho to it, possibly to keep the phenyl ring twisted out of plane with the pyrazole ring. This was in agreement with the structure-activity previously observed with bifenthrin analogs (4, 5). The lower activity of these analogs relative to pyrethroid standards such as bifenthrin may be the result of not only steric changes, but also the result of lower lipophilicities due to the pyrazole ring. At the time this work was being carried out, Plummer (5, 17) et al. reported that in other heterocyclic analogs of bifenthrin that changes in lipophilicities could have a marked influence on the insecticidal activity. Those results are in agreement with our work which also demonstrated that heterocyclic modifications to the alcohol portion of the bifenthrin molecule could have a significant impact on the level of insecticidal activity.

Acknowledgments

The author wishes to thank Diane Stanley and Michael Primiani who carried out the biological testing and Marilisa Wirt and James Beck for technical assistance with the chemistry.

Literature Cited

1. Elliot, M. "Synthetic Pyrethroids" ACS Symp. Ser. Series No. 42, American Chemical Society, Washington, D.C., 1977, p. 1 and references cited therein.
2. Arlt, D; Jautelat, M.; Lantzsch, R. Angew. Chem., Int. Ed. Engl. 1981, 20, 703 and references therein.
3. Janes, N. F. "Recent Advances in the Chemistry of Insect Control," Proc. Roy. Soc. No. 53, The Royal Society of Chemistry, Burlington House, London, 1984, p. 133-192.
4. Engel, J. F.; Plummer, E. L.; Stewart, R. R.; VanSaun, W. A.; Montgomery, R. E.; Cruickshank, P. A.; Harnish, W. N.; Nethery, A. A.; Crosby, G. A. "Pesticide Chemistry: Human Welfare and the Environment" Proceedings of the 5th International IUPAC Congress of Pesticide Chemistry, Miyamoto, J; Kearney, P. C., Eds., International Union of Pure and Applied Chemistry, Pergamon Press, 1982, p. 101.
5. Plummer, E. L. and Stewart, R. R. J. Agric. Chem. 1984, 32, 1116.
6. Claisen, L. Justus Liebigs Ann. Chem. 1897, 297, 1.
7. Jones, R. G. J. Am. Chem. Soc. 1951, 73, 3684.
8. Claisen, L. Justus Liebigs Ann. Chem. 1896, 295, 301.
9. Stein, R. G. U.S. Patent 4,151,293 (1979), Chem. Abstr. 91: 56999d. Although this patent generically covered pyrethroid 9, the compound was not actually prepared.
10. Finar, I. L.; Hurlock, R. J. J. Chem. Soc. 1958, 3259.
11. Tensmeyer, L. G.; Ainsworth, C. J. Org. Chem. 1966, 31, 1878.

12. Libermann, D.; Rist. N.; Grumbach, F.; Cals, S.; Moyeux, M. and Rouaix, A. Bull. Soc. Chim. Fr. 1958, 687.
13. Büchi, J.; Meyer, H. R.; Hirt, R.; Hunziker, F.; Eichenberger, E., and Lieberherr, R. Helv. Chim. Acta 1955, 38, 670.
14. Sjollema, B. Justus Liebigs Ann. Chem. 1894, 279, 248.
15. Alberti, C. Gazz. Chim. Ital. 1957, 87, 729.
16. Elguero, J.; Jacquier, R. Bull. Soc. Chim. Fr. 1966, 2832.
17. Plummer, E. L. J. Agric. Food Chem. 1983, 31, 718.

RECEIVED May 15, 1987

Chapter 16

Insecticidal Substituted Biphenylmethyl Oxime Ethers

Thomas G. Cullen, Charles J. Manly, Philip A. Cruickshank, and Sandra M. Kellar

Agricultural Chemical Group, FMC Corporation, P.O. Box 8, Princeton, NJ 08543

Replacement of the normal pyrethroid ester by alternative linkages usually leads to diminution of biological activity. One important exception to this general phenomena is several oxime ether derivatives, in particular, 3-phenoxybenzyl derivatives of various alkyl aryl ketones. Pyrethroid esters derived from certain 2-substituted-[1,1'-biphenyl]-3-methanols have been shown to possess initial and residual activity surpassing that of esters derived from 3-phenoxybenzyl alcohol. Now it has been demonstrated that the same enhancement of activity was observed for alkyl aryl oxime ethers of certain [1,1'-biphenyl]-3-methanols compared to the corresponding 3-phenoxybenzyl alcohol derived oximes. The synthesis, biological activity, including soil activity, structure-activity relationships and toxicity of several of these biphenylmethyl oxime ethers are described.

Many synthetic pyrethroids with excellent insecticidal activity have been discovered through modification of the acid and alcohol moieties of the natural pyrethrins. However, replacement of the pyrethroid ester linkage with an alternative linkage usually leads to compounds of diminished biological activity(1). One exception to this trend of lower activity is the class of compounds wherein the oxime linkage is introduced in place of the ester linkage in the fenvalerate series. Additionally, only the E-isomer of the alkyl aryl oxime ethers is reported to be insecticidal(2-4).

Pyrethroid esters derived from [1,1'-biphenyl]-3-methanol have been of interest at FMC(5-7). It has been reported that [1,1'-biphenyl]-3-methanol esterified with both cis-3-(2-chloro-3,3,3-trifluoro-1-propenyl)-2,2-dimethylcyclopropanecarboxylic acid and cis-3-(2,2-dichloroethenyl)-2,2-dimethylcyclopropanecarboxylic acid produced esters which have initial and residual activity surpassing that of permethrin against a number of insects. It occurred to us that this same enhancement of activity might be observed with alkyl

0097-6156/87/0355-0173$06.00/0
© 1987 American Chemical Society

aryl methanone oxime ethers of 2-substituted-[1,1-biphenyl]-3-methanols compared to those alkyl aryl methanone oxime ethers derived from 3-phenoxybenzyl alcohol. We wish to report on the synthesis, biological activity, mammalian toxicology, and structure-activity relationships of alkyl aryl methanone oxime ethers derived from 2-methyl[1,1'-biphenyl]-3-methanol.

MATERIALS AND METHODS

Nuclear magnetic resonance (^1H NMR) spectra were recorded on either a Varian T-60 or a Varian FT-80A with Me_4Si as an internal standard. Infrared spectra were obtained on a Perkin-Elmer 735B infrared spectrophotometer. All boiling points and melting points are uncorrected. Thin layer chromatography (TLC) utilized silica gel 60 F-254 chromatoplates (0.2-5 mm thickness).

Chemicals

(4-Chlorophenyl)cyclopropyl Ketone. Under a dry nitrogen atmosphere, a mixture of 1.6 g (0.066 mole) of magnesium, 7.9 g (0.066 mole) of cyclopropyl bromide, 20 mL of anhydrous diethyl ether and 60 mL of anhydrous tetrahydrofuran was heated at reflux for 2.5 hours. The stirred mixture was cooled to room temperature and a solution of 9.04 g (0.066 mole) of 4-chlorobenzonitrile in 40 mL of anhydrous tetrahydrofuran was added over one hour. After complete addition, the mixture was heated at reflux for two hours, then cooled to room temperature. A 100 mL portion of 2N hydrochloric acid was added slowly to the mixture and stirred for one hour. The mixture was extracted with three 100 mL portions of diethyl ether. The combined extracts were washed with one 25 mL portion of water, dried over anhydrous magnesium sulfate and filtered. The filtrate was concentrated under reduced pressure to give an oil which was distilled to give 3.9 g of product. The ^1H NMR was consistent with the proposed structure.

(E,Z)-(4-Chlorophenyl)cyclopropyl Methanone Oxime. A mixture of 25.0 g (0.138 mole) of (4-chlorophenyl)(cyclopropyl)ketone, 15.0 g (0.216 mole) of hydroxylamine hydrochloride, 27.6 g (0.69 mole) of sodium hydroxide, 50 mL of 95% ethanol and 7 mL of water was refluxed for ten minutes. After cooling, the contents were poured into a solution of 500 mL of 1.6 N hydrochloric acid. The resulting oil was extracted with three 100 mL portions of diethyl ether. The combined extracts were washed with one 50 mL portion of water, dried over anhydrous magnesium sulfate and filtered. The filtrate was concentrated under reduced pressure to give 11.7 g of E,Z-oxime. The ^1H nmr was consistent with the proposed structure.

(E)-(4-Chlorophenyl)(cyclopropyl) Methanone Oxime. A solution of 25.42 g (0.13 mole) of (E,Z)-(4-chlorophenyl)(cyclopropyl)-methanone oxime in 100 mL of anhydrous diethyl ether was treated with anhydrous hydrogen chloride. The resultant precipitate was filtered and washed with three 50 mL portions of anhydrous diethyl ether. The precipitate was collected and added to 500 mL of an aqueous 10% sodium carbonate solution to yield 23.5 g of E-oxime. The ^1H NMR was consistent with the proposed structure.

(E)-(4-Chlorophenyl)(cyclopropyl)methanone O-[2-Methyl[1,1'-biphenyl]-3-yl)methyl]oxime. To a solution of 0.23 g (0.01 mole) of sodium ethoxide in 10 mL of ethanol was added 1.96 (0.01 mole) of (E)-(4-chlorophenyl)(cyclopropyl)methanone oxime. After stirring at room temperature for one hour, the mixture was evaporated to dryness. The residue was dissolved in a minimum amount of solvent consisting of N,N-dimethylformamide and t-butanol (9:1 ratio) and treated with 2.16 g (0.01 mole) of 3-chloromethyl-2-methyl[1,1'-biphenyl]. The mixture was stirred overnight at room temperature and then poured into 50 mL of water. The resulting oil was extracted with three 50 mL portions of toluene. The combined organic layers were washed with one 10 mL portion of aqueous 10% sodium hydroxide, one 10 mL portion of water and dried over anhydrous magnesium sulfate. The filtrate was concentrated under reduced pressure and the residue was purified by column chromatography on silica gel, eluting with toluene to give 0.83 g of E-oxime ether as an oil; ^{1}H NMR ($CDCl_3$) δ 0.5-0.95 (m,5H), 2.10 (s,3H); 5.25 (s,2H); 7.08-7.42 (m,12H).

Biological Methods

The compounds were evaluated for insecticidal and acaricidal activity against the following species: cabbage looper (*Trichoplusia ni* [Hubner]), Mexican bean beetle (*Epilachna varivestis* Muls), southern armyworm (*Spodoptera eridania* [Cram]), pea aphid (*Acyrthosiphon pisum* [Harris]), twospotted spider mite (*Tetranychus urticae* [Koch]) and southern corn rootworm (*Diabrotica undecimpunctata* Howardi).

The activity against Mexican bean beetle (MBB), southern armyworm (SAW) and cabbage looper (CL) was determined by spraying the upper and lower surfaces of the leaves of pinto bean plants with test solution until run-off and infesting with third instar larvae (ten larvae for each of two replicates for each compound) after the foliage had dried.

The activity against pea aphid (PA) was determined in similar fashion, except that broad bean plants were used and the leaves were infested with adult aphids.

The activity against mites (TSM) was determined on pinto bean plants. The bean leaves were infested with adult mites (about 75 mites for each of two replicates for each compound), then sprayed until the run-off with test solution. The pinto bean plants were infested by placing sections of plants from earlier infested plants onto the leaves of the test plants.

To prevent escape of the insects from the test site, the test plant or the incised leaves were placed in capped paper cups or other appropriate containers. The tests were transferred to a holding room at 25°C and 50% relative humidity for an exposure period of 48 hours. At the end of this time the dead and living insects/mites were counted and the percent mortality was calculated.

The relative potency of each compound was calculated as the ratio of the LD_{50} of cypermethrin (included in all tests as the standard) to that of the experimental compound.

The activity against the southern corn rootworm (SCR) was determined in a soil environment at testing rates of 10, 4, 2 and 0.5 ppm in soil and for residual periods of 7, 14 and 28 days.

For a testing rate of 10 ppm, 15 mg of test compound was dissolved in 100 ml of an acetone-water-surfactant stock solution (1:9 acetone-water, one drop of octylphenoxypolyethoxyethanol surfactant for each 100 ml of acetone-water) to give a stock solution containing 150 ppm of test compound, and 2 ml of the 150 ppm stock solution was thoroughly mixed with 30 ml of air-dried topsoil in a 120 mL plastic cup to give a concentration of test compound in the soil of 10 ppm. For a testing rate of 4 ppm, 2 mL of a 60 ppm stock solution of test compound in acetone-water-surfactant was admixed with 30 mL of air-dried topsoil in a plastic cup. Similarly, 2 mL of a 30 ppm test compound stock solution mixed with 30 mL of air-dried soil gave a testing rate of 2 ppm, and 2 mL of a 7.5 ppm test compound stock solution mixed with 30 mL of dry topsoil gave a testing rate of 0.5 ppm.

Each cup of treated topsoil was capped with a plastic lid and stored for 7, 14, and 28 days. On the terminal day of the storage period, the cups were infested with southern corn rootworm larvae (10 specimens for each of the two replicates for each compound), and a kernel of germinating corn was added to each cup as a food supply. The cups were recapped and returned to storage for three days. At the end of this time the dead and living rootworms were counted and the percent mortality was calculated.

RESULTS AND DISCUSSION

Chemistry. The majority of the alkyl aryl methanone oxime ethers were synthesized as shown in Figure 1. The alkyl aryl methanones were prepared by either of two methods. In the first method, the appropriately-substituted benzonitrile was treated with the desired alkylmagnesium halide to give the desired ketone(8). The second approach involved the appropriately substituted benzoic acid and conversion to the acid chloride. Subsequently, the acid chloride is treated with O,N-dimethylhydroxylamine hydrochloride(9). This methoxymethylbenzamide is treated with an alkylmagnesium halide to give the alkyl aryl methanone. These ketones were purified by distillation.

The ketones were converted to the E,Z-alkyl aryl methanone oximes by a variety of methods. Most commonly, the ketone and hydroxylamine hydrochloride were suspended in ethanol and two equivalents of pyridine added. After isolation, the oximes were treated with anhydrous hydrogen chloride gas to give the hydrogen chloride salt of the E-alkyl aryl methanone oxime(10). The resulting salt was treated with dilute sodium bicarbonate to yield the desired E-alkyl aryl methanone oxime. Earlier literature reports indicated that E-aldoxime was converted to the Z-aldoxime under similar conditions(11).

The alkyl aryl methanone oximes can be converted to oxime ethers by several methods. The usual alkylation procedure utilized was a phase transfer catalyzed alkylation wherein the E-alkyl aryl

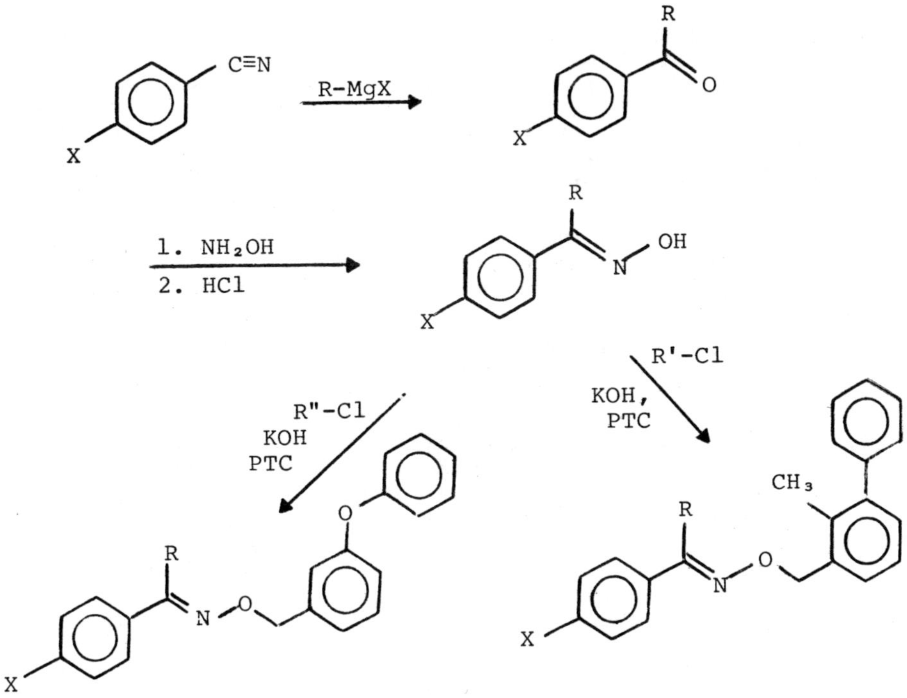

R-MgX

1. NH_2OH
2. HCl

R'-Cl
KOH,
PTC

R"-Cl
KOH
PTC

R = alkyl, cycloalkyl
R' = [1,1'-biphenyl]-2-methyl-3-yl
R" = 3-phenoxybenzyl

Figure 1. Synthesis of Alkyl Aryl Methanone Oxime Ethers.

oxime, 3-chloromethyl-2-methyl-[1,1'-biphenyl], powdered potassium hydroxide and tetrabutylammonium bromide were refluxed in tetrahydrofuran. After work-up, the E-alkyl aryl methanone oxime ether was purified by column chromatography(12). Table I lists the alkyl aryl methanone oxime ethers prepared in this study.

Biology. The alcohol portion of most pyrethroids contains two centers of unsaturation separated by a bridging atom. In allethrin and resmethrin this structural feature is represented by the carbon atom of the methylene groups, while in permethrin, the bridging group is oxygen. Qualitative discussions of structure-activity relationships of pyrethroids have generally pointed to this feature as a requirement for insecticidal activity. More recently it had been suggested that the lack of coplanarity between the centers of unsaturation, that results from the presence of the bridging group, provides optimum fit at the active site. A series of monosubstituted benzyl alcohols prepared at FMC revealed that insecticidal activity can be obtained when the substituent has two centers of unsaturation even if it lacks an atom bridging those centers(5). In this work it was reported that the biological activity and residual properties of biphenyl-3-ylmethyl (1R,S)-cis-3-(2,2-dichlorovinyl)-2,2-dimethylcyclopropanecarboxylate were about one-half that of the corresponding 3-phenoxybenzyl ester. The preparation of a series of substituted derivatives of biphenyl-3-ylmethyl (1R,S)-cis-3-(2,2-dichlorovinyl)-2,2-dimethylcyclopropanecarboxylates resulted in esters with significantly greater insecticidal activity and broader spectrum of biological activity than the conventional pyrethroid insecticides(7). The 2-monosubstituted derivatives were found to be the most active compounds in this series with the 2-methyl compound being the most active. This result encouraged us to combine these biphenyl-3-ylmethyl compounds with alkyl aryl methanone oximes.

The replacement of the ester linkage of pyrethroids by alternatives was known to lead to compounds of diminished biological activity. Thiol esters and amides are two such isosteric replacements that lead to a loss in biological activity(13,14). The exception to this trend was the replacement by the oxime functionality(2,3). The alkyl aryl oxime ethers are not susceptible to alkaline hydrolysis and esteric attack as are the pyrethroid esters(15). The present study details our investigation of the biological activity of [1,1'-biphenyl]-3-methanols when combined with alkyl aryl methanone oximes.

The objectives of this study were to determine the effect on the biological activity by varying the alkyl portion of the oxime, changing the para-substituent of the aryl group and varying the E,Z ratio. The foliar activity of these compounds is reported in Table II. Table III reports the soil insecticidal activity of the compounds of interest.

The first question of interest was to compare 2-methyl[1,1'-biphenyl]-3-methanol with 3-phenoxybenzyl alcohol when combined with the oximes of certain alkyl aryl ketones. The enhancement in

Table I. Alkyl Aryl Oxime Ethers

Cmpd No.	Isomer	X	R	R^1
1	E	4-Cl	isopropyl	PB
2	E	4-Cl	isopropyl	BPM
3	E	4-Cl	cyclopropyl	PB
4	E	4-Cl	cyclopropyl	BPM
5	E	4-F	cyclopropyl	BPM
6	E	4-F	cyclopropyl	PB
7	E,Z	4-Br	isopropyl	BPM
8	E	4-Br	isopropyl	BPM
9	E,Z	4-Br	cyclopropyl	BPM
10	E	4-Br	cyclopropyl	BPM
11	E	4-CF_3	cyclopropyl	BPM
12	E,Z	4-CF_3	isopropyl	BPM
13	E	4-CF_3	isopropyl	BPM
14	E,Z	4-OCF_3	cyclopropyl	BPM
15	E	4-OCF_3	cyclopropyl	BPM
16	E,Z	4-OCF_3	isopropyl	BPM
17	E,Z	4-OCF_3	ethyl	BPM
18	E	4-OCF_3	ethyl	BPM
19	E,Z	4-OCF_3	methyl	BPM
20	E	4-SCF_3	cyclopropyl	BPM
21	E,Z	4-SCF_3	cyclopropyl	BPM
22	E	4-SC_2H_5	cyclopropyl	BPM
23	E,Z	4-SC_2H_5	cyclopropyl	BPM
24	E	4-OC_2F_4H	cyclopropyl	BPM
25	E,Z	4-OC_2F_4H	cyclopropyl	BPM
26	E	4-$CH(CH_3)_2$	cyclopropyl	BPM
27	E	4-C_2H_5	cyclopropyl	BPM
28	E	4-$C(CH_3)_3$	cyclopropyl	BPM
29	E	4-OCF_2H	cyclopropyl	BPM
30	E	4-I	cyclopropyl	BPM

PB = 3-Phenoxybenzyl
BPM = [1,1'-Biphenyl]-2-methyl-3-yl

Table II. Foliar Activity of Alkyl Aryl Oxime Ethers

Cmpd No.	MBB		SAW		TSM	
	LC_{50}[a]	RP[b]	LC_{50}	RP	LC_{50}	RP
1	35.0	0.1	19.0	0.1	I[c]	-
2	13.9	0.1	14.0	0.1	I	-
3	100.0	0.1	11.2	0.3	I	-
4	2.4	0.6	1.3	0.9	10.3	0.6
5	10.1	0.2	84.0	0.3	I	-
6	I	-	I	-	I	-
7	55.0	0.1	ND[d]	ND	I	-
8	14.0	0.1	42.0	0.1	I	-
9	6.0	0.2	6.0	0.2	I	-
10	5.3	0.2	5.7	0.2	ND	ND
11	15.4	0.1	28.7	1.2	5.3	1.1
12	40.0	0.1	10.0	0.2	50.0	0.1
13	15.0	0.1	16.8	0.1	ND	ND
14	22.9	0.1	4.9	0.3	1.3	4.4
15	5.3	0.2	2.2	0.4	1.2	4.4
16	45.0	0.1	50.0	0.1	45.0	0.1
17	7.3	0.1	3.4	0.5	ND	ND
18	6.0	0.8	6.0	0.3	4.0	1.1
19	I	-	55.0	0.1	I	-
20	4.5	0.2	4.6	0.3	2.7	1.5
21	17.5	0.1	5.7	0.2	3.7	0.4
22	6.0	0.2	24.0	0.1	48.0	0.1
23	3.0	0.4	32.0	0.1	ND	ND
24	3.2	0.2	0.1	4.5	0.3	3.4
25	11.4	0.1	4.5	0.3	3.4	0.4
26	3.5	0.2	I	-	ND	ND
27	2.4	0.3	71.5	0.3	I	-
28	4.1	0.2	ND	ND	6.5	1.0
29	0.9	0.8	1.2	0.9	5.8	1.0
30	38.1	0.1	4.8	0.3	38.2	0.1

a LC_{50} (ppm)
b RP = vs cypermethrin
c I = Inactive
d ND = No data

Table III. Soil Activity of Alkyl Aryl Oxime Ethers

	SCR		Residual Activity (% control)		
Cmpd No.	LC_{50}	RP	7 day	14 day	28 day
1	I[a]	-	-	-	-
2	I	-	-	-	-
3	I	-	-	-	-
4	0.6	0.5	80	50	30
5	I	-	-	-	-
6	I	-	-	-	-
7	I	-	-	-	-
8	I	-	-	-	-
9	I	-	-	-	-
10	I	-	-	-	-
11	0.5	0.6	100	10	10
12	I	-	-	-	-
13	I	-	-	-	-
14	0.4	0.7	100	70	90
15	0.5	0.6	100	40	40
16	I	-	-	-	-
17	I	-	-	-	-
18	2.1	0.2	30	-	-
19	I	-	-	-	-
20	3.7	0.2	40	25	-
21	4.1	0.1	25	-	-
22	2.1	0.3	64	40	-
23	3.5	0.2	75	15	-
24	1.3	0.3	100	15	-
25	2.5	0.1	50	5	-
26	2.5	0.2	65	35	5
27	2.4	0.2	75	85	65
28	I	-	-	-	-
29	0.8	0.4	90	40	0
30	1.6	0.3	35	25	-

[a]I = Inactive at 4 ppm - No further testing

activity with the biphenyl alcohol can be seen in Table IV. In both cases, the aryl alkyl oxime ethers derived from 2-methyl[1,1'-biphenyl]-3-methanol were consistently more active than those derived from 3-phenoxybenzyl alcohol.

Next, the effect on activity with respect to the size of the alkyl group in our series compared to that disclosed in the literature (2,4) was of interest. The effectiveness of alkyl groups is reported to be cyclopropyl > isopropyl > ethyl > methyl. In fact, this trend was followed in the [1,1'-biphenyl]-2-methyl-3-methanol derived alkyl aryl oxime ethers. This is illustrated with the (E,Z)-4-trifluoromethoxyphenyl(alkyl)methanone oxime ethers, Compounds 14, 16, 19 (Table V). The activity of this series increases with increasing size of the alkyl group. However, when cyclobutyl was incorporated, activity was lost. The cyclopropyl was the most effective while the isopropyl group was somewhat less effective. Other alkyl changes resulted in a rapid loss of activity.

The activity of the 3-phenoxybenzyl alkyl aryl oxime ethers is reported to reside in the E-isomer. The activity of the E-isomer was compared with the activity of the E,Z alkyl aryl oxime ethers for this new series. This trend also occurs in the biphenylmethylmethyl alkyl aryl oxime ethers (Table VI).

The discovery of biological activity against the southern corn rootworm (*Diabrotica undecipunctata* Howardii) was an unanticipated result from this research program. The trends in biological activity of the alkyl aryl methanone oxime ethers derived from 3-chloromethyl-2-methyl[1,1'-biphenyl] closely paralleled the oxime ethers derived from 3-phenoxybenzyl chloride. The major difference was the enhanced biological activity against a wider variety of insects by the biphenylmethyl derivatives. When these compounds were tested in a soil environment against the southern corn rootworm, the methylbiphenylmethyl oxime ethers were active. None of the 3-phenoxybenzyl oxime ethers were active at the rates tested against this soil-borne insect (Table III).

QSAR. An analysis of the activity of oxime ethers was undertaken to further our understanding of the SAR in this system. All analyses were performed utilizing a FMC proprietary Quantitative Structure Activity Relationships (QSAR) software system. Parameters for structure-activity studies were obtained as previously

Table IV. Comparison of BPM vs PB Alkyl Aryl Oxime Ethers

			LC_{50} (ppm)		
Cmpd No.	R	Ar	MBB	SAW	TSM
1	isopropyl	PB	35.0	19.0	I
2	isopropyl	BPM	13.9	14.0	I
3	cyclopropyl	PB	100	11.2	I
4	cyclopropyl	BPM	2.3	1.3	10.3

described (5). A description of the techniques used in the structure-activity studies has been described (8). Biological activity used for QSAR analysis was foliar activity against southern corn rootworm expressed as LC_{50} in units of ppm. The set of compounds studied represents substitution in the aromatic ring for the cyclopropyl compounds shown in Table VII.

Interestingly, only the *para* monosubstituted compounds displayed activity, suggesting some strict activity requirements, perhaps steric in nature, at the *ortho* and *meta* positions.

Discriminant analysis was performed on all 22 compounds. Compounds were assigned to the "active" set if the activity was LC_{50} = 5 ppm or lower. All others were designated "inactive". Stepwise discriminant analysis BMDP-7M (16) was performed using the following physicochemical descriptors as variables: pi, (17) Hammett σ, F, R, (18) and molar refractivity. The sum over substituted positions for each of these parameters was used for multiply-substituted compounds. A set of linear classification functions in the summation of R was found to be statistically significant at the 5% level, but the classification of these 22 compounds was only 73 percent correct, missing 3 of the active set.

$$\text{active} \quad f(\Sigma R) = -2.53\ \Sigma R - 0.76$$
$$\text{inactive} \quad f(\Sigma R) = -10.4\ \Sigma R - 1.93$$
$$F_{1,20}(\text{approx.}) = 7.75\ (<0.05)$$

Two-dimensional plots of the 22 compounds were made for these physicochemical parameters *vs*. each other using the above set

Table V. Foliar Activity of (E,Z)-4-Trifluoromethoxyphenyl-(alkyl)methanone Oxime Ethers

Cmpd No.	R	LC_{50} (ppm) MBB	SAW	TSM
14	cyclopropyl	22.9	1.5	1.3
16	isopropyl	45.0	50.0	45.0
19	methyl	I	55.0	I

Table VI. Comparison of E vs E,Z Isomers

Cmpd No.	Isomer	LC_{50} (ppm; Foliar) MBB	SAW
7	E,Z	55.0	I
8	E	14.0	42.0
11	E,Z	40.0	10.0
13	E	15.0	16.8

definitions of active/inactive, and inspection of these plots suggested that the "active" region of parameter space could be defined by approximately the following ranges: $0.6 > \Sigma\sigma > -0.2$ and $\Sigma\pi > 0.3$. Further, the five most active compounds fell in the range $0.5 > \Sigma F > 0.3$, and all of the active compounds were in the range defined by $\Sigma F < 0.5$ and $\Sigma R > -0.3$. Electronic character appeared to be one of the important factors relating to biological activity.

Using discriminant analysis, the following non-linear classification functions were generated in $\Sigma\sigma$ space also allowing discrimination between active and inactive sets. However, the parabolic functions in $\Sigma\sigma$ were no more statistically significant than the functions in ΣR and classification was still only 73 percent correct, missing two of the active set. (19)

$$\text{active} \quad f(\Sigma\sigma) = 2.51\ \Sigma\sigma - 2.09\ \Sigma\sigma^2$$
$$\text{inactive} \quad f(\Sigma\sigma) = -4.98\ \Sigma\sigma + 10.81\ \Sigma\sigma^2$$
$$F_{2,19}(\text{approx.}) = 5.40\ (<0.05)$$

It should be noted that while a range of σ may be important, mono, para-subsitution would also appear to be an important determinant of biological activity, and it is difficult to assess the relative importance of these two factors for this set of compounds.

Table VII. Chemical Structure, Biological Activity and Physicochemical Properties

COMPOUND	$\Sigma\pi$	$\Sigma\sigma$	ΣF	ΣR	ΣMR	L-para	B1-para	B4-para	LC_{50}
4 t-butyl	1.98	-0.20	-0.07	-0.13	23.74	4.11	2.59	2.97	
2,4 dimethyl	1.12	-0.30	-0.09	-0.24	14.39	3.00	1.52	2.04	
2,5 dimethyl	1.12	-0.20	-0.09	-0.16	14.39	2.06	1.00	1.00	
4 F	0.14	0.06	0.43	-0.34	5.04	2.65	1.35	1.35	
H (unsubstituted)	0.00	0.00	0.00	0.00	5.15	2.06	1.00	1.00	
3,4 dimethyl	1.12	-0.24	-0.08	-0.18	14.39	3.00	1.52	2.04	
2,4 dichloro	1.42	0.90	0.92	-0.28	15.15	3.52	1.80	1.80	
3,5 dichloro	1.42	0.74	0.80	-0.10	15.15	2.06	1.00	1.00	
4 Br	0.86	0.23	0.44	-0.17	13.00	3.83	1.95	1.95	
3,4 dichloro	1.42	0.60	0.81	-0.20	15.15	3.52	1.80	1.80	
4 $OCH_2CH_2CH_3$	1.05	-0.25	0.22	-0.45	21.18	6.05	1.35	4.30	
2,6 difluoro	0.28	0.94	1.08	-0.58	4.93	2.06	1.00	1.00	
4 CF_3	0.88	0.54	0.38	0.19	9.14	3.30	1.98	2.61	0.50
4 OCF_3	1.04	0.35	0.38	0.00	11.98	4.57	1.35	3.33	0.52
4 Cl	0.71	0.23	0.41	-0.15	10.15	3.52	1.80	1.80	0.61
4 OCF_2H	0.58	0.18	0.35	-0.14	11.98	4.99	1.35	4.15	0.75
4 OCF_2CF_2H	1.78	0.25	0.36	-0.08	14.96	5.23	1.35	3.94	1.32
4 I	1.12	0.18	0.40	-0.19	18.06	4.23	2.15	2.15	1.57
4 SCH_2CH_3	1.07	0.03	0.23	-0.18	22.54	5.24	1.70	3.97	2.05
4 ethyl	1.02	-0.15	-0.05	-0.10	14.42	4.11	1.52	2.97	2.37
4 isopropyl	1.53	-0.15	-0.05	-0.10	19.10	4.11	2.04	3.16	2.49
4 SCF_3	1.44	0.50	0.35	0.18	17.93	4.89	1.70	3.69	3.68

The subset of compounds showing activity LC_{50}< 5 ppm (all para substituted) were submitted to regression analysis. Plots of $\log(1/LC_{50})$ *vs.* each physicochemical parameter (π, σ, F, R, molar refractivity (MR), L, B1, B4) (20) revealed several promising relationships, and it appeared that σ was important although the 4-SCF_3 compound was identified as an "outlier" in the analysis. (21)

$$\log(1/LC_{50}) = -0.50\ (0.24)\ \pi + 0.45$$
$$n = 10,\ s = 0.27,\ r = 0.59,\ F_{1,8} = 4.32\ (0.07)$$

$$\log(1/LC_{50}) = 0.579\ (0.42)\ \sigma - 0.22$$
$$\text{(with 4-}SCF_3\text{)}$$
$$n = 10,\ s = 0.30,\ r = 0.44,\ F_{1,8} = 1.89\ (0.21)$$

$$\log(1/LC_{50}) = -0.059\ (0.015)\ MR + 0.79$$
$$n = 10,\ s = 0.19,\ r = 0.82,\ F_{1,8} = 16.29\ (0.0038)$$

Exclusion of the 4-SCF_3 compound from the regression revealed a more statistically significant equation in σ.

$$\log(1/LC_{50}) = 1.11\ (0.23)\ \sigma - 0.23$$
$$n = 9,\ s = 0.14,\ r = 0.88,\ F_{1,7} = 23.94\ (0.0018)$$

Although it might be imagined that the -SCF_3 group could easily be oxidized, this does not adequately distinguish this group from, for example, the -SCH_3 compound and therefore cannot, alone, form a rationale for exclusion of only the -SCF_3 compound. It is interesting to note that one property which might distinguish the -SCF_3 functionality is the potential for homologous cleavage for the bond between the sulfur and trifluoromethyl in this group.

Stepwise multiple regression (BMDP-2R) of this set of nine compounds (excluding the -SCF_3 compound) yielded the equation in σ and molar refractivity shown below:

$$\log(1/LC_{50}) = 0.734\ (0.219)\ \sigma - 0.029\ (0.011)\ MR + 0.138$$
$$n = 9,\ r = 0.95,\ s = 0.10,\ F_{2,6} = 26.0\ (<0.01)$$

The corresponding equation with π instead of molar refractivity resulted in a less statistically significant correlation. Table XIII shows the correlation matrix for para parameters for the para substituted compounds.

$$\log\ (1/LC_{50}) = 1.01\ (0.19)\ \sigma - 0.247\ (0.114)\ \text{pi} + 0.049$$
$$n = 9,\ r = 0.93,\ s = 0.12,\ F_{2,6} = 20.6\ (<0.01)$$

Toxicology. The mammalian toxicity of the alkyl aryl oxime ethers was unknown. Compound 15, which had good foliar and soil insecticidal activity, was chosen for an acute toxicological study.

The results of the oral screen on rats resulted in a qualitative rating of extremely toxic. All five rats dosed at 5 mg/kg died. Clinical signs included tremors and chronic convulsions.

Table VIII. Correlation Matrix for Para Parameters for Para Substituted Compounds (n = 9, excluding 4-SCF_3)

		Biological Activity log ($1/LC_{50}$)	π	σ	F	R	MR	L	B1	B4
		1	2	3	4	5	6	7	8	9
	1	1.0000								
π	2	-0.5328	1.0000							
σ	3	0.8797	-0.2601	1.0000						
F	4	0.7581	-0.3097	0.8559	1.0000					
R	5	0.5540	-0.0353	0.6390	0.1492	1.0000				
MR	6	-0.8385	0.4862	-0.6510	-0.4394	-0.5903	1.0000			
L	7	-0.3226	0.3307	-0.2323	0.0243	-0.4723	0.5233	1.0000		
B1	8	-0.2155	0.0345	-0.0562	-0.0966	0.0291	0.2529	-0.6044	1.0000	
B4	9	-0.1999	0.2501	-0.1668	-0.1503	-0.0854	0.3159	0.8523	-0.6630	1.0000

Therefore, this compound was rated extremely toxic when administered orally.

The preliminary dermal toxicity and irritation study led to the conclusion that Compound 15 was non-irritating and moderately toxic. Clinical signs in the individuals tested included loss of muscle control, tremors, and nasal discharge.

An Ames assay was conducted with Compound 15 using five tester strains of Salmonella typhimurium (TA98, TA100, TA1535, TA1537 and TA538) both with and without metabolic activation by Aroclor 1254 induced rat liver microsomes. No significant increase in the number of revertants per plate was found for any of the tester strains in either the presence or absence of metabolic activation. Therefore, it was concluded that this compound was not mutagenic.

CONCLUSIONS

The replacement of the 3-phenoxybenzyl alcohol fragment by 2-methyl[1,1'-biphenyl]-3-yl leads to an increase in initial and residual foliar activity in the alkyl aryl oxime ethers. An unanticipated result was the activity of these oxime ethers as soil insecticides. The corresponding 3-phenoxybenzyl alcohol oxime ethers were inactive as soil insecticides. The results of a structure activity relationship study revealed biological activity is enhanced by electron withdrawing substituents.

The results show that 2-methyl[1,1'-biphenyl]-3-methanol is an effective pyrethroid alcohol. It has been shown that this is true not only for pyrethroid esters but also for their isosteric replacements such as oxime ethers.

ACKNOWLEDGMENTS

The authors thank Jacob J. Vukich for his contributions to the synthesis of compounds reported in this paper. They also thank Susan E. Burkart, John H. Leigh, Albert C. Lew and Robert R. Stewart; and Sara J. Renna for manuscript preparation.

LITERATURE CITED

1. Elliott, M.; Farnham, A.W.; Janes, N.F.; Johnson, D.M.; and Pulman, D.A.; Pestic. Sci. 1980, 11, 513.

2. Bull, M.J.; Davies, J.H.; Searle, R.J.G.; and Henry, A.C.; Pestic. Sci. 1980, 11, 249.

3. Nanjyo, K.; Katsuyama, N.; Kariya, A.;Yamamura, S.B.; Suzuki, A.; and Tamura, S.; Agric. Biol. Chem. 1983, 31, 1091.

4. Paul, J.H. and Strong, J.G., European Patent Application 4,754, 1979.

5. Plummer, E.L. and Pincus, D.S.; J. Agric. Food Chem. 1981, 29, 1118.

6. Plummer, E.L.; J. Agric. Food Chem. 1983, 31, 718.

7. Plummer, E.L.; Cardis, A.B.; Martinez, A.J.; Van Saun, W.A.; Palmere, R.M.; Pincus, D.S.; and Stewart, R.R.; Pestic. Sci. 1983, 14, 560.

8. Plummer, E.L.; In Pesticide Synthesis Through Rational Approaches, Edited by Magee, P.S.; Kohn, G.K.; and Menn, J.J.; American Chemical Society: Washington, D.C., 1984.

9. Weinreb, S.M. and Nahm, S.W.; Tetrahedron Lett. 1981, 3815.

10. Paul, J.H.; United States Patent 4,158,015, 1979.

11. Hauser, C. R. and Hoffenberg, D. s.; J. Org. Chem. 1955, 20, 1491.

12. Cullen, T.G. and Cruickshank, P.A.; United States Patent 4,434,182, 1984.

13. Elliott, M. and Janes, N.F.; Chem. Soc. Rev. (London), 1978, 7, 473.

14. Bertau, P.E. and Casida, J.E.; J. Agric. Food Chem. 1969, 17, 931.

15. Brown, M.A.; Gammon, D.A.; and Casida, J.E.; J. Agric. Food Chem. 1983, 31, 1091.

16. BMDP Statistical Software, University of California Press, Berkeley, CA, 1985.

17. Hansch-Fujita substituent constant characterizing hydrophobicity. Fujita, T., Iwasa, J., Hansch, C., J. Am. Chem. Soc. 1964, 86, 5175. Leo, A., Hansch, C., Elkins, D., Chem. Rev. 1971, 71, 525.

18. F and R are parameters reflecting electronic effects, Swain, C. Gardner and Lupton, Elmer C., J. Am. Chem. Soc. 1968, 90, 4328-4337. Norrington, F.E. and Williams, S.G., J. Am. Chem. Soc. 1976, 98, 508-516.

19. Limited numbers of compounds precluded usage of a second set for evaluation of the classification functions.

20. STERIMOL parameters: Verloop, A., Hoogenstraaten, W. and Tipker, J., "Development and Application of New Steric Substituent Parameters in Drug Design", Drug Design, Vol VII, Ariens, E.J., ed., Academic Press, New York, 1976.

21. In all regression equations: n is the number of compounds, r is the correlation coefficient, s is the standard deviation, F is the F ratio of the correlation, and P is the significance (tail probability). Numbers in parenthesis after regression coefficients represent standard error. Numbers in parentheses after F statistics indicate significance level.

RECEIVED July 20, 1987

Chapter 17

Synthesis of Synthetic Pyrethroids

Stereoselection in the Synthesis of Cyclopropane Carboxylates

William A. Kleschick

Agricultural Products Department, Dow Chemical Company, Walnut Creek, CA 94598

A discussion of approaches to the stereoselective synthesis of 3-(dichlorovinyl)-2,2-dimethylcyclopropane carboxylic acid through intramolecular alkylation of an enolate ion is presented. Principles for achieving good control of the relative stereochemistry about the cyclopropane ring will be described. The control of the absolute stereochemistry on the ring was accomplished through the use of a chiral enolate.

The synthetic pyrethroids represent an important class of compounds for insect control in modern agriculture (1). These materials owe their success to their high insecticidal activity combined with their low mammalian toxicity. Some examples of these compounds include permethrin (2), cypermethrin (2), DOWCO 417 (3) and deltamethrin (2) shown in Figure 1. A key structural element of these materials is the 3-(dihalovinyl)-2,2-dimethylcyclopropane-carboxylic acid. The relative and absolute stereochemistry about the cyclopropane ring influences both the level and spectrum of insecticidal activity exhibited by these compounds (1,2). In general the cis diastereomers are more active than the trans, and the component of the racemate of R-configuration at the carboxyl stereocenter is the more active. Consequently, methods for the stereoselective synthesis of these cyclopropanecarboxylic acids are highly desirable.

We chose 1R,3R-3-(dichlorovinyl)-2,2-dimethylcyclopropane-carboxylic acid as our initial synthetic target. A number of imaginative approaches to the synthesis of pyrethroid cyclopropane-carboxylic acids have been reported (4). Conceptually, one of the simplest approaches to these materials involves an intramolecular alkylation of an enolate anion to form the cyclopropane ring as illustrated in Figure 2. The starting materials for such approaches are readily available through methodology based on [3,3] sigmatropic rearrangements followed by free radical initiated addition of polyhaloalkanes to olefins. We chose to reexamine this route from the standpoint of stereocontrol.

0097–6156/87/0355–0189$06.00/0
© 1987 American Chemical Society

Some measures of stereocontrol had previously been observed in approaches to pyrethroid acids involving intramolecular enolate alkylation. As outlined in Figure 3, workers at Sumitomo have investigated the cyclization of a methyl ketone enolate (5). They obtained a 9:1 ratio of cis:trans products upon ring closure initiated by sodium hydroxide. The methyl ketone was subsequently converted to the corresponding carboxylic acid via the haloform reaction.

An additional example (Figure 4) of stereochemical control was observed by workers at FMC in cyclization of ester enolates (6). Cyclization of the ethyl ester initiated by sodium t-butoxide in hexane produced a 12:88 ratio of cis:trans cyclopropanes. Repeating this experiment in the presence of the polar aprotic solvent, HMPA, reversed the stereoselection in the ring closure. The ratio of cis:trans isomers was 74:26. One obvious interpretation of these results can be derived from observations of Ireland regarding the influence of HMPA on the stereoselection in the formation of ester enolates (7). Based on Ireland's work, in hexane the E-enolate would be formed preferentially and in the presence of HMPA the Z-enolate would be the major diastereomeric intermediate. It follows that E-enolates cyclize selectively to form trans cyclopropanes, and Z-enolates selectively produce cis products (Figure 5).

We chose to explore the intramolecular alkylation of amide enolates as a potential stereoselective route to cis pyrethroid cyclopropane carboxylates. If the relationship between the stereoselection in enolate formation and ring closure is operable, amide enolates would be an excellent means of developing a stereoselective synthesis of cis products (8). Furthermore, recent progress in achieving enantioselection in the intermolecular alkylation of chiral amide enolates would provide a means of obtaining optically active pyrethroid acids (Figure 6) (9-13).

Our initial efforts were aimed at examining the stereoselection of the cyclization of enolates from simple N,N-dialkyl amides. To this end we prepared N,N,3,3-tetramethyl-4-pentenamide in 77% yield using the Meerwein-Eschenmoser variant of the Claisen rearrangement (Figure 7) (14). However, we met with considerable difficulty upon attempts to functionalize the olefin. Repeated attempts at free radical initiated addition of CCl_4 or $CBrCl_3$ under standard conditions resulted in recovery of starting material. Upon going to more vigorous conditions the formation of a lactone was observed (15). The lactone presumably arises from an intramolecular alkylation of the initial CCl_4 addition product. We also attempted epoxidation as a means of functionalizing the olefin. Again we observed a lack of reactivity. Ultimately we found that reaction occurred with 2-hydroperoxyhexafluoro-2-propanol (16), but again a lactone derived from intramolecular epoxide opening was the product.

After our initial attempts to test our idea in a model compound met with failure, we chose to examine a system which more closely resembled one of interest for our ultimate goal. We prepared the product of the Claisen rearrangement of 3-methyl-2-buten-1-ol adduct with triethylorthoacetate (Figure 8). The resulting unsaturated ester was hydrolized to the corresponding

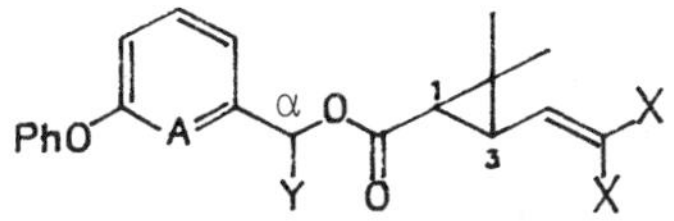

Permethrin	A=CH, X=Cl, Y=H
Cypermethrin	A=CH, X=Cl, Y=CN
DOWCO 417	A=N, X=Cl, Y=CN
Decamethrin	A=CH, X=Br, Y=CN (1R, 3R, α S)

Figure 1. Some examples of synthetic pyrethroid insecticides

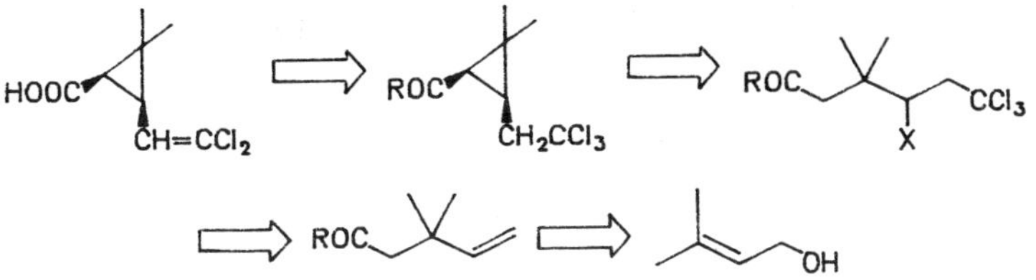

Figure 2. Retrosynthetic analysis

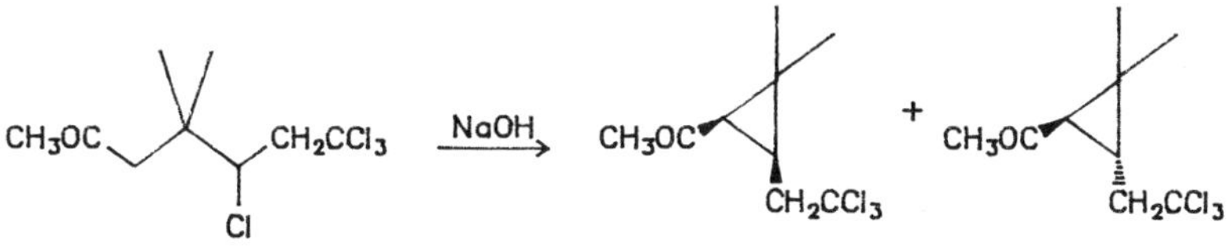

NaOH

cis: trans = 9:1

Figure 3. Stereoselection in the cyclization of the methyl ketone enolate

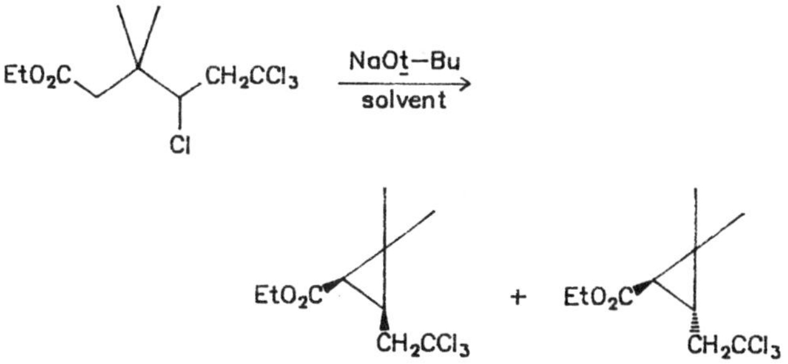

NaO*t*–Bu / solvent

solvent	cis: trans
hexane	12: 88
hexane–HMPA	74: 26

Figure 4. Stereoselection in the cyclization of the ester enolate

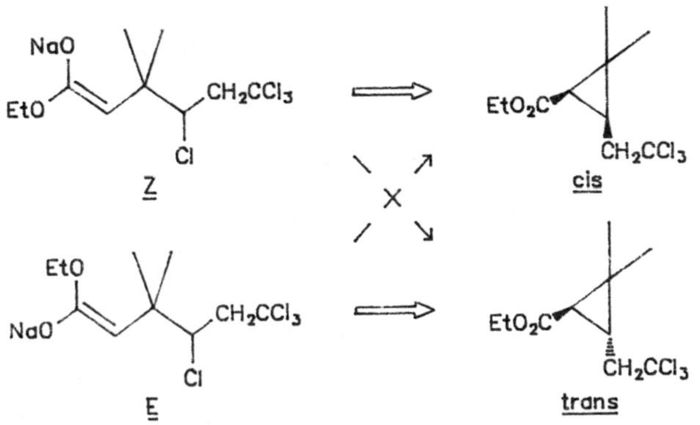

Figure 5. Stereoselection in cyclopropane formation as a function of enolate stereochemistry

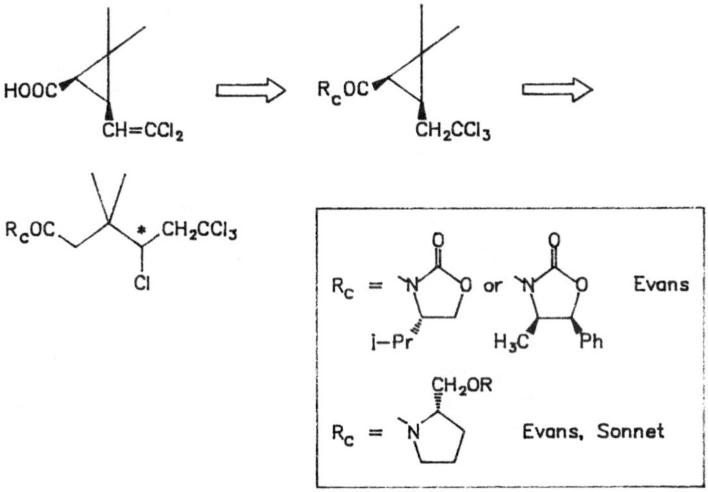

Figure 6. Retrosynthetic analysis for the asymmetric synthesis

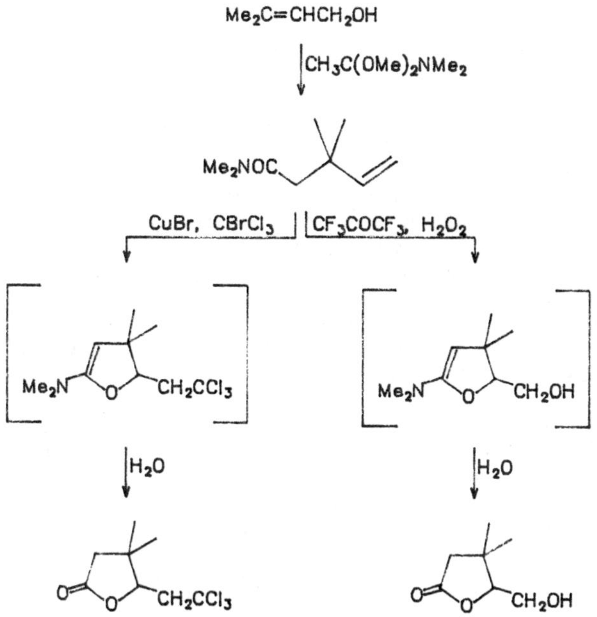

$Me_2C{=}CHCH_2OH$

$CH_3C(OMe)_2NMe_2$

Me_2NOC

CuBr, $CBrCl_3$ | CF_3COCF_3, H_2O_2

Me_2N O CH_2CCl_3 | Me_2N O CH_2OH

H_2O | H_2O

O O CH_2CCl_3 | O O CH_2OH

Figure 7. Attempted synthesis via the N,N-dimethylamide

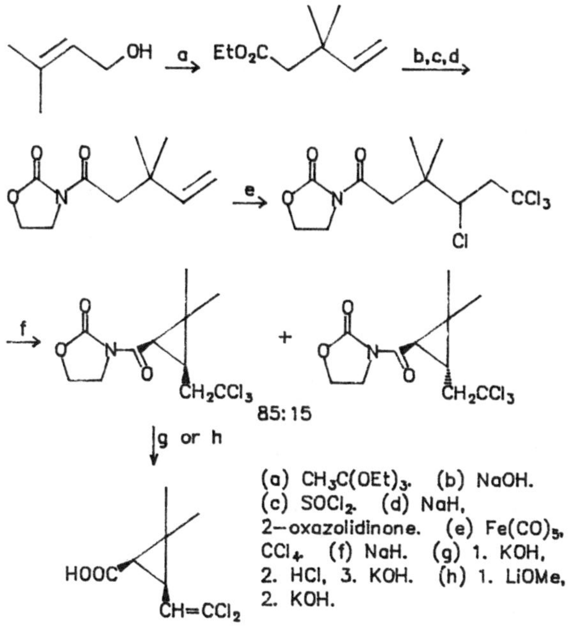

OH a EtO_2C b,c,d

O O O N e O O O N CCl_3 Cl

f O O N O CH_2CCl_3 + O O N O CH_2CCl_3

85:15

g or h

HOOC $CH{=}CCl_2$

(a) $CH_3C(OEt)_3$. (b) NaOH. (c) $SOCl_2$. (d) NaH, 2-oxazolidinone. (e) $Fe(CO)_5$, CCl_4. (f) NaH. (g) 1. KOH, 2. HCl, 3. KOH. (h) 1. LiOMe, 2. KOH.

Figure 8. Stereoselective synthesis of cis-3-(2,2-dichlorovinyl)-2,2-dimethylcyclopropanecarboxylic acid

carboxylic acid (17), and the acid was converted to the acid chloride. Reaction of the acid chloride with the sodium salt of 2-oxazolidinone produced the desired imide. Functionalizing the olefin in this material also proved difficult. After much experimentation we found that reaction with CCl_4 catalyzed by iron pentacarbonyl at reflux produced the desired CCl_4 adduct in excellent yield. Cyclization of this material was accomplished by treatment with sodium hydride. Other bases could also be used to bring about cyclization, however the desired products were contaminated with minor products from dehydrohalogenation or oxazolidinone ring opening. The ratio of cis to trans cyclopropanes was 85:15. The stereochemistry of the major product was confirmed by separation and conversion to a sample of the cis carboxylic acid. No scrambling of the carboxyl stereocenter was detected during the hydrolysis and dehydrohalogenation reactions involved in the conversion.

Having established the stereoselection in the cyclization of a simple imide, we began to explore a chiral imide system. The starting material for the ring closure was prepared by a straightforward extension of the route described above (Figure 9). The starting point for this material was R-valine. R-valine was reduced with borane-methyl sulfide to the corresponding amino alcohol without any loss of stereochemical integrity (18). This was verified by conversion of the amino alcohol to the Mosher's amide and examination of the ^{19}F NMR spectrum and HPLC chromatographic properties (19). The imidazolidinone was prepared by reaction of the amino alcohol with carbonyl diimidazole. In this reaction sequence, CCl_4 addition to the olefin produced two diastereomeric products. As expected the stereoselection in this addition was low due to the great distance between the resident stereocenter and the newly created one. The two CCl_4 addition products were nearly identical in all respects. Identification of the stereostructure of the major diastereomer was accomplished by single crystal X-ray analysis.

The stereoselection in the cyclization of each diastereomer was examined independently. The stereochemical outcome of the cyclization should be predictable based on our assumption regarding the relationship between enolate stereochemistry and cyclopropane stereochemistry, the principles of asymmetric, intermolecular alkylation of optically active amides (9-13) and the assumption that the mechanism of cyclopropane formation involves a straightforward back-side, S_N2 reaction. In the case of the major diastereomer, the natural tendency of the enolate to produce the cis-cyclopropane will oppose the facial preference for the alkylation of the chiral enolate. Consequently, poorer stereochemical control would be expected in the ring closure. In the minor diastereomer these two forces are working in tandem, and high degrees of stereocontrol should result.

Cyclization of the major diastereomer produced a mixture of all four possible products in a ratio of 1:23:74:2 (Figure 10). The stereochemical assignment (Figure 10) was based on conversion to dihalovinyl acid. Ratios of cis to trans products were established by ^1H NMR, and assignment of absolute configuration was made based on comparison of the optical rotation with literature

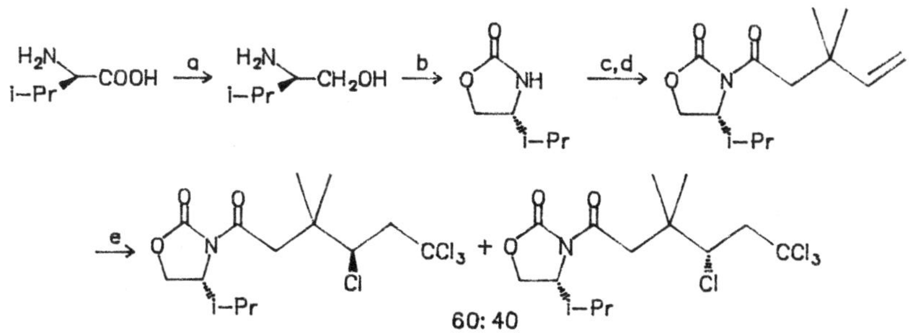

(a) $BH_3 \cdot SMe_2$, $BF_3 \cdot OEt_2$. (b) carbonyldiimidazole. (c) NaH.
(d) $ClOCCH_2C(CH_3)_2CH{=}CH_2$. (e) $Fe(CO)_5$, CCl_4.

Figure 9. Synthesis of cyclization precursor for the asymmetric synthesis

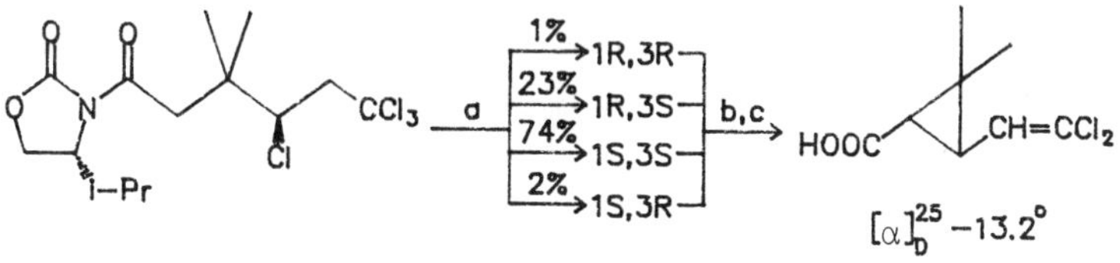

(a) NaOH (b) LiOMe (c) KOH

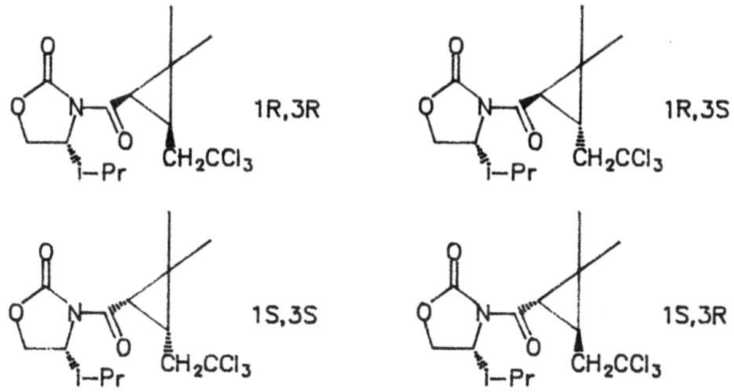

Figure 10. Stereoselection in the cyclization of the major diastereomer

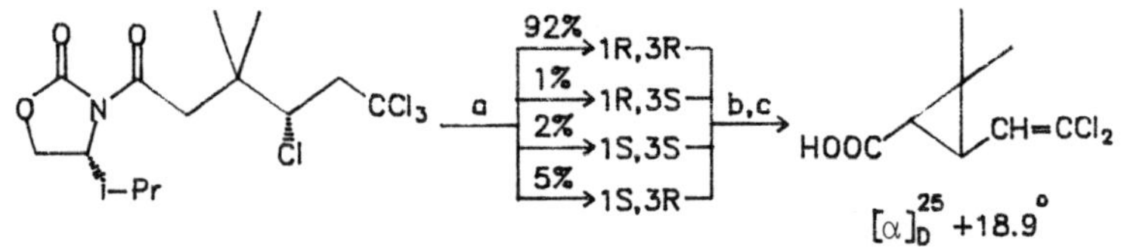

(a) NaOH (b) LiOMe (c) KOH

Figure 11. Stereoselection in the cyclization of the minor diastereomer

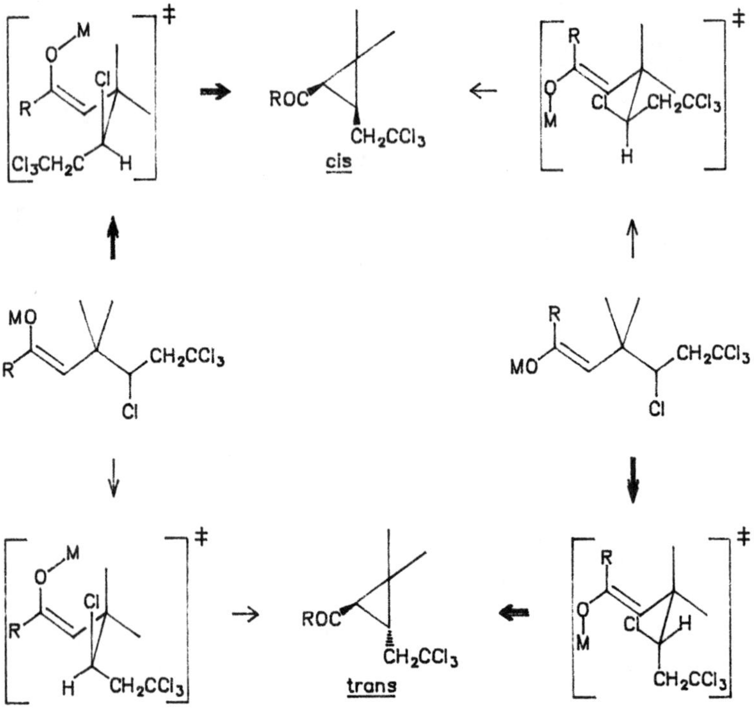

Figure 12. Transition state model for the cyclization

values (2). When the minor diastereomer was reacted with sodium hydride again all four possible diastereomers were produced (Figure 11). However, the ratio of diastereomers was 92:1:2:5 with the 1R,3R predominating. These results are in accord with our prediction.

One potential explanation for the stereochemical outcome of these cyclopropane ring forming reactions is presented in Figure 12. We examined two possible transition state conformations for the cyclization of enolates in which -OM (M = metal) is *cis* to the side chain containing the leaving group. In each of these conformations the leaving group and the metal associated with the leaving group are kept in close proximity. A major distinguishing feature in these two conformations involves the interactions of the trichloroethyl group. In the transition state leading to the *cis* product an eclipsed interaction with the enolate double bond is present, and in the other transition state an eclipsed interaction with a methyl group is evident. It would be expected that that the former interaction leading to *cis* product would be of lower energy. This expectation is based on studies of the preferred conformations of 1-butene (20). A similar argument involving gauche interactions in the transition state conformations for the ring closure of the other enolate diastereomer supports the observation of the preference to form a *trans* cyclopropane.

The results presented here illustrate some basic principles for achieving good measures of stereocontrol in the formation of cyclopropanecarboxylate derivatives *via* intramolecular enolate alkylation. They also represent an additional example of the important role that stereoselection in enolate formation plays in stereoselective synthesis (21, 22).

Acknowledgments

I would like to acknowledge Michael W. Reed who assisted with the synthetic work and Professor Jon Bordner for the X-ray structure analysis described in this report. I would also like to thank Professor Andrew S. Kende for many helpful discussions and for providing 400 MHz ^{1}H NMR spectra.

Literature Cited

1. Elliott, M. *Pestic. Sci.* 1980, *11*, 119.
2. Burt, P. E.; Elliott, M.; Farnham, A.; Janes, N. F.; Needham, P. H.; Pulman, D. A. *Pestic. Sci.* 1974, *5*, 791.
3. Malhotra, S. K.; VanHeertum, J. C.; Larson, L. L.; Ricks, M. J. *J. Agric. Food Chem.* 1981, *29*, 1287.
4. For an excellent review of this subject, see: Arlt, D.; Jautelat, M.; Lantzsch, R. *Angew. Chem. Int. Ed. Engl.* 1981, *20*, 703.
5. Itaya, N.; Matsuo, T.; Ohno, N.; Mizutani, T.; Fujita, F.; Yoshioka, H., In *Synthetic Pyrethroids*; Elliott, M., Ed.; ACS Symposium Series No. 42; American Chemical Society: Washington, D.C., 1977; p 45.
6. Kondo, K.; Takashima, T.; Negishi, A.; Matsui, K.; Fujimoto, T.; Sugimoto, K.; Hatch, C. E., III; Baum, J. S. *Pestic. Sci.* 1980, *11*, 180.

7. Ireland, R. E.; Mueller, R. H.; Willard, A. K. J. Am. Chem. Soc. 1976, 98, 2868.
8. For a discussion and leading references to stereoselection in enolate formation, see: Moreland, D. W.; Dauben, W. G. J. Am. Chem. Soc. 1985, 107, 2264.
9. Evans, D. A.; Takacs, J. M.; McGee, L. R.; Ennis, M. D.; Mathre, D. J.; Bartroli, J. Pure Appl. Chem. 1981, 53, 1109.
10. Evans, D. A. Aldrichimica Acta 1982, 15, 23.
11. Evans, D. A.; Takacs, J. M. Tetrahedron Lett. 1980, 4233.
12. Sonnet, P. E.; Heath, R. R. J. Org. Chem. 1980, 45, 3137.
13. Evans, D. A.; Ennis, M. D.; Mathre, D. J. J. Am. Chem. Soc. 1982, 104, 1737.
14. For a leading reference, see: Hill, R. K.; Soman, R.; Sawada, S. J. Org. Chem. 1972, 37, 3737.
15. For an account of similar results observed by other workers, see: Kropp, R.; Fisher, M.; Halbritter, K. U.S. Patent 4 320 062, 1982. Kropp, R.; Fisher, M.; Halbritter, K. U.S. Patent 4 324 725, 1982.
16. Heggs, R. P.; Ganem, B. J. Am. Chem. Soc. 1979, 101, 2484.
17. Jager, V.; Gunther, H. J. Tetrahedron Lett. 1977, 2543.
18. Lane, C. F. U.S. Patent 3 935 280, 1976.
19. Dale, J. A.; Dull, D. L.; Mosher, H. S. J. Org. Chem. 1969, 34, 2543.
20. Eliel, E. L.; Allinger, N. L.; Angyal, S. J.; Morrison, G. A. Conformational Analysis; Wiley-Interscience: New York, 1966; Chapter 1.
21. For a more complete account of a portion of this work, see: Kleschick, W. A. J. Org. Chem. 1986, 51, 5429.
22. For a more detailed account of the portion of this work dealing with asymmetric synthesis, see: Kleschick, W. A.; Reed, M. W.; Bordner, J. J. Org. Chem. 1987, 52, 0000.

RECEIVED May 15, 1987

Chapter 18

Heterobicyclic Oxime Carbamates

Thomas A. Magee[1], Lawrence E. Limpel[1], Robert D. Battershell[2], Stephen B. Bowlus[1,3], Susan E. Branchick[1], William W. Brand[1,4], Russell Buchman[1], Hsiao-Chiung Chen[1], H. Glenn Corkins[1,5], Arthur J. Friedman[1,6], Andrew W. W. Ho[1,7], J. Lawrence Holodnak[1,8], Eva M. Marczewski[1], Kimberly S. Monti[1], John R. Nicklas[1], Edmond R. Osgood[1], Larry J. Powers[1], and Louis Storace[1]

[1]Ricerca, P.O. Box 1000, Painesville, OH 44077
[2]Fermenta Plant Protection, P.O. Box 348, Painesville, OH 44077

Carbamates of bicyclic hydroximidates and thiolhydroximidates show contact and systemic activity against insects, mites, and nematodes with a spectrum and/or level of activity somewhat different from the known art. The active thiolhydroximidates are exceptionally powerful inhibitors of cholinesterase. Most of the compounds were synthesized from the reaction products of cyclic dienes with (a) thiophosgene or (b) chlorosulfonylisocyanate. Analogous bicyclic amidoxime derivatives were devoid of activity.

Carbamates of acyclic hydroximidates and thiolhydroximidates have been reported to exhibit insecticidal and nematicidal activity (1-5). Included among these are the commercial materials methomyl and oxamyl. Derivatives of monocyclic thiolhydroximidates have also been described (6). We wish to report a series of carbamates of bicyclic hydroximidates, thiolhydroximidates, and amidoximes which exhibit broad activity as insecticides and nematicides (7).

CHEMISTRY

The bicyclic thiolhydroximidates were prepared by the reaction of hydroxylamine with *gem*-dichlorothiabicycloalkenes which are readily obtained by the Diels-Alder reaction of thiophosgene with the appropriately substituted cyclic 1,3-diene (8,9). A more detailed report of this chemistry will be published elsewhere.

[3]Current address: Sandoz AG, Basel, Switzerland
[4]Current address: ICI Americas, Wilmington, DE 19897
[5]Current address: Nepera, Inc., Harriman, NY 10926
[6]Current address: Sandoz Crop Protection, Chicago, IL 60018
[7]Current address: Chevron Chemical Company, Richmond, CA 94804
[8]Current address: Occidental Chemical Corporation, Ashtabula, OH 44004

0097-6156/87/0355-0199$06.00/0
© 1987 American Chemical Society

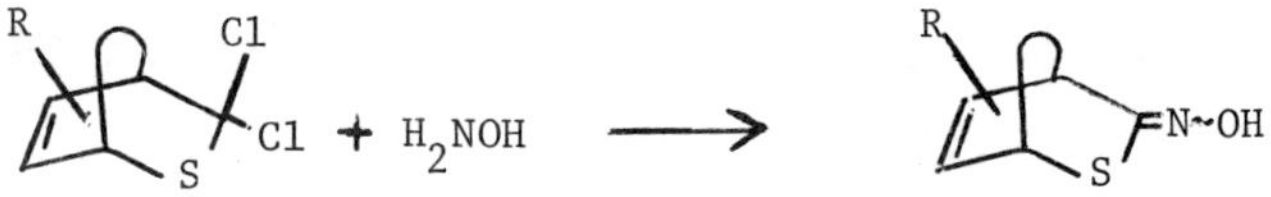

Most of the bicyclic hydroximidates were prepared by the reaction of hydroxylamine with oxabicyclic N-chlorosulfonylimines which are products of the reaction of chlorosulfonyl isocyanate with cyclic 1,3-dienes (10,11).

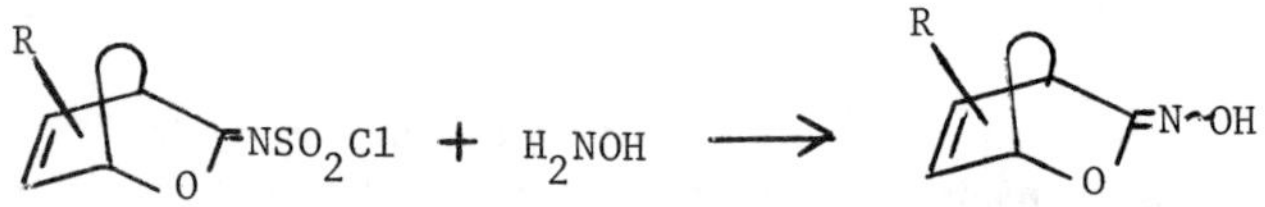

This reaction is not useful for synthesis of the [2.2.1] oxabicyclic system; attempts to prepare this system by alternate approaches have been unsuccessful. Again, a more detailed report of this chemistry will be published elsewhere.

The [3.2.1] bicyclohydroximidates were prepared by reaction of the thionolactone with hydroxylamine. The lactones were prepared by standard methods (12,13) and converted to the thionolactones with Lawesson's reagent. These carbamates were viscous oils which could not be obtained analytically pure; their structures are based on spectral evidence.

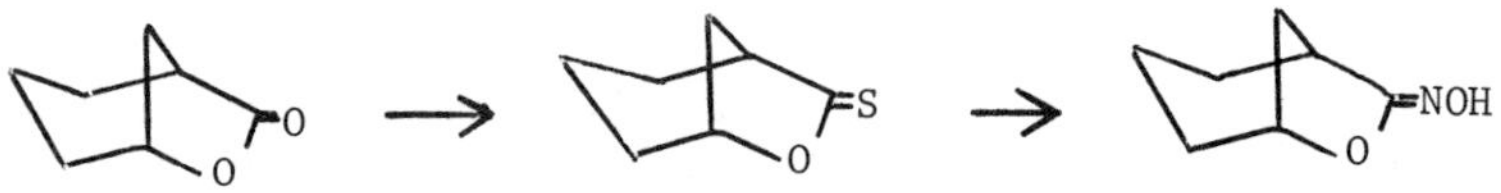

The amidoximes were prepared by modifications of literature procedures.

These hydroximidates and thiolhydroximidates may exist in E and Z forms. Both isomers were isolated only with the unsubstituted [2.2.1] thia system, although the presence of both isomers in other reaction mixtures cannot be excluded. Compounds **1** and **39** were shown to be the Z-isomer by single crystal x-ray crystallography. The Z-form has been shown to be the stable isomer of methomyl (14-16). The more stable isomer of methyl acetohydroximidate and related compounds possesses the E-configuration (17). We have no information on the isomeric configuration of the present bicyclic hydroximidates other than that they appear to be single isomers.

Carbamates were prepared from the hydroxylic compound and methyl isocyanate by standard methods. Dichloromethane was the solvent of choice.

BIOLOGICAL TESTING

The compounds were screened for insecticidal or acaricidal activity against five species: Mexican bean beetle larvae

(*Epilachna varivestis*), Southern armyworm larvae (*Spodoptera eridania*), adult housefly (*Musca domestica*), two-spotted spider mite (*Tetranychus urticae*), and black bean aphid (*Aphis fabae*). Contact activity was determined against all five; systemic activity against the mite and aphid was also measured. The fly, mite and aphid were sprayed directly; the beetle and armyworm larvae were placed onto previously sprayed leaf surfaces. Details of these procedures have been published (18). Screening for activity against soil phytopathogenic nematodes was conducted with the root knot nematode (*Meloidogyne incognita*)(7).

Anticholinesterase activity was measured against electric eel acetylcholinesterase by the method previously described (19).

DISCUSSION

The oxa- and thiabicyclic carbamates exhibit contact and/or stomach poison activity against all five species tested; significant soil applied foliar systemic activity is shown only by the oxa compounds; the azabicyclics are essentially inactive. Nematicidal activity is restricted primarily to the thia series and is variable. The data are contained in Tables I-III.

No significant structure activity patterns stand out for the unsubstituted oxa or thia compounds. Neither ring size, degree of unsaturation, nor nature of the heteroatom has a dramatic effect on contact activity. Substitution in the thia compounds exhibits a stronger effect on activity. With the unsaturated [2.2.2] series, a small substituent at the four bridgehead position affords optimum results. Based on only two examples, a small substituent at the one bridgehead position reduces activity against the armyworm without affecting control of the other test organisms. A larger group at either the one or four bridgehead position lowers activity. Substitution on the unsaturated bridge of the thiabicycloalkenes is tolerated; substitution on the saturated bridge lowers activity. With the thiabicycloalkanes, *exo* substitution essentially abolishes activity while *endo* substituents or planar groups (e.g. carbonyl) are tolerated; again a small substituent at the four bridgehead position maximizes activity.

The small number of substituted examples in the oxa series limits interpretation. The [3.2.1] series (**67-70**) suggests that a small substituent at the bridgehead adjacent to the oxime function is again beneficial.

Where both *E* and *Z* isomers were available (**1** and **2**, **28** and **29**), the *Z* isomers were significantly more active. Oxidation of the sulfur atom in the thiabicyclic compounds generally lowered insecticidal activity.

Good nematicidal activity was found only in the thia series. The highest activity, $\geq$ four times the standards, was shown by the [2.2.2] compounds with a small electronegative group at the four bridgehead position.

The thiabicyclic compounds as a group show very high activity as inhibitors of cholinesterase, causing 50% inhibition at 10^{-8} to 10^{-10} moles/liter. The oxa compounds were two to four orders of magnitude less active as esterase inhibitors while showing similar contact insecticidal effectiveness. Felton (3) has suggested for

Table I. [2.2.1]Thiabicyclic N-Methylcarbamates

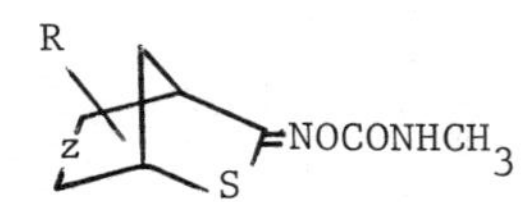

Cpd No.	z[(a)]	R	Melting Range in °C	LC_{50} in ppm: BB[(b)]	AW[(b)]	HF[(b)]	M[(b)]	LC_{50} in kg/ha: A[(b)]	RKN[(b)]	I_{50} mol/L x 10^7
1[c]	d		118-9	8.2	47	4.3	19	4.6	0.43	0.40
2[d]	d		89-91	110	>128	54	71	16	>8	---
3	s		121-2	45	61	35	19	2.7	0.60	0.072
4	d	2-(O)	118 (dec)	26	>128	>128	>128	45	---	0.005
5	d	2,2-$(O)_2$	132 (dec)	>128	>128	>128	>128	>128	>16	0.11
6	s	2-(O)	oil	23	>128	45	>128	16	---	0.034
7	d	4-CH_3	86-8	18	6.4	5.0	2.3	1.8	0.25	0.18
8[e]	d	1(5)(6)-CH_3	oil	25	>128	16	8.8	1.8	---	1.3
9	d	1-$COOCH_3$	102-6	>128	>128	>128	>128	>128	3.0	>100
10[f]	d	4-$COOCH_3$	112-3	>128	>128	>128	>128	>128	>16	66
11[f]	d	4-$COOCH_3$	oil	34	>128	>128	>128	42	1.1	---
12	d	5(6)-Cl	oil	14	84	26	7.1	4.5	3.2	---

13	d	7-Br	87-92	103	>128	100	45	>128	>16	34
14	s	exo-6-Cl	130-3	>128	>128	>128	80	>128	---	41
15	s	endo-5-Cl	125-7	3.7	>128	70	5.6	2.8	---	2.3
16	s	endo-5(6)-CH_3	oil	30	56	>128	11	5.5	---	0.55
17	s	6-(OH)	159-64	>128	>128	>128	>128	>128	---	>100
18	s	6,6-(=O)	oil	4.2	30	12	70	14	---	1.3
19	s	6,6-$(OCH_3)_2$	oil	6.0	102	7.6	>128	24	---	---
20	s	6,6-(=NOH)	oil	7.4	45	16	>128	35	---	>100
21[f]	s	6,6-(=$NOCH_3$)	oil	2.0	16	3.5	7.6	5.8	---	---
22[f]	s	6,6-(=$NOCH_3$)	oil	4.3	64	4.3	8.0	12	---	10
23	s	7-Cl-6,6-(=O)	150	14	107	31	21	33	---	0.29
24	s	5,6-Cl_2	137-8	46	>128	93	8.6	110	---	2.3
25	s	6,7-Br_2	163	>128	>128	>128	>128	>128	>16	1300
26	s	5,6-$(OH)_2$	98-101	>128	>128	>128	>128	>128	>16	170
27	s	5,6-OC(O)O-	190-2	>128	>128	>128	>128	>128	>16	---
		Methomyl		1.2	12	2.2	128	8.8	>16	10[g]
		Aldicarb		38	>128	7.5	32	1.3	1.1	100[h]

(a) d = double bond; s = single bond; (b) BB = Mexican bean beetle; AW = southern armyworm; HF = housefly; M = two-spotted spider mite; A = bean aphid; RKN = root knot nematode; (c) Z isomer; (d) E isomer; (e) Mixed positional isomers; (f) Conformational isomers; (g) Reference 20; (h) Reference 21.

Table II. [2.2.2]Thiabicyclic N-Methylcarbamates

Cpd No.	z[a]	R	Melting Range (°C)	$BB^{(b)}$	$AW^{(b)}$	LC_{50} in ppm $HF^{(b)}$	$M^{(b)}$	$A^{(b)}$	LC_{50} in kg/ha $RKN^{(b)}$	I_{50} mol/L x 10^7
28[c]	d		112-4	5.8	32	13	12	1.1	0.4	0.20
29[d]	d		122-4	70	>128	11	28	24	1.9	0.58
30	s		115-6.5	6.0	42	16	4.1	1.2	0.42	0.015
31	d	1-CH_3	88-90	36	128	---	11	8	---	0.20
32	d	4-CH_3	100-2	5	22	---	3.8	1.5	---	---
33	d	4-COOH	157-8	>128	>128	>128	>128	>128	---	>100
34	d	1(4)-$COOCH_3$	122-5	>128	>128	>128	>128	45	>16	52
35	d	7(8)-$COOCH_3$	139-42	11	>128	>128	90	41	>16	2.6
36	d	1(4)-$COOC_2H_5$	123-5	>128	>128	>128	>128	22	3.6	2.3
37	d	4(1)-$COOC_2H_5$	oil	33	>128	>128	114	42	2.8	0.057
38	d	4-$CONH_2$	175-6	24	>128	>128	>128	>128	---	5.9
39	d	4-CN	153-7	2.1	30	28	3.2	6.8	0.16	0.005
40	d	4-CN-2-(O)	178-9 dec	7.5	110	>128	5.4	12	---	0.38
41	d	4-CN-2,2-$(O)_2$	196-8 dec	>128	>128	64	>128	>128	---	0.12
42	s	4-CN	178-80	2.1	17	29	1.2	1.6	0.08	0.014
43	s	4-CN-2-(O)	188-90 dec	15	>128	76	8	>128	---	---

44	d	5-CN	139-40	6.8	64	12	6	22	---	0.27
45	d	6-CN	134-5	10	105	42	33	11	---	0.34
46	d	4-Cl	104-6	2.7	20	12	1.2	1.0	0.25	>0.001
47[e]	d	5(6)-Cl	oil	11	66	14	2.7	4.4	0.7	0.01
48[e]	d	5(6)-Cl	61-4	4.0	32	50	5.2	3.8	1.0	0.003
49[e]	d	6(5)-Cl	101-4	18	74	66	17	2.7	1.1	0.006
50	d	5(6)-Br	oil	6.6	>128	32	14	7.8	1.4	0.024
51	d	6(5)-Br	87-9	6.4	80	50	23	4.6	3.3	0.005
52	d	5(6)-$(CH_3O)_2P(O)O$	oil	<128	>128	>128	>128	>128	---	27
53	d	1-CH_3-4-CN	138-40	4.5	>128	29	5.6	3.7	---	0.12
54	d	4-CN-6-CH_3	115-6.5	1.9	23	60	2.8	5.0	---	0.10
55	d	7,8-CH_2	124-5	12	>128	17	12	20	1.0	1.8
56	s	7,8-CH_2	124-5	14	>128	>128	15	52	0.8	2.1
57	d	7,8-CH(CN)	125	11	>128	>128	32	>128	9.0	26
58	s	5,6-$(HO)_2$	123-5	>128	>128	>128	>128	>128	>16	---
59	s	5,6-$(CH_3O)_2$	156-7	>128	>128	>128	>128	>128	>16	37
60	s	5,6-OCH_2O	126-8	100	>128	>128	>128	>128	>16	---
		Methomyl		1.2	12	2.2	128	8.8	>16	10[f]
		Aldicarb		38	>128	7.5	32	1.3	1.1	100[g]

(a) d = double bond; s = single bond; (b) BB = Mexican bean beetle; AW = southern armyworm; HF = housefly; M = two-spotted spider mite; A = bean aphid; RKN = root knot nematode; (c) Z isomer; (d) E isomer; (e) positional and conformational isomers; (f) Reference 20; (g) Reference 21.

Table III. Miscellaneous Bicyclic N-Methylcarbamates

Cpd No.	A	x	y	R	Melting Range °C	$BB^{(a)}$	LC_{50} in ppm $AW^{(a)}$	$HF^{(a)}$	$M^{(a)}$	$A^{(a)}$	LC_{50} in kg/ha MS^{a}	AS^{a}	I_{50} mol/L x 10^7
61	NH	-CH=CH-	$-CH_2-$		98-10	>128	>128	>128	>128	>128	---	---	81
62	O	-CH=CH-	$-CH_2CH_2-$		103-4	6.1	17	4.7	13	1.1	>4	0.06	1.7
63	O	$-CH_2CH_2-$	$-CH_2CH_2-$		111-2	4.2	22	6.8	28	2.4	2.5	0.034	1.4
64	O	-CH=CH-	$-CH_2CH_2-$	6-Br	oil	1.6	64	17	11	1.7	>4	0.18	---
65	NH	-CH=CH-	$-CH_2CH_2-$		128-9	>128	>128	36	>128	>128	---	---	48
66	NCH_3	$-CH_2CH_2-$	$-CH_2CH_2-$		oil	>128	>128	>128	>128	35	---	---	---
67	O	$-(CH_2)_3-$	$-CH_2-$		oil	6	32	9	5.4	0.25	>4	0.034	1.2
68	O	$-(CH_2)_3-$	$-CH_2-$	$1-CH_3$	oil	6.5	>128	23	4	0.6	0.6	0.12	1.7
69	O	$-(CH_2)_3-$	$-CH_2-$	1-Cl	oil	1.2	58	4.5	1.5	0.6	0.34	0.048	---
70	O	$-(CH_2)_3-$	$-CH_2-$	$1-CH_3O$	oil	4	100	26	15	1	2.0	0.13	---
71	S	$-(CH_2)_3-$	-CH=CH-		oil	4.2	59	12	1.2	1.5	---	---	0.007
72	S	$-(CH_2)_3-$	$-CH_2CH_2-$		112-4	5.2	60	25	2.9	1.4	---	---	0.011
73	O	$-(CH_2)_3-$	-CH=CH-		oil	7	70	15	12	1.6	2	0.25	---

74	O	$-(CH_2)_3-$	$-CH_2CH_2-$	110-2	8	90	48	11	0.4	2	0.07	---
75	S	$-OCH_2CH_2-$	-CH=C(Cl)-	140-2	2.0	>128	22	5.0	24	---	---	0.82
76	O	-CH=CH-CH=CH-	$-CH_2-$	137-8	6.9	99	26	26	8.1	>4	0.14	0.79
77	O	$-CH=CH-CH_2CH_2-$	$-CH_2-$	oil	5	20	25	23	1	>4	0.38	---
78	O	$-(CH_2)_4-$	$-CH_2-$	oil	7.8	>128	46	45	1.8	>4	0.18	---
79	S	$1,2-C_6H_4-$	$1,2-C_6H_4-$	172-4	23	>128	>128	>128	>128	---	---	>100
		Methomyl			1.2	12	2.2	128	8.8	>4	0.6	10[b]
		Aldicarb			38	>128	7.5	32	1.3	0.68	0.014	100[c]

(a) BB = Mexican bean beetle; AW = southern armyworm; HF = housefly; M = two-spotted spider mite; A = bean aphid; MS = mite systemic; AS = aphid systemic; (b) Reference 20; (c) Reference 21.

a group of linear thiolhydroximidates that high lipophilicity leads to increased anticholinesterase activity but also renders the compound more susceptible to detoxification by the insect. Whatever the cause, the very high anticholinesterase activity of the thiabicyclics is not translated well into insecticidal effectiveness.

Many of these bicyclic carbamates showed high acute oral toxicity to rats; they were relatively safe by dermal or inhalation exposure. An extensive program of derivatization, especially sulfenylation, of the carbamates was carried out. Ten fold or greater increases in acute oral safety were obtained; this was usually accompanied by significant loss of contact insecticidal activity.

LITERATURE CITED

1. Buchanan, J. B. British Patent 1 138 349, 1965.
2. Addor, R. W. J. Agric. Food Chem. 1965, 13, 207-9.
3. Felton, J.C. J. Sci. Food Agri. Supp. 1968, 33-8.
4. Davies, J. H.; Davis, R. H. Canadian Patent 846 846, 1970.
5. Weiden, M. H. J. J. Sci. Food Agri. Suppl. 1968, 19-31.
6. Addor, R. W. U. S. Patent 3 223 585, 1965.
7. Magee, T. A.; Battershell, R. D.; Limpel, L. E.; Ho, A. W.; Friedman, A. J.; Corkins, H. G.; Brand, W. W.; Buchman, R.; Storace, L.; Osgood, E. R. U. S. Patent 4 424 213, 1984.
8. Middleton, W. J. J. Org. Chem. 1965, 30, 1390-4.
9. Reich, H. J.; Trend, J. E. J. Org. Chem. 1973, 38, 2637-40.
10. Moriconi, E. J.; Hummel, C. F. J. Org. Chem. 1976, 41, 3583-6.
11. Malpass, J. R.; Tweddle, N. J. J. Chem. Soc. Perkin I, 1977, 874-84.
12. Grewe, R.; Heinke, A.; Sommer, C. Chem. Ber. 1956, 89, 1978-88.
13. Kato, M.; Kageyama, M.; Tanaka, R.; Kuwahara, K.; Yoshikoshi, A. J. Org. Chem. 1975, 40, 1932-41.
14. Davies, J. H.; Davis, R. H.; Kirby, P. J. Chem. Soc. (C), 1968, 431-5.
15. Waite, M. G.; Sim, G. A. J. Chem. Soc. (B) 1971, 752-6.
16. Takusagawa, F.; Jacobson, R. A. J. Agri. Food Chem. 1977, 25, 577-81.
17. Kjaer, A.; Larsen, I. K.; Silvertsen, P. Acta. Chem. Scand. Ser. B 1977, 31, 415-23.
18. Magee, T. A.; Limpel, L. E. J. Agri. Food Chem. 1977, 25, 1376-82.
19. Corkins, H. G.; Osgood, E. R.; Storace, L.; Limpel, L. E.; Simcox, P. D. J. Agric. Food Chem. 1980, 28, 1108-15.
20. Weiden, M. H. J. Bull. W. H. O. 1971, 44, 203-13.
21. Payne, L. K., Jr.; Stansbury, H. A., Jr.; Weiden, M. H. J. J. Agric. Food Chem. 1966, 14, 356-65.

RECEIVED May 15, 1987

Chapter 19

Synthesis, Insecticidal Activity, and Field Performance of Some S-Cyanoalkyl Phosphorodithioates

J. R. Sanborn[1], R. L. Sagaser, D. Marsden[1], T. A. Andrea[1], and B. T. Grayson[2]

Biological Sciences Research Center, Shell Agricultural Chemical Company, P.O. Box 4248, Modesto, CA 95352

This report summarizes the synthesis, insecticidal activity, and field performances of some S-cyanoalkyl phosphorodithioates related to terbufos. Replacement of one of the methyl groups of terbufos with a nitrile yielded an insecticide more active than terbufos but lacking its soil persistence. However, addition of a methyl group to the carbon between the two sulfur atoms of this S-cyanoalkyl phosphorodithioate produced a compound that was almost as active as Terbufos as an insecticide and gave economic control of corn rootworms at 1 lb/A.

The incorporation of a nitrile group into atrazine yielded Bladex as shown below:

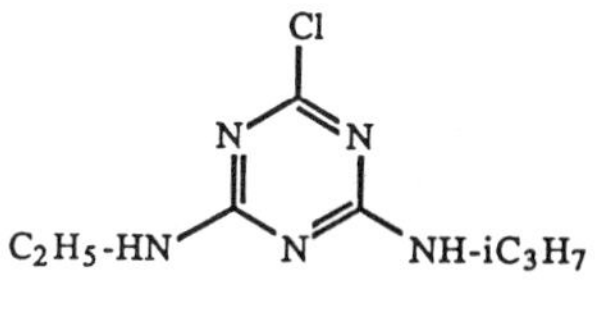

Cl, N, N, C_2H_5-HN, N, NH-iC_3H_7

Atrazine

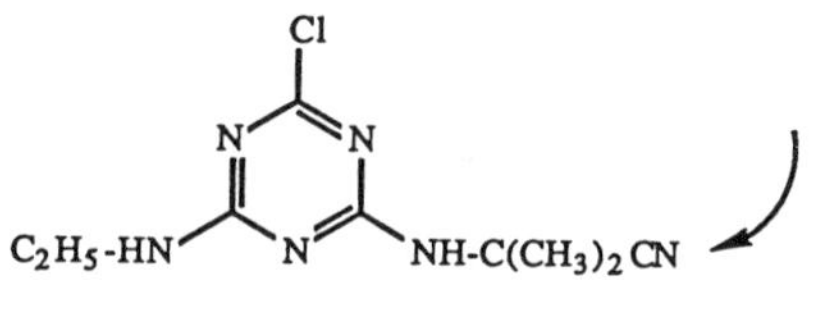

Cl, N, N, C_2H_5-HN, N, NH-C$(CH_3)_2$CN

Bladex

an herbicide with slightly different physical and biological characteristics. Perhaps the most significant change in the molecule is its decreased soil persistence, which is related to the ability of the nitrile moiety to undergo hydrolysis and afford significantly less herbicidal products.

[1]Current address: E. I. du Pont de Nemours & Co., Wilmington, DE 19898
[2]Current address: Shell Biosciences Laboratory, Sittingbourne, England

0097-6156/87/0355-0209$06.00/0
© 1987 American Chemical Society

This feature allows the farmer to plant other triazine susceptible crops if his first crop is lost because of environmental factors. Other physical properties that are changed because of the presence of the cyano group are a nearly 5-fold increase in water solubility (Atrazine=33ppm, Bladex=160 ppm) and an approximate 200-fold decrease in the vapor pressure (Atrazine=3.0×10^{-7} mm, Bladex=1.6×10^{-9} mm).

Since a nitrile group addition to the triazine herbicide Atrazine did not significantly detract from its field performance, we decided to examine what effect a nitrile group might have on the insecticidal and field performance of the highly successful corn rootworm insecticide (1,2), terbufos, whose structure is shown below:

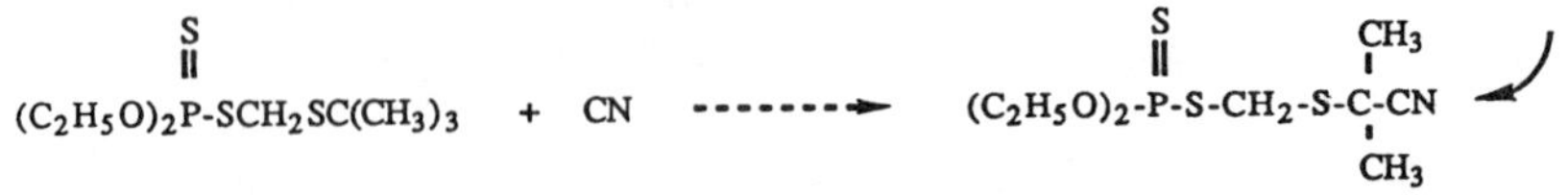

$$(C_2H_5O)_2\overset{S}{\overset{\|}{P}}\text{-}SCH_2SC(CH_3)_3 \quad + \quad CN \quad \dashrightarrow \quad (C_2H_5O)_2\text{-}\overset{S}{\overset{\|}{P}}\text{-}S\text{-}CH_2\text{-}S\text{-}\underset{CH_3}{\overset{CH_3}{C}}\text{-}CN$$

The following questions come to mind as to what might happen to the physical properties and insecticidal activity of terbufos if a nitrile group was incorporated into it:

1. Is the vapor pressure reduced?
2. Will the soil persistence be less and therefore the field efficacy be reduced?
3. Will the insect spectra be changed compared to terbufos which only controls corn rootworms?
4. How will the incorporation of a nitrile affect the economics of the manufacture of the compound compared to other corn-soil insecticides?

Patent Background

Since, organophosphorus insecticides have been articles of commerce for about 35-40 years, it was necessary to carefully examine the patent literature to determine if there was prior art germane to this work. There were two related patents in this area (3,4) and they are associated with the structures shown below.

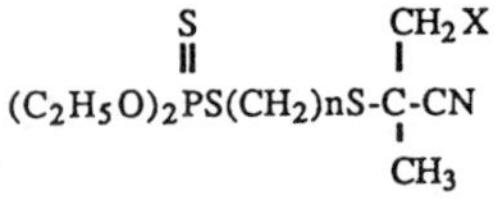

$$(C_2H_5O)_2\overset{S}{\overset{\|}{P}}S(CH_2)nS\text{-}\underset{CH_3}{\overset{CH_2X}{C}}\text{-}CN$$

X=halogen, n=1 Ref. 3
X=H, n=2 Ref. 4

Synthetic Route

In order to prepare the desired product, the intermediate in below was required.

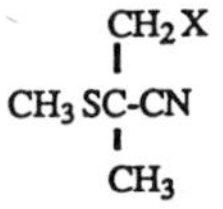

$$CH_3SC\underset{CH_3}{\overset{CH_2X}{}}\text{-}CN$$

X=H or halogen

For these intermediates, the three routes depicted below were utilized for the preparation of both the novel compounds as well as those required for the prior art examples.

$$1.\quad CH_3SNa + (CH_3)_2(CN)CX \xrightarrow[PhCH_3\ PTC]{DMF\ or} (CH_3)_2(CN)C\text{-}SCH_3$$

X = Br OR Mesyl

$$2.\quad (CH_3)_2CHCN \xrightarrow[2)\ CH_3SSCH_3]{1)\ LDA\ -78^\circ C} (CH_3)_2C(CN)SCH_3$$

$$3.\quad H_2C{=}CCH_3CN + CH_3SCl \xrightarrow{CH_2Cl_2} ClH_2S\text{-}C(CH_3)(SCH_3)\text{-}CN$$

For the first reaction scheme, the bromo nitrile was prepared via radical bromination of the appropriate nitrile, and the mesityl ester was prepared by treatment of acetone cyanohydrin. With mesityl chloride in the presence of an amine base. The next two routes are sufficiently clear to require no further explanation.

Final synthesis of the desired product is shown via the two equation reaction sequence shown below.

$$CH_3SC(CH_3)_2 + SO_2Cl_2 \text{ or NCS} \xrightarrow{CH_2Cl_2} \underset{\mathbf{I}}{ClCH_2SC(CH_3)_2CN}$$

$$\mathbf{I} + (C_2H_5O)_2\text{-}\overset{S}{\overset{\|}{P}}\text{-}SNa \xrightarrow{THF} (C_2H_5O)_2\text{-}\overset{S}{\overset{\|}{P}}\text{-}SCH_2SC(CH_3)_2CN$$

Primary Insecticide Screening Data

The laboratory testing of these molecules was carried out on four insects, the housefly, *Musca domestica*, M.d., the pea aphid, *Acrythosiphon pisum*, A.P., the corn earworm, *Heliothis zea*, H.z., and the two-spotted spidermite, *Triticum urticae*, T.u. In all toxicity test evaluations, parathion was employed as a standard. Therefore, any compound having a Toxicity Index (TI) of 100 is equal to parathion. The data for the laboratory toxicity evaluation of these molecules are collected in Tables 1 and 2.

Examination of the data shows that the first entry in the Table 1 had exceptionally high activity on aphids and mites with TI values of 1750 and 3192, respectively. For houseflies and corn earworms this compound was less active than the standard parathion. Increases in size of the substituent R significantly reduced the activity against all insects except the corn earworm where a major reduction only occurred when the hydrogen was replaced by ethyl and larger groups.

The molecules in Table 2 shown below have a substituent beta to the nitrile group. For comparison, two of the molecules from Table 1 have been included.

Table 1. Insecticide Evaluation of some S-cyanoalkyl Phosphorodithioates

$$(C_2H_5O)_2\text{-}\overset{\overset{\displaystyle S}{\|}}{P}\text{-}S\underset{\underset{\displaystyle R}{|}}{C}H\text{-}SC(CH_3)_2CN$$

R	Toxicity Index (parathion = 100) M.d.	A.p.	H.z.	T.u.
H	56	1750	16	3192
CH_3	13	66	16	496
C_2H_5	8	56	5	438
n-C_3H_7	4	46	+	120
SCH_3	2	103	0	68
terbufos	19	85	14	617

Table 2. Insecticide Evaluation of some S-cyanoalkyl Phosphorodithioates

$$(C_2H_5O)_2\text{-}\overset{\overset{\displaystyle S}{\|}}{P}\text{-}S\underset{\underset{\displaystyle X}{|}}{C}HSC(CH_3)(CN)CH_2Y$$

X	Y	Toxicity Index (parathion = 100) M.d.	A.p.	H.z.	T.u.
H	H	56	1750	16	3192
H	Cl	19	60	3	3341
CH_3	H	13	66	16	496
CH_3	Cl	3	28	4	112
CH_3	C_2H_5	12	32	6	106
H	SCH_3	15	309	+	267
terbufos		19	85	14	617

In general compounds possessing a substituent (Cl, C_2H_5, SCH_3) beta to the nitrile substituent are less active against these insects than compounds with only hydrogens in this position. The only exception is for the first two entries in Table 2 where the chlorinated derivative appears to be somewhat more active on mites than its unchlorinated analogue.

Laboratory Diabrotica jar test

Since these molecules were initially prepared to be used as a soil insecticide, it was necessary to evaluate them in a laboratory bioassay to determine if any of them had sufficient activity to merit a field evaluation as a soil insecticide for control of insects injurious to field corn in the Midwest. The protocol to evaluate potential soil insecticides follows that described previously(5). Briefly, it consists of a 4 oz. jar containing 20 g of insecticide treated soil containing two cornseeds moistened by damp vermiculite. Into this jar are placed 20 eggs of the Southern corn rootworm, *Diabrotica undecimpunctata howardi*. After about 10 days the jar contents are examined for the presence of live larvae. A secondary assessment of feeding damage by the hatched larvae to the roots of the germinated corn seedlings is also made. In order to quantitate the results, comparisons are made with number of live larvae in the untreated control. For example, if the number of larvae in a treated jar is equal to the number in the untreated control than a score of 4 is given. If a treated jar has no live larvae then a score of 0 is given. Numerical values therefore, of 1-3 are given for treated jars that have live larvae in them that are less than the untreated check but greater than zero. To determine the persistence of a new compound, the soil is aged for periods of time up to 8 weeks.

Since terbufos is utilized broadly in the Midwest to control *Diabrotica* species associated with corn, it served as the standard in the laboratory assay. Table 3 gives data for the performance of terbufos in the laboratory bioassay at 1.0 and 0.3 ppm.

Table 3. Performance of Terbufos in a Laboratory *Diabrotica* Jar Test

Concentration	Time (weeks)			
(ppm)	0	2	4	8
1.0	0	0	0	0
0.3	0	0	0	1

Only at the end of the eighth week are there a few live larvae as indicated by a numerical value of 1.

In Table 4 below are data for evaluation of the three best compounds in the *Diabrotica* jar test.

Table 4. Performance of Three S-Cyanoalkyl Phosphorodithioates in a Laboratory Jar Test

$$(C_2H_5O)_2\text{-}\overset{\overset{\displaystyle S}{\|}}{P}\text{-}S\underset{\underset{\displaystyle X}{|}}{C}HSC(CH_3)(CN)CH_2Y$$

Concentration P.P.M.	Time (weeks) 0	2	4	8	Structure X	Y
1.0	0	4	-	-	H	H
0.3	-	-	-	-		
1.0	0	0	0	0	CH_3	H
0.3	0	0	1	4		
1.0	0	0	0	0	CH_3	Cl
0.3	2	3	3	3		

Examination of these data clearly shows that none of the three compounds is as effective as terbufos in the jar test. Perhaps the most interesting aspect of this data is the relative soil efficacy of the second compound compared to the first. The substitution of a methyl group for a hydrogen between the two sulfur atoms greatly enhances the soil activity of this molecule. Quantitation of the relative soil stability of these three molecules as measured by the bioassay data are collected in Table 5 using a pseudo first order kinetic analysis of the data.

Table 5. Estimated Soil Persistence of Three S-Cyanoalkyl Phosphorodithioates

$$(C_2H_5O)_2\text{-}\overset{\overset{\displaystyle S}{\|}}{P}\text{-}S\underset{\underset{\displaystyle R}{|}}{C}H\text{-}SC(CH_3)_2X$$

Structure R	X	Soil Half Life $T_{1/2}$ (days)
H	CH_3	>35
H	CN	5
CH_3	CN	10
C_2H_5	CN	20

Clearly terbufos, the first entry in the Table, is the most persistent with a $T_{1/2}$ of more than 35 days. Alkyl substitution on the carbon between the sulfur atoms of those molecules containing a nitrile group increases the soil persistence. Still, none are as persistent as terbufos. Therefore, the presence of a nitrile in these molecules, as was previously discussed for the Atrazine/Bladex-triazine relationship, decreases the soil persistence of these organophosphorodithioates compared to terbufos.

Field Evaluation

Despite their weaker performance in the laboratory Diabrotica jar test when compared to terbufos, two of the best compounds of Table 4 were taken to the Midwest for evaluation as soil insecticides for control of corn rootworm. The compounds were placed in the soil at planting as a band application at 1 lb/A. During late July and early August the roots were evaluated for corn rootworms damage. A summary of those tests is collected in Table 6 along with terbufos as a standard.

Table 6. Field Performance of Two S-Cyanoalkyl Phosphorodithioates and Terbufos

$$(C_2H_5O)_2\text{-}\overset{\overset{\displaystyle S}{\|}}{P}\text{-}S\underset{\underset{\displaystyle X}{|}}{C}HSC(CH_3)(CN)CH_2Y$$

Structure		Site				
X	Y	1	2	3	4	5
CH_3	H	2.7	2.9	2.4	2.0	2.7
CH_3	Cl	2.9	3.2	---	2.4	3.1
terbufos		2.5	3.5	2.5	2.3	2.4
Untreated		3.2	4.3	5.2	5.2	5.6

Two conclusions can be drawn from the data in the table. Firstly, the nitrile containing phosphorodithioates of this study gave insect control in the order previously estimated from the laboratory screen in that the nonhalogenated molecule gave slightly better control than its halogenated analogue. Secondly, the nonhalogenated nitrile derivative gave control that was comparable to terbufos. In all cases, root ratings for the first compound in the table averaged below 3.0 which is considered to be the economic threshold for this insect.

Conclusions

This work reports on the effect of incorporation of a nitrile group in to terbufos and what effect this group had on its laboratory insecticidal activity and field performance. With respect to the question regarding efficacy, we demonstrated that the addition of a nitrile moiety did not markedly reduce the field performance as compared to terbufos. This was despite a significantly shorter soil half-life as estimated from the laboratory data in the Diabrotica jar test. With respect to the question of the effect on the vapor pressure of incorporation of a nitrile into terbufos, the compound $(C_2H_5O)_2P(S)SCH(CH_3)SC(CH_3)_2CN$, had an estimated vapor pressure which is 10-fold lower (3.0×10^{-5} mm) than the measured vapor pressure of terbufos. With respect to alteration of insect spectra, especially those insects injurious to Midwest field corn, laboratory studies indicated that like terbufos, only corn rootworms would be expected to be controlled. Finally, with regards to the estimated cost of manufacture, the addition of a nitrile group to terbufos increases the cost to approximately $2-2.25/lb. This is greater than that for the manufacture of terbufos, but is still competitive with the other corn-soil insecticides in current use today.

Literature Cited

1. Sanborn, J. R. U.S. Patent 4 505 904 1985.
2. Sanborn, J. R. U.S. Patent 4 536 497 1985.
3. Hoffmann, H.; Hammann, I. U. S. Patent 3 706 820 1972.
4. Godfrey, K. L.; Saul, G.A. U.S. Patent 2 908 604 1959.
5. Gemrich II, E. G.; Goldsberry, D.M. J. Econ. Ent. 1982, 220-222.

RECEIVED May 12, 1987

Chapter 20

Diphenylchloronitroethane Insecticides

Joel R. Coats, Laura L. Karr, Rebecca L. Fryer, and Hunter S. Beard

Department of Entomology, Iowa State University, Ames, IA 50011

Insecticidal activity of chloronitroalkanes was predicted on the basis of structure-activity relationships. Two series of new bis(substituted-phenyl) chloronitroalkanes were synthesized and evaluated for insecticidal activity. The synthetic pathway proceeded through phenylnitroethanols and diphenylnitroethanes as intermediates. Final products were 1,1-bis (substituted-phenyl)-2-chloro-2-nitroethanes and 1,1-bis(substituted-phenyl)-2,2-dichloro-2-nitroethanes. Aromatic substituents were selected from alkyl, alkoxy, and halogen moieties. Following purifications and confirmation of structures, the compounds were bioassayed against insects. The two series were compared for potency, as were various combinations of X and Y substituents. Adult female house flies (*Musca domestica*), mosquito larvae (*Aedes aegypti*), western corn rootworm (*Diabrotica virgifera virgifera*) and German cockroach (*Blattella germanica*) have been tested. In general, the mono-chloro series is more toxic than the di-chloro series. Five of the mono-chloro analogs are 8-10 times more potent than pyrethrins and 6-7 times more toxic than methoxychlor to the house fly.

Insecticides of the "DDT-type" have potent excitatory activity in the peripheral nervous system of insects (Narahashi, 1979). For DDT, X = Y = R_1 = R_2 = R_3 = Cl in the structure below.

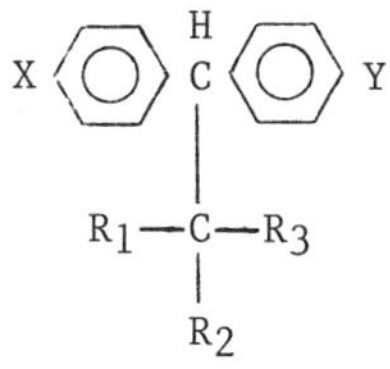

X–C₆H₄–C(H)–C₆H₄–Y, with the central C bonded to R_1—C—R_3 (with R_2 below)

0097-6156/87/0355-0217$06.00/0
© 1987 American Chemical Society

Many analogs have been made since the initial disclosure of insecticidal activity (Müller, 1940). Major synthetic efforts have been made over the years (reviewed by Coats, 1982) and several commercially successful compounds were discovered, e.g., methoxychlor, perthane, rhothane, dicofol. The nitroalkanes prolan (or 1,1-bis-bis(p,p'-dichlorophenyl)-2-nitropropane), bulan and dilan were among the commercial products.

Structure-activity studies have indicated that X and Y groups of proper size and shape with appropriate combinations of R_1, R_2, and R_3 groups act as good insecticides. However, steric factors alone may not account for optimal potency. Neurotoxicological studies on insect nerve indicate that increasing electronegativity in the aliphatic moiety may enhance insecticidal activity (Brown et al., 1981). Nitroalkane analogs possess excellent activity as do chloro, dichloro, and trichloro alkanes, while pure alkanes are only moderately good compounds. Trifluoro, pentafluoro, or chlorodifluoro alkanes are rather poor insecticides, apparently too electronegative of an aliphatic moiety or too polar to penetrate the insect cuticle well (Abu-El-Haj et al., 1979). Combinations of nitro and halogen groups R_1, R_2, and R_3 have been attempted by Hass et al. (1951) and by Skerrett and Woodcock (1952). The latter group made 3 p,p'-dichlorophenyl haloalkanes with disappointing results: the 2-chloro-2-nitroethane and 2,2-dichloro-2-nitroethane were not insecticidal, but the 2-chloro-2-nitropropane was as effective as the 2-nitropropane. Deactivation via dehydrochlorination of the aliphatic moiety occurs more rapidly when the X and Y aromatic substituents are e^- withdrawing but occurs much more slowly with e^- donating aromatic groups (Metcalf and Fukuto, 1968). Electron donating substituents (at least one) on the rings also provide for greater insecticidal potency (Holan, 1969; Metcalf et al., 1971; Coats et al., 1977). Hence, the only 2-chloro-2-nitroethane synthesized by Skerrett and Woodcock lacked insecticidal activity, probably due to poor stability and low intrinsic toxicity, both resulting from the p,p'-dichloro substituents. Hass et al. (1951) also made some 2-chloro-2-nitroethanes with chlorophenyl-, tolyl-, or unsubstituted phenyl rings, but they gave no data on insecticidal activity.

Other synthesis and structure-activity progress with diphenylnitroalkane insecticides include work by Jacob et al., 1951; Holan 1971a; 1971b; Boehner et al., 1974; Kaufman and Strong, 1975; Lee et al., 1977; and Coats, 1983.

Synthesis Pathway

A 3-step reaction pathway was followed, using reactions previously described. Reactions I and II are described by Lee, et al., 1977. Reaction III was adapted from Tindall (1943; 1946).

Reaction I

$$X\text{-}C_6H_4\text{-}CHO + CH_3NO_2 \xrightarrow[\text{DMSO}]{\text{r.t., DBN}} X\text{-}C_6H_4\text{-}CH(OH)\text{-}CH_2\text{-}NO_2$$

Reaction II

$$X\text{-}C_6H_4\text{-}CH(OH)\text{-}CH_2NO_2 + C_6H_5\text{-}Y \xrightarrow[H_2SO_4/HOAc]{0°C} X\text{-}C_6H_4\text{-}CH(C_6H_4\text{-}Y)\text{-}CH_2NO_2$$

Reaction III

$$X\text{-}C_6H_4\text{-}CH(C_6H_4\text{-}Y)\text{-}CH_2NO_2 \xrightarrow[Cl_2/4°C]{KOH/CH_3OH\ aq.} X\text{-}C_6H_4\text{-}CH(C_6H_4\text{-}Y)\text{-}CH(Cl)NO_2$$

Series 1

In Reaction I, a large excess of nitromethane was added to maximize efficient use of the benzaldehyde and minimize clean up of the crude reaction mixture (an aqueous $NaHSO_3$ wash helped remove any unreacted benzaldehyde).

The base used by Lee et al. (1977) and Coats (1983) was 1,5-diazabicyclo-[4.3.0] non-5-ene (DBN); numerous other bases have also been utilized, e.g., sodium methoxide, sodium bicarbonate, triethylamine, KOH, pyridine (Worrall, 1934; Hass et al., 1951; Kamlet, 1939). The carbinol intermediates were not purified prior to use in the condensation reaction. The acid used was a mixture of conc. sulfuric and glacial acetic acids (ratios ranged from 4:1 to 1:3).

In Reaction II, the crude carbinol was mixed with a 3-6 fold excess of the substituted benzene and dripped into cold acid mixture, with stirring. A 4:1 ratio of sulfuric (conc.) and acetic (glacial) acids was determined to be optimal for most condensations attempted. The reaction was allowed to warm to room temperature after 1 h, and it was then poured over ice. Following extraction with diethyl ether, washing with $NaHCO_3$, drying with anhydrous Na_2SO_4, filtration, and rotary evaporation, the product was purified and characterized before further use.

Reaction III was initiated by dissolving the diphenyl-nitroethane in methanol and adding it to an aqueous solution of KOH. Chlorine gas was introduced at 4°C (Tindall, 1943; 1946), and was added until the pH of the reaction fell to 5-6. Mixtures of mono- and di-chloro nitroethanes were formed, often requiring separation by silica gel column chromatography.

Purification

Every nitrocarbinol, nitroethane, chloronitroethane and dichloro-nitroethane synthesized was worked up to eliminate the solvent and as much of the unreacted materials as possible. Diethyl ether/water extractions were utilized, with a $NaHSO_3$ wash of the carbinol to remove excess benzaldehyde, or a $NaHCO_3$ wash of the diphenylnitroethane to remove excess acetic acid. Anhydrous Na_2SO_4 was used to dry the ether extract. Column chromatography with silica gel and hexane/diethyl ether or hexane/benzene solvent systems were used to obtain pure samples of the insecticides in Series 1 and Series 2.

Characterization

Three techniques were used to determine the structure of each chemical made. For each new analog, an ^{1}H NMR (nuclear magnetic resonance) analysis of a 25 mg sample was run on a Nicolet 300 MHz NMR spectrometer. The sample was dissolved in $CDCl_3$ with tetramethylsilane (TMS) as a reference.

^{1}H-NMR information is provided here for the aliphatic protons on the central nitroethane skeleton, for 1-p-ethylphenyl-1-p-ethoxyphenyl-2-nitroethane, its monochloro derivative (compound 1e) and its dichloro derivative (compound 2e) as typical of the compounds synthesized. Ethylphenyl ethoxyphenyl-2-nitroethane: α-H at δ 4.7-4.9 (triplet), β-H's at δ 4.9-5.0 (doublet); 1e: α-H at δ 4.6-4.8 (2 doublets); β-H at δ 6.4 (doublet); 2e: α-H at δ 4.8 (singlet).

Two uncorrected melting points observed were for 1,1-bis(p-ethoxyphenyl)-2,2-dichloro-2-nitroethane at 75-77°C and for 1-(p-methylphenyl)-1-(p-ethoxyphenyl)-2,2-dichloro-2-nitroethane at 51-54°C.

After a chemical structure had been confirmed, TLC (thin layer chromatography) was used to monitor the purity of the chemicals. The TLC solvent systems hexane and diethyl ether (8:2) or hexane and benzene (1:1) best separated chemicals on F_{254} silica gel TLC plates. The Series 2 compounds had the highest R_fs, followed by the Series 1 compounds, and then the nitroethanes. The TLC plates were then sprayed with a solution made from zinc chloride and diphenylamine (1:1), dissolved in acetone. After the plates were sprayed, they were placed in a 125°C oven overnight. Generally, carbinols turned green, nitroethanes turned pink, Series 1 and Series 2 compounds turned purple. Color and R_f on the plate confirmed the identity of a product.

Mass spectrometry was also employed to confirm the structure of one Series 1 and one Series 2 compound, utilizing a Finnegan 4000 direct exposure probe mass spectrometer.

Bioassay

Toxicity of the compounds was examined in four types of insects: house fly (*Musca domestica*), mosquito (*Aedes aegypti*), corn rootworm beetles (*Diabrotica virgifera virgifera* and *Diabrotica undecimpunctata howardi*) and the German cockroach (*Blattella* germanica). Topical toxicities were determined for adult female house flies (susceptible Orlando Regular stock) and field-collected adult western corn rootworms (D. v. virgifera). Toxicity to fourth instar Aedes aegypti (Liverpool strain) larvae was also investigated.

In examining topical toxicity, known concentrations of the compounds were applied in one µl of acetone solution to the abdominal venters of anesthesized insects using a syringe micro-applicator. Ten insects received each treatment, and treatments were replicated three times. The standards for comparison were pyrethrins and methoxychlor for house flies. Carbaryl and methoxychlor were used for rootworms, and chlorpyrifos was used against the cockroach. Mortality was recorded at 24 h following exposure. Insects were considered dead when a tactile stimulus produced no significant movement. LD_{50} values were computed using the Spearman-Karber procedure (Hamilton et al., 1977).

Toxicity to larval mosquitoes was examined by applying known concentrations of the compounds in one ml of acetone solution to 4-oz. glass jars containing 100 ml of distilled water and 20 early fourth-instar mosquito larvae. Treatments were replicated three times and chlorpyrifos was used as a standard for comparison. Mortality was recorded at 24 h following initial exposure to the compounds. Larvae were considered dead when tapping on the glass containers failed to elicit swimming movements. LC_{50} values were computed by the Spearman-Karber procedure.

Results and Discussion

The results of the insect bioassay trials are presented in Tables I and II. The data show that the monochloro derivatives (Series 1 - Table I) are much more active than the dichloro compounds (Series 2 - Table II). In both series, the p,p'-dichlorophenyl analogs, made earlier by other investigators, listed above, were the poorest insecticides of the series. Deployment of an ethoxy group on one ring resulted in insect toxicity increases of 10-20 fold. The best compounds were the Cl-OC_2H_5, the CH_3-OC_2H_5, the C_2H_5-OC_2H_5, and the C_2H_5O-OC_2H_5 analogs. The poorest insecticides, other than the Cl-Cl derivatives, were the F-OC_2H_5 analogs.

Comparison of the monochloro series with standard compounds indicate that several of the new chemicals possess insecticidal activity comparable or superior to some commercial products.

Toxicity to house fly is obviously quite good. Moderate efficacy is demonstrated against the corn rootworm beetles and mosquito larvae. For an insecticide of the prolan/DDT class, the potency demonstrated against the wild strain German cockroach is quite remarkable. Preliminary tests on the larval stage corn rootworm revealed soil activity of a monochloro compound, unlike most previously reported chemicals in this class. Overall, the spectrum of activity is quite broad, although other categories of insect pests must still be tested (e.g., lepidopteran larvae).

The physical properties of these compounds are somewhat different from prolan, DDT, methoxychlor, perthane, and other related chemicals. Water solubility and polarity are considerably

Table I. Toxicity of monochloronitroethanes to insects by topical application or in water

Series 1

$$X\text{-}C_6H_4\text{-}CH(C_6H_4\text{-}Y)\text{-}CHCl\text{-}NO_2$$

No.	X	Y	24 h-LD_{50} (μg/insect) House fly	Corn rootworm beetle	Cockroach	24 h-LC_{50} (ppm) Mosquito larva
1a	F	OC_2H_5	0.20	2.71	34	0.22
1b	Cl	OC_2H_5	0.08	0.58	6.3	0.04
1c	Br	OC_2H_5	----	----	---	0.02
1d	CH_3	OC_2H_5	0.07	0.54	6.3	0.03
1e	C_2H_5	OC_2H_5	0.08	0.25	1.5	0.01
1f	$CH(CH_3)_2$	OC_2H_5	0.07	0.29	2.5	0.03
1g	$C(CH_3)_2$	OC_2H_5	0.54	----	---	0.46
1h	OC_3H_3	OC_2H_5	0.05	0.18	2.0	0.03
1i	Cl	Cl	1.8	2.55	---	----
	pyrethrins		0.69	----	0.89	------
	methoxychlor		0.50	0.35	>100	------
	chlorpyrifos		----	----	0.86	0.0026
	carbaryl		>10	0.02	>100	------

Table II. Toxicity of bis(substituted phenyl) dichloronitroethanes to insects by topical application or in water

Series 2

X–C₆H₄–CH(–C₆H₄–Y)–C(Cl)₂–NO_2

No.	X	Y	24 h-LD_{50} (µg/insect) House fly	Corn rootworm beetle	Cockroach	24 h-LC_{50} (ppm) Mosquito larva
2a	F	OC_2H_5	10	100	>100	0.46
2b	Cl	OC_2H_5	0.55	59	>100	0.38
2c	Br	OC_2H_5	1.71	23	>100	0.19
2d	CH_3	OC_2H_5	0.63	5.4	>100	0.07
2e	C_2H_5	OC_2H_5	0.86	4.0	>100	0.06
2f	$CH(CH_3)_2$	OC_2H_5	1.13	4.3	>100	1.13
2g	OC_2H_5	OC_2H_5	0.50	4.3	>100	0.06
2h	Cl	Cl	2.95	24	---	----
	pyrethrins		0.69	----	0.89	------
	methoxychlor		0.50	0.35	100	------
	chlorpyrifos		----	----	0.86	0.0026
	carbaryl		10	0.02	100	------

higher, with lower lipophilicity apparent as well. These properties may approach a more effective optimum for rapid and thorough penetration through insect cuticle, combined with charge distribution and steric dimensions for excellent insecticidal potency at the site of action (sodium gate in the peripheral nervous system).

Research remains to be done on the residual activity and mammalian toxicity of the chloronitroethane insecticides, but our initial studies on design, directed synthesis, and bioassay indicate there is clearly potential for those compounds in insect control.

Acknowledgments

The authors thank the Iowa High Technology Council for funding portions of this research. Tracy Hageman and Wael Mahmoud are cited for valuable technical assistance on this project.

Literature Cited

1. Abu-El-Haj, S.; Fahmy, M. A. H.; Fukuto, T.R. J. Agric. Food Chem. 1979, 27, 258-261.
2. Boehner, B.; Dawes, D.; Meyer. Ger. Offen. 2 404 914 (to Ciba Geigy, A. G.), 1974.
3. Brown, D. D.; Metcalf, R. L.; Sternburg, J. G.; Coats, J. R. Pestic. Biochem. Physiol. 1981, 15, 43-57.
4. Coats, J. R. In Insecticide Mode of Action; Coats, J. R., Ed.; Academic: New York, 1982; p 29-43.
5. Coats, J. R. J. Environ. Sci. Health 1983, B 18, 173-188.
6. Coats, J. R.; Metcalf, R. L.; Kapoor, I. P. J. Agric. Food Chem. 1977, 25, 859-868.
7. Hamilton, M. A.; Russo, R. C.; Thurston, R. V. Environ. Sci. Technol. 1977, 11, 714-719. Correction 1978, 12, 417.
8. Hass, H. B.; Neher, M. B.; Blickenstaff, R. T. Ind. Eng. Chem. 1951, 43, 2875-2878.
9. Holan, G. Nature (London) 1969, 221, 1025-1029.
10. Holan, G. Bull. W. H. O. 1971a, 44 355-362.
11. Holan, G. Nature (London) 1971b, 232, 644-647.
12. Jacob, T. A.; Backman, G. B.; Hass, H. B. J. Org. Chem. 1951, 16, 1572-1576.
13. Kamlet, J. U.S. Patent 2 151 517, 1939.
14. Kaufman, H. A.; Strong, J. G. Ger. Offen. 2 451 137 (to Mobil Oil Corp.), 1975.
15. Lee, A.; Metcalf, R. L.; Williams, J. W.; Hirwe, A. S.; Sanborn, J. R.; Coats, J. R.; Fukuto, T. R. Pestic. Biochem. Physiol. 1977, 7, 426-436.
16. Metcalf, R. L.; Fukuto, T. R. Bull. W. H. O. 1968, 38, 633-647.
17. Metcalf, R. L.; Kapoor, I. P.; Hirwe, A. S. Bull. W. H. O. 1971, 44 363-374.
18. Müller, P. Swiss Patent 226 180 (to J. R. Geigy, A. G.), 1940.
19. Narahashi, T. In Neurotoxicology of Insecticides and Pheromones; Narahashi, T., Ed.; Plenum: New York, 1979; p 211-243.

20. Skerrett, E. J.; Woodcock, D. Insecticidal activity and chemical constitution. Part V. Synthesis of some di-p-chlorophenyl-alkanes; J. Chem. Soc., 1952; p 3308-3312.
21. Tindall, J. B. U.S. Patent 2 309 806 (to Commercial Solvents Corp.), 1943.
22. Tindall, J. B. U. S. Patent 2 397 384 (to Commercial Solvents Corp.), 1946.
23. Worrall, D. E. J. Am. Chem. Soc. 1934, 56 1556-1558.

RECEIVED May 15, 1987

Chapter 21

Fluorinated Sulfonamides

A New Class of Delayed-Action Toxicants for Fire Ant Control

Robert K. Vander Meer, Clifford S. Lofgren, and David F. Williams

Agricultural Research Service, U.S. Department of Agriculture, Insects Affecting Man and Animals Research Laboratory, P.O. Box 14565, Gainesville, FL 32604

Fluorinated sulfonamides were discovered to have the delayed toxic activity required to control the fire ant, *Solenopsis invicta*, a medical and agricultural pest ant species. The large number of fluorinated sulfonamide analogues and derivatives available offer a wide variety of activities (delayed and rapid) and solubilities (water to soybean oil). These compounds were effective against fire ants in laboratory and field tests and one of the compounds is being commercialized. Certain compounds have been demonstrated to be good control agents against other ant species, cockroaches, and mosquitoes.

The fire ants, *Solenopsis richteri* and *S. invicta*, were accidentally imported from South America, (probably through the port of Buenos Aires) into the Mobile, Alabama area around 1910 and 1935, respectively. Fire ants normally infest new areas through mating flights during which the queens may fly up to 12 miles (1). However, it was evident from early surveys (2) that spread of the fire ants was accelerated greatly by man through the transportation of nursery stock. Soil on plants harbored new queens or incipient colonies and these were transported throughout the southern United States. Once isolated populations were established they spread locally through mating flights until all the infestations coalesced. *S. richteri* proved to be less competitive or adaptable than *S. invicta* and now occupies only a small enclave in northeastern Mississippi and northwestern Alabama. In spite of federal-state quarantines, recent discoveries of *S. invicta* infestations in Tennessee, Oklahoma and New Mexico highlight the fact that this fire ant has not yet reached the limit of its northern or western expansion (Homer Collins, APHIS, USDA, personal communication, 1987). A further complicating factor in determining the fire ant's spread was the discovery of hybridization between the two imported fire ants (3). The reproductively viable hybrid has a large, but as yet undefined, range in northern Mississippi, Alabama, and Georgia (Ross, K. G., Vander Meer, R. K., Fletcher, D. J. C., and Vargo,E.

This chapter is not subject to U.S. copyright.
Published 1987, American Chemical Society

L., Evolution, in press; and *Diffie, S., +Vander Meer, R. K., and *Bass, M. H., *University of Georgia and +USDA). How the hybrid strain will affect the limits of fire ant expansion is under investigation.

Medical Impact. Fire ants have been likened to weeds since they have a high reproductive capacity and their ecology and biology are ideally suited to take advantage of disturbed ecosystems (4). Since man is the greatest disturber of the environment, it follows that man-ant interactions are inevitable. Essentially, everywhere man lives and plays (backyards, playgrounds, parks, golf courses, etc.) or works (gardens and all types of agriculture) become disturbed habitats. The fact that a mound may contain as many as 230,000 workers, and many infested areas commonly have 125 to 150 mounds per hectare insures that there will always be a great deal of contact between fire ants and people in the infested areas (5).

The common name "fire ant" is derived from its painful sting, which causes a burning sensation followed by the formation of a sterile pustule within 24 hours. Approximately 30% of the people in the infested areas are stung by fire ants in a given year (6) and of these 0.61% experience systemic anaphylaxis (7). The venom of fire ants is composed primarily of 2-methyl 6-alkyl or alkenyl piperidine alkaloids (8). These alkaloids cause pustule formation because they are necrotoxic but they also have many other physiological effects (9). Less than 1% of the venom is protein but this small amount can cause severe allergic reactions and occasionally death (5,7,10).

Economic Impact. It is believed that fire ant damage to agricultural crops was masked before the late 1970's because of the prior use of residual insecticides, such as chlordane for control of other insect pests. Since these chemicals are highly toxic to fire ants, they undoubtedly kept these fields free of infestations (6). Current research indicates that fire ants cause economically important losses of soybeans, potatoes, citrus, eggplants, okra, and other vegetable crops. In addition, fire ants have killed newborn calves, pigs, and chickens, attacked the young or eggs of numerous bird species, amphibians and rabbits, damaged highways, and electrical equipment; and can be a pest in homes and hospitals (11).

Control Requirements. Historically, the control of the imported fire ants, S. invicta and S. richteri, in the United States dates back to 1938 when calcium cyanide dust treatments were used to treat individual colonies infesting agricultural land near Mobile, AL (12). A concern with fire ants escalated along with their population until, in 1957, the United States Congress appropriated money for a Federal-State Imported Fire Ant Control Program. The first chemicals used in this program were residual applications of heptachlor or dieldrin (13). These toxicants were replaced in 1963 because of environmental concerns with a bait toxicant system using mirex, which required the use of much less active ingredient (13). Unfortunately, registrations of mirex were cancelled at the end of 1977 because of residues in environmental organisms and possible carcinogenicity (14). This regulatory action resulted in an intensive search for other toxicants suitable for fire ant baits (15).

The difficulty in finding suitable insecticides for use in baits for fire ants is directly related to the behavior and ecology of the insect. Foraging worker ants represent only a small fraction of a colony's population. Once a foraging ant locates food, other workers are recruited to the food source with the trail pheromone (16). The foraging ants store food in their crops, and through regurgitation and food exchange (trophallaxis), they quickly disperse the material to other members of the colony (5). Because of this system of food gathering which is followed by ingestion, storage and regurgitation, two major qualifications for a toxicant become apparent. If the toxicant acts too quickly, the foraging workers will die before they can distribute the material to other members of the colony and ultimately to the queen. Therefore, delayed toxicity is required. Tests with dyed soybean oil indicated that complete colony distribution is achieved within 24-72 hr. Secondly, the process of trophallaxis greatly dilutes a toxicant (a mature colony may contain more than 230,000 workers) making it necessary to have delayed toxicity over a wide range of dosages (preferably > 100) (17).

TABLE 1. Classification System for Imported Fire Ant Bait Toxicants

Class	Definition
I	Compounds that give insufficient kill at the preliminary concentrations (less than 90% at the end of the test period).
II	Compounds that kill too quickly at the higher concentrations but give insufficient kill at the lower concentrations, that is, higher concentrations give 15% or more kill after 24 hr and 90-100% at the end of the test period, but lower concentrations give less than 90% kill at the end of the test period.
III	Compounds that show no greater than a 9-fold difference between the minimum and maximum concentrations that exhibit delayed toxicity.[a]
IV	Compounds that showed at least a 10-fold but not greater than 99-fold difference between the minimum and maximum concentrations that exhibited delayed toxicity.
V	Compounds that show at least a 100-fold difference between the minimum and maximum concentrations that exhibit delayed toxicity.

[a]Delayed toxicity is defined as mortality of less than 15% after 24 hr and more than 89% at the end of the test period.

As of the end of 1986, our laboratory had screened 6,882 chemicals for the delayed toxicity required for fire ant baits. The following procedures were used: The toxicant was dissolved to the desired concentration in either soybean oil or honey-water (1:1) depending on its solubility. Test groups of 20 worker ants were allowed to feed for 24 hr on cotton swabs saturated with the formulation. After 48 hr, the ants were fed unadulterated soybean oil. Mortality counts were made at 1, 2, 3, 6, 8, 10, 14, 17, and 21 days after the initial exposure. Each material was tested at 3 concentrations: 1, 0.1, and 0.01% (18).

All chemicals tested were classified according to the scheme shown in Table I. Class I compounds are inactive while Class II materials are good toxicants but do not have the required delayed toxicity. Class III compounds have delayed action, but the concentration range of their activity is too narrow. The type of activity we are looking for in a toxicant is exemplified by a Class IV or V response, i.e., it exhibits delayed toxicity over a wide range of concentrations.

As expected, most (86.6%) of the 8,662 compounds screened fell into the non-toxic Class I category. Less than 0.5% were Classes IV and V.

Fluoroaliphatic Sulfonamide Insecticidal Activity

In the search for delayed-action formulations we experimented with several controlled release techniques (19). One of these projects involved pendant toxicants, in which a fast acting insecticide was chemically bonded to a polymer backbone (20). The polymer-pesticide linkage was in theory supposed to deactivate the toxicant until the organism released the free toxicant via metabolic processes. Few insecticides have functional groups suitable for this purpose; however, our screening program had uncovered several fluorinated primary alcohols active against fire ants (21). One of these compounds was used as a model insecticide to test the pendant-toxicant technique. Poor solubility of the products in soybean oil led to the use of commercially available fluorinated surfactants to aid in the dissolution of the pendant-toxicant. Standard control bioassays uncovered the fact that the fluorinated surfactants themselves had delayed-action toxicity against fire ants. Further investigation led to the discovery of fluorinated sulfonamides, a new class of insecticide with the general structure $R_fSO_2NR_1R_2$.

Several fluorine containing compounds have been shown to have delayed-action toxicity against the fire ant (21,22). One of these, tetrahydro-5,5-dimethyl-2(IH)-pyrmidinone(3-(4-trifluoromethylphenyl)-1-(2-(4-trifluoromethyl) phenyl)ethenyl)-2-propenylidene) hydrazone, has been commercialized (23). In another approach fluoroacetyl derivatives and analogues were designed as pro-insecticides (24). Although there is precedence for delayed-action fluorine containing insecticides, the discovery of the fluorinated sulfones provides a class of compounds with tremendous structural diversity (25).

Synthesis of Fluorinated Sulfonamides. All compounds presented in this paper were prepared and provided by 3M Company. The general class of compound has been known for many years as surfactants (26,27). The general synthetic scheme is as follows:

$$R_fSO_2F + R_1R_2NH \text{ ---------- } R_fSO_2NR_1R_2$$

The amine can be aliphatic or heterocyclic. If one of the R-groups is a hydrogen, then further derivatization can be made by reaction of the sulfonamide sodium salt with a halide; i.e.

$$R_fSO_2NHR_1 \xrightarrow[\text{2) } ClCH_2CH_2OH]{\text{1) } CH_3ONa} R_fSO_2NR_1CH_2CH_2OH$$

The variety of possible reactants provided a large number of compounds for primary screening against fire ants (28).

Primary Delayed-Action Bioassay Results

Over 250 compounds of the general formula, R_fSO_2A, were tested for toxicity against fire ants, where R_f is a fluoroaliphatic radical and A is any compatible chemical structure. The majority of the compounds were fluorinated sulfonamides, $R_fSO_2NR_1R_2$, where R_1 and R_2 can be any compatible structure and $R_f = C_8F_{17}$-. The following is a summary of results for R- groups of like functionality. Unless specified R_f was held constant (C_8F_{17}-).

Alkyl-Substituted Sulfonamides. Class III delayed activity was observed in the methyl-(II), ethyl-(III), isopropyl-(IV), and diethyl-(VI) substituted sulfonamides; however, the t-butyl-analog (V) showed no toxicity (Table 2). The cause of its inactivity is unknown but may be related to increased steric bulk. The active members of this group were close to being in the highly desirable Class IV category.

Unsaturated Hydrocarbon-Substituted Sulfonamides. N-substituents containing double bonds gave either fast or delayed action at 1% concentration (Table 3). Double bonds directly attached to the nitrogen (phenyl (X) and vinyl (VII)) gave fast kill at 1%, whereas the methylene interrupted allyl (VIII), and benzyl (XI) substituents gave excellent delayed activity. The allyl (VIII) analog had Class IV activity.

Aliphatic Alcohol-Substituted Sulfonamides. Several monohydroxy alcohols were tested (Table 4) and gave Class III or IV delayed activity; however, the toxicity was delayed to a greater extent than the corresponding compound without the alcohol group. (Compare XII with III and XIV with II). Because of the combination of N-alkyl and alcohol substituents, it was difficult to draw conclusions about structure-activity relationships. If the R-groups contained two hydroxyls, in any combination, activity was lost (XV).

Polyether-Substituted Sulfonamides. In general the polyether group, either ending in a hydrogen or capped with a methyl group, moderated the activity of the analogous unsubstituted compound in a way similar to the alcohol-substituted sulfonamides (Table 5). In one example, activity was diminished from Class III (III) to

Table 2. Toxicity of Alkyl Substituted Sulfonamides to Fire Ant Workers

Compound	$C_8F_{17}SO_2NR_1R_2$ R1	R2	Conc. %	% Mortality at specified days[a] 1	2	3	6	8	10	14	17	21
I	-H	-H	0.01	0	0	0	3	7	7	10	20	23
			0.1	0	0	0	2	33	77	92	95	98
			1.0	43	85	98	100					
II	-H	$-CH_3$	0.01	0	0	2	3	7	7	7	23	40
			0.1	0	0	7	88	97	98	100		
			1.0	17	93	100						
III	-H	$-C_2H_5$	0.01	0	0	0	0	2	2	10	22	50
			0.1	0	0	2	80	97	97	98	98	100
			1.0	25	100							
IV	-H	$-CH(CH_3)_3$	0.01	2	2	2	2	2	3	5	27	65
			0.1	0	0	10	75	93	98	100		
			1.0	83	97	100						
V	-H	$-C(CH_3)_3$	1.0	0	0	0	0	0	0	5		
VI	$-C_2H_5$	$-C_2H_5$	0.01	0	0	0	2	5	10	20	50	60
			0.1	0	7	13	78	92	98	100		
			1.0	30	100							

[a]Percentages are the mean of three replicates. The soybean oil control had <15% mortality at the end of the test, and the mirex standard had normal delayed activity.

Table 3. Toxicity of Unsaturated Sulfonamides to Fire Ant Workers

$C_8F_{17}SO_2NR_1R_2$ Compound	R1	R2	Conc. %	% Mortality at specified days[a] 1	2	3	6	8	10	14	17	21
VII	$-CH_3$	$-CH=CH_2$	0.01	0	0	0	8	8	13	25	37	57
			0.1	0	7	33	77	90	92	100		
			1.0	100								
VIII	-H	$-CH_2CH=CH_2$	0.01	2	2	2	2	2	2	12	37	75
			0.1	3	3	3	48	60	78	93	98	100
			1.0	13	53	80	100					
IX	-H	$-CH_2C{\equiv}CH$	0.01	5	5	5	5	5	5	15	15	30
			0.1	2	2	2	2	3	5	43	73	87
			1.0	83	87	88	95	97	97	100		
X	-H	$-C_6H_5$	0.01	0	0	0	2	3	3	7	17	27
			0.1	0	2	2	8	53	70	93	95	98
			1.0	83	87	88	95	97	100			
XI	$-C_2H_5$	$-CH_2C_6H_5$	1.0	0	0	0	0	0	3	3	3	3
			0.1	0	0	0	2	2	3	8	18	42
			1.0	0	0	0	2	42	83	100		

[a]Percentages are the mean of three replicates. The soybean oil control had <15% mortality at the end of the test.

Table 4. Toxicity of Mono- and Di-alcohol-substituted Sulfonamides to Fire Ant Workers

$C_8F_{17}SO_2NR_1R_2$ Compound	R1	R2	Conc. %	% Mortality at specified days[a] 1	2	3	6	8	10	14	17	21
XII	$-C_2H_5$	$-C_2H_4OH$	0.01	0	0	2	2	2	2	2	2	3
			0.1	0	0	0	0	2	2	8	40	60
			1.0	0	0	0	45	67	88	98	100	
XIII	$-C_4H_9$	$-C_2H_4OH$	0.01	0	0	0	0	0	0	0	0	2
			0.1	0	2	2	3	3	3	25	48	78
			1.0	0	0	0	0	0	40	92	98	100
XIV	$-CH_3$	$-C_4H_8OH$	0.01	0	0	2	5	8	8	8	10	13
			0.1	0	0	0	2	5	30	75	85	92
			1.0	0	2	10	83	85	95	100		
XV	$-C_2H_4OH$	$-C_2H_4OH$	0.01	0	0	0	2	5	10	35		
XVI	$-CH_3$	$-CH_2CH(OH)CH_2OH$	1.0	0	0	0	2	2	2	5		

[a]See footnote a Table 2.

Class I (XVIII). No trends in activity could be distinguished based on the length of the polyether or whether it contained ethoxy or propoxy units.

Miscellaneous Active Compounds. Many active sulfonamide derivatives did not fall into a convenient functional group category or there were only one or two examples of a category. Results for several of these compounds are shown in Table 6. Compounds XXII to XXVI show a diversity of nitrogen substitutions that in most cases gave excellent delayed activity. Compound XXV gave rapid kill at the 1.0 percent level. We view XXII to XXVI as lead compounds that may be useful in discovering more effective toxicants both in terms of delayed action for fire ant control and fast action for the potential control of other insect pests. Compound XXII is an intriguing example where the nitrogen of the sulfonamide is utilized directly in the imidazole ring. Many other derivatives could be prepared that incorporate the sulfonamide nitrogen into a ring system; i.e. oxazole, piperidine, and pyrrole.

Substituents that Inactivate the Sulfonamides. Only a few of the previously discussed compounds did not have either delayed-action or rapid kill. Table 7 illustrates sulfonamide nitrogen substituents that resulted in inactivity. Substituents containing an amino (XXVII), amide (XXVIII), phosphate (XXIX), or an aromatic carboxylic acid (XXX) group showed no toxicity.

Structural Features Important to Toxicity

Effects of Decreasing the Length of R_f. Of the compounds available, five had an unsubstituted sulfonamide moiety and decreasing fluorocarbon chain lengths. Table 8 illustrates that decreasing the length of R_f decreases the toxicity of the compound compared to $R_f = C_8F_{17}$-. The best activity was obtained when R_f equaled C_6F_{13}- (XXXIV) or C_8F_{17}-(I). Compound XXXI showed some activity, but did not rank higher than Class 1. No corresponding compounds were available that had R_f chains greater than C_8. When the fluoraliphatic portion of the molecule was sandwiched between two methyl sulfonamides, $(CH_3NHSO_2C_4F_8-)_2$, activity was lost, which emphasizes the importance of an unencumbered R_f group.

The Importance of the Fluorocarbon and Sulfone Moiety to Toxicity. The importance of R_f (Table 9) to the toxicity of the fluorinated sulfonamide structure was tested using the hydrogen analogue of compound I. When the fluorines were replaced by hydrogens (XXXV) all activity was lost. The activity found in compound XXXI was diminished by the removal of one of the three fluorines (XXXVI). Similarly when the sulfone moiety was replaced with a carbonyl group (XXXVII), activity was lost. Interestingly, bioassays of the corresponding sulfonic acid (XXXVIII) or its potassium salt (XXXIX) in honey water (required because of a lack of solubility in soybean oil) gave very good delayed activity. Although these water soluble compounds are not suitable for fire ant control, they offer potential for the control of other insect pests, especially those associated with water. These results point out

Table 5. Toxicity of polyether-substituted sulfonamides to Fire Ant Workers

Compound	$C_8F_{17}SO_2NR_1R_2$ R1	R2	Conc. %	% Mortality at specified days[a] 1	2	3	6	8	10	14	17	21
XVII	$-C_2H_5$	$-(C_2H_4O)_3H$	0.01	0	0	0	0	3	7	7	13	20
			0.1	0	0	0	0	0	0	3	7	27
			1.0	0	0	2	52	87	98	99	100	
XVIII	$-C_2H_5$	$-C_2H_4O(C_3H_6O)_8H$	0.01	0	0	0	0	0	0	0	0	0
			0.1	0	0	0	0	0	0	0	3	17
			1.0	0	0	0	3	5	23	37	45	60
XIX	$-C_4H_9$	$-C_2H_4O(C_3H_6O)_8$	0.01	0	0	2	2	2	2	2	2	2
			0.1	0	0	0	0	0	3	3	15	45
			1.0	0	2	2	2	2	40	87	97	100
XX	$-C_2H_5$	$-(C_2H_4O)_7CH_3$	0.01	2	3	3	3	3	5	8		
			0.1	5	5	8	15	20	23	40		
			1.0	2	5	5	38	57	80	88		
XXI	C_2H_5	$-(C_2H_4O)_{17}CH_3$	0.01	0	0	0	3	7	7	10	13	17
			0.1	0	0	0	2	3	5	10	25	48
			1.0	0	0	32	100					

[a]See footnote a Table 2.

Table 6. Toxicity of Some Miscellaneous Active Sulfonamides to Fire Ant Workers

Compound	$C_8F_{17}SO_2NR_1R_2$ R1	R2	Conc. %	% Mortality at specified days[a] 1	2	3	6	8	10	14	17	21
XXII	-CH=CHN=CH-		0.01	2	3	3	8	8	8	13	15	18
	(imidazole)		0.1	0	2	3	10	10	52	67	80	88
			1.0	0	2	17	92	100				
XXIII	-H	CH_2CH_2	0.01	0	0	0	0	0	0	0	0	
		$-CH_2N$ O	0.1	0	0	0	0	0	10	30	73	
		CH_2CH_2	1.0	7	35	50	50	92	97	100		
XXIV	-H	$-C(=O)NHC_6H_{11}$	0.01	0	0	0	2	2	7	10		
		(cyclic)	0.1	0	0	0	28	40	60	85		
			1.0	2	5	18	62	70	93	100		
XXV	-H	$-C_2H_4Cl$	0.01	0	0	0	0	3	3	5	23	47
			0.1	0	0	2	22	83	95	97	100	
			1.0	57	87	98	100					
XXVI	-H	$-SCCl_3$	0.01	0	0	2	2	2	2	7		
			0.1	0	2	5	43	45	70	80		
			1.0	7	25	97	100					

[a]See footnote a Table 2.

Table 7. Toxicity of Inactive Substituted Sulfonamides to Fire Ant Workers

Compound	$C_8H_{17}SO_2NR_1R_2$ R1	R2	Conc. %	% Mortality (days) 1	2	3	6	8	10	14
XXVII	-H	$C_2H_4NH_2$	1.0	2	2	2	2	2	2	10
XXVIII	$-CH_3$	$C_2H_4C(=O)NH_2$	1.0	0	0	0	0	3	5	10
XXIX	$-C_2H_5$	$C_2H_4OPO_3H$	1.0	2	3	3	3	3	3	10
XXX	$-C_2H_5$	$CH_2-C_6H_4-CO_2H$	1.0	0	0	0	0	2	2	2

[a]See footnote a Table 2.

Table 8. Effects of Decreasing the Fluorocarbon Chain Length on Toxicity to Fire Ant Workers

Compound	Structure	Conc. %	% Mortality at specified days[a] 1	2	3	6	8	10	14	17	21
XXXI	$CF_3SO_2NH_2$	0.01	0	0	0	3	3	5	7	8	17
		0.1	3	3	3	5	5	5	17	27	58
		1.0	2	8	18	33	42	50	67	73	82
XXXII	$C_2F_5SO_2NH_2$	1.0	3	17	22	35	40	45	50		
XXXIII	$C_4F_9SO_2NH_2$	0.01	0	0	0	3	3	3	5		
XXXIV	$C_6F_{13}SO_2NH_2$	0.01	0	0	0	2	2	2	2	5	12
		0.1	3	7	7	7	7	17	63	77	92
		1.0	0	3	30	67	75	87	95	98	100
I	$C_8F_{17}SO_2NH_2$	0.01	0	0	0	3	7	7	10	20	23
		0.1	0	0	0	2	33	77	92	95	98
		1.0	43	85	98	100					

[a]See footnote a Table 2.

Table 9. Importance of Fluorocarbon and Sulfone Moiety of Molecules on Toxicity

Compound	Structure	Conc. %	% Mortality at specified days[a] 1	2	3	6	8	10	14	17	21
XXXV	$C_8H_{17}SO_2NH_2$	1.0	5	7	8	12	12	12	12		
XXXVI	$HCF_2SO_2NH_2$	1.0	0	2	2	13	18	20	30		
XXXVII	$C_7F_{15}C(=O)NH_2$	1.0	0	0	0	2	2	2	2		
XXXVIII	$C_8F_{17}SO_3H$[b]	1.0	0	37	62	95	100				
XXXIX	$C_8F_{17}SO_3H$[b]	1.0	2	2	23	87	100				

[a]See footnote a Table 2
[b]Formulated in honey water.

that the insecticidal activity of this class of compounds resides in the basic R_fSO_2A formula, and that the sulfonamide structure was useful because it allowed a great deal of structural variability to be built into the molecule.

Laboratory Colony and Field Evaluation

Twelve fluorinated sulfonamides (I, II, III, IV, VI, VII, VIII, IX, X, XXII, XXV, XXIV) were selected for evaluation against laboratory colonies of the fire ant. The materials were fed to queenright colonies formulated in soybean oil absorbed on a corn grit carrier (18). The queens in all colonies were either sick or dead by 21 days, and in most cases within 7 to 14 days. All of the compounds produced good delayed kill (1 to 24% after 2 to 3 days).

Although the laboratory colony results indicated that all the compounds warranted field tests, these tests are expensive, time consuming, and labor intensive (29), thus, other factors important to eventual commercialization, such as oil solubility, bait acceptance, and availability, were considered. Consequently, XXII, which was not very soluble in soybean oil and showed the lowest worker mortality was not tested. Compound X did not kill all of the queens in the four replicates and was also omitted.

Field assays of the 10 remaining compounds were conducted in Florida and Georgia. All chemicals were dissolved in once-refined soybean oil at concentrations of 1.0-2.5% (w/w). The oil solution was absorbed onto pregelled defatted corn grits 30% by weight of total formulation to yield baits containing 0.30, 0.60, or 0.75% active ingredient (AI). All baits were applied with a tractor-mounted auger applicator at 3.3, 4.9, or 8.1g AI/ha (29). Amdro fire ant bait (0.88% AI) was applied at the label recommendation rate of 10.4g AI/ha. Each treatment was replicated 3 times. Pretreatment and post-treatment evaluations were made at 6 and 12 wks. The pre-and post treatment population levels were used to calculate the percent control. Untreated plots similar in size to treated plots were monitored as controls.

The results demonstrated that several of the fluoro- aliphatic sulfones (I, II, III, XXV, and XXXIV) are suitable as bait-toxicants for control of the fire ant and have activity comparable to the currently available bait toxicant (Amdro).

Activity Against Other Insects

Social Insects. The same rationale for delayed-action toxicants against fire ants can be applied to other social insect pest species. Also, the potential for this class of compounds in the control of social insects is enhanced because their structural variety provides water and oil soluble compounds with a range of activities. Many of the compounds developed for fire ant control have been tested for efficacy against other ant pests (30,31) and several of the fluorinated sulfonamides were tested against the leaf-cutting ant, *Acromyrmex octospinosus* Reich. Four of these latter compounds (I, IV, VIII, and XXXVIII) showed excellent results in laboratory tests (Kermarrec, A., Centre de Recherches Agronomiques, Petit-Borg, Guadeloupe). Other social insect pests such as, Pharoah's ants, the Argentine ant, the Formosan termite, and the Africanized honey bee, may be prime targets for this class of compounds.

Cockroaches, Mosquitoes and Houseflies. Initial tests against the American (*Periplaneta americana*) and German (*Blattella germanica*) cockroaches involved five fluorosulfonamides, (I, II, III, XIV, and XXII) that gave excellent delayed-action against the fire ant. The cockroach bait was composed of the toxicant formulated in a mixture of cornmeal and powdered sugar (32). For the American cockroach marked delayed activity was observed, with a mean mortality of only 5 percent after 24 hours. However, by 10 days all replicates had 100 percent mortality. In contrast, there was rapid mortality against the German cockroach (mean of 85 percent by the first day, 94 percent at day 2, and 100 percent by day seven). In both cases the trichlorfon standard gave 100 percent kill after 24 hours (25). In the control of cockroaches, delayed activity is not a necessary feature of potential control methods. Among the many fluorinated compounds tested several displayed rapid kill (IV, VIII, X, and XXV) and these compounds are currently being tested.

The same five fluorinated sulfonamides were screened as mosquito larvicides against *Anopheles quadrimaculatus*. Preliminary results showed that all of the compounds tested except XXII, had good to excellent larvicidal activity. Compound I compared well with the standard larvicide, temephos, with an LC-50 of 0.0029 ppm. In 24 hour mortality tests, all compounds except XXII gave 100 percent kill at 10 ppm and compound II gave 78 percent kill at 0.1 ppm (25). In the case of mosquito larvicide action, water solubility may be an important feature of the toxicant. Again the fluorinated sulfonic acids and their salts (XXXVIII and XXXIX) have greater water solubility. Tests with these compounds in the field have shown outstanding persistence and remarkable species selectivity (25; Roberts, R., USDA, Gainesville, Fl).

Compounds I, II, III, XIV, and XXII, were tested for insecticidal activity against houseflies (*Musca domestica*). The insecticide-resistant strain of housefly was fed a food bait containing 1 percent of the test compounds. After 3 days, compounds II, III, and XIV showed no mortality and compounds I and XXII gave only 80 and 60 percent mortality, respectively (25). As in the case of cockroaches, the faster acting analogues may provide a more acceptable level of control.

Conclusion

As illustrated in the previous discussion, this new class of insecticide was serendipitously discovered to have the very specialized delayed-activity over a wide range of concentrations required for fire ant control. These same properties may well broaden the use of these compounds to the control of other social insect pests. The wide range of chemical functional types, toxic activity and solubilities broaden the potential use of this class of compound to a wide variety of insect pests. Compound III is currently under commercial development by Griffin Corporation, Valdosta, Georgia, for fire ant control. If the compound passes the strict toxicological requirements of the EPA, the future of these chemicals for insect control will be very exciting.

Literature Cited

1. Banks, W. A., B. M. Glancey, C. E. Stringer, D. P. Jouvenaz, C. S. Lofgren, and D. E. Weidhaas. J. Econ. Entomol. 1973, 66, 785-789.
2. Culpepper, G. H. USDA, Agric. Res. Admin., Bur. Entomol. Pl.Quar. 1953, E-867.
3. Vander Meer, R. K., C. S. Lofgren, and F. M. Alvarez. Fla. Entomol. 1985, 68, 501-506.
4. Tschinkel, W. R. In Fire Ants and Leaf-Cutting Ants: Biology and Control; C. S. Lofgren and R. K. Vander Meer, Eds.; Westview Press: Boulder, CO, 1986, pp. 72-87.
5. Lofgren, C. S., W. A. Banks, and B. M. Glancey. Ann. Rev. Entomol. 1975, 29, 1-30.
6. Lofgren, C. S. and C. T. Adams. In The Biology of Social Insects; Westview Press: Boulder, CO, 1982; pp. 124-128.
7. Paull, B. R. Postgrad. Med. 1984, 76; 155-161.
8. MacConnell, J. G., M. S. Blum, and H. M. Fales. Tetrahedron. 1971, 26, 1129-1139.
9. Lockey, R. F. In Advances in Allergology and Clinical Immunology; Pergamon Press: New York, 1979, pp. 441-448.
10. James, F. K. J. Asthma Res. 1976, 13, 179-183.
11. Lofgren, C. S. In Economic Import and Control of Social Insects; S. B. Vinson, Ed.; Praeger Publishers, NY, 1986; pp. 227-256.
12. Eden, W. G., and F. S. Arant. Alabama J. Econ. Entomol. 1949, 42, 976-979.
13. Lofgren, C. S. In Fire Ants and Leaf-Cutting Ants: Biology and Control; C. S. Lofgren and R. K. Vander Meer, Eds.; Westview Press: Boulder, CO, 1986; pp. 36-47.
14. Johnson, E. L. Fed. Regist. 41: 56694-56704. Administrator's decision to accept plan of Mississippi Authority and order suspending hearing for the pesticide chemical mirex.
15. Lofgren, C. S. In Fire Ants and Leaf-Cutting Ants: Biology and Control; C. S. Lofgren and R. K. Vander Meer, Eds.; Westview Press: Boulder, CO, 1986; pp. 369-377.
16. Vander Meer, R. K. In Fire Ants and Leaf-Cutting Ants: Biology and Control; C. S. Lofgren and R. K. Vander Meer, Eds.; Westview Press: Boulder, CO, 1986; pp. 201-210.
17. Stringer, C. F., C. S. Lofgren, and F. J. Bartlett. J. Econ. Entomol. 1964, 57, 941-945.
18. Williams, D. F. Fla. Entomol. 1983, 66, 162-172.
19. Vander Meer, R. K., C. S. Lofgren, D. H. Lewis, and W. E. Meyers. In Controlled Release of Bioactive Materials; R. Blake, Ed.; Academic Press, Inc., New York, 1980; pp. 251-256.
20. Meyers, W. E., Lewis, D. H., Vander Meer, R. K., Lofgren, C. S. Controlled Release of Bioactive Materials; Lewis, D. H., Ed.; Plenum Press, New York, 1981, pp. 171-190.
21. Vander Meer, R. K., Williams, D. F., Lofgren, C. S. Insect. Acar. Tests; 1983, 8, 252-253.

22. Vander Meer, R. K., Lofgren, C. S., Williams, D. F. Pestic. Sci.; 1986, 17, 449-455.
23. Lovell, J. B. Proc. Br. Crop. Prot. Conf. - Pests Dis. 1979,No. 2, 575-582.
24. Kochansky, J. P., Robbins, W. E., Lofgren, C. S., Williams, D. F. J. Econ. Entomol. 1979, 72, 655-658.
25. Vander Meer, R. K., Lofgren, C. S., Williams, D. F. U. S. Patent Application No. 758,856, 1985.
26. Ahlbrecht, A. H., Brown, H. A. U. S. Patent 2 803 656, 1957.
27. Brice, T. I., Trott, P. W. U. S. Patent 2 732 398, 1956.
28. Vander Meer, R. K., Lofgren, C. S., Williams, D. F. J. Econ. Entomol.; 1985, 78, 1190-1197.
29. Williams, D. F., Lofgren, C. S., Plumley, J. K., and Hicks, D. M. J. Econ. Entomol. 1983. 76, 395-397.
30. Su, T. H., Beardsley, J. W., McEwen, F. L. J. Econ. Entomol. 1980. 73, 755-756.
31. Barth, P. W. J. Econ. Entomol. 1986. 79, 1632-1636.
32. Burden, G. S. Pest Control, 1980, 48, 22-24.

RECEIVED May 15, 1987

Chapter 22

Synthesis, Insecticidal Activity, and Anticholinesterase Activity of Some Oxadiazolones

J. R. Sanborn[1], Kurt H. Pilgram, E. J. Ayers, and Richard D. Skiles

Biological Sciences Research Center, Shell Agricultural Chemical Company, Modesto, CA 95352

This report summarizes the synthesis, insecticidal activity, and anticholinesterase activity of some novel N-dihydrobenzofuranyl oxadiazolones. The compounds were primarily aphicides with reduced activity on houseflies, corn earworms and two-spotted spider mites. Some of these compounds were potent anticholineterases (I_{50} values 1-10x10^{-8}M) that were slowly reversible. There was little relationship between *in vitro* anticholinesterase activity and *in vivo* activity.

A synthesis program was initiated to optimize the insecticidal activity of the following molecules that are related to RP 32861, a substance reported to be insecticidal against sucking insects(1).

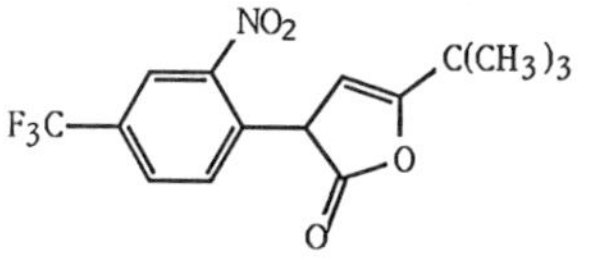

Housefly TI*=6 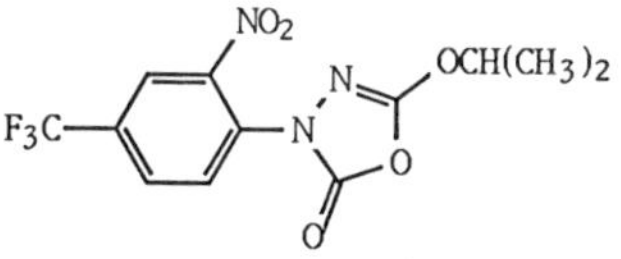 Aphid TI*=4 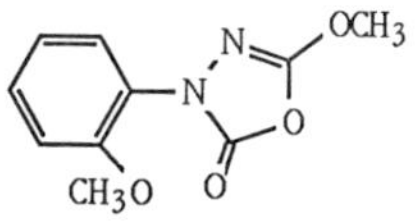 RP 32861

*Parathion TI=100

The new molecules had the following generalized structure(2):

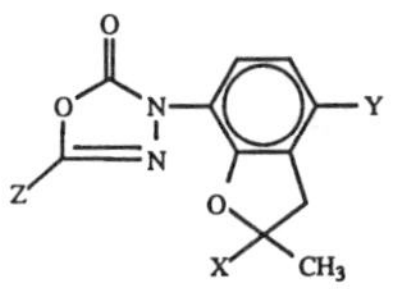

Where X = H or CH_3
Y = H, halogen or alkyl
Z = alkoxy, aryloxy alkyl or aryl

[1]Current address: E. I. de Pont de Nemours & Co., Wilmington, DE 19898

0097-6156/87/0355-0241$06.00/0
© 1987 American Chemical Society

Synthesis

The synthesis of these molecules can be broken down into two parts. The first segment consisted of preparation of the dihydrobenzofuranylhydrazines from which the oxadiazolones were eventually prepared. These hydrazines were prepared as follows: the appropriate *o*-nitrophenol was treated with the desired allylic halide under alkaline conditions to yield an allyl ether. This was rearranged and ring-closed at elevated temperatures under acidic conditions to yield the 7-nitro substituted dihydrobenzofuran. Reduction with hydrogen over palladium on carbon and diazotization of the 7-aminodihydrobenzofuran with sodium nitrite yielded a diazonium salt that was reduced with sodium dithionite to give the 7-hydrazinodihydrobenzofuran sulfonic acid. Treatment of this sulfonic acid in ethanol with hydrochloric acid yielded the desired 7-hydrazinodihybenzofurans.

Construction of the oxadiazolone ring from the aforementioned hydrazine is illustrated below:

$$\text{*ArNHNH}_2 \quad + \quad \text{ClC(O)R} \xrightarrow[\text{-HCL}]{} \text{ArNHNHC(O)R} \quad \text{(I)}$$

$$\text{(I)} \quad + \quad \text{Cl}_2\text{C(O)} \xrightarrow[\text{-HCL}]{} \text{ArN(C(O)Cl)NHC(O)R} \quad \text{(II)}$$

$$\text{(II)} \xrightarrow[\text{-HCL}]{\Delta} \text{R–C}{=}\text{N–N(Ar)–C(=O)–O– (oxadiazolone ring)}$$

*Ar = 7-substituted benzofuran
R = alkoxy, aryl or alkyl

Treatment of the 7-hydrazinodihydrobenzofuran with either a chloroformate or an acyl chloride in the presence of *N*,*N*-diisopropylethylamine yielded the *N*-acylated product. Treatment of this intermediate *N*-acylated 7-dihydrobenzofuranyl hydrazine with phosgene followed by treatment of the intermediate chlorocarbonyl compound with an equivalent of base yielded the insecticidal molecules to be discussed in this report.

Insecticidal Activity

The molecules of this report were evaluated on four insects: the housefly, *Musca domestica* (M.d.), the pea aphid, *Acyrthosiphon pisum* (A.p.), the corn earworm, *Heliothis zea* (H.z.) and two-spotted spidermite *Triticum urticae* (T.u.). Using parathion as the standard for each insect, it is given a value of 100, so other molecules with toxicity index values (TI) of 100 are as toxic as parathion. Higher TI values represent greater toxicity and so forth.

Table 1. Effect of Ring Substituents at 4-Position on the Toxicity of Dihydrobenzofuranyl Oxadiazolones

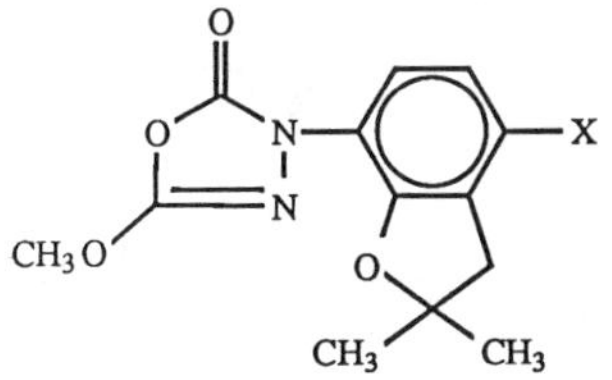

Structure	Toxicity Index (parathion=100)			
X	M.d.	A.p.	H.z.	T.u.
H	68	714	34	53
CH_3	18	988	23	38
$i\text{-}C_3H_7$	36	91	13	37
Cl	2	554	+	20
F	13	546	36	2

Table 1 contains insecticidal toxicity information on five compounds which differ only in their substituents at the 4-position of the dihydrobenzofuranyl ring. With the exception of aphids, the most broadly active compound was unsubstituted at this position. Other substituent at this site had no enhancing effect and in some cases (Cl on houseflies and corn earworms and F on mites) a strong deleterious effect resulted. The only case where a substituent, CH_3, increased the activity was with aphids.

Table 2. Effects of Methyl Substituents at the 2- and 4-Positions on the Insecticidal Toxicity of the Dihydrobenzofuranyl Oxadiazolones

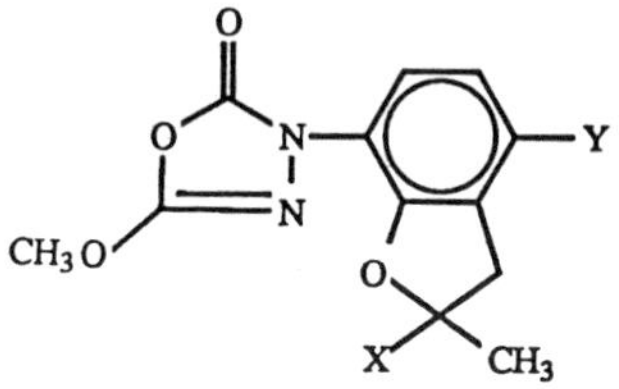

Structure		Toxicity Index (parathion=100)			
X	Y	M.d.	A.p.	H.z.	T.u.
H	H	22	243	19	20
CH_3	H	68	714	34	53
H	CH_3	11	479	16	0
CH_3	CH_3	18	988	23	38

Maximal activity for all insects was obtained when the molecules contained two methyl groups at the 2-position of the dihydrobenzofuranyl ring. If the molecule had only one methyl group at the 2-position and methyl group at the 4-position, this substituent pattern conferred inferior toxicity as compared to molecules containing gem dimethyls at the 2-position of the dihydrobenzofuranyl ring. See Table 2.

Table 3. Effect of Alkyl or Aryl Substituents at the 5-Position of Oxadiazolone Ring on the Insecticidal Toxicity

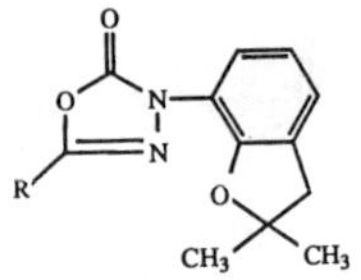

R	M.d.	A.p.	H.z.	T.u.
CH_3	0	0	0	0
C_3H_5	0	1	0	0
C_6H_5	0	0	0	0

Examination of the data in Table 3 clearly points out the necessity of having some type of an alkoxy substituent in the 5-position of the oxadiazolone ring as most of the compounds were inactive against the insects in the primary screen. Only one of the compounds, ($R=C_3H_5$) had marginal activity (TI=1) against aphids.

Table 4. Effect of a Phenoxy Group at 5-position of the Oxadiazolone Ring on Insecticidal Toxicity

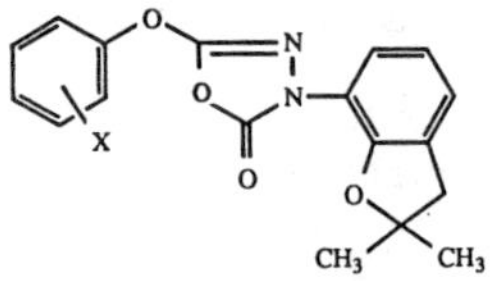

X	M.d.	A.p.	H.z.	T.u.
H	0	20	0	0
2-F	0	8	+	0
4-Cl	0	6	0	0
3,4,5 CH_3	0	8	0	0

The presence of a phenoxy or a substituted phenoxy group at the 5-position of the oxadiazolone ring yields molecules that possess low level activity on aphids in the primary screen. The most active compound is the unsubstituted phenyl molecule (TI=20), and any other substituent on the phenyl ring (2F, 4-Cl or 3,4,5-CH_3) reduces the activity on aphids compared to the unsubstituted phenyl compound. See Table 4.

Anticholinesterase Activity

The anticholinesterase activity of the oxadiazolones of this report was measured using housefly heads as the enzyme source and the method of Ellman(3) was utilized to determine the enzyme activity. The conditions for the enzyme inhibition studies are shown below:

Anticholinesterase Activity Conditions	
Enzyme Source:	Housefly heads, Electric eel
Incubation Time:	30 minutes
Temperature:	30°C
Enzyme Activity:	Ellman's Reagent
pH:	8

In Table 5 are the molar I_{50} values for oxadiazolones that differ only in their substituents at the 4-position of the dihydrobenzofuran ring. The potency of these molecules is in the order CH_3> F> i-C_3H_7>H>Cl. This was not the order of whole insect toxicity, which was H> i-C_3H_7>CH_3>F>Cl. Since studies were not performed with synergists, it is not possible to characterize the reasons the poor correlation between *in vitro* anticholinesterase activity and whole insect toxicity. What is clear from the studies is that two of the molecules, 4-CH_3 (I_{50}=1.6x10^{-8}M) and 4-F (I_{50}-4.4x10^{-8}M) represent a potent new class of anticholinesterase agents unlike the known organophosphates or carbamates.

Table 6 contains data that show the effects of methyl groups at the 2,4-positions of the dihydrobenzofuranyl ring on the anticholinesterase potency of these molecules. Clearly, from an anticholinesterase perspective, it is best (I_{50}=1.6x10^{-8}M) to have methyl groups present in the 2 and 4 positions of the benzofuranyl ring. The next best arrangement of methyl groups for anticholinesterase activity is to have a methyl group at each of the 2 and 4 positions (I_{50}=9.8x10^{-8}M) followed by the molecule with a single methyl group at the 2-position (I_{50}=1.7x10^{-7}M).

From an anticholinesterase/*in vivo* toxicity point of view, these molecules are perhaps the most interesting. They are as effective in some cases (2-F, I_{50} 2.1x10^{-8}M) as the best 5-methoxy compound (I_{50} 1.6x10^{-8}M), and yet their whole insect toxicity on houseflies is less. Again, without studies incorporating synergists into the toxicity evaluations, it is not possible to determine the reasons for the discrepancy between the *in vitro* and *in vivo* activity. See Table 7.

Table 5. Anticholinesterase Activity of 4-Substituted Dihydrobenzofuranyl Oxadiazolones

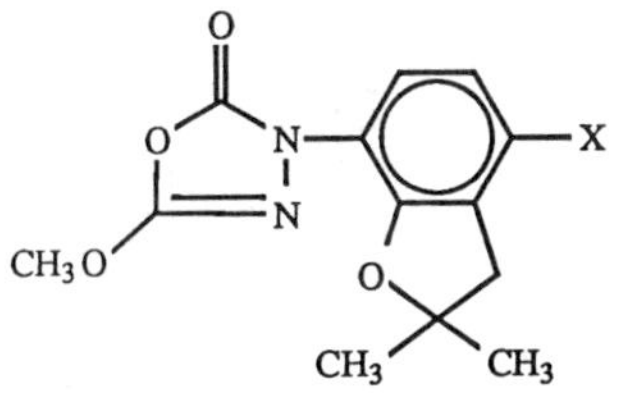

Structure X	Enzyme Activity I_{50} (M x10^{8})
H	25
CH_3	1.6
i-C_3H_7	15
Cl	183
F	4.4

Table 6. Anticholinesterase Activity of 2-and 4-Methyl Substituented Dihydrobenzofuranyl Oxadiazolones

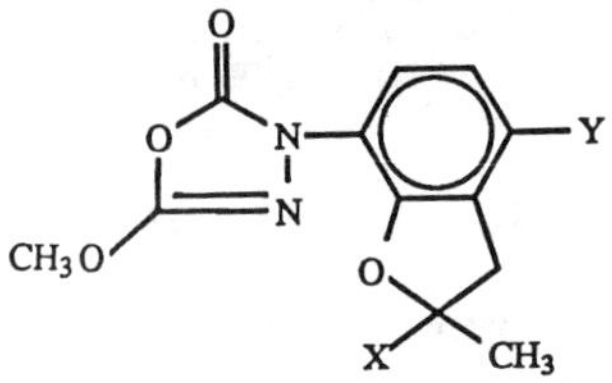

Structure X	Y	Enzyme Activity I_{50} (M x10^8)
H	H	17
CH_3	H	25
H	CH_3	9.8
CH_3	CH_3	1.6

Table 7. Anticholinesterase Activity of Oxadiazolones Containing 5-Phenoxy Substituent

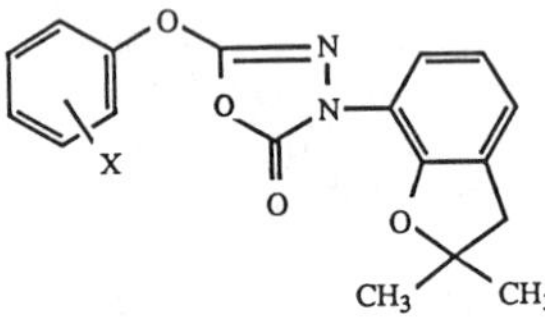

Structure X	Enzyme Activity I_{50} (M x 10^8)
H	5.8
2-F	2.7
4-Cl	9.1
3,4,5-CH_3	15

These molecules, which are also inactive on houseflies in the primary screen, have molar I_{50} values which are 100-710,000 less than that of the most potent molecules of this report, perhaps indicating that a leaving group at the 5-position on the oxadiazolone ring is requisite for the active anticholinesterases. See Table 8.

Nature of the molecularity of the interaction of benzofuranyl oxidiazolones with housefly head acetylcholinesterase

For determination of how these inhibitors interact with housefly acetyl cholinesterase the method of Aldridge and Davidson(3) was employed. The log % residual activity is plotted against (molar concentration)(incubation time). When straight line results, it is interpreted that the enzyme-inhibitor interaction is governed by pseudo first order kinetics and is a bimolecular reaction. For the

Table 8. Anticholinesterase Activity of 5-Alkyl or 5-Aryl Oxadiazolones

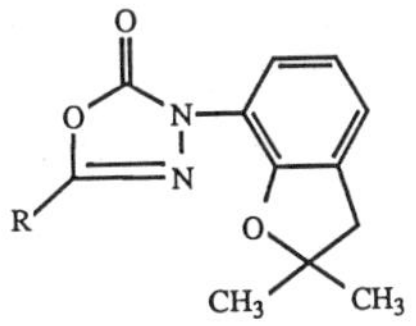

Structure R	Enzyme Activity I_{50} (M x10^{8})
CH_3	110
C_3H_5	3,000
Ph	710,000
p-Cl Ph	5,800

molecule in Figure 1, the bimolecular rate constant was found to be 5.9×10^{5} l.mol.$^{-1}$ min^{-1}. The observation that these oxadiazolones react with acetyl cholinesterase in a bimolecular fashion puts them in the same category as the better known organophosphate acetyl cholinesterase inhibitors. While the reactive center in an organophosphate inhibitors is characterized, the mechanistic details of how these oxadiazolones inhibit this enzyme are unknown and await further investigation.

Reversibility of the enzyme - inhibitor complex

It was of interest to determine the whether these oxadiazolones were irreversible inhibitors like many organophosphates or reversible inhibitors like carbamates. Since acetyl cholinesterase enzyme from *Electrophorus electricus* was more stable, it was chosen as the enzyme for these regeneration studies. The enzyme was inhibited to about 36% of its activity, requiring 30 min. Then the test solution was placed in dialysis tubing to retain the enzyme and allow inhibitor to pass through into the dialysis solution. Subsequently, aliquots were taken from the test solution to measure increase in activity resulting from decomposition of the enzyme-inhibitor complex. This regeneration study was only carried out for seven hours as breakdown of the enzyme became significant. During the seven hour experiment adequate controls ensured that increase in enzyme activity was due to regeneration of the enzyme. Examination of Figure 2, allows the calculation of a $T_{1/2}$ for regeneration of approximately 43 hours.

Conclusions

This report briefly summarizes the synthesis, insect toxicity and anticholinesterase activity of some novel dihydrobenzofuranyl oxadiazolones, a class of insecticides whose major strength lies in their toxicity to aphids with reduced activity on houseflies, two-spotted spider mites and corn earworms. This is similar to the previously reported RP 32,861, which also was most active on sucking insects. The molecule with the broadest toxicity spectrum

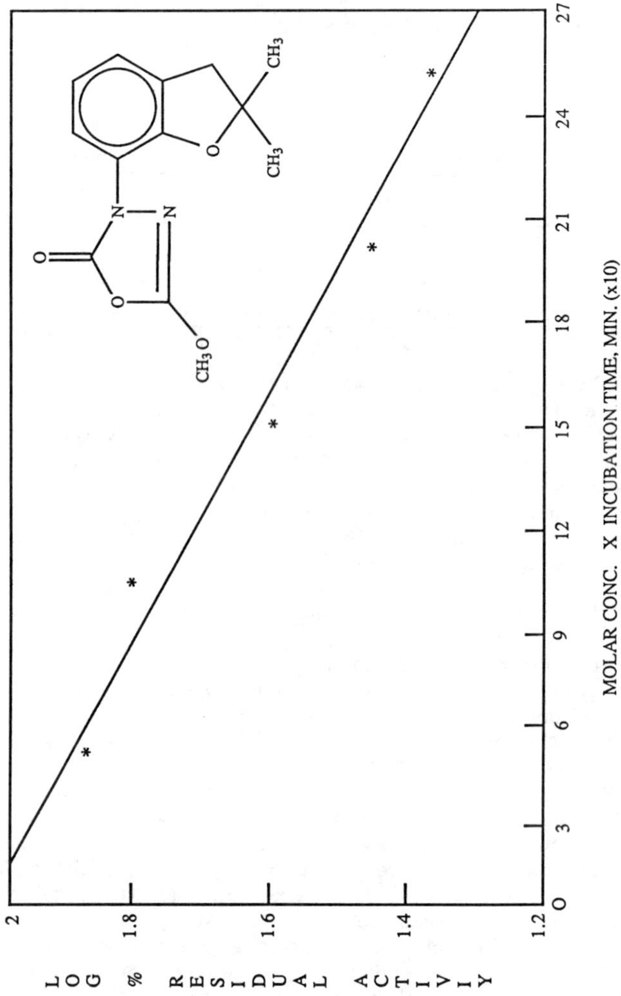

Figure 1. Bimolecular rate constant.

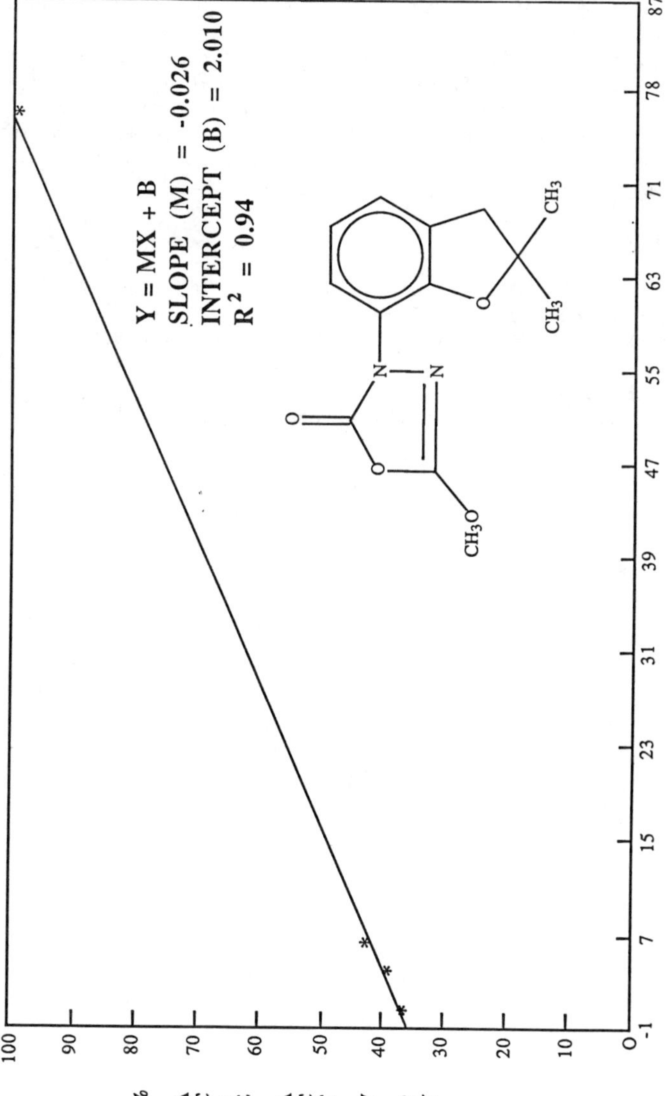

Figure 2. Increase in enzyme activity due to regeneration of the enzyme.

contained the 2,2-dimethyl dihydrobenzofuranyl ring system. The most toxic molecule to aphids had an additional methyl in the 4 position of the dihydrobenzofuranyl ring. Enzyme inhibition studies with housefly acetyl cholinesterase demonstrated that these molecules were potent anticholinesterases (30 min I_{50} values $1\text{-}10 \times 10^{-8}$ M for the most active molecules). However, the correlation between their *in vitro* enzyme inhibitory potency and their *in vitro* activity on houseflies was poor, indicating the importance of other factors that determine whole insect toxicity of these molecules. Further work must be carried out to determine the exact nature of the mechanism by which these molecules inhibit acetyl cholinesterase.

Literature Cited

1. Ambrosi, D.; Bic, G.; Desmoras, J.; Gallinell, G; Roussel, G. Proc Br. Crop Prot. Conf. Pests. Dis. 1979, (2) 533.
2. Pilgram, K. H., Skiles, R. D. U. S. Patent 4 406 910, 1983.
3. Ellman, G. L., Courtney, K. D., Andres, V., Jr., Feather stone, R.M. Biochemical J. 1961, 7, 62-70.
4. Aldridge, W. N., Davison, A.N. Biochem. J., 1952, 51, 62-70.

RECEIVED August 5, 1987

Chapter 23

Synthetic Approaches to Milbemycin Analogs

G. I. Kornis, S. J. Nelson, and F. E. Dutton

Upjohn Company, Kalamazoo, MI 49001

The milbemycins are a family of 16 membered lactones produced by Streptomyces hygroscopicus. The structures are characterized by a 5.5 spiroketal unit, a side chain with eight carbon atoms, and a complex cyclohexene carboxylic acid. A synthetic route for the spiroketal and connecting chain, and an approach to a southern portion analog via Diels Alder Chemistry are described.

The milbemycins (1) are a family of naturally occurring macrocyclic lactones showing high efficacy against arthropods and nematodes, with milbemycin D, 1 (Figure 1) currently being developed by the Sankyo Company against heartworms in dogs (2). Milbemycin D is closely related to Ivermectin 2, a semi-synthetic antibiotic (3), derived from the avermectin family and marketed by Merck, as a highly efficacious nematocide. The milbemycins are characterized by a 5.5 spiroketal, a rigid 16 membered lactone and a southern portion which, in the α series consists of a hexahydrobenzofuran as shown in 1. In the β_{1-2} series, the furan ring is open, while in the β_3 series the cyclohexene ring is aromatic. The members within each series differ by changes at positions 4, 5, 22, 23 and 25.

While milbemycin β_3 has been synthesized by several workers (4), a total synthesis of the α milbemycins or the avermectins has not been achieved to date. Our aim is the construction of a somewhat less complex molecule with a biological spectrum similar to that of the milbemycin/avermectin complex.

SPIROKETAL SYNTHESIS

The literature (4) contains a considerable number of methods for the construction of the 1,7-dioxaspiro(5.5)undecane system. Our synthetic sequence shown in Scheme 1, starts with the commercially available 5-hexyne-1-ol 3, which on treatment with dilute sulfuric acid in the presence of mercuric oxide yields a mixture of the

0097-6156/87/0355-0251$06.00/0
© 1987 American Chemical Society

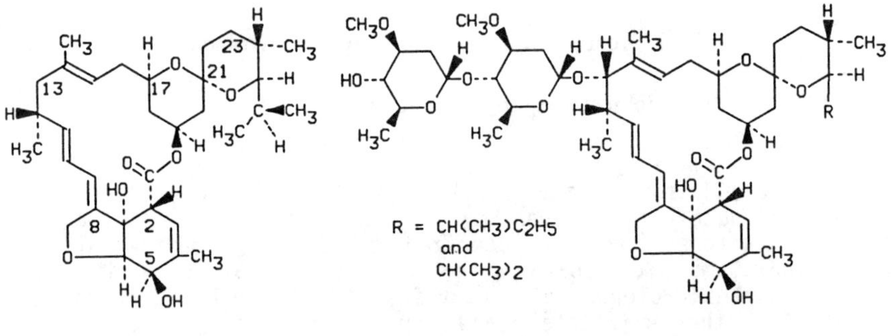

R = CH(CH3)C2H5 and CH(CH3)2

Figure 1. Structures of milbemycin D 1 and ivermectin 2.

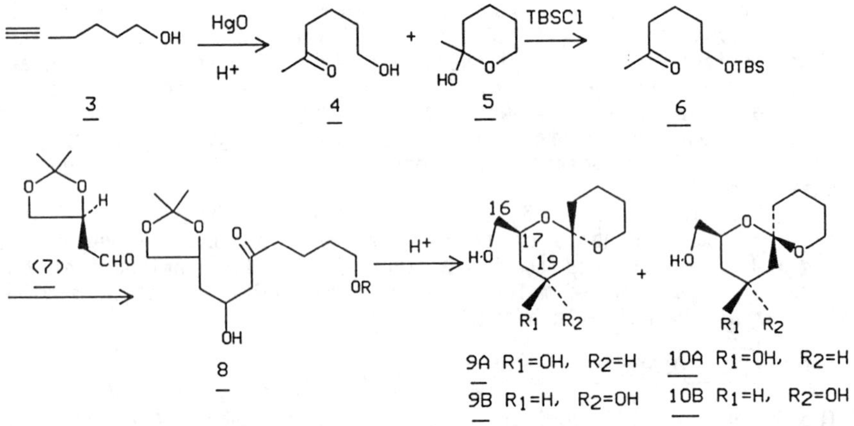

9A R_1=OH, R_2=H
9B R_1=H, R_2=OH
10A R_1=OH, R_2=H
10B R_1=H, R_2=OH

SCHEME 1

desired alcohol 4 and the cyclic hemiacetal 5 in a ratio of 82:18. Silation of the mixture of 4 and 5 with t-butyldimethylsilyl chloride (TBSCl) gave the ketone 6 in about 80% yield. Aldehyde 7 was prepared from the acetonide of racemic 1,2,4-butanetriol in 60% yield; optically active 7 could also be obtained form l-malic acid.

Treatment of ketone 6 with lithium diisopropylamide (LDA) followed by the addition of the racemic aldehyde 7 yielded the aldol 8, purified by chromatography, to give an unseparable mixture of epimers. Treatment of 8 with fluoroboric acid in ether led to a precipitate within minutes, and by simple filtration the desired spiroketal 9A was obtained in a 40-50% yield, with correct relative stereochemistry at all three optical centers. The mothers liquors provided additional 9A, a second diastereoisomer 9B and an inseparable mixture (10% of the total) of 10A and 10B. The combined yield of spiroketal products was 85% with a ratio of isomers of 7.86:3.43:1 for 9A, 9B and 10A + 10B respectively.

Proof of structure for 9A is provided by the high resolution pmr spectrum of the corresponding C_{16} monobenzoate and comparison with spectra of the 24,25-dimethyl spiro-ketals kindly provided by Professor D. Williams of Indiana University. Based on spin decoupling experiments, absorptions due to H-17 and H-19 are readily assigned. The coupling constants clearly indicate that these protons are both axial, hence the hydroxyl and the hydroxymethyl are cis and have the desired equatorial configuration. Assignment of configuration at C_{21} was made through comparison with the spectra provided by Professor Williams.

Jones oxidation of the C_{16} monobenzoate of 9A and 9B gave the same ketone, therefore they must be epimeric at C_{19}. The mixture of 10A and 10B shows a single parent ion in the mass spectrum and is considered to be a mixture of spiroketals epimeric with the C_{16} benzoates of 9A and 9B at C_{21}. The product ratio of 2.3 to 1 for 9A and 9B can be explained by chelation effects as described for β-alkoxy aldehydes(5).

SIDE CHAIN SYNTHESIS

The introduction of the side chain containing carbon atoms 16 to 11 was accomplished as shown in Scheme 2. Selective tosylation of 9A followed by displacement with cyanide ion and protection of the C-19 alcohol with tert-butyldimethylsilyl (TBS) chloride gave 11. Subsequent reduction with diisobutylaluminum hydride (DIBAL) and hydrolysis gave the aldehyde 12. Wittig reaction of 12 with (carbethoxyethylidene)triphenlyphosphorane provided the α,β unsaturated ester 13 in high yield. Only the E isomer was detected by nmr and tlc. Reduction of 13 to the alcohol 14 with DIBAL followed by oxidation with pyridinium chlorochromate (PCC) gave aldehyde 15. Attempts to reduce 13 directly to 15 always gave a mixture of 13, 14 and 15. Utilizing the procedure of Heathcock(6), an aldol condensation of 15 with 2,6-dimethylphenyl propionate provided the aldol product 16, which was converted to the corresponding methoxymethyl ether giving 17 as an inseparable mixture of anti-isomers (substituents at C_{12} and C_{13} being α, as

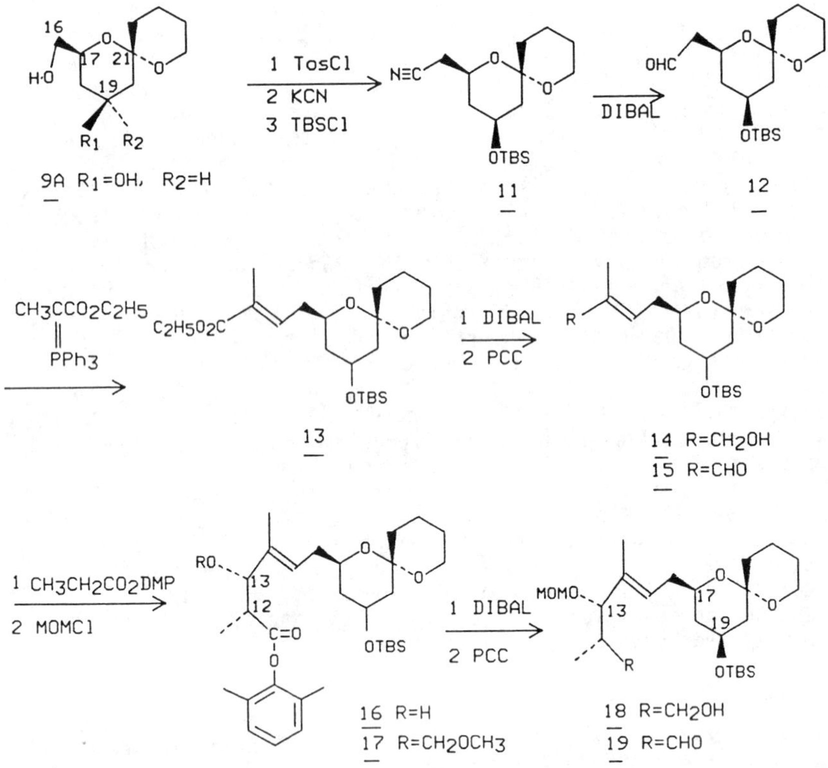

16 17 21 19 H·O O O R_1 R_2

9A R_1=OH, R_2=H

1 TosCl
2 KCN
3 TBSCl

N≡C O O OTBS

11

DIBAL

OHC O O OTBS

12

$CH_3CCO_2C_2H_5$ ‖ PPh_3

$C_2H_5O_2C$ O O OTBS

13

1 DIBAL
2 PCC

R O O OTBS

14 R=CH_2OH
15 R=CHO

1 $CH_3CH_2CO_2DMP$
2 MOMCl

RO 13 12 C=O O O O OTBS

16 R=H
17 R=CH_2OCH_3

1 DIBAL
2 PCC

MOMO 13 17 19 R O O OTBS

18 R=CH_2OH
19 R=CHO

SCHEME 2

shown, and β) in a 55/45 ratio based on the nmr spectra. That the products from the reaction are exclusively anti is clear from the coupling constant(7) of 10.5 Hz for H_{12-13}. The syn isomers were not detected. Reduction of the ester 17 to the alcohol 18 proved unexpectedly troublesome. Lithium aluminum hydride gave rise to a complex mixture of products in which the methoxymethyl ether had been cleaved. A similar result was obtained with DIBAL at room temperature. At -78° however, DIBAL cleanly gave the alcohol 18. PCC oxidation then gave the target aldehyde 19.

SOUTHERN PORTION

Our first synthesis of a simplified southern portion was based on work done by Buchi (8) (Scheme 3). Protection of the dimer of acrolein 20 as a Schiffs base with t-butylamine, followed by proton abstraction with a Grignard reagent and methylation and deprotection gave 21. Reaction with trimethylphosphonoacetate (TMP) in the presence of sodium hydride gave the α, β unsaturated ester 22, which at 200° underwent a Claisen rearrangement to give the aldehyde ester 23 as a mixture of trans and cis isomers. The cis isomer in the presence of base epimerized mainly to the trans form.

A shorter sequence was developed starting with methacrolein 24, which underwent a Wadsworth Emmons reaction with trimethylphosphonoacetate (TMP) to give the diene ester 25 in 80% yield. A Diels Alder reaction with acrolein 26A, at 200°, gave 27A, identical in all respects with the trans aldehyde obtained by Buchi. The methyl ketone, 27B was obtained in the same way by replacing acrolein with methyl vinyl ketone 26B. The yield averaged 75%, and only one regio isomer was formed.

Introduction of functionality at C_5 was also achieved by the above procedure, albeit in a low yield (Scheme 3). Thus treatment of the diethylacetal of propionaldehyde with sulfanilic acid followed by fractional distillation gave a mixture of the cis and trans vinyl ether 28 which, on treatment with triethyl orthoformate in the presence of a catalytic amount of BF_3/etherate, gave 2-methyl-1,3-tetraethoxypropane 29, in a 55% yield(9). Further heating at 80° with a catalytic amount of p-toluenesulfonic acid(10), gave in a 85% yield the unsaturated aldehyde 30. This in turn was reacted with trimethylphosphonoacetate and base to give the ethoxy diene ester 31, which then underwent a Diels Alder reaction with acrolein to give a mixture of the regioisomers 32 and 33 in an unacceptably low yield.

ELABORATION OF THE SIDE CHAIN

Introduction of the 8,9 double bond was achieved by reacting the methyl ketone 27B with t-butyldimethylphosphonoacetate to give the ester 34A in a yield of 80% (Scheme 4). Brief treatment at room temperature with formic acid gave the unsaturated acid 34B in quantitative yield. Attempted reduction with thexylchloroborane-dimethyl sulfide (11) to the desired aldehyde 35C gave only starting material. Treatment of 34B with t-butyldimethylsilyl

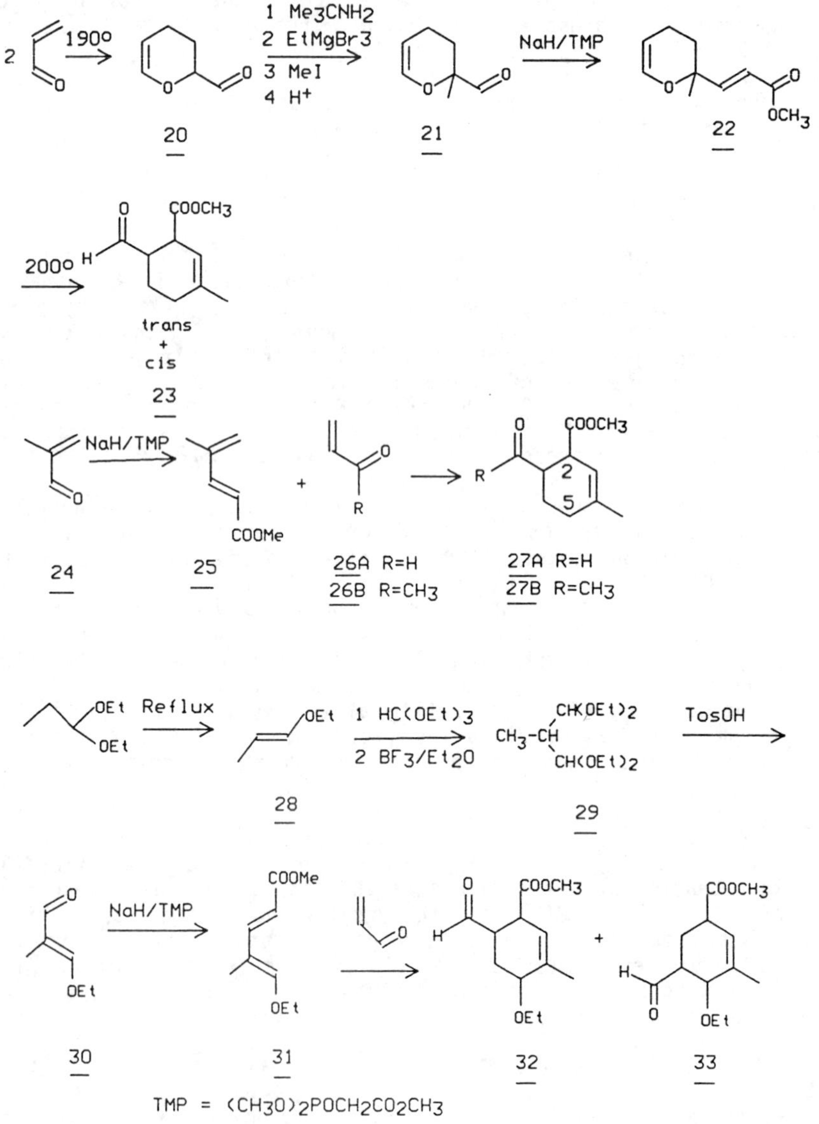

2 → 190° → 20 → 1 Me_3CNH_2; 2 $EtMgBr_3$; 3 MeI; 4 H^+ → 21 → NaH/TMP → 22 (O, OCH_3)

200° → 23 (O, $COOCH_3$, H; trans + cis)

24 (O) → NaH/TMP → 25 (COOMe) + 26A R=H, 26B R=CH_3 (O, R) → 27A R=H, 27B R=CH_3 (O, $COOCH_3$, R, 2, 5)

(OEt, OEt) → Reflux → 28 (OEt) → 1 $HC(OEt)_3$; 2 BF_3/Et_2O → 29 (CH_3-CH($CH(OEt)_2$)($CH(OEt)_2$)) → TosOH →

30 (O, OEt) → NaH/TMP → 31 (COOMe, OEt) + (O) → 32 (O, H, $COOCH_3$, OEt) + 33 ($COOCH_3$, H, O, OEt)

TMP = $(CH_3O)_2POCH_2CO_2CH_3$

SCHEME 3

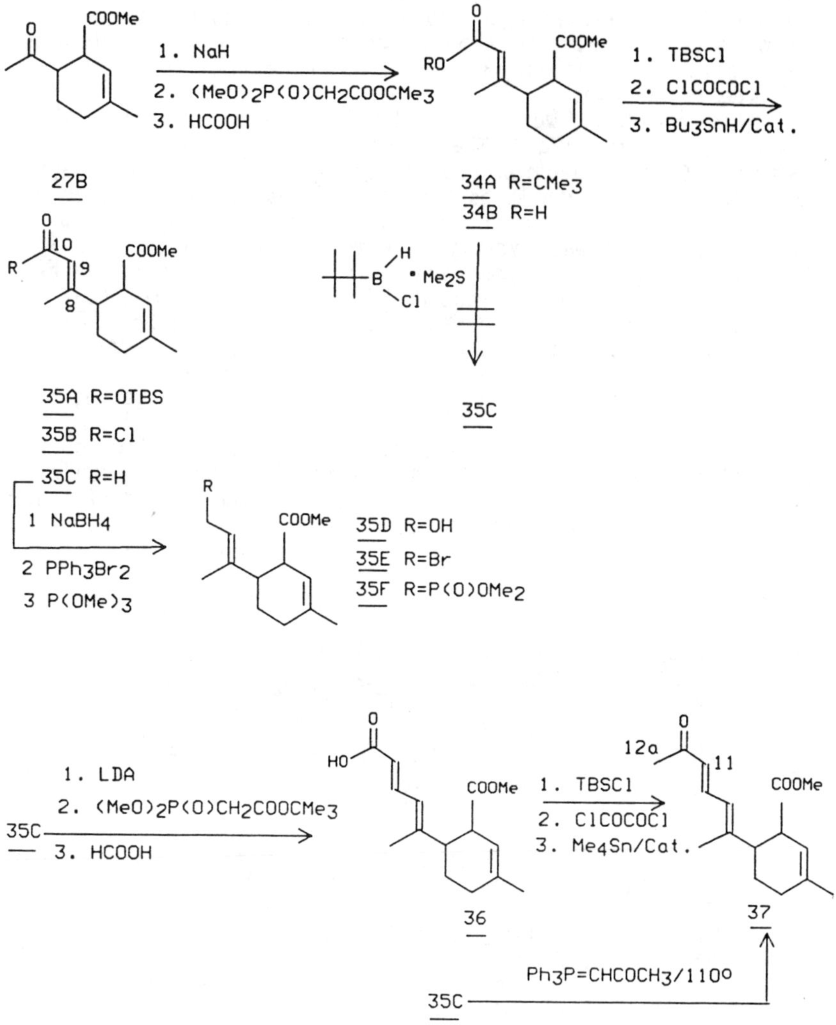
COOMe
1. NaH
2. (MeO)2P(O)CH2COOCMe3
3. HCOOH
27B
RO
COOMe
1. TBSCl
2. ClCOCOCl
3. Bu3SnH/Cat.
34A R=CMe3
34B R=H
10
9
8
R
COOMe
Me2S
Cl
35C
35A R=OTBS
35B R=Cl
35C R=H
1 NaBH4
2 PPh3Br2
3 P(OMe)3
COOMe
35D R=OH
35E R=Br
35F R=P(O)OMe2
1. LDA
2. (MeO)2P(O)CH2COOCMe3
3. HCOOH
35C
HO
COOMe
36
1. TBSCl
2. ClCOCOCl
3. Me4Sn/Cat.
12a
11
COOMe
37
Ph3P=CHCOCH3/110°
35C

SCHEME 4

chloride (TBSCl) gave the ester 35A which was reacted with oxalyl chloride to give 35B. Reduction with tributyltin hydride (12) catalysed by tetrakis(triphenylphosphine)palladium(0) gave 35C in an overall yield of 70% starting with 34A. Unfortunately the aldehyde 35C did not undergo the Wittig reaction under the conditions tried. 35C was also reduced with sodium borohydride to the alcohol 35D, which was then treated with dibromotriphenyl phosphorane to give the bromo compound 35E. An Arbuzov reaction with trimethyl phosphite gave the Wittig reagent 35F which again failed to react with the aldehyde 19 (R=CHO).

Two procedures were developed for the introduction of carbon atoms 11, 12, and 12a. The first procedure was a repeat of the Wadsworth Emmons reaction previously described. Thus, reaction of 35C with t-butyldimethylphosphonoacetate and LDA at -78°, or at room temperature with lithium chloride (13) and DBU, gave the expected t-butyl ester which was hydrolysed with formic acid to give 36, then silated with TBSCl, reacted with oxalyl chloride (14) to the acid chloride, and finally treated with tetramethyltin (15) and a catalytic amount of benzylchlorobis(triphenylphosphine)-palladium(II) to yield the 12-methyl ketone 37. An alternate procedure using the stabilized Wittig reagent of acetone and heating under reflux in toluene for 24 hours, also provided the ketone 37 in 70% yield.

To summarize then, procedures for the synthesis of the spiroketal, the side chain, and a simplified southern portion are available. Their joining together to form the macrocyclic lactone present in the milbemycins and avermectins will be the subject of a future communication.

LITERATURE CITED

1. Mishima, H.; Kurabayashi, M.; Tamura, C.; Sato, S.; Kuwano, H.; Saito, A. Tetrahedron Letters 1975, 711-714.
2. Mishima, H.; Ide, J.; Muramatsu, S.; Ono, M. J. of Antibiotics. 1983, 36, 980.
3. Chabala, J.C.; Mrozik, H.; Tolman, R. L.; Eskola, P.; Lusi, A.; Peterson, L. H.; Woods, M. F.; Fisher, M. H.; Campbell, W. C.; Egerton, J. R.; Ostlind, D. A. J. Med. Chem. 1980, 23, 1134-1136.
4. Barrett, A. G. M.; Carr, R. A. E.; Attwood, S. V.; Richardson, G.; Walshe, N. D. A. J. Org. Chem. 1986, 51, 4840-4856 and references therein.
5. Masamune, S.; Ellingboe, J. W.; Choy, W. J. Amer. Chem. Soc. 1982, 104, 5526.
6. Heathcock, C. H.; Pirrung, M. C.; Montgomery, S. H.; Lampe, J. Tetrahedron 1981, 37, 4087.
7. Heathcock, C. H.; Pirrung, M. C.; Sohn, J. E. J. Org. Chem. 1979, 44, 4294.
8. Buchi, G.; Powell, J. E. J. Amer. Chem. Soc. 1970, 92, 3126.
9. Zeller, P.; Bader, F.; Lindlar, H.; Montavon, M.; Muller, P.; Ruegg, R,; Ryser, G.; Saucy, G.; Schaeren, S. F.; Schwieter, U.; Stricker, K.; Tamm, R.; Zurcher, P.; Isler, O. Helv. Chim. Acta 1959, 42, 481.

10. Ruegg, von R.; Lindlar, H.; Montavon, M.; Saucy, G.; Schaeren, S. F.; Schwieter, U.; Isler, O. Helv. Chim. Acta 1959, 42, 847.
11. Brown, H. C.; Cha, J. S.; Nazer, B.; Yoon, N. M. J. Am. Chem. Soc. 1984, 106, 8001-8002.
12. Four, P.; Guibe, F.; J. Org. Chem. 1981, 46, 4439-4445.
13. Blanchette, M. A.; Choy, W.; Davis, J. T.; Essenfeld, A. P.; Masamune, S.; Roush, W. R.; Sakai, T. Tetrahedron Letters 1984, 25, 2183-2186.
14. Wissner, A.; Grudzinskas, C. V.; J. Org. Chem. 1978, 43, 3972.
15. Milstein, D.; Stille, J. K. J.Org. Chem. 1979, 44, 1613.

RECEIVED May 15, 1987

Chapter 24

Nonterpenoid *S*-Benzyl Thiolcarbamates with Juvenile Hormonelike Activity

Structure—Activity Relationships

Albert B. DeMilo, Stephen B. Haught, and Thomas J. Kelly

Insect Reproduction Laboratory, U.S. Department of Agriculture, Agricultural Research Center, Beltsville, MD 20705

A novel class of nonterpenoid juvenoids based on *S*-benzylthiolcarbamate chemistry is described. Juvenile hormone(JH)-mimicking activity of the lead thiolcarbamate was increased 500-fold as a result of synthesis of 42 analogs that were required for a systematic structure-activity relationship study conducted with the large milkweed bug, *Oncopeltus fasciatus* (Dallas). Typical of the morphological effects elicited by classical JH mimics, the most potent analog synthesized, the *S*-(1-phenylethyl) ester of 2,4-dichlorophenylcarbamothioic acid, caused 5th-stage *O. fasciatus* nymphs to molt to supernumerary 6th-instars rather than to normal adults when applied topically at a dose of 5 ng/nymph. Studies designed to elucidate the physiological role of thiolcarbamate juvenoids in *O. fasciatus* are described.

Over the last two decades, virtually thousands of juvenile hormone (JH) mimics have been synthesized and assessed for biological activity in numerous insect species, and a few of the exceptional compounds are already in or near commercial use (1). It is widely acknowledged that the majority of synthetic mimics are derived from a terpene template characteristic of the naturally occurring hormones. Throughout the intensive developmental period, many innovative changes were made on the terpene template. These modifications led to the discovery of new juvenoids that were, from a structural point of view, more terpene-inspired than terpene-derived (2,3). In addition to the classical JH mimics, a small collection of compounds (4,5,6) exists which elicit classical JH morphological effects in insects, yet they fail to fit the terpene template in any obvious way (Figure 1). Regardless of their potency, compounds

This chapter is not subject to U.S. copyright.
Published 1987, American Chemical Society

like those in Figure 1, whose structures differ widely from the terpenes and sesquiterpenes, are extremely important because they stimulate additional research geared to probing the biochemical and physiological mechanisms through which they operate.

Recently we discovered that a fluorine substituted thiolcarbamate, **5**, 2,4-difluorophenylcarbamothioic acid, *S*-(phenylmethyl) ester (Figure 2) elicited typical JH-morphological effects when large milkweed bug (*Oncopeltus fasciatus* (Dallas)) nymphs were treated topically with this material. Although **5** was only moderately effective against the large milkweed bug, the fact that its structure was strikingly simple and non-terpenoid motivated us to continue studies with this material.

Optimization of Biological Activity

Synthesis of Compounds. Thiolcarbamates and dithio=carbamates were synthesized by adding the appropriate phenyl isocyanate or phenyl isothiocyanate to a methylene chloride or benzene solution containing the benzyl mercaptan (ca. 1*M*) and a catalytic amount of triethylamine. When the reaction was complete (1-18hr at ambient temperature), the solvent was removed and the residue recrystallized from a suitable aprotic solvent. Satisfactory analyses ($\pm$ 0.4% of calculated values) for carbon and hydrogen were obtained for new compounds.

Biological Tests. Biological activity of candidate mimics were assessed by a JH-morphogenetic bioassay (*7*). Briefly, the test material, dissolved at the appropiate concentration in acetone, was applied topically to the last ventral abdominal segments of a newly emerged 5th-stage nymph (5 nymphs/test concentration). Treated insects were held on a normal diet of milkweed seed and water for approximately 1 week and then were scored for specific morphological changes, reflecting the degree of retention of juvenile characteristics in newly molted forms. Insects that partially ecdysed were also scored by surgically removing the old, outer cuticle and then assessing the morphology of the newly formed inner cuticle. *Scoring system:* 0 = normal adult (no JH effect); 1 = normal adult but some nymphal color on the abdomen; 2 = adult with smaller wings plus retention of nymphal color on the abdomen; 3 = supernumerary nymph (maximum JH effect). To facilitate comparison between compounds, lowest effective doses causing JH scores of $\geq$ 2.0 are reported in tables. Insects rated with JH scores $\geq$ 2.0 did not reach reproductive maturity and were considered non-viable.

Structure-Activity Relationships

Initial tests with thiolcarbamate **5** indicated only moderate JH-like activity in *O. fasciatus*; topical

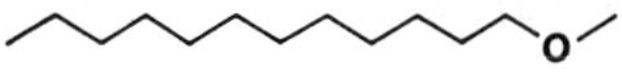

Figure 1. Structures of Nonterpenoid juvenoids. 1, dodecyl methyl ether; 2, piperonyl butoxide; 3, Niagara 16388; 4, ethyl 4-[2-(*tert*-butylcarbonyloxy)butoxy]benzoate, ETB. Structures are based on information in References 4-6.

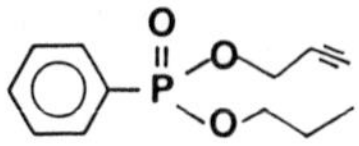

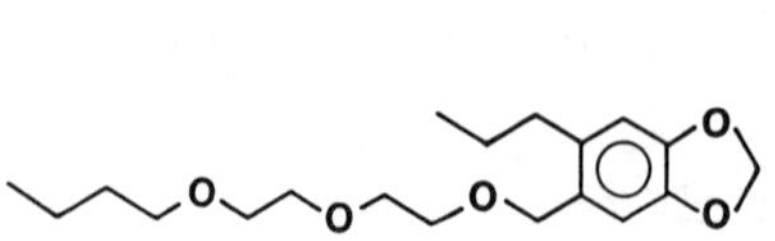

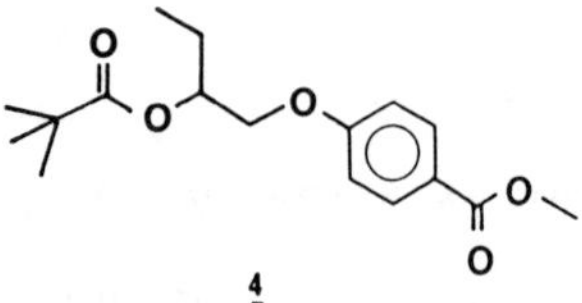

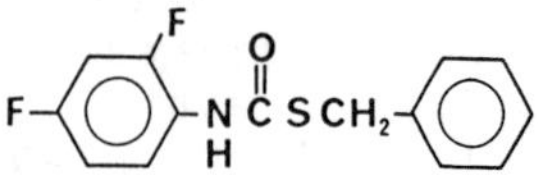

Figure 2. JH-active thiolcarbamate.

application of 5 (5 μg/nymph) to 5th instars caused insects to molt to supernumerary nymphs rather than to normal adults. Third instars, however, were unaffected by similar treatment with 5 (10 μg/nymph) and molted normally to 4th instars. Adults were also unaffected by 5 in topical treatments at doses as high as 100 μg per insect; mortality was low (ca. 7 %, 10 days posttreatment), and oviposition and egg hatch indices of treated insects were comparable to those of controls.

Initial activity of 5 encouraged us to synthesize analogs for optimization of activity and to define structure-activity relationships (SAR) within this unusual class of JH mimics. However, prior to the synthesis of analogs, the potential hydrolysis products of 5, benzyl mercaptan and 2,4-difluoroaniline (8), were tested. Both compounds were morphogenetically ineffective.

One of the most important steps in the SAR study was to assess the optimal arrangement of sulfur and oxygen atoms in the carbamoyl moiety. Data in Table I show that compounds 5 and 6, both thiolesters, were most effective. Clearly, the complete loss of activity in carbamate 8 highlighted the importance of sulfur in the molecule.

Table I. Influence of Carbamoyl Moiety on Activity

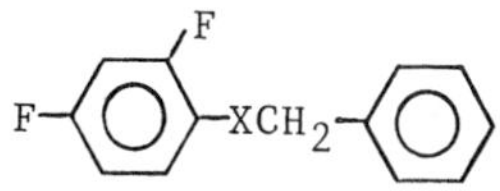

2,4-difluorophenyl–XCH_2–phenyl

No.	X	Lowest Effective Dose[a] (μg/nymph)
5	NHC(=O)S	2.5
6	NHC(=S)S	10
7	NHC(=S)O	25
8	NHC(=O)O	n.a.[b]

[a] Causing JH score of ≥ 2.0. [b] No activity at highest dose tested (50 μg).

The importance of the benzyl group in 5 as a requirement for activity can be seen from data presented for analogs listed in Table II. Interestingly, while substitution of the benzylic ring with various electron withdrawing or donating moieties caused complete or near complete loss of activity, α-methyl substitution caused appreciable enhancement of activity. Because 9 lacked juvenoid activity (growth-inhibition effects were observed at high doses) no further consideration was given to alkyl thiolester analogs of 5.

Table II. Influence of Various Thiols on Activity

(General structure: 2,4-difluorophenyl–NHC(O)SR)

No.	R	Lowest Effective Dose[a] (μg/nymph)
5	$CH_2C_6H_5$	2.5
9	n-C_3H_7	n.a.[b]
10	C_6H_5	n.a.[b]
11	$CH_2CH_2C_6H_5$	>50
12	$CH(CH_3)C_6H_5$	0.05
13	$CH_2C_6H_4(4\text{-}CH_3O)$	25
14	$CH_2C_6H_4(4\text{-}CH_3)$	n.a.[b]
15	$CH_2C_6H_4(4\text{-}Cl)$	n.a.[b]
16	$CH_2C_6H_4(4\text{-}NO_2)$	n.a.[b]

[a] Causing JH score of ≥2.0. [b] No activity at highest dose tested (50 μg).

Table III shows data for a series of thiolcarbamates and dithiocarbamates containing various single or multiple substituents on the aniline moiety. Because lead compound 5 contained fluorine, the selection of compounds chosen for this segment of the SAR study was biased toward halogen containing analogs. For thiolcarbamates, the only effective halogenated analog was 22: the 2,4-dichloro analog of 5. Surprisingly, a single fluorine or chlorine substituent at either the ortho or para position of the aniline ring caused loss of activity. Positional isomers, 2,6- and 2,5-difluoro analogs of 5, were also tested but were ineffective. The increased activity of the 4-methoxy analog 27 over 5 indicated that activity was not exclusively restricted to compounds bearing halogen substituents.

Table III. Effects of Substituents on the Aniline Moiety

R-C6H4-NHC(=X)-SCH2-C6H5

R	Thiolcarbamate X=O, Lowest Effective Dose[a] No.	Thiolcarbamate X=O, Lowest Effective Dose[a] (µg/nymph)	Dithiocarbamate X=S, Lowest Effective Dose[a] No.	Dithiocarbamate X=S, Lowest Effective Dose[a] (µg/nymph)
2,4-F_2	5	2.5	6	10
2-F	17	n.a.[b]	--	--
4-F	18	n.a.[b]	32	>50
3-F	19	n.a.[b]	--	--
2,6-F_2	20	n.a.[b]	--	--
2,5-F_2	21	n.a.[b]	--	--
2,4-Cl_2	22	1.0	33	2.5
2-Cl	23	n.a.[b]	34	n.a.[b]
4-Cl	24	n.a.[b]	35	5
3-Cl	25	n.a.[b]	36	n.a.[b]
3,4-Cl_2	26	n.a.[b]	37	2.5
4-CH_3O	27	0.5	38	0.1
4-CH_3S	28	n.a.[b]	--	--
4-CH_3	29	n.a.[b]	39	10
H	30	n.a.[b]	--	--
4-NO_2	31	>50	40	50

[a] Causing JH score of $\geq$2.0. [b] No activity at highest dose tested (50 µg).

Although fewer dithiocarbamates were investigated, results from those studied suggest that structure-activity correlations derived for thiolcarbamates were only partly applicable to dithiocarbamates. Differences between thiolcarbamates and dithiocarbamates were clearly highlighted from the lack of parallel activity between three analog pairs 24 and 35, 26 and 37, 29 and 39.

Since attachment of a methyl group at the alpha position of 5 (Table II) improved activity substantially, several racemic S-α-(methyl)benzyl thiolcarbamates and dithiocarbamates were synthesized and assessed for activity. Data in Table IV show that, except for 41 and 47, α-(methyl)benzyl analogs were more effective than their benzyl counterparts. Data also show that α-methyl substituted thiolcarbamates were consistently more effective than their corresponding dithiocarbamates. The chiral center in α-(methyl)-benzyl analogs poses a question regarding its influence on activity. Since only racemic samples were evaluated in this study, future studies should include evaluation of appropriate enantiomers.

Table IV. Activity of α-(Methyl)benzyl Analogs

R-C₆H₃(ring)-NHC(=X)SCH(CH₃)-C₆H₅

No.	R	X	Lowest Effective Dose[a,b] (μg/nymph)	
12	2,4-F_2	O	0.05	(2.5)
41	2,4-F_2	S	>50	(10)
42	2,4-Cl_2	O	0.005	(1.0)
43	2,4-Cl_2	S	0.5	(2.5)
44	3,4-Cl_2	O	0.05	(n.a.)[c]
45	3,4-Cl_2	S	1.0	(2.5)
46	4-CH_3O	O	0.1	(0.5)
47	4-CH_3O	S	0.5	(0.1)

[a] Causing JH score of ≥2.0. [b] Values in parentheses are lowest effective doses for corresponding S-benzyl analogs. [c] No activity at highest dose tested (50 μg).

Physiological Studies With Thiolcarbamates

Although thiolcarbamates are a well known class of herbicides (9), little is known regarding their juvenoid effects in insects. Certain JH-active bisthiolcarbam=ates (10) and phenoxyphenoxy-substituted thiolcarbamates (11) are known, but structures representing these juvenoids suggest *a priori* that activity may be owed to the fact that these compounds had terpene-inspired origins (10,12,13). In studies (14,15) to elucidate the mode of action of a bisthiolcarbamate juvenoid, *N*-ethyl-1,2-bis=(isobutylthiocarbamoyl)ethane, a herbicidally active *S*-benzyl thiolcarbamate, *S*-(4-chlorobenzyl) *N,N*-diethyl=thiocarbamate (thiobencarb), and its sulfoxide were shown to inhibit JH biosynthesis *in vitro*. However, neither thiobencarb nor its sulfoxide elicited *in vivo* JH-antagonistic activity. Interestingly, in our studies the bisthiolcarbamate elicited JH-mimicking activity in *O. fasciatus* at 1.0 µg/nymph while thiobencarb, a compound structurally resembling **5**, was morphogenetically inactive at the highest dose tested (50 µg/nymph).

Juvenile hormone or related compounds are important factors promoting yolk uptake in developing ovarian follicles in *O. fasciatus* (16). To determine if thiol=carbamates **5** and **42** behaved physiologically similar to a known JH mimic, female *O. fasciatus*, maintained for 4 days on protein-free diet of 3% glucose, were topically treated with the thiolcarbamates over a wide range of doses (including doses presumably exceeding physiological levels). At 4 days posttreatment their ovaries were examined under a low-power dissecting microscope and scored (16) for the presence or absence of stage C (vitellogenic) ovaries (i.e., ovaries containing 1-3 large yellow follicles per ovariole). A parallel experiment was run for 2,6-difluoro-*N*-[[4-[(3-fluorophen=yl)methoxy]phenyl]methyl]benzenamine (AI3-63604), a JH mimic with known effectiveness against *O. fasciatus* (17).

Data in Table V show that ovaries from AI3-63604 treated females were, as expected, vitellogenic. However, data obtained from insects treated with **42** or **5** were conflicting; i.e., ovaries from **42**-treated females were vitellogenic at high doses (suggestive of normal JH behavior) while ovaries from **5**-treated females were non-vitellogenic (compared to controls) over the entire dose range (suggestive of non-JH behavior). Two explanations could account for the widely different results. First, thiolcarbamates **42** and **5** may have different modes of action (unlikely, since **42** and **5** have similar structures). Second, the more active the compound (**42**>>**5**) the easier it would be to reach JH-responsive tissues to induce JH-like effects.

Methoprene, when topically applied to newly emerged 5th-stage *O. fasciatus*, shortens the duration of the 5th stadium by approximately 36 hours, causes supernumerary nymph formation, and accelerates the onset of molting hormone secretion (18). Two of these phenomena, i.e., shortening of the 5th stage and supernumerary nymph formation, were readily observed for **5** in morphogenetic

Table V. Effects of Compounds on Ovarian Development

Compound[a]	Treatment Dose (μg/Adult Females)	% Females with Vitellogenic Eggs[b]
JH mimic	1.0	74 (0)
(AI3-63604)	1.0	88 (30)
5	500	20 (30)
	250	20 (30)
	100	33 (30)
	10	30 (30)
42	10	100 (0)
	1.0	85 (0)
	0.1	74 (0)
	0.01	0 (0)

[a] Structure in text. [b] Numbers in parentheses are for controls (acetone treated only).

tests. To investigate the influence of 5 on the ecdysteroid secretion, hemolymph from topically treated (10 μg/nymph), newly emerged, 5th-instar O. fasciatus females was periodically removed and analyzed for ecdysteroid content by radioimmunoassay (19). Ecdysteroid titer profiles (Figure 3) for 5th-stage O. fasciatus females, treated with 5 (10 μg/nymph) or JH mimic AI3-63604 (1 μg/nymph), show that both compounds accelerate onset of ecdysteroid secretion with peak titers occuring approximately 2 days earlier than those observed for untreated insects. The striking resemblance of the ecdysteroid profiles of 5 to that of AI3-63604 and methoprene (18) suggests, more clearly than the results obtained in the ovarian development bioassay, that thiolcarbamate 5 may indeed mimic the behavior of known juvenoids. Although bisthiolcarbamate, N-ethyl-1,2-bis(isobutylthiolcarbamoyl)ethane, inhibited JH biosynthesis (14,15), we found no evidence during the course of our studies to suggest that thiolcarbamates related to 5 were antagonistic to JH synthesis. Other experiments will undoubtedly be required to elucidate the mechanism by which thiolcarbamates elicit their juvenoid effects in O. fasciatus. However, since the exact nature of the juvenile hormones in O. fasciatus is still uncertain, meaningful experiments to determine the mode of action of thiolcarbamates are difficult to design at present.

Effects of Compounds on Different Insect Species

Most of the compounds were evaluated in larval development screens for three other species: *Musca domestica* L., *Plodia interpunctella* (Hübner), and *Spodoptera frugiperda* (J. E. Smith). A few compounds elicited

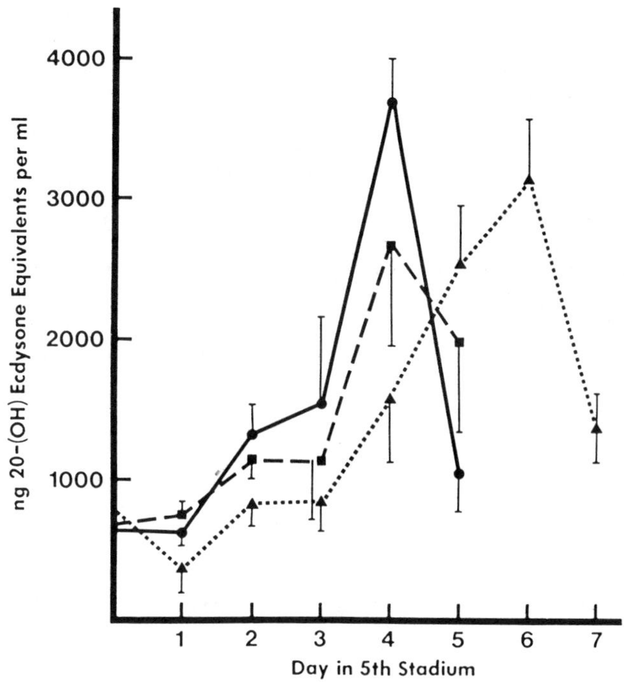

Figure 3. Ecdysteroid titers of female 5th-stage O. fasciatus treated topically with compounds. Circles, thiolcarbamate 5 treated; squares, JH-mimic AI3-63604 treated; triangles, acetone treated (controls).

moderate larvicidal effects in *M. domestica* and *P. interpunctella*, but none of the compounds evaluated were larvicidal against *S. frugiperda*. Except for a single test with **12** in *P. interpunctella*, highly active thiolcarbamates **12**, **42**, and **44** were ineffective as larvicides for these species.

In *M. domestica* tests, only dithiocarbamates **6**, **32**, **35**, **38**, **39**, **43**, and **45** were larvicidal; all caused 100% mortality to immatures when incorporated in a larval diet at 100 ppm. At 10 ppm none of the compounds were active.

Again, dithiocarbamates were prominent when tested as larvicides against *P. interpunctella*. While **12**, **39**, **43**, and **45** were moderately toxic at 1000 ppm, **38**, and **47** were completely toxic at the same concentration.

Although none of the compounds tested were larvicidal against *S. frugiperda*, several compounds (mostly dithiocarbamates) inhibited reproduction of adults that survived the larval treatment. For example, adults that emerged from a larval medium, dosed with **32**, **34**, **35**, **41**, **46**, or **47** at 100 ppm, oviposited after mating, but eggs failed to hatch. In addition to preventing egg hatch, **41**, **46**, and **47** reduced oviposition substantially.

Summary

Although the effects of thiolcarbamates in *M. domestica*, *P. interpunctella*, and *S. frugiperda* were considered marginal, the exceptional morphogenetic activity of thiolcarbamates in *O. fasciatus*, combined with the uniqueness of their structure, makes this class of compounds worthy of further investigation, particularly in economically important hemipterans. Structure modifications investigated in this study were highly successful in increasing activity 500-fold over lead compound **5**. The most active compound **42**, *S*-(1-phenylethyl) ester of 2,4-dichlorophenylcarbamothioic acid, was topically active against *O. fasciatus* at a dose as low as 5 ng per insect. It is not unreasonable to assume that further modifications may lead to even more potent juvenoids than those identified in this study.

Clearly, more physiological studies will be required to elaborate the mechanism through which *S*-benzyl thiolcarbamates act. Studies in plants and animals provide ample evidence to show that thiolcarbamates are metabolically oxidized to sulfoxides (*20*,*21*) that are capable of carbamoylating critical thiol sites on enzyme cofactors such as coenzyme A and gluthione (*22*). Carbamoylation of thiol sites of enzymes or cofactors regulating lipid or terpene biosynthesis has been suggested as a possible mechanism of action of bisthiolcarbamate juvenoids (*14*,*23*). Accordingly, it is tempting to speculate here that the biochemical role for *S*-benzyl thiolcarbamates identified in this study may well involve carbamoylation of thiol sites in cellular metabolites that regulate JH titers during critical stages of the insect's development.

Acknowledgments

Thanks are due to Robert E. Redfern, retired, (Livestock Insects Laboratory, USDA-ARS, Beltsville, Maryland) for providing test results for the fall armyworm. Thanks are also due to Suzanne M. Spalding for technical assistance and to Richard T. Brown, previously affiliated with this laboratory, for synthesizing many of the compounds used in this study. Finally, thanks are due to the Chevron Chemical Company for providing a sample of thiobencarb and to the Zoecon Corporation for providing a sample of the bisthiolcarb= amate.

Literature Cited

1. Menn, J.J; Henrick, C.A.; In Agricultural Chemicals of the Future; Hilton, J.L., Ed.; BARC Symposium Series VIII, Rowman and Allenheld, Totowa, New Jersey, 1985, 248-265.
2. Sláma, K.; Romaňuk, M.; Šorm, F. In Insect Hormones and Bioanalogues; Springer-Verlag, New York/Wien, 1974, 137-213.
3. Henrick, C. In Insecticide Mode of Action; Coats, J. R., Ed; Academic Press, New York, 1982, 315-402.
4. Bowers, W. S.; Thompson, M. J. Science 1963, 142, 1469-1470.
5. Bowers, W. S. Science 1968, 161, 895-897.
6. Staal, G. B. Scri. varia pont. Acad. Sci. 1977, 41, 353-377.
7. Redfern, R. E.; McGovern, T. P.; Sarmiento, R.; Beroza, M. J. Econ. Entomol. 1971, 64, 374-376.
8. Melnikov, N.N. In Residue Reviews; 1971, 36, Chapt. 17., Chemistry of Pesticides.
9. Jäger, G. In Chemistry of Pesticides; Büchel, K.M., Ed.; John Wiley & Sons, Inc., New York, 1983, 315-405.
10. Pallos, M. F.; Letchworth, P. E.; and Menn, J. J. J. Agric. Food Chem. 1984, 24, 218-221.
11. Kisida, H.; Hatakoshi, M.; Itaya, N., Nakayama, I. Agric. Biol. Chem. 1984, 48, 2889-2891.
12. Karrer, F; Farooq, S. Proc. Int'l. Conf. Regulation of Insect Development and Behavior; Sehnal, F.; Zabza, A.; Menn, J. J.; Cymborowski, E.; Eds., Wroclaw Techn. University Press, Wroclaw, 1981, 289-302.
13. Franke, v.A.; Mattern,G.; Traber, W. Helv. Chem. Acta 1975, 58, 268-296.
14. Kramer, S. J.; Tsai, L. W.; Lee, S. F.; Menn, J. J. Pestic. Biochem. Physiol. 1982, 17, 134-141.

15. Kramer, S. J.; Baker, F. C.; Miller, C. A.; Cerf, D. C.; Schooley, D. A.; Menn, J. J. Proc. 5th Int'l. Cong. Pestic. Chem., Human Welfare and the Environment, Miyamoto, J.; Kearney, P., Eds.; Pergaman Press, Oxford, 1983, 177-82.
16. Kelly, T. J.; Davenport, R. J. Insect Physiol., 1976, 22, 1381-1393.
17. DeMilo, A. B.; Redfern, R. E. J. Agric. Food. Chem., 1979, 27, 760-762.
18. Smith, W. A.; Nijhout, H. F. J. Insect Physiol. 1981, 27, 169-173.
19. Kelly, T. J.; Woods, C. W.; Redfern, R. E.; Borkovec, A. B. J. Exp. Zool. 1981, 218, 127-132.
20. Hubbell, J. P.; Casida, J. E. J. Agric. Food Chem. 1977, 25, 404-413.
21. Casida, J. E. In Symposium on Environmental Transport and Transformation of Pesticides; Duttweiler, D. W. Ed., U. S. Environmental Protection Agency, Athens, Georgia, 1978, 163.
22. Lay, M. -M.; Hubbell, J. P.; Casida, J. E. Science 1975, 189, 287-289.
23. Menn, J. J. In Approaches to New Leads for Insecticides; v. Keyserlingk et al., Eds., Springer-Verlag Berlin Heidelberg, 1985, 38-46.

RECEIVED May 15, 1987

Chapter 25

Larvicidal and Fungicidal Activity of Compounds with Hydrazinecarboxamide and Diazenecarboxamide Moieties

Albert B. DeMilo [1], Stephen B. Haught [1], and Hugh D. Sisler [2]

[1]Insect Reproduction Laboratory, Agricultural Research Center, U.S. Department of Agriculture, Beltsville, MD 20705
[2]Department of Botany, University of Maryland, College Park, MD 20742

Based on the effectiveness of N-(2,4-difluoro=phenyl)-2-(2-fluorophenyl)-hydrazinecarboxamide in house fly larvicidal tests, 53 analogs were synthesized and structure-activity relationships (SAR) defined. The most potent larvicide identified from this study was 2-(2-fluorophenyl)=-N-[2-(trifluoromethyl)phenyl]-hydrazinecarbox=amide. This compound caused > 90% mortality to early instars, when administered in a larval diet at a concentration of 1-5 ppm. As part of the SAR study, nine diazenecarboxamides were synthesized and evaluated. Activity of diazenecarboxamides paralleled that observed for corresponding hydra=zinecarboxamides. Three hydrazinecarboxamides and three diazenecarboxamides were highly (< 5.0 ppm) fungitoxic to one or more plant pathogens: *Pyricularia oryzae*, *Botrytis cinerea*, and *Monilinia fructicola*. SAR defined from fungicide tests appear to parallel those defined from larvicide tests. The most potent larvicides and fungicides possessed fluorine or fluorine-containing substituents on the benzene rings.

Because of their ability to induce sterility in insects, hydrazine-derived compounds have long been of interest to us in our search for new reproduction inhibitors (1-4). In this context, we recently evalu=ated compound 1, N-(2,4-difluorophenyl)-2-(2-fluoro=phenyl)-hydrazinecarboxamide (Figure 1), and found that it inhibited oviposition in house flies (*Musca domestica* L.) when administered orally to adults. However, since infertility was accompanied by excessive adult mortality, failure to lay eggs was probably symptomatic of nonspecific toxic effects rather than effects directed at the reproduction pathway. Consistent with toxicity exhibited in adults, 1 was

0097-6156/87/0355-0273$06.00/0
© 1987 American Chemical Society

also toxic to house fly larvae reared on a diet containing this material.

Although the parent compound 2 (Figure 1), *N*,2-diphenylhydrazinecarboxamide, (nomenclature prior to 1972: 1,4-diphenylsemicarbazide) is a known larvicide (5-9), and related compounds 3 and 4 were described (10) as having similar activity, little is known regarding the larvicidal effectiveness of fluorine analogs in this class of compounds.

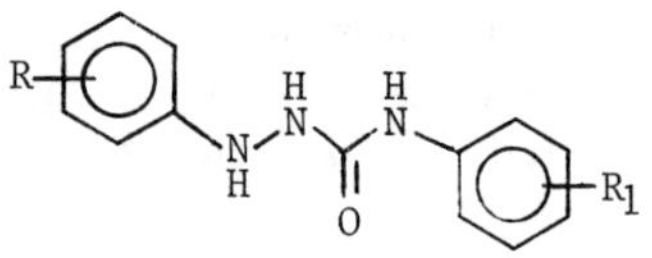

1, R=2-F; R_1=2,4-F_2 3, R=H, R_1=4-C_2H_5
2, R=R_1=H 4, R=4-Cl, R_1=4-C_2H_5

Figure 1. Structures of *N*,2-diphenylhydrazinecarboxamides

Because this information is lacking and because 1 resembled some recently reported larvicidal thiosemicarbazones (11,12), we decided to study 1 in detail. Also, since 2 (13) and related chlorine derivatives (14,15) are fungitoxic, we evaluated 1 and analogs against selected plant pathogenic fungi.

Synthesis of Compounds

The *N*,2-diphenylhydrazinecarboxamides were readily synthesized in moderate to excellent yields. Briefly, the method involved addition of a substituted phenyl isocyanate to a solution or slurry containing the appropriately substituted phenylhydrazine. When reaction was complete, the product was isolated by filtration (if precipitated) or by evaporation of the solvent and recrystallization of the residue.

Diazenecarboxamides 40-48 (Table IV) were synthesized by oxidizing the corresponding hydrazinecarboxamides with ferric chloride (16). Although oxidizing agents such as bromine, *N*-bromoacetamide and chromic acid provided products in acceptable yields, ferric chloride was the reagent of choice. To illustrate the procedure, the synthesis of 42, 2-(2-fluorophenyl)-*N*-[2-(trifluoromethyl)phenyl]-diazenecarboxamide, follows. To a solution of the precursor 16 (2.0 g) in methanol (30 ml) was rapidly added an aqueous solution containing ferric chloride hexahydrate (3.4 g) in water (8 ml). Within seconds the color of the oxidant dissipated and the product precipitated. After 0.5 hr at room temperature, the mixture was poured into water (25 ml) and the product collected by filtration. Recrystallization from cyclohexane afforded 1.6 g (79%) of 42, mp 102-105°C.

All new compounds gave satisfactory (± 0.4%) combustion analyses for carbon, hydrogen and nitrogen. Compounds submitted for bioassay were >98% pure.

Larvicidal Effects of Compounds

Bioassays. House fly larvicide tests required a modified (17), semi-defined (18) synthetic diet to rear larvae. A brief description of the test method follows. Fifty freshly deposited eggs (from NAIDM strain of flies) were placed on top of a gel matrix comprised of water (8 ml), synthetic house fly diet (1.5 g), vitamin mixture (0.5 ml), and test compound at the required concentration. Resulting larvae were allowed to develop in the gel (held at 27°C for the duration of the test) to the pupal stage and pupae that survived treatment were counted. From counts, percent inhibition of pupation was calculated. Scoring system (based on percent inhibition of pupation): 0, normal pupation at 100 ppm; +, <90% inhibition at 100 ppm; ++, >90% inhibition at 50-100 ppm; +++, >90% inhibition at 10-50 ppm; ++++, >90% inhibition at 5-10 ppm; +++++, >90% inhibition at 1-5 ppm.

A brief description of the yellow fever mosquito (*Aedes aegypti* (L.)) larvicide test follows. An acetone solution (0.5 ml) containing the appropriate amount of test compound was added to a mixture of distilled water (49.5 ml), Tween 80 (25 mg), and a single pellet of rabbit chow (Ralston-Purina). Twenty late-4th instars (5-6 days posthatch) were added to this medium and the medium was incubated at 27°C. The test was terminated when all larvae died or when adults emerged from surviving pupae.

Previously described methods were used to assess larvicidal activity in the fall armyworm, *Spodoptera frugiperda* (J.E. Smith) (19) and in the Indian meal moth, *Plodia interpunctella* (Hübner) (20).

Structure-Activity Relationships. Effects caused by initial structural modifications in the lead compound are shown in Table I. Replacement of the oxygen in 1 with sulfur caused complete loss of activity. Replacement of the phenyl moiety at the 2-position with benzyl, hydrogen, or alkyl gave inactive analogs 6-9. Similary, replacement of *N*-phenyl with hydrogen, alkyl, or cycloalkyl gave inactive analogs 10-12. Clearly, larvicidal activity is restricted to compounds with *N*,2-diphenyl substitution. Activity also appears enhanced by fluorine substituents.

To further define structure-activity relationships, two series of compounds (13-22 and 23-30) were synthesized and evaluated (Table II). Because 1 was highly fluorinated, compounds selected for this part of

Table I. Activity of hydrazinecarboxamides in *Musca*

R–NH–NH–C(=X)–NH–R$_1$

No.	R	X	R$_1$	Graded Larvicidal Activity[a]
1	2-F-C_6H_4	O	2,4-F_2-C_6H_3	+ + + +
2	C_6H_5	O	C_6H_5	+ + +
3	"	O	4-(C_2H_5)-C_6H_4	+ +
4	4-Cl-C_6H_4	O	"	+
5	2-F-C_6H_4	S	2,4-F_2-C_6H_3	0
6	2-F-$C_6H_4CH_2$	O	"	0
7	H	O	"	0
8	CF_3CH_2	O	"	0
9	$NCCH_2CH_2$	O	"	0
10	2-F-C_6H_4	O	H	0
11	"	O	*n*-C_3H_7	0
12	"	O	*c*-C_6H_{11}	0

[a] Assessed from percentage of pupae surviving larval treatment (corrected for controls). See bioassay methods for key to activity scale.

Table II. Larvicidal activity of N,2-diphenylhydrazine=carboxamides in *Musca*

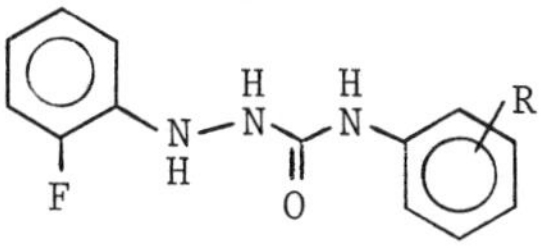

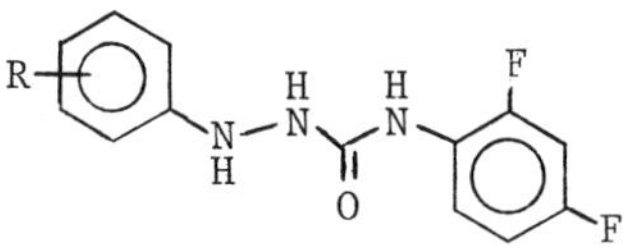

No.	R	Graded Activity[a]	No.	R	Graded Activity[a]
1	2,4-F_2	+ + + +	1	2-F	+ + + +
13	2,5-F_2	+ + + +	23	2,4-F_2	+ + +
14	2,6-F_2	+ + +	24	3,5-$(CF_3)_2$	0
15	2-F	+ + +	25	2,3,4,5,6-F_5	0
16	2-CF_3	+ + + + +	26	2-CN,3-F	0
17	3-CF_3	+ + +	27	4-CH_3O	+ + + +
18	4-CF_3	+ + +	28	H	+ + + +
19	4-Cl	+ +	29	4-Cl	+ + + +
20	H	+ + +	30	4-NO_2	+
21	4-CH_3	+ + +			
22	4-CH_3O	+			

[a] Assessed from percentage of pupae surviving larval treatment. See bioassay methods for key to activity scale.

the study were admittedly biased toward those with fluorine substituents. In analogs 13-22, the 2-fluoro=phenyl moiety of 1 was kept intact, and substituent changes were made in the N-phenyl moiety. Conversely, in analogs 23-30, the 2,4-difluorophenyl moiety in 1 was kept intact and substituent changes were made in the 2-phenyl moiety. Data from analogs 13-22 supported the conclusion that activity was influenced by the type (compare 18,19 and 22) and location (compare 16,17,18 and 1,13,14) of the substituent. Since all analogs in this series were active, structural variations in this area of the molecule did not appear to have a significant influence on activity.

Activities of analogs 27-30, however, indicated a lack of correlation with *para* substitution (low activity of 30 may be due to its poor solubility). Clearly, none of the substituent modifications improved activity over 1. Interestingly, even unsubstituted 28 had appreciable activity.

To further increase activity, analogs (31-34) were prepared. This series (Table III) combined optimum substitution (2-trifluoromethyl) for the N-phenyl moiety with optimum substitution (4-chloro, 4-methoxy, etc.) for the 2-phenyl moiety. None of the compounds reflecting this approach exceeded activity obtained for 16. Again, data from 35-39 support the conclusion suggested by analogs 27-30: activity can not be correlated with the electronic properties of the *para* substituent on the N-phenyl moiety.

During their synthesis, some hydrazinecarboxamides appeared sensitive to air oxidation. Because of this and because certain related phenyldiazenecarboxamide-derived fungicides are more toxic than their corresponding hydrazines (21), nine (40-48) diazene (= azo) analogs of 1 were evaluated as potential larvicides. Data in Table IV show that five azo analogs were larvicidal and, except for 44, were equal in effectiveness to their hydrazine counterparts. In no case involving azo/hydrazine pairs was activity exceeded by the azo analog. This parallel activity is suggestive of a single mode of action for the similar but distinctly different compounds.

Evidence to further support the single mode of action concept was obtained in closely monitored parallel tests with a cognate pair 16 and 42. Results from these tests (at lethal and sublethal doses) showed 16 and 42 were essentially indistinguishable in their effects on larval, pupal, and adult stages of development. Because azo analogs were no more effective than their hydrazine counterparts and because alkylation of 33 (at the 2-position) with methyl provided an analog (incapable of azo formation) equal to 33 in effectiveness, synthesis of azo analogs was discontinued.

Analogs 49-54 (Table V) show additional modifications investigated. All compounds in Table V were

Table III. Activity of *N*,2-diphenylhydrazinecarboxamides in *Musca*

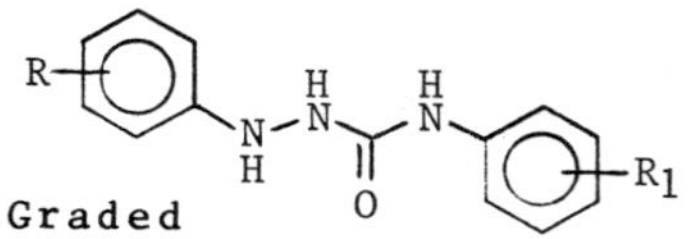

No.	R	R_1	Graded Larvicidal Activity[a]	No.	R	R_1	Graded Larvicidal Activity[a]
31	2,4-F_2	2-CF_3	+ + +	35	2-Cl	2-F	+ + +
32	4-CH_3O	2-CF_3	+ + + +	36	4-CH_3O	2-F	+ + + +
33	H	2-CF_3	+ + + +	37	H	2-F	+ + + +
34	4-Cl	2-CF_3	+ + + +	38	4-Cl	2-F	+ + + +
				39	4-NO_2	2-F	0

[a] Assessed from percentage of pupae surviving larval treatment (corrected for controls). See bioassay methods for key to activity scale.

Table IV. Activity of diazenecarboxamides in *Musca*

R–C_6H_4–N=N–C(=O)–NH–R_1

No.	R	R_1	Larvicidal Activity: L.E.D.[a] Causing >90% Inhibition of Pupation (ppm)
40	2-F	2,4-F_2-C_6H_3	10(10)[b]
41	2-F	2,5-F_2-C_6H_3	10(10)[b]
42	2-F	2-(CF_3)-C_6H_4	5-10(5)[b]
43	2-F	2-F-C_6H_4	10-50(10-50)[b]
44	2-Cl	2-F-C_6H_4	n.a.[c](50)[b]
45	2-F	C_6H_5	50(50)[b]
46	2-F	*n*-C_3H_7	n.a.[c](n.a.)[b,c]
47	2-F	H	n.a.[c](n.a.)[b,c]
48	H	*c*-C_6H_{11}	n.a.[c](n.a.)[b,c]

[a] Lowest effective dose. [b] Number in parenthesis represents activity of hydrazinecarboxamide precursor. [c] n.a. = No activity at 100 ppm.

Table V. Ineffective hydrazinecarboxamides and related compounds[a]

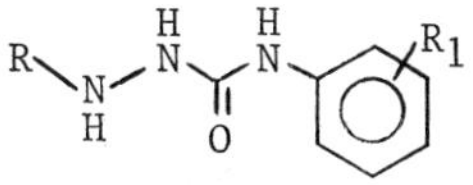

No.	R	R_1
49	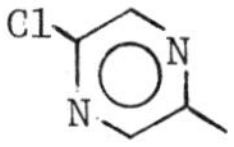 Cl, N, N	2,4-F_2
50	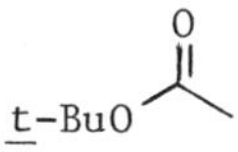 t-BuO, O	2,4-F_2
51	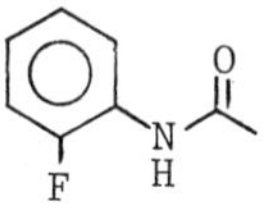 O, NH, F	2,4-F_2
52	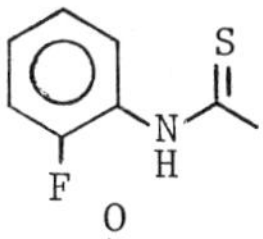 S, NH, F	2,4-F_2
53	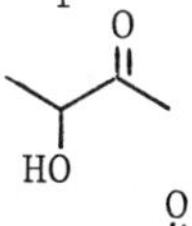 O, HO	4-Cl
54	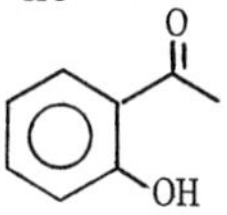 O, OH	4-Cl

[a] Inactive at 100 ppm in *Musca* larvicide bioassay.

inactive in Musca at the highest concentration tested. Although little can be said here about the effects of heterocyclic substitution (only the pyrazine analog 49 was tested), lack of activity in analogs 50-54 clearly emphasizes the importance of phenyl substitution at the 2-position.

Effects of Compounds in Other Species. Three analogs (16, 36 and 42) effective against Musca were evaluated in the Aedes developmental bioassay. Hydrazinecarboxamides 16 and 36 elicited strong larvicidal effects at the highest concentration (10 ppm) tested; 24-hr posttreatment mortalities were 92% and 100%, respectively. Although mortality decreased at 1 ppm (22% for 16 and 47% for 36), adult emergence was completely inhibited by 36. Unlike results in Musca, 42 (azo analog of 16) was ineffective at 10 ppm in Aedes. Inactivity of 42 was surprising in light of activity in Aedes previously reported (12) for N,2-diphenyldiazenecarboxamide.

In Plodia, hydrazinecarboxamides 1, 13 and 16 were toxic to larvae when administered in a larval diet at 1000 ppm. However, at 100 ppm all analogs were nontoxic and larvae surviving treatment produced normal adults. Reproduction indices (oviposition, egg hatch) observed from matings of surviving adults were also normal. Azo analogs of 1, 13 and 16 were evaluated in Plodia and except 42 (nontoxic at 100 ppm), elicited effects identical to their hydrazine counterparts.

Azo-azine pairs 1 and 40, 13 and 41, and 16 and 42 were also evaluated in the Spodoptera bioassay. With only minor deviations, a uniform profile of effects was observed when these analogs were added to a larval diet. For example, at 100 ppm 16 caused a substantial (20-30%) decrease in size and weight of pupae (low larval mortality) and severely inhibited egg production of adults that survived larval treatment. Invariably, eggs deposited by females, whose oviposition was severely affected, did not hatch. At 10 ppm, 16 had no effect on larval growth and development, and no effect on reproduction. Although it is not known how reproduction is inhibited by 16 and related compounds, the correlation between pupal size and egg production suggests that pupal health and vigor are major contributing factors.

Fungicidal Effects of Compounds

Fungitoxicity Tests. Fungitoxicity was determined by measuring inhibition of linear growth of fungi in malt-extract agar medium on 100 x 15 mm petri plates incubated at 25 ^{o}C. An acetone solution of the test compound was added to the molten agar (50 ^{o}C) and the hot medium was then poured onto the plates. Final concentration of acetone in the control and fungicide treatments was 0.5%. After solidification, the medium was inoculated with a 6 mm hyphal disc cut from an agar culture of the fungus. To facilitate comparison between compounds, doses (ED_{50}) causing half-maximal linear growth inhibition were determined.

Structure-Activity Relationships. Toxicity tests were conducted with 3 hydrazinecarboxamides and 5 diazenecarboxamides on 3 plant pathogenic fungi, *Pyricularia oryzae*, *Botrytis cinerea*, and *Monilinia fructicola*. Data in Table VI show that, except for **46**, all compounds are fungitoxic. Five compounds elicited exceptional activity (<1 ppm) in two species: *P. oryzae* (**13**,**40**,**41** and **42**) and *M. fructicola* (**16**,**41** and **42**). Test results with **16**, **41**, **42**, and **46** show *P. oryzae* and *M. fructicola* are equal in their susceptibility but both are more susceptible than *B. cineria*.

Data in Table VI support the following structure-activity relationships: fungicidal activity roughly parallels larvicidal activity and diazenecarboxamides are consistently more toxic than corresponding hydrazine analogs. However, since the number of compounds tested was small, correlations derived should be regarded as tentative.

Summary

Structure-activity relationships were defined in the house fly for a series of highly fluorinated and larvicidally active *N*,2-diphenylhydrazinecarboxamides. The most effective larvicide identified from the study was **16**, 2-(2-fluorophenyl)-*N*-[2-(trifluoromethyl)phenyl]-hydrazinecarboxamide. Compound **16** completely inhibited larval development at 1-5 ppm in the diet. As a part of this study, nine related diazenecarboxamides were synthesized and evaluated. Five of these were effective larvicides. Structure-activity correlations defined for this series of compounds may serve as a useful guide for future development of hydrazine-derived larvicides. Little information was gained in *Musca* tests to determine how **1** and related compounds work (early instars reared on a diet containing **1** appeared to molt normally but vigor and food consumption were severely decreased). Clearly, future work with hydrazine- and diazenecarboxamides should include physiological and biochemical studies designed to elucidate their mode of action.

Fungicidal activity of these compounds was striking; several hydrazine- and diazenecarboxamides were effective in one or more plant pathogenic fungi below 1 ppm. Although only eight analogs were evaluated, it appears that fluorine or trifluoromethyl substituents

Table VI. Toxicity of selected hydrazine and diazenecarboxamides against three plant pathogenic fungi

No.	X	R	ED$_{50}$ (ppm[b]) *P. oryzae*	*B. cinerea*	*M. fructicola*
1	NHNH	2,4-F_2-C_6H_3	2.4	>10	-
40	N=N	"	0.45	4.5	-
13	NHNH	2,5-F_2-C_6H_3	0.45	9.0	-
41	N=N	"	0.35	6.8	0.30
16	NHNH	2-(CF_3)-C_6H_4	1.5	2.2	0.93
42	N=N	"	0.39	1.7	0.40
46	N=N	*n*-C_3H_7	>10	>10	>10
47	N=N	H	5.8	>10	-

[a] Dose that inhibited linear growth to 50% of that of controls (based on means of duplicate samples from two experiments). [b] Also µg A.I./ml medium.

provide a high potential for fungicidal activity. We consider this information important and speculate that further investigations of highly fluorinated compounds related to those in this study will lead to promising fungicides.

Little is known about the mode of action of hydrazinecarboxamide-derived fungicides. Since diazene formation is involved in the fungitoxic action of phenylthiosemicarbazide (22) and is implicated in a glutathione-oxidation mechanism to account for fungitoxicity of similarly structured compounds (21), it is conceivable that diazenes described in this study may well play a critical role in the action of fluorine-substituted hydrazinecarboxamide fungicides and perhaps larvicides as well.

Acknowledgments

Thanks are due to Robert E. Redfern (retired), Livestock Insects Laboratory, USDA, ARS, Beltsville, MD, for providing bioassay data for *Spodoptera*. Thanks are also due to Lydia Rodriguez-Castro and Richard T. Brown for synthesizing some of the compounds.

Literature Cited

1. Crystal, M.M. *J. Econ. Entomol.* 1970, 63, 491-492.
2. DeMilo, A.B.; Crystal, M.M. *J. Econ. Entomol.* 1972, 65, 594-595.
3. DeMilo, A.B.; Fye, R.L.; Borkovec, A.B. *J. Econ. Entomol.* 1973, 66, 1007-1008.
4. DeMilo, A.B.; Fye, R.L. *Botyu-Kagaku* 1976, 41, 195-197.
5. Gahan, J.B.; Swingle, M.C.; Phillips, A.M. *U.S. Bur. Ent. and Plant Quar.* U.S. Department of Agriculture, 1941, E-549, pp. 1-11.
6. Freeman, A.F. U.S. Patent 2 272 047, 1942.
7. McGovran, E.R. *J. Econ. Entomol.* 1944, 37, 336-338.
8. Swingle, M.C.; Gahan, J.B.; Phillips, A.M. *U.S. Bur. Ent. and Plant Quar.* U.S. Department of Agriculture, 1947, E-730, pp. 1-57.
9. Mayer, E.L.; McGovran, E.R. *U.S. Bur. Ent. and Plant Quar.* U.S. Department of Agriculture, 1949, E-768, pp. 1-16.
10. Pedersen, L.-E.K. *Proc. XVII Int'l. Congr. Entomol.* 1984, Abstr. S21.1.6, p 861.
11. DeMilo, A.B.; Redfern, R.E.; Borkovec, A.B. *J. Agric. Food Chem.* 1983, 31, 713-718.
12. Pedersen, L.-E.K.; Svendsen, A. Klemmensen, P.D. *Pestic. Sci.* 1984, 25, 462-470.
13. Meng, J.; Sun, W.; Ou, C.; Pan, R.; Feng, Z.; Lu, S. *Acta Microbiol. Sinica* 1981, 21, 350-362.
14. Usui, Y.; Matsumura, C. *Yakugaku Zasshi* 1967, 87, 43-65; *Chem. Abstr.* 1967, 67, 32382a.

15. Kakui, Y.; Murakami, S. Japanese Patent 70 03 771, 1970; Chem. Abstr. 1970, 72, P121208u.
16. Jalles, E.; Bini, B. Gazz. Chim. Ital. 1938, 68, 510-515; Chem. Abstr. 1939, 33, 545.
17. Dutky, R.C.; Robbins, W.E.; Shortino, T.J.; Kaplanis, J.N.; Vroman, H.E. J. Insect Physiol. 1967, 13, 1501-1510.
18. Monroe, R.E. Ann. Entomol. Soc. Amer. 1962, 55, 140.
19. DeMilo, A.B.; Ostromecky, D.M.; Chang, S.C.; Redfern, R.E.; Fye, R.L. J. Agric. Food Chem. 1978, 26, 164-166.
20. Cohen, C.F.; Marks, E.P. Southwest. Entomol. 1979, 4, 294-297.
21. Kosower, E.M.; Miyadera, T. J. Med. Chem. 1972, 15, 307-312.
22. Sijpesteyn, A.K.; Pluijers, C.W.; Verloop, A.; Tempel, A. Ann. Appl. Biol. 1968, 61, 473-479.

RECEIVED May 27, 1986

FUNGICIDES

Chapter 26

Biologically Active Organosilicon Compounds

Fungicidal Silylmethyltriazoles

William K. Moberg, Gregory S. Basarab, John Cuomo, and Paul H. Liang

Agricultural Products Department, E. I. du Pont de Nemours & Co., Experimental Station, Building 402, Wilmington, DE 19898

Silylmethyltriazoles represent a new, highly active class of triazole fungicides, whose success in a wide variety of crops and climatic conditions confirms the utility of organosilicon compounds as agrichemicals. This paper describes their discovery, synthesis, and structure-activity relationships. Based on the results of worldwide field evaluations, some of which are presented, a member of this class, DPX-H6573, is being developed as a broad spectrum foliar fungicide.

Research at Du Pont on silicon-containing agrichemicals has provided a new class of triazole fungicides, the silylmethyltriazoles (1, 2). We describe herein the discovery and optimization of this class, concluding with some field results for DPX-H6573 (proposed common name: flusilazole), an active ingredient in the new fungicides Nustar®, Punch®, Triumph™, and Olymp®.

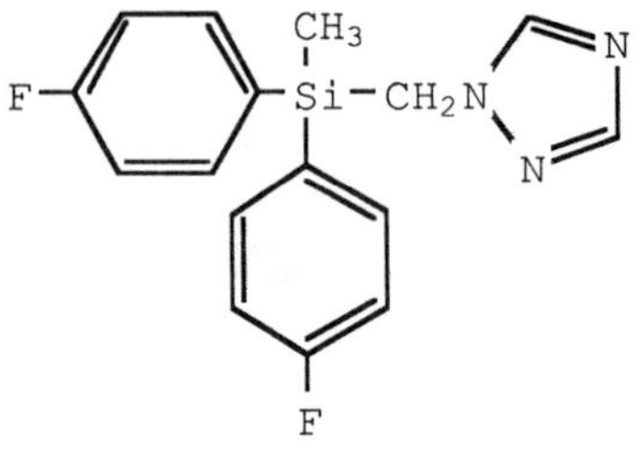

DPX-H6573

0097-6156/87/0355-0288$06.00/0
© 1987 American Chemical Society

Discovery

Silylmethyltriazoles combine a little-explored area, that of silicon-containing agrichemicals, with a well known area, that of triazole fungicides. We begin by considering each facet separately, then show how they came together to provide the initial discovery that eventually produced DPX-H6573.

Incorporating Silicon Into Agrichemicals. This concept attracted us for several reasons. First, it was relatively unexplored. Industrial interest in silicon has concentrated almost entirely on polymers, and to our knowledge the only silicon compounds ever commercialized as agrichemicals are chloroethylsilanes such as etacelasil [2-chloroethyl-tris(2-methoxyethoxy)silane; Ciba-Geigy] (3), which are used as plant growth modifiers. However, these compounds act by decomposing in plants to release the hormone ethylene. Thus, although they represent a very clever application of silicon chemistry, they are not active *per se*, and the active principle they release no longer contains silicon. Second, there was a vast literature on organosilicon chemistry going back almost 100 years, and academic work in the area has been extensive in recent years. Fortunately for us, however, in virtually all contemporary studies silicon is used to facilitate chemical transformations, and it disappears gracefully as the desired product is formed. Thus there was an excellent background of synthetic literature, but still relatively little interest in the biological activity of organosilanes. Third, thanks to the polymer research mentioned earlier, there were several simple but highly functionalized building blocks available in bulk and at reasonable cost: the monomers for silicone polymers. Finally, there was the scientific interest of working with an element whose chemical properties are practically unique in the periodic table.

Triazole Fungicides. At the same time, we had an independent interest in the area of triazole fungicides. These compounds, which act by interfering with steroid biosynthesis in sensitive fungi (4, 5), show high activity against a broad spectrum of economically important plant diseases. The area was pioneered by Bayer and Janssen in the early 1970's, and two of the most successful compounds to emerge from this work are triadimefon, invented and developed by Bayer, and propiconazole, invented by Janssen and licensed to Ciba-Geigy for development.

Discovery Strategy. Our discovery began with the observation that these and related compounds from other companies shared common structural features (Figure 1). Each has a triazole ring; a two-atom spacer, with or without heteroatoms and variously substituted at either position; and a benzene ring, usually substituted. The common elements are represented schematically, with X and Y as the bridging atoms.

In considering this structural template, it occurred to us that we might use it to test the organosilicon strategy, by making X or Y silicon. We initially ruled out Y, since N-silylazoles are known to hydrolyze readily. This left X as silicon, and we set out to prepare the simplest structure fitting this template, compound I.

Figure 1. Discovery Strategy

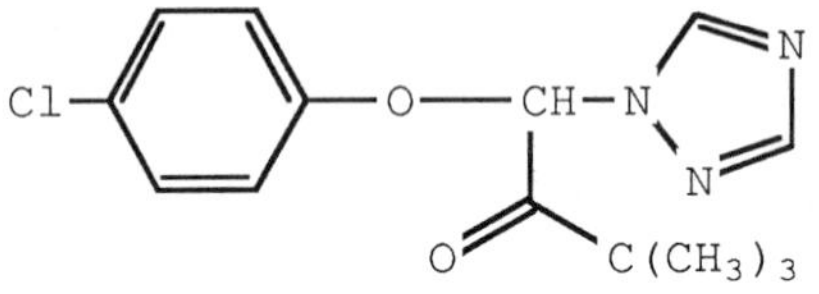

Triadimefon

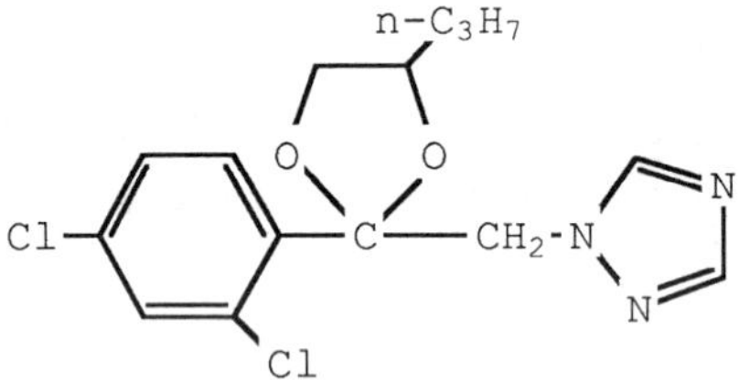

Propiconazole

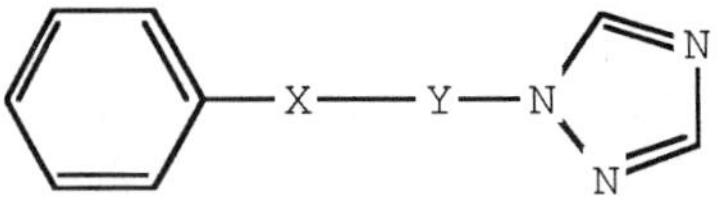

Common Structure

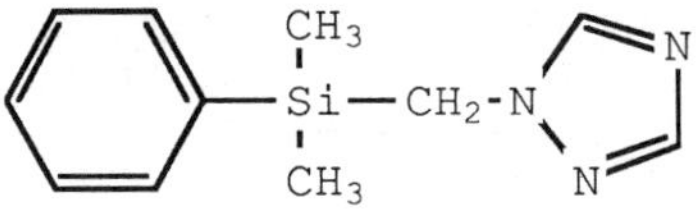

Compound I

Of course, we were aware of potential pitfalls in this sort of reasoning. One often starts with an apparent insight that turns out to be faulty, and even with a biochemically accurate insight such a drastic modification seldom leads to active compounds. Furthermore, in this case there was the added uncertainty that little is known about the stability of organosilanes in biological systems. And there were quite specific negative precedents, such as the work of Fukuto on DDT analogs (6), where replacement of a trichloromethyl group with trimethylsilyl completely destroyed activity. Finally, there was even some question as to whether I could be prepared, since the literature on chloromethylsilane displacement chemistry has many examples of undesired carbon-silicon bond cleavage intervening. However, the idea had one very attractive feature: it was easy to test.

In the event, we were pleasantly surprised to find that I could be made, and even more surprised (and pleased) to find that it was a classic chemical lead. Its activity was relatively modest and its spectrum relatively narrow, but it had the kind of activity we were hoping for, and it showed other desirable properties such as the ability to move systemically in plant tissues and some ability to cure established fungal infections. Equally important, it was a very simple structure that could be modified at several sites. We therefore undertook a synthesis program aimed at optimizing this activity, and every portion of the molecule except the silicon atom was varied systematically.

Chemistry

We alluded earlier to the fact that several polymer intermediates are readily available as starting materials, and these formed the basis for our work. The entire series of silanes in which silicon bears varying numbers of chlorines and methyl groups is produced in the industrial process for making dichlorodimethylsilane, the prototypical starting material for silicone polymers. These compounds arise from direct reaction of metallic silicon and chloromethane, catalyzed by copper (Equation 1).

$$Si^{\circ} \xrightarrow[Cu]{MeCl} ClSiMe_3 + Cl_2SiMe_2 + Cl_3SiMe \qquad (1)$$

For eventual introduction of a triazole ring, one methyl group must be functionalized selectively, and this is readily accomplished by light-catalyzed photochlorination, as illustrated in Equation 2 for dichlorodimethyl silane. The other methylchlorosilanes can be monochlorinated in the same way.

$$Cl_2SiMe_2 \xrightarrow[\text{light}]{Cl_2} Cl_2Si(CH_3)CH_2Cl \quad (2)$$

Introducing Substituents About Silicon. With displaceable chlorine atoms at all the required positions, we took advantage of the unique chemistry of silicon to introduce a wide variety of substituents about the silicon atom, since the Si-Cl bonds are much more reactive than the C-Cl bond. Typically, organometallic reagents are used, and since the chlorines on silicon can be replaced stepwise, the synthesis offers considerable flexibility (Equation 3).

$$Cl_3SiCH_2Cl \xrightarrow{R^1Li} \xrightarrow{R^2Li} \xrightarrow{R^3Li} R^2\text{-}Si(R^1)(R^3)\text{-}CH_2Cl \quad (3)$$

This chemistry was generally uneventful, but two findings useful from the preparative point of view deserve mention. First, below -60°C lithium-halogen exchange between aryl bromides and alkyllithiums is so much faster than reaction of alkyllithiums with chlorosilanes that *in situ* metalation is possible. The aryl bromide and chlorosilane are simply mixed together, then coupled by dropwise addition of alkyllithium. This has advantages when the desired aryllithium tends to precipitate from the reaction mixture, and it also allows us to work with unstable alpha-haloaryllithiums that could form benzyne, since the aryllithium reacts with the chlorosilane as fast as it is generated. This reaction can even be used to introduce two different substituents in one pot. For example (Equation 4), when an equimolar mixture of a dichlorosilane and an aryl bromide is treated with two equivalents of n-butyllithium, the first equivalent forms the aryl-silicon bond and the second reacts with the remaining silicon-chlorine bond, producing the fully substituted silane in useable yield after distillation.

$$2,4\text{-}Cl_2C_6H_3Br + Cl_2Si(CH_3)CH_2Cl \xrightarrow[-60^\circ C]{2\ n\text{-}BuLi} 2,4\text{-}Cl_2C_6H_3\text{-}Si(CH_3)(n\text{-}C_4H_9)CH_2Cl \quad (4)$$

The second finding was that aryl Grignard reagents were significantly more selective than aryllithiums in reactions with polychlorosilanes. For example, when chloromethyltrichlorosilane was treated with three equivalents of 4-fluorophenyllithium, the triarylsilane was formed as expected. However, the corresponding Grignard reagent introduced only two aryl groups, no matter how many equivalents were used, giving cleanly compounds with one silicon-chlorine bond remaining for further transformation. This chemistry is illustrated in Scheme I.

Scheme I. Organometallic Selectivity

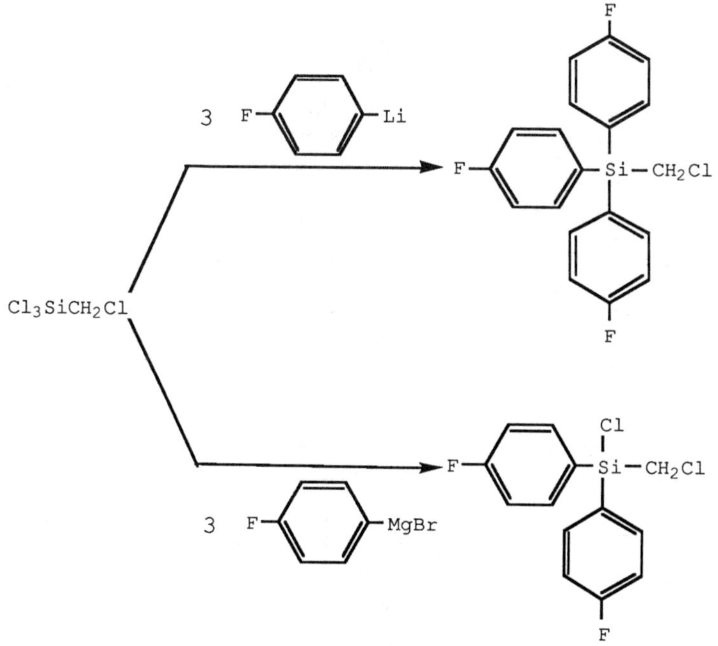

Cl_3SiCH_2Cl + 3 F–C_6H_4–Li → $(4\text{-}FC_6H_4)_3Si–CH_2Cl$

Cl_3SiCH_2Cl + 3 F–C_6H_4–MgBr → $(4\text{-}FC_6H_4)_2Si(Cl)–CH_2Cl$

Introducing the Triazole Ring. The final step of the synthesis was displacement of the carbon-bound chlorine with triazole salts. Once again, silicon made life easy for us, since it activates such hindered systems toward displacement. The corresponding all-carbon compounds react very sluggishly with triazole salts. Luckily, silicon-carbon bond cleavage is not observed, provided water or other oxygen nucleophiles are excluded. The displacement reaction is illustrated in Equation 5 for DPX-H6573.

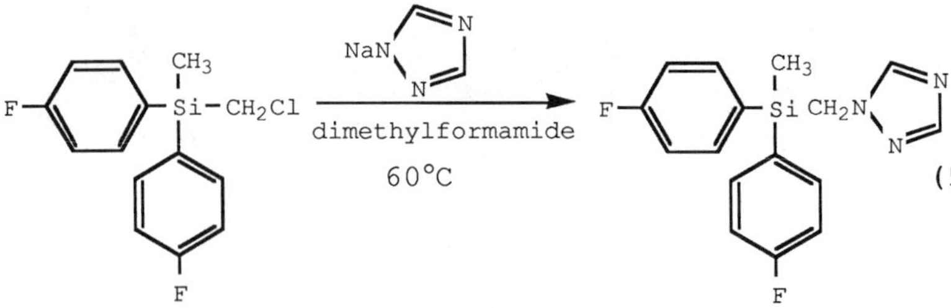

(5)

Oxygenated Silanes. Controlled introduction of oxygen substituents onto silicon is an interesting special case, since several syntheses are possible. For mono-oxygenated compounds, one can simply react a chloro-(chloromethyl)silane with two equivalents of triazole and then displace the labile silicon-bound triazole with water or an alcohol. However, a better alternative in practice is to introduce first an alcohol and then triazole. In this case, the hydroxy compound can be prepared by hydrolysis of the silyl ether with aqueous acid. Scheme II outlines these options.

Scheme II. Mono-oxygenated Silanes

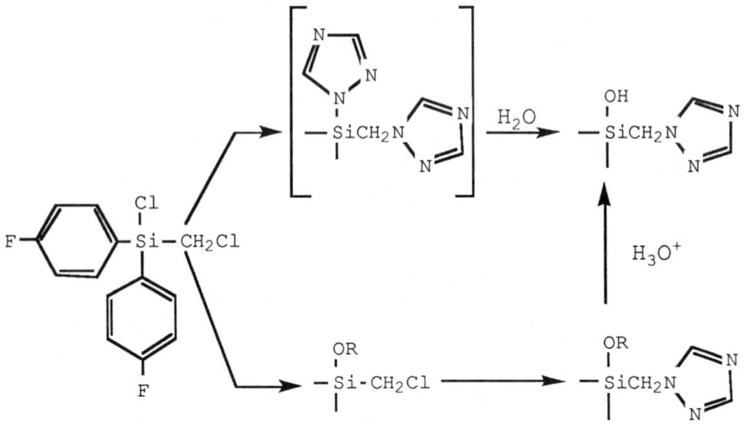

Dioxygenated compounds are formed similarly, except here it is often advantageous to exchange chloride for iodide before doing the triazole displacement. Cyclic derivatives can then be prepared by an exchange reaction (Scheme III).

Scheme III. Dioxygenated Silanes

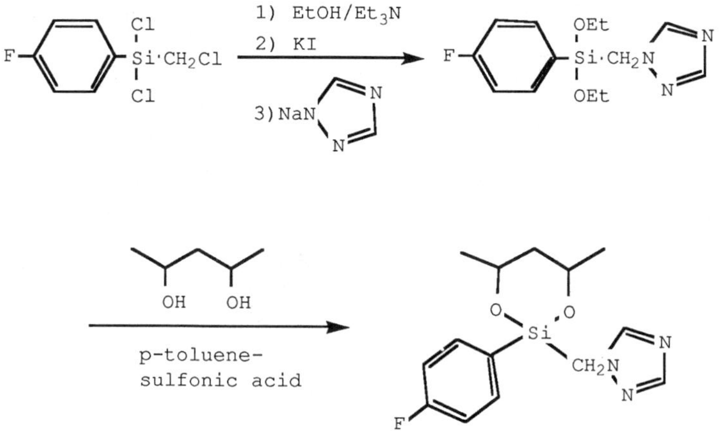

F–C$_6$H$_4$–Si(Cl)$_2$·CH$_2$Cl
1) EtOH/Et$_3$N
2) KI
3) NaN(triazole)
F–C$_6$H$_4$–Si(OEt)$_2$·CH$_2$N(triazole)

OH OH
p-toluene-sulfonic acid
O Si O CH$_2$N N N F

Structure-Activity

With this chemistry in hand, we set out to define the structure-activity relationships of silylmethyltriazoles.

Primary Testing. Table I presents initial greenhouse test results for some compounds having alkyl and aryl substituents about silicon. In these tests, compounds were applied to foliage at a concentration of 100 parts per million and evaluated for preventive control of cucumber powdery mildew (CPM), apple scab (APS), peanut early leaf spot (PCA), and wheat leaf rust (WLR). These pathogens represent all the major families of economically important foliar pathogens, except for Phycomycetes such as tomato late blight and grape downy mildew. As is expected in view of their mode of action, silylmethyltriazoles do not show appreciable activity against this pathogen family, since Phycomycetes do not require ergosterol for their cell membranes.

Starting with our lead compound (first entry of Table I), we began by adding substituents to the phenyl ring. Moving a chlorine around the ring showed that a 4-substituent gave a dramatic boost in activity, a 2-substituent gave a moderate boost, and a 3-substituent was not helpful. These trends were confirmed as we surveyed other substituents, and the 4-phenyl and 2,4-

dichloro analogs were found to be particularly effective. Other examples in Table I show that extension of the alkyl groups on silicon, or substitution of naphthyl or cyclohexyl for the phenyl moiety, failed to improve activity.

Although some compounds from the monoaryl series were active enough to warrent field evaluation, replacement of one of the methyl groups with a second aryl moiety provided even better activity. As in the monoaryl series, para-halogenation gave the best potency. Extending this series to triarylsilanes caused activity to drop off again, as shown in the last entry of Table I.

Table I. Structure-Activity of Aryl/Alkyl Silanes

$$R^1-Si(R^2)(R^3)-CH_2N$$ (1,2,4-triazol-1-yl)

R^1	R^2	R^3	Percent Control at 100 ppm CPM	APS	PCA	WLR
Ph	Me	Me	100	0	0	90
2-ClPh	Me	Me	100	90	100	0
3-ClPh	Me	Me	0	60	0	0
4-ClPh	Me	Me	100	100	90	100
4-PhPh	Me	Me	100	100	100	100
2,4-diClPh	Me	Me	100	100	100	90
4-ClPh	n-Bu	Me	100	100	0	80
1-Naphthyl	Me	Me	100	50	90	0
Cyclohexyl	Me	Me	100	0	0	0
Ph	Ph	Me	100	100	100	0
4-FPh	Ph	Me	100	100	100	90
4-FPh	4-FPh	Me	100	100	100	100
4-FPh	4-FPh	4-FPh	0	60	90	90

Structure-activity for oxygenated silanes is presented in Table II. Mono-oxy compounds were highly active, but those with two oxygens attached to silicon were less interesting.

Table II. Structure-Activity of Oxygenated Silanes

	Percent Control at 100 ppm			
	CPM	APS	PCA	WLR
$(F-C_6H_4)_2-Si(OH)CH_2N$ (1,2,4-triazol-1-yl)	100	100	100	100
$(F-C_6H_4)_2-Si(OCMe_3)-$	100	100	100	80
$F-C_6H_4-Si(OEt)_2-$	100	0	0	0
$F-C_6H_4-Si-$ (cyclic dioxasilinane)	100	0	50	100

<u>Secondary Testing</u>. Primary tests separated the mediocre from the good, but secondary testing was needed to separate the good from the excellent. In Table III, this process is illustrated for the diaryl series. Here efficacy is expressed by ED90 values, the amount of compound in grams per hectare required to give 90% control. Thus, the lower the number, the higher the activity. It should be noted that these data are derived from dosage response curves obtained under controlled greenhouse conditions, and therefore do not translate directly to field rates; however, they are a good tool for comparing compounds to each other, and the trends they indicate have been borne out in field testing.

Compared to the unsubstituted case, one para-fluorine boosts activity substantially, and a second fluorine (DPX-H6573) takes the activity to excellent levels across the board. ED90 values rise again when the fluorines of DPX-H6573 are replaced by chlorine. This analog also showed reduced mobility in plant tissues.

Table III. Structure-Activity of Diarylsilanes

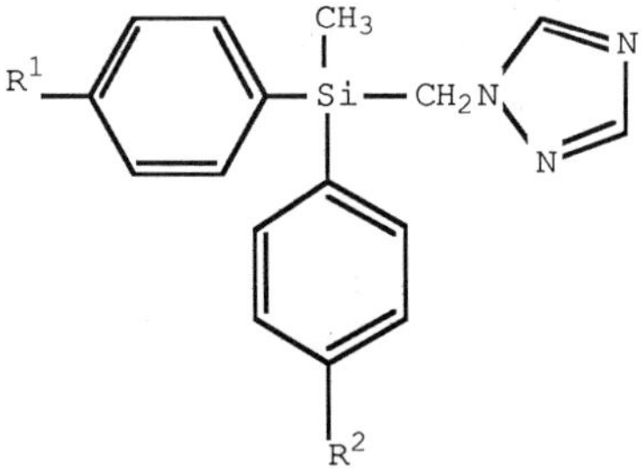

R^1	R^2	ED90 (G/Ha) CPM	APS	PCA	WLR
H	H	12	100	70	75
F	H	4	5	30	120
F	F	0.5	3	10	15
Cl	Cl	9	7	25	60

Tests such as these, along with extensive field evaluation worldwide, led to the selection of DPX-H6573 for development as a foliar fungicide.

Field Results

DPX-H6573 controls many important pathogens of crop plants at low rates, and a sampling of diseases for which good efficacy has been demonstrated in field testing is shown in Table IV, organized by crops. In most instances, multiple pathogens are controlled on a given crop. We conclude with some representative field results.

Cereals. Table V summarizes the results of trials in France on diseases of wheat and barley. The commercial standards, propiconazole for foliar diseases and carbendazim and prochloraz for *Pseudocercosporella* foot rot, are taken at recommended field rates. The dashes, which indicate that the standard is not generally used to control the disease in question, make a point: there are

Table IV. Field Efficacy of DPX-H6573

Crops	Diseases Controlled
Cereals	Powdery Mildew, Rusts, Foot Rot, Septoria, Helminthosporium, Rhyncosporium
Apples	Scab, Powdery Mildew, Rust
Grapes	Powdery Mildew, Black Rot
Sugar Beets	Cercospora Leafspot, Powdery Mildew
Bananas	Yellow and Black Sigatoka
Coffee	Rust
Peanuts	Early and Late Leafspots
Stone Fruit	Brown Rot

currently no compounds effective against both such a broad range of leaf diseases and against foot rot.

We have looked closely at foot rot, since this is a serious problem for which few control measures are available. Benzimidazole fungicides such as carbendazim have been very successful against this fungus over the years, but it is always dangerous to have only one mode of action available for controlling any pathogen, since fungi are so adept at developing resistance. Among sterol inhibitors, only prochloraz has shown promise of complementing benzimidazoles. Table VI shows the results of additional trials, this time in England. These tests and many others suggest that DPX-H6573 offers a uniquely broad spectrum of control for cereal diseases, at rates comparable to or less than those of the best commercial standards.

Peanuts, Sugarbeets. Pathogens bearing some taxonomic relationship to foot rot cause leafspot diseases of these crops. Table VII presents results of field trials in the southeastern United States on late leafspot, using the non-systemic protectant fungicide chlorothalonil as standard. There are no sterol inhibitors currently registered for this market. In addition to good control at dramatically lower rates of application, DPX-H6573 offers the added advantage of systemic movement into new growth and curative action against established infections; it is also effective against early leafspot at these rates. Good control of sugarbeet leafspot, especially by combinations with protectant fungicides, is reported in Reference 2.

Fruits. DPX-H6573 is also effective for controlling a broad range of fruit diseases. Table VIII illustrates control of grape powdery mildew at rates of 1-2 grams active ingredient per 100 L of spray. The black rot pathogen of grapes is also controlled at these rates.

For tree fruits such as apples (Table IX), low rates of 2-4 grams active ingredient per 100 liters of spray give near-perfect control of both major diseases, scab and powdery mildew; excellent cedar apple rust control is also observed at these rates. Standards for these tests include both sterol inhibitors (fenarimol and bitertanol) and non-systemic protectant fungicides (sulfur and captan).

Table V. Cereal Trials (France, 1983)

		Percent Control			
		Barley	Wheat		
	G/Ha	Mildew	Rust	Septoria	Foot Rot
DPX-H6573	80	88	91	78	--
	160	92	98	80	--
	240	--	--	--	76
Propiconazole	125	91	96	81	--
Carbendazim	200	--	--	--	82
Prochloraz	750	--	--	--	76

Table VI. Wheat Foot Rot Trials (England, 1983)

	G/Ha	Percent Control
DPX-H6573	100	51
	200	59
	400	75
Carbendazim	250	30
Prochloraz	400	54

Table VII. Peanut Late Leafspot Trials (U.S., 1983)

	G/Ha	Percent Control
DPX-H6573	70	76
	140	86
Chlorothalonil	1240	75

Table VIII. Grape Powdery Mildew Trials (France, 1983)

	G/100L	Percent Control
DPX-H6573	1	78
	2	96
	4	98
Fenarimol	1.2	83
Sulfur	1000	58

Table IX. Apple Trials (France, 1983)

	G/100L	Percent Control: Scab Foliage	Scab Fruit	Powdery Mildew Foliage
DPX-H6573	2	86	92	95
	4	96	95	97
Fenarimol	4	75	61	96
Bitertanol	19	76	87	82
Captan	150	72	62	54

Summary

DPX-H6573 is a new fungicide of great promise. From the chemical point of view, it is to our knowledge the first agrichemical or pharmaceutical commercialized that contains silicon in the active form of the molecule, and we feel it confirms the utility of organosilicon compounds in agriculture. From the biological point of view, it is at least as active as the best commercial standards, sterol inhibitors or otherwise, for many diseases of important crops, and for several of these crops it is either more active than any standard or controls a broader range of diseases.

Acknowledgments

We acknowledge with gratitude the many Du Pont biologists, in Wilmington and in the field, who have worked so closely with us in developing this discovery, and Ray Luckenbaugh, the supervisor who provided the atmosphere in which these ideas could take root. We are also grateful to Cathy Kershaw and Joyce Granger for preparing the manuscript. Finally, we thank Joe Fenyes and Don Baker for their work in establishing this symposium series.

Literature Cited

1. Moberg, W. K. U. S. Patent 4 510 136, 1985.
2. Fort, T. M.; Moberg, W. K. British Crop Protection Conference - Pests and Diseases 1984, Vol. 2, p 413.
3. British Patent 1 371 804, 1974.
4. Davidse, L. L.; de Waard, M. A. Adv. Plant Pathology 1984, 2, 191.
5. Langcake, P.; Kuhn, P. J.; Wade, M. Prog. Pestic. Biochem. Toxicol. 1983, 3, 1.
6. Fahmy, M. A. H.; Fukuto, T. R.; Metcalf, R. L.; Holmstead, R. L. J. Agr. Food Chem. 1973, 21, 585.

RECEIVED May 27, 1987

Chapter 27

Synthesis and Fungicidal Activity of Triazole Tertiary Alcohols

Paul A. Worthington

Department of Chemistry, Imperial Chemical Industries PLC, Plant Protection Division, Jealott's Hill Research Station, Bracknell, Berkshire, RG12 6EY, England

Using a knowledge of the mode of action of the plant growth regulator paclobutrazol, it has been possible to design a series of 1,2,4 triazole containing tertiary alcohols which have high levels of plant fungicidal activity. From this group flutriafol and hexaconazole have been introduced into crop protection.

Since their discovery in the late 1960s several compounds from the chemical class of 1-substituted imidazoles and 1,2,4-triazoles have been developed and successfully used for the control of plant diseases and for the treatment of human fungal infections. The first commercial triazole compound was triadimefon (1), introduced by Bayer in 1973 for the control of powdery mildew, rusts, and seed-borne diseases of cereals. Since that time many other so called "azole-fungicides" have been introduced into crop protection (2) and others are still being developed.

These 1,2,4-triazole fungicides share a common mode of action by inhibiting the C-14α-demethylation step in ergosterol biosynthesis (Figure 1) (3), between 24-methylenedihydrolanosterol and 4,4-dimethylergosta-8,14,24(28)-trienol.

Paclobutrazol was the first 1,2,4-triazole containing compound to be introduced in agriculture as a broad-spectrum plant growth regulator (4). In addition it possesses good fungicidal activity.

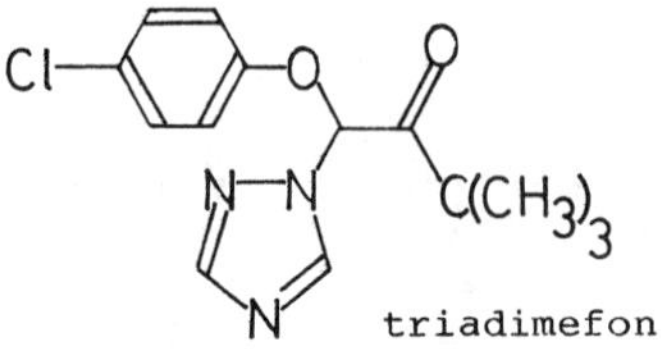

triadimefon

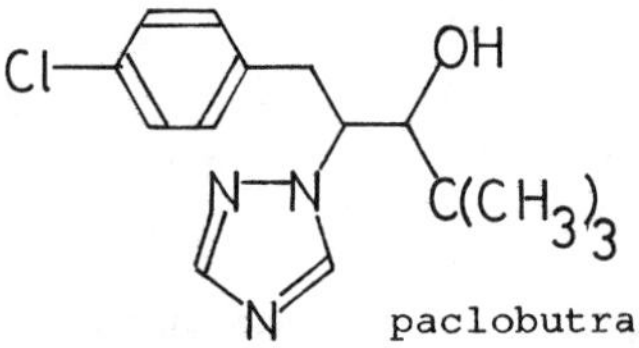

paclobutrazol

0097-6156/87/0355-0302$06.00/0
© 1987 American Chemical Society

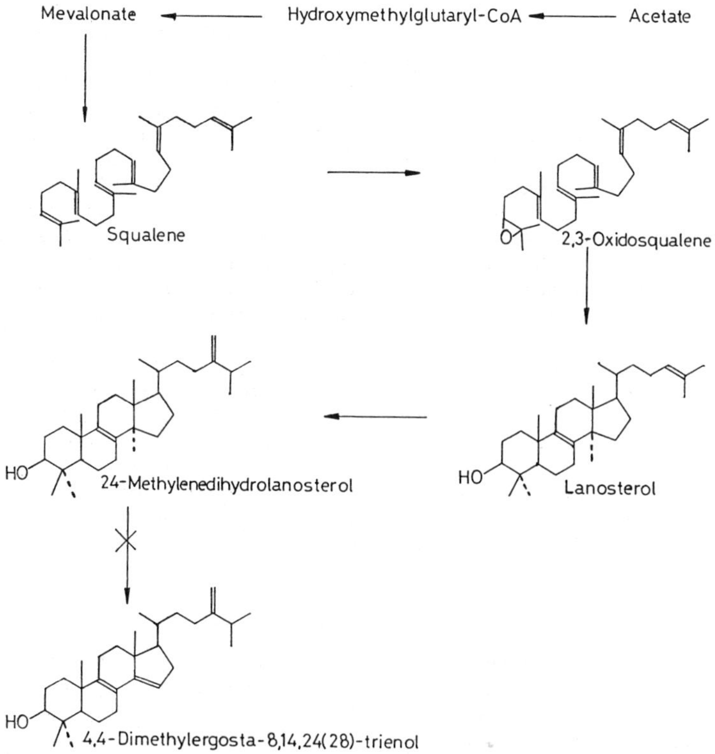

Figure 1. Inhibition of 14α-demethylation in ergosterol biosynthesis

This plant growth regulatory activity is due to inhibition of the biosynthesis of gibberellins (5), at the three oxidation steps between ent-kaurene and ent-kaurenoic acid (Figure 2).

The synthesis of paclobutrazol starting from pinacolone is shown in Figure 3 and the final reduction step with sodium borohydride is highly stereoselective, giving only the 2RS, 3RS diastereoisomer (6). Reduction using n-butylmagnesium bromide gives the other diastereoisomer, 2RS, 3SR, which has less biological activity. This high stereoselectivity observed in the sodium borohydride reduction can be explained by the delivery of hydride from the least hindered direction in the uncomplexed (Cram) transition state (Figure 4a). In contrast reduction using the Grignard reagent might be expected to go through a six-membered chelated transition state, with attack by the hydride species preferentially from one direction (Figure 4b). Resolution of 2RS, 3RS paclobutrazol has shown that the (+) 2R, 3R enantiomer possesses good fungicidal activity and that the plant growth regulatory properties reside with the (-) 2S,3S enantiomer.

The useful biological properties of paclobutrazol have inspired further chemical synthesis of azole structures, culminating with the discovery of a series of tertiary alcohol compounds. The original synthetic strategy was conceived as a disconnection and reconnection analysis from paclobutrazol (Figure 5). These early compounds were good fungicides and further optimisation in this area has led to the commercial introduction of two products flutriafol and recently hexaconazole.

Computer Graphic Studies and Chemical Synthesis

The 14α-demethylase enzyme involved in sterol biosynthesis has been shown to be dependent on an iron heme-containing cytochrome P450 for the initial oxidation of the $-CH_3$ to $-CH_2OH$, which is the rate determining step (7). Using computer graphics procedures that have been developed (8) it is possible to align RR paclobutrazol, a good inhibitor, with 24-methylene-24, 25-dihydrolanosterol which is the normal sterol substrate for the 14α-demethylase enzyme. With RR paclobutrazol in a computed minimum energy conformation, the 4-chlorobenzyl group is over the sterol side chain at the active site (Figure 6). The N-4 of the 1,2,4-triazole ring lies perpendicularly above the heme, and the tert-butyl group folds over the A and B rings of lanosterol in its extended form.

From this analysis it is possible to represent the general structural requirements for an inhibitor of the 14α demethylase enzyme by Figure 7. In this model the lipophilic groups A,B,C and D may be any substituents which on rotation of the carbon-carbon bond will allow the gauche conformation between the polar function and the triazole.

In paclobutrazol A and D of Figure 7 are substituted, producing a stabilised gauche conformation. By substituting at A and B, but leaving C and D as hydrogen it is possible to generate tertiary alcohol compounds with all the correct requirements for

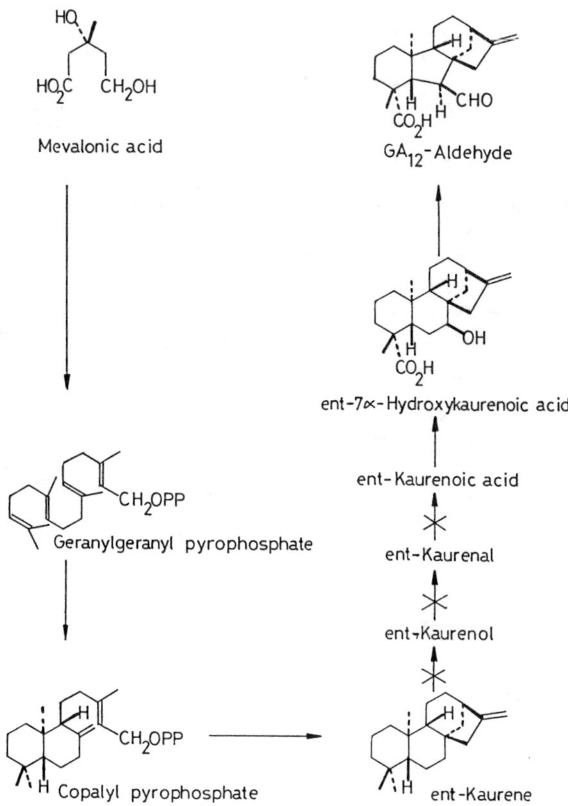

Figure 2. Inhibition of gibberellin biosynthesis with paclobutrazol

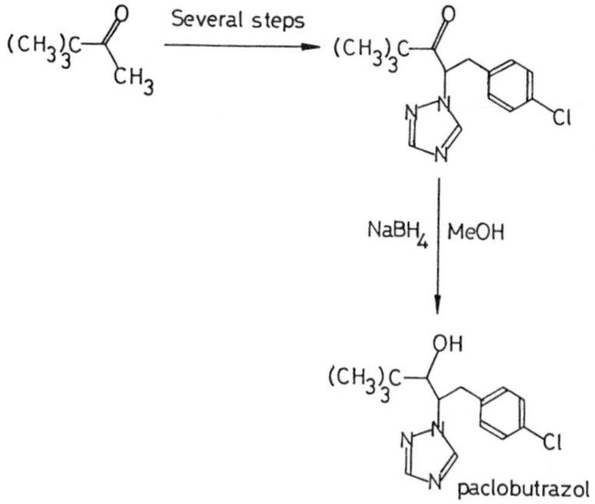

Several steps

$NaBH_4$ | MeOH

paclobutrazol

Figure 3. Synthesis of paclobutrazol

biological activity and yet different in overall appearance. The tertiary alcohol (Figure 5, A is tertiary butyl and B is 4-chlorobenzyl), which is isomeric with paclobutrazol, was synthesised from pinacolone in three steps (Figure 8). This compound showed good activity against mildews and apple scab. Further chemical synthesis demonstrated that the tertiary alcohol series in which A and B are halophenyl have good fungicidal properties. The fungicide flutriafol (9) introduced in 1983 for the control of important cereal diseases including powdery mildews, rusts, Septoria spp., and Rhynchosporium secalis belongs to this family. It was originally synthesised by the addition of the appropriate aryl Grignard reagent to a substituted phenacyl chloride followed by reaction of the intermediate chlorohydrin

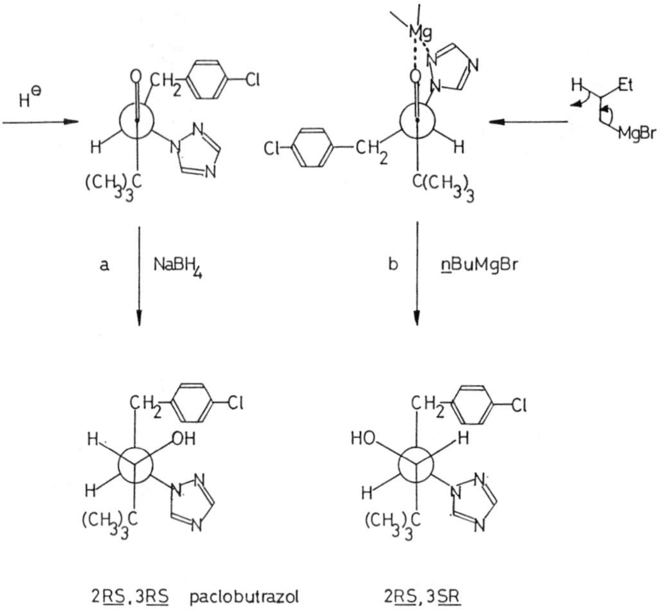

Figure 4. Stereoselective reduction of 1,2,4-triazol-1-yl ketone

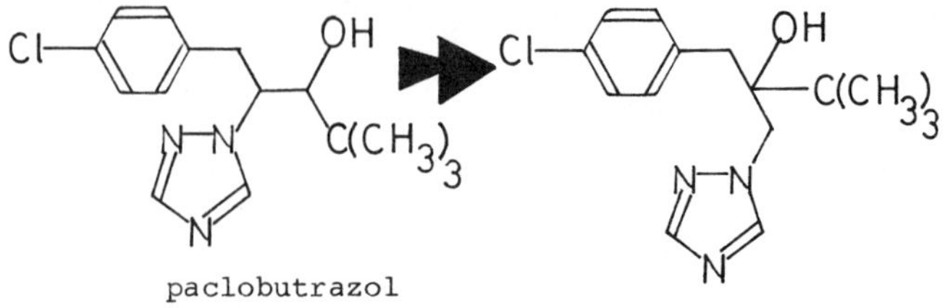

Figure 5. Tertiary alcohol derived from paclobutrazol

with 1,2,4-triazole (Figure 9). In order to explore the structure activity relationships for this group of compounds efficiently and for large quantities of material to be prepared for development work, two other synthetic routes were established starting from 2,4'-difluorobenzophenone (Figure 10).

In the computer graphic study, the fit of flutriafol does not correspond to 24-methylene-24,25-dihydrolanosterol, in the extended conformation, but with the side chain of the sterol

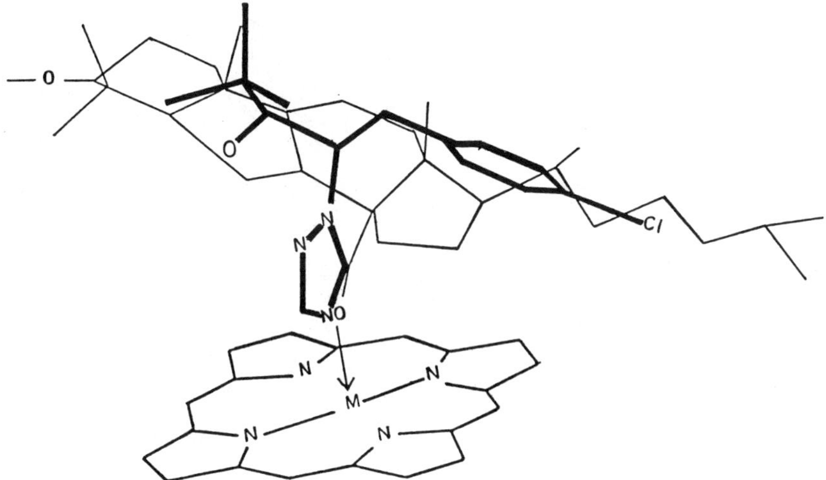

Figure 6. Computer graphic model showing the binding of lanosterol and RR paclobutrazol with heme of cytochrome P-450

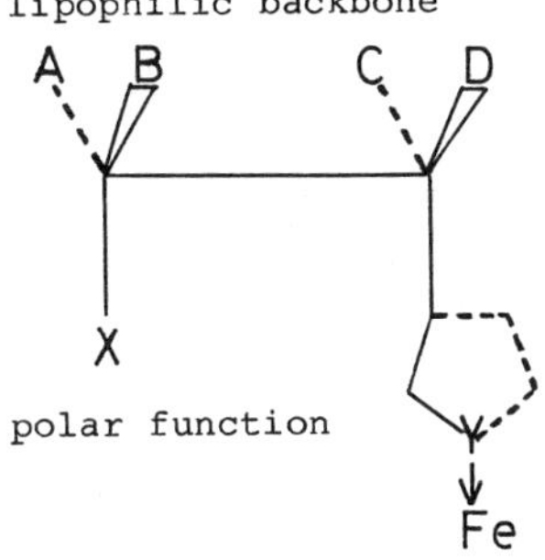

Figure 7. Model of requirement for 14-demethylase inhibitor.

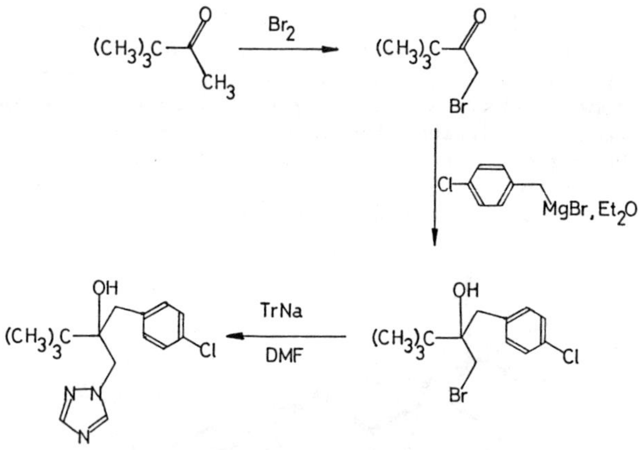

Figure 8. Synthesis of a tertiary alcohol compound

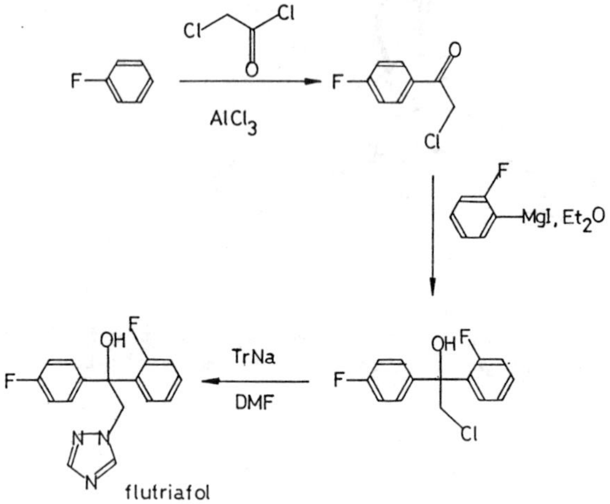

Figure 9. Synthesis of flutriafol

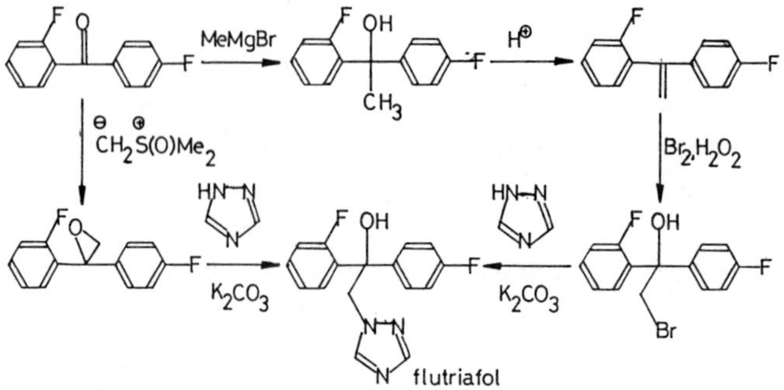

Figure 10. Other routes to flutriafol

rotated to the position shown in Figure 11. It is now possible to closely align flutriafol and RR paclobutrazol with the lanosterol substrate(10). Both the R and S isomers of flutriafol fit the computer graphic model, and show fungicidal activity. Further inspection of this model suggested that it should also be possible to replace one of the aryl rings in the flutriafol structure by other groups, with appropriate adjustments of the physical properties, and retain good biological activity. From this group of compounds we have recently introduced hexaconazole (PP523)(11) which shows outstanding protectant activity, combined with curative, translaminar, antisporulant and systemic properties against a range of diseases of vines, apples, peanuts and coffee. A synthetic route to hexaconazole and its analogues has been used. (Figure 12).

A number of other 1,2,4-triazole containing tertiary alcohols (Figure 13) are being developed for crop protection e.g. BAY HWG 1608(12) and SAN 619F(13), and fluconazole(14) is in clinical trials for the oral treatment of human fungal infections.

Biological Activity and Structure Activity Relationships

It is possible to correlate the fungicidal properties of the halogen containing flutriafol type tertiary alcohols with octanol/water partition coefficients (log P). Using the protectant breakpoint data on wheat rust, and in general the results on barley and wheat powdery mildews run parallel, there is an increase in biological activity with increasing log P (Figure 14). This is consistent with the accepted model for 1,2,4-triazole compounds of hydrophobic binding at a lipophilic receptor site. The data would also suggest that there is an upper limit of about log P = 3.3 above which the biological activity will not increase. A similar pattern is seen with the protectant activity against apple powdery mildew but the dependence on log P is less steep and it shows a tendency to plateau at a log P above 2 (Figure 15). Also the 2 and 4 halogen substituted compounds were intrinsically more active than many others that were tested but are not included in the graph.

It became clear from the relationships, particularly on the cereal diseases, that further synthesis aiming at high levels of both protectant and systemic activity must take log P into account. On cereals the range was approximately 2.4-3.3 with an optimum value depending on the balance of protectant and systemic activity required. For diseases of top fruit the requirements were less stringent except that if high systemic activity was required the upper log P limit was lower than on cereals.

For flutriafol the measured log P of 2.3 was low and indicates that the compound should have high systemic properties. It is now being used as a seed treatment in mixture with ethirimol and thiabendazole for the control of seed-, soil-, and air-borne diseases of cereals.(15)

In the case of hexaconazole the log P was 3.9 which is high but the compound gives good protectant(11) and systemic(16) control of diseases of vines and apples. For example in field

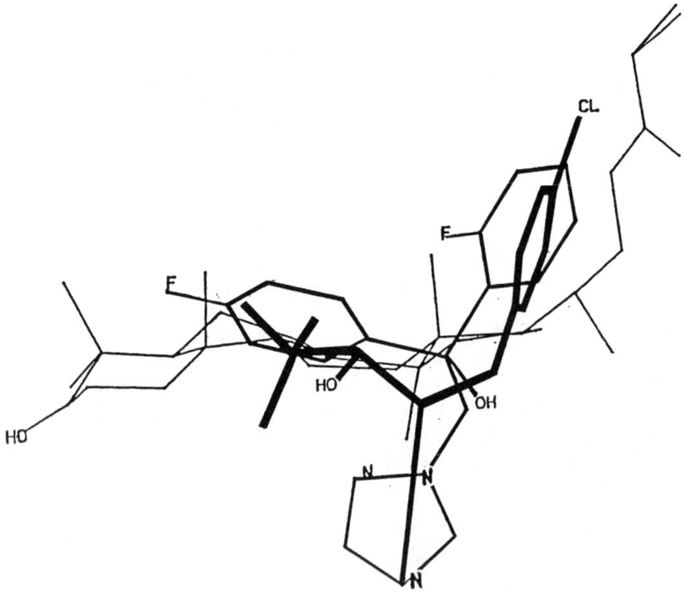

Figure 11. Computer graphic overlap of RR paclobutrazol and flutriafol with lanosterol

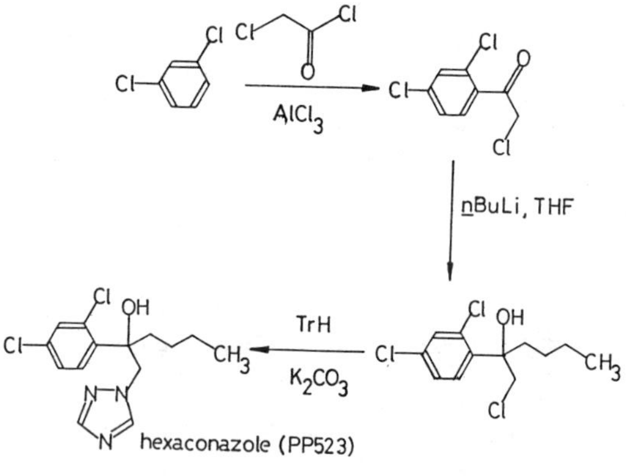

Figure 12. Synthesis of hexaconazole

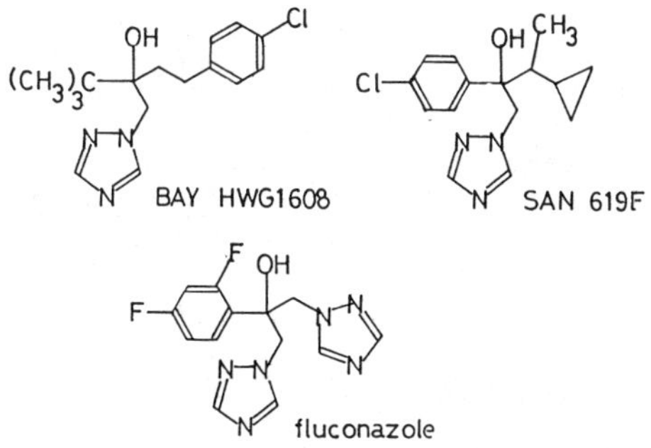

BAY HWG1608

SAN 619F

fluconazole

Figure 13. Other 1,2,4,-triazole tertiary alcohols

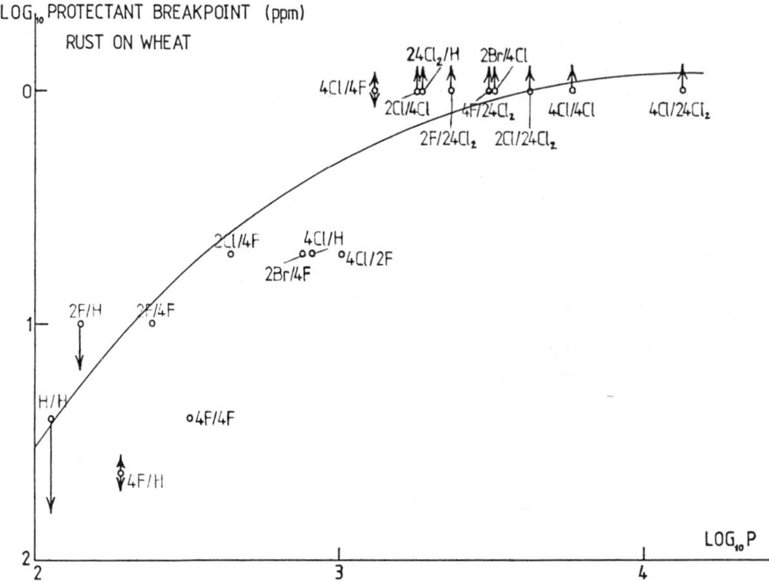

Figure 14. Plot log protectant activity (wheat rust) against log P for flutriafol compounds

trials on vines over a 5 year period, the control of powdery mildew on leaves and bunches was outstanding (Figure 16). Coupled with this, the activity against black rot (Guignardia bidwellii) was higher than with any of the standards (Figure 17). A dose of 15-20 ppm (ai) was adequate to control a heavy epidemic of either disease. On apples, hexaconazole at 10-20 ppm (ai), alone or in a mixture with dithiocarbamate, gave excellent control of apple mildew (Podosphaera leucotricha) (Figure 18) and apple scab (Figure 19). In a trial in the USA, cedar apple rust (Gymnosporangium juniperi-virginianae) was also controlled very effectively with 10 ppm (ai) of hexaconazole.

Synthesis of Analogues of Hexaconazole

Having identified hexaconazole as a fungicide development compound it was important to synthesise any closely related compounds that may also possess good fungicidal activity. In particular, we have investigated the importance of the hydroxyl group and the nature of the normal butyl side chain in the molecule on the biological activity.

It had been shown in the early stages of this work that it was possible to deoxygenate hexaconazole using a dehydration and reduction sequence (Figure 20). These compounds have some fungicidal activity and are closely related in structure to the top-fruit fungicide, penconazole (17). The compound in which the hydroxyl function of hexaconazole was replaced by a methyl group was also prepared (Figure 21) and has fungicidal properties.

In going from the flutriafol structure to hexaconazole we have demonstrated that it is possible to replace one of the aryl rings by a normal butyl group and retain useful fungicidal activity. We have developed chemical synthetic methods to prepare other compounds, related to hexaconazole, in which the butyl group is replaced by other functional groups. These methods include, the opening of an epoxide with 1,2,4 triazole, the addition of an appropriate carbanion to a 1,2,4-triazol-1-yl ketone, and various functional group transformations.

It is possible to construct tertiary alcohols in a one-step process from an α-1,2,4-triazol-1-yl ketone with a suitable carbanion (Figure 22). In this case the ester enolate generated using lithium diisopropylamide gives a much better yield than the product of the Reformatsky reaction.

The 1,2 dione and 1,2 diol were prepared starting from 2,4-dichlorobenzyl propyl ketone using a modification of the Mannich reaction and epoxidising the intermediate enone with basic hydrogen peroxide. Opening of the epoxide with 1,2,4-triazole followed by reduction completes the synthesis. (Figure 23).

The synthesis of the 1,3 dione and 1,3 diol was accomplished in an efficient two-step process. Base promoted addition of ethyl methyl ketone to the substituted 1,2,4-triazol-1-yl acetophenone gives the intermediate kinetic aldol product which was reduced using sodium borohydride to the required compound (Figure 24).

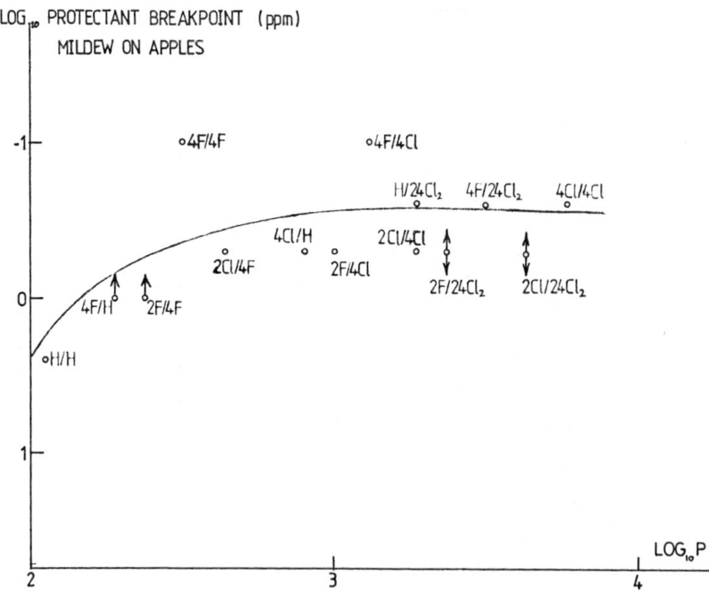

Figure 15. Plot log protectant activity (apple mildew) against log P for flutriafol compounds

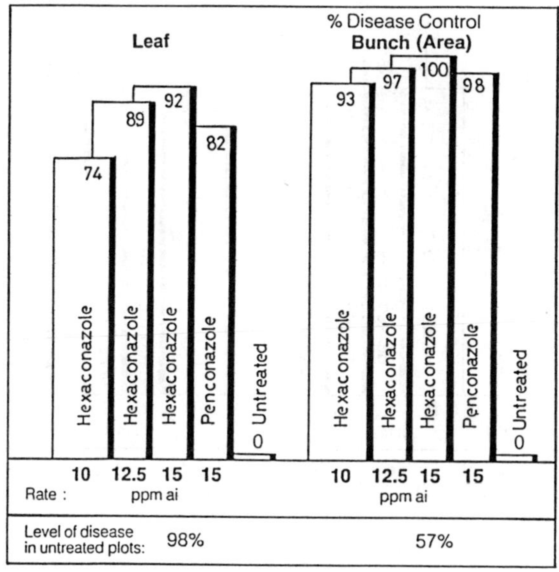

Figure 16. Control of vine powdery mildew, France 1984

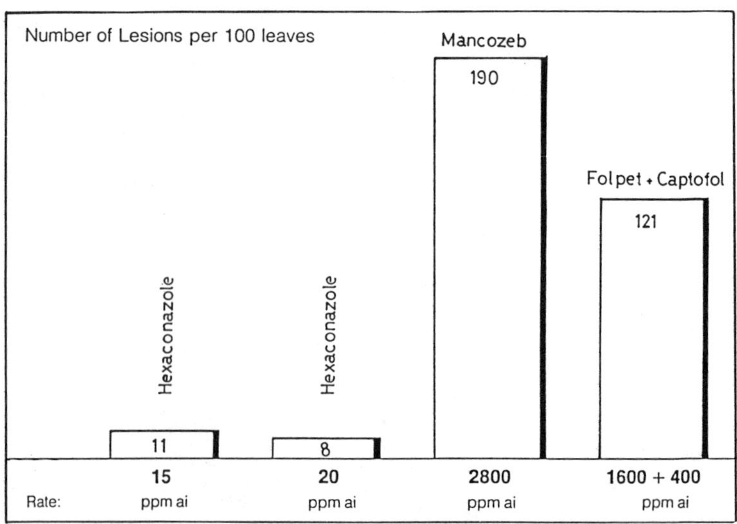

Figure 17. Control of black rot, France 1984

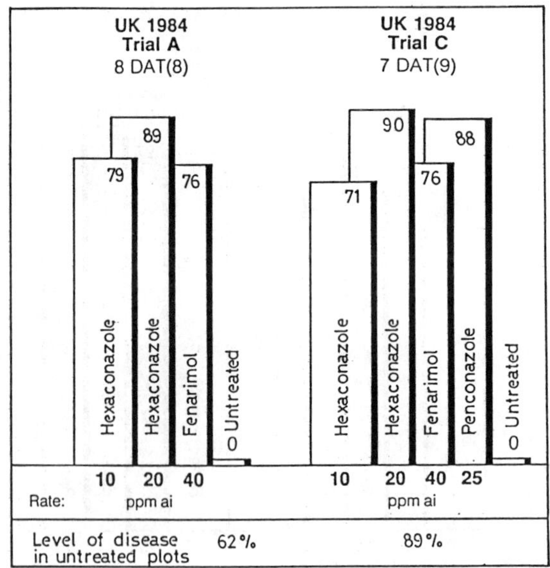

Figure 18. Control of apple powdery mildew

Treatment	Rate ppm ai	West Germany 1984 10 DAT (7) Leaf Scab	Fruit Scab	France 1984 18 DAT (8) Leaf Scab	Fruit Scab	Holland 1984 28 DAT (10) Leaf Scab	Fruit Scab
Hexaconazole	15	96	91	80	84	99	100
Hexaconazole	20	100	96	84	89	100	100
Bitertanol	125	-	-	-	-	100	99
Fenarimol	36	95	85	-	-	-	-
Fenarimol	40	-	-	84	88	-	-
Untreated	-	0	0	0	0	0	0
Level of disease in untreated plots		19^+	6^+	22^+	7^{++}	91^x	68^{xx}

\+ % leaf area infected; ++ % fruit area infected; x % of leaves infected; xx % of fruit infected

Figure 19. Control of apple scab

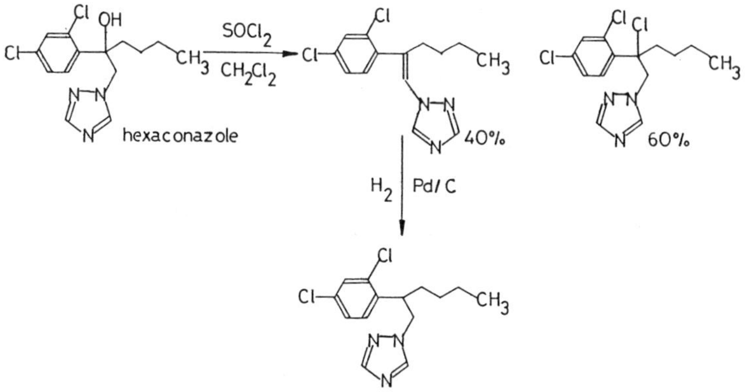

Figure 20. Deoxygenation of hexaconazole

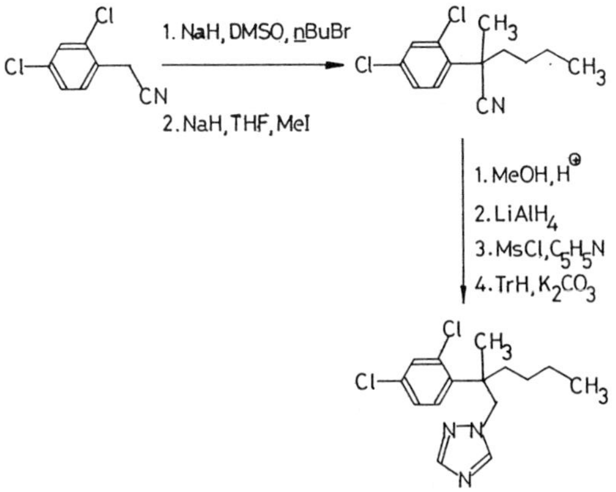

Figure 21. Methyl replacement of hydroxy in hexaconazole

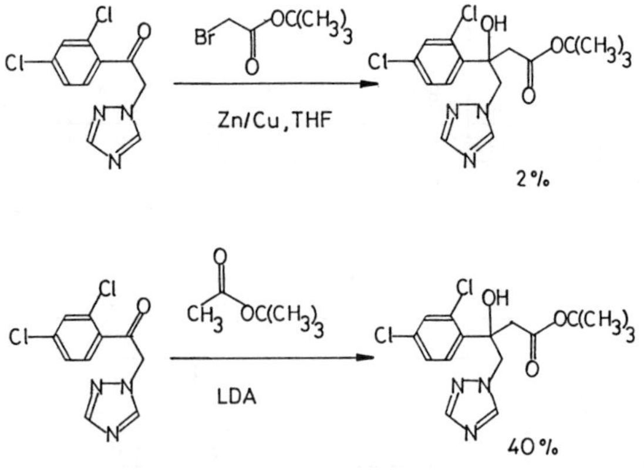

Figure 22. Synthesis of β-hydroxy esters

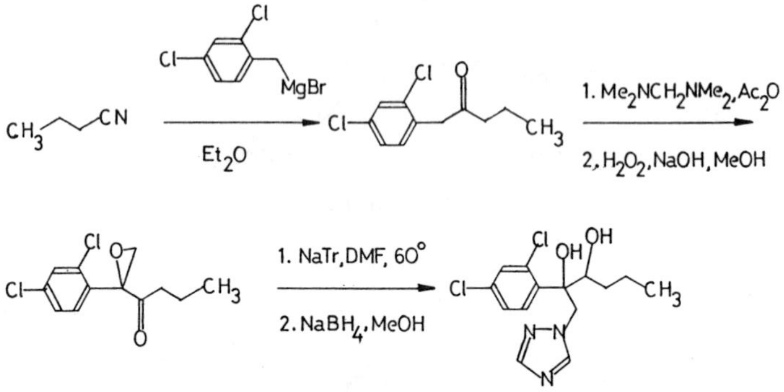

Figure 23. Synthesis of the 1,2 diol

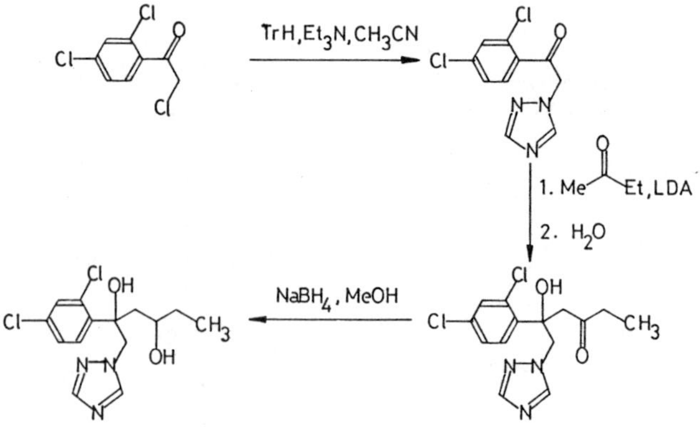

Figure 24. Synthesis of the 1,3 diol

Conclusions

From a knowledge of the mode of action of known inhibitors of the 14α-demethylase enzyme and the use of computer graphic techniques it has been possible to identify a series of novel 1,2,4-triazole tertiary alcohol structures which have high fungicidal activity. From this group of structures, two compounds flutriafol and hexaconazole have been developed for use on diseases of cereals and top-fruit respectively. Hexaconazole contains a normal butyl chain and this can be replaced by other functional groups to give compounds which have useful fungicidal properties.

Other 1,2,4-triazole containing tertiary alcohols are being developed as fungicides, and it is likely that further compounds from this family, with useful biological properties, will be discovered.

Literature Cited

1. Grewe, F.; Buchel, K.H. Mitt. Biol. Bundesanst. Land-Forstwirtsh. Berlin, 1973, 151, p208
2. Worthington, P.A. Proc. Br. Crop. Protect. Conf. Pests Dis., 1984, 3, p955.
3. Baldwin, B.C. Biochemical Society Transactions 1983, 11, 659-663.
4. Lever, B.G.; Shearing S.J.; Batch, J.J. Proc. Br. Crop. Protect Conf. Weeds, 1982, 1, p3.
5. Dalziel, J.; Lawrence, D.K. Br. Plant Growth Regulator Group, Monograph 11, 1984, p43.
6. Sugavanam, B. Pestic. Sci. 1984, 15, 296-302.
7. Gibbons, G.F.; Pullinger C.R.; Mitropoulos, K.A. Biochem. J. 1979, 183, 309-315.
8. Marchington, A.F. 10th Int. Cong. Plant Protn., 1983, 1, p201.
9. Skidmore, A.M.; French, P.N.; Rathmell, W.G. 10th Int. Cong. Plant Protn., 1983, 1, p368.
10. Baldwin, B.C.; Wiggins, T.E.; Marchington, A.F.; Worthington, P.A. Med. Fac. Landbouww. Rijksuniv. Gent, 1984, 49/2a, p303.
11. Shephard, M.C.; Noon, R.A.; Worthington, P.A.; McClellan, W.D.; Lever, B.G. Proc. Br. Crop. Protect. Conf. Pests Dis., 1986, 1, p19.
12. Reinecke, P.; Kaspers, H.; Scheinpflug, H.; Holmwood, G. Proc. Br. Crop Protect. Conf. Pests Dis., 1986, 1, p41.
13. Gisi, U.; Schaub, F.; Wiedmer, H.; Ummel, E. Proc. Br. Crop Protect. Conf. Pests Dis., 1986, 1, p.33.
14. Richardson, K.; Brammer, K.W.; Marriott, M.S.; Troke, P.F. Antimicrob. Agents Chemother., 1985, 27, p832.
15. Northwood, P.J.; Paul, J.A.; Gibbard, M.; Noon, R.A. Proc. Br. Crop. Protect. Conf. Pest Dis., 1984, 1, p47.
16. Heaney, S.P.; Atger, J.C.; Roques, J.F.; Proc. Br. Crop Protect. Conf. Pests Dis., 1986, 1, p363.
17. Eberle, J.; Ruess, W.; Urech, P.A. 10th Int. Cong. Plant Protn., 1983, 1, p376.

RECEIVED May 15, 1987

Chapter 28

Successful Exploitation of 2-Cyano Arylethyltriazoles as Agricultural Fungicides

T. T. Fujimoto, S. H. Shaber, H. F. Chan, J. A. Quinn, and G. R. Carlson

Rohm and Haas Company, 727 Norristown Road, Spring House, PA 19477

The utilization of phenylacetonitriles as a starting point for the preparation of 2-substituted-2-cyano-phenethylazoles, led to the discovery of a class of compounds with high antifungal activity. Through systematic structure-activity investigations, the antifungal activity of α-butyl-α-(4-chlorophenyl)-1H-1,2,4-triazole-1-propanenitrile was discovered. This compound, whose common name is myclobutanil, has been successfully introduced as an agricultural fungicide by Rohm and Haas Co., under the trademark Systhane.

The first strongly active, broad spectrum, ergosterol biosynthesis inhibiting fungicide we prepared was 2-(2,4-dichlorophenyl)-1-(1-imidazolyl) hexane, 1, and we began a synthesis program in this area of chemistry in an attempt to obtain an

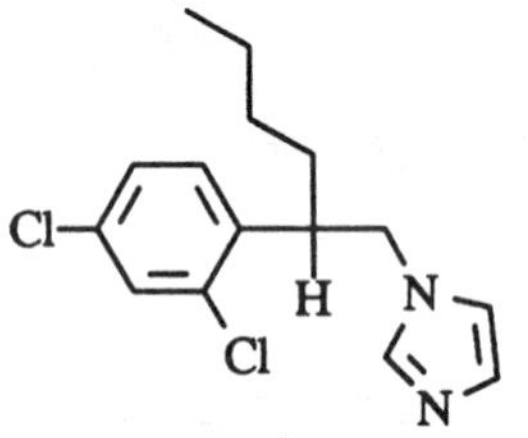

Cl H N N Cl

1

agricultural fungicide. A related series, the α-alkoxyalkyl phenethyl imidazoles was patented by Janssen Pharmaceuticals (1), who, subsequently, also reported its preparation (2).

However, for an agricultural chemical, structures which are more synthetically accessible are desirable, and alternative structures were sought. Conceptually, it appeared that a small biologically neutral, chemical activating group which allowed either nucleophilic or electrophilic attachment of substituents would be an ideal substituent to have on the benzylic carbon. The cyano moiety seemed to have the best potential and it was found that phenylacetonitrile was

0097–6156/87/0355–0318$06.00/0
© 1987 American Chemical Society

readily alkylated in a sequential manner to introduce an alkyl fragment, and a methylene bromide fragment, which could subsequently be converted to a methylene imidazole.

This series of compounds turned out to be highly active, and RH-2161, 2-butyl-2-cyano-phenethylimidazole, 2, was selected to undergo field evaluation. RH-2161 was superceded by the triazole counterpart, RH-5781F, 3, which had better residual activity in the field. However, the efficacious rate of RH-5781F was found to be too high for cost-effective use.

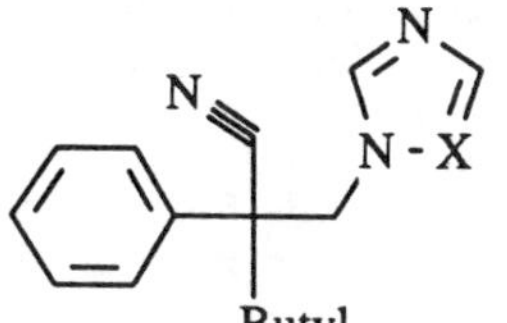

Butyl

	X	
2	C	(RH-2161)
3	N	(RH-5781F)

Though the literature (3) claimed that o, p-dichloro subsitution on phenyl is optimum in the phenethylazoles and our own experiences had supported this claim, the QSAR study of the 2-cyano-phenethyltriazoles we conducted indicated otherwise. The QSAR analysis of the aryl ring substitution in conjunction with modifications of the alkyl substituent in the 2-position indicated that the best compound should have only a p-chloro as the aryl substituent; the o-chloro being detrimental to activity. The best 2-alkyl substituent was predicted to be a 4 to 5 carbon alkyl chain. (T.T. Fujimoto, J.A. Quinn, A.R. Egan, S.H. Shaber and R.R. Ross, to be published). The compound with the alkyl group equal to butyl was made, and had superior activity over the corresponding unsubstituted, and o,p-dichloro substituted phenyl, phenethyltriazoles. Further structure-activity studies on the alkyl group as well as investigation of aryl substitution showed this compound to have the best overall level of activity, and in 1986, α-butyl-α-(4-chlorophenyl)-1H-1,2,4-triazole-1-propanenitrile was introduced as a commercial product in France under the trademark Systhane.

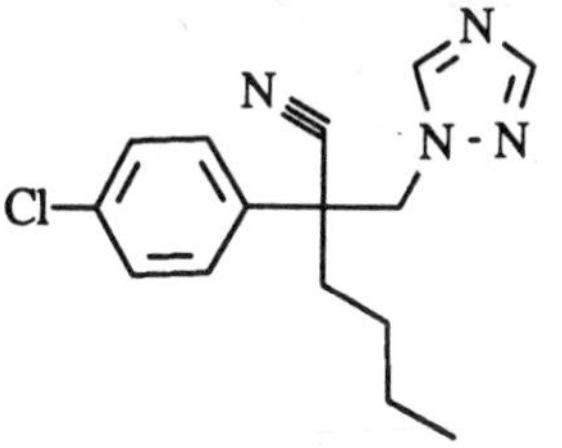

Systhane
(myclobutanil)

Chemical Synthesis

The synthesis of phenethylimidazole 1 proceeded by alkylation of ethyl 2,4-dichlorophenylacetate with n-butyl chloride under basic conditions to give the ethyl ester 4, which was reduced to 5, and activated as the mesylate 6. Treatment with imidazole gave the desired final product as shown in Figure 1.

The 2-substituted-2-cyano-arylethyltriazoles were prepared by sequential alkylation of substituted phenylacetonitriles (4) as shown in Figure 2. The alkylation of phenylacetonitriles were performed under a variety of basic conditions. Alkylation by phase transfer catalysis, (PTC), (5) using NaOH, catalyst and toluene or with NaOH in DMSO, proceeded smoothly at room temperature with alkyl chlorides. For less reactive phenylacetonitriles and for NaOH sensitive alkylating reagents, NaH or KH was utilized. The methylene fragment was appended by using CH_2Cl_2 or CH_2Br_2 in NaOH/DMSO or via PTC conditions and gave 9 in high yield. Completion of the synthesis proceeded by displacement of the neopentyl halide with imidazole or potassium triazole at elevated temperatures. In the displacement using imidazole, the reaction proceeded cleanly without preparation of the salt. An alternative and more efficient preparation of 10a involves the reaction of the intermediate 8 with chloromethyltriazole hydrochloride or its corresponding free base as shown in Figure 3. Chloromethyltriazole hydrochloride (6) was prepared in a two step sequence from triazole via paraformaldehyde followed by treatment with $SOCl_2$. The coupling with chloromethyltriazole and 8 proceeded by using hydride bases in DMF or by using NaOH in DMSO.

The alkylation of phenylacetonitriles can result in significant quantities of dialkylated products, especially with reactive alkylating reagents (7). Therefore, for the preparation of α-benzyl substituents, the facile two step procedure shown in Figure 4 was employed, which eliminated the dialkylation problem. Reaction of phenylacetonitriles with benzaldehydes in MeOH with NaOH as the base gives the acrylonitriles, 11, in quantitative yield. Reduction with $NaBH_4$/EtOH then gives pure monoalkylated α-benzyl intermediates 12, which are subjected to the sequences described in Figures 2 and 3.

Two procedures have been utilized for attaching α-alkoxy functionality at the 2-position affording the desired intermediate 14. Both involve the acetals of substituted benzaldehydes as a starting point. As shown in Figure 5, reaction of acetal 13 with trimethylsilyl cyanide and $SnCl_2$ gave the alkoxy nitrile directly (9), while a two step procedure with pyridine/ acetyl chloride (α-chloro ether formation) followed by NaCN (10) displacement also afforded 14. Again, completion of the synthesis to the desired triazoles proceeded as described in Figures 2 and 3.

In the preparation of 2-cyano-2-(fluoroalkyl) phenethyltriazole derivatives the fluorinated alkyl halides, e.g. 4,4,4-trifluorobutyl bromide, were employed, whenever possible, in alkylations with phenylacetonitriles. The desired triazoles were obtained by continuing the synthesis as described above. Other fluorinated and chlorinated side chains were prepared by incorporating the halogens to complete the synthesis. In these cases, alkylation using an alkyl halide containing a protected carbonyl or hydroxyl group was used. This functionality was then unprotected and converted to the appropriate fluorinated material. For terminal halogen substituents, the terminal protecting group differed between the propyl and butyl series. The compounds in the following discussion are shown in Table I.

In the propyl series, the diethyl acetal was the protecting group with 3-chloropropionaldehyde diethyl acetal serving as the alkylating reagent for 4-chlorophenylacetonitrile. After conversion to triazole 15, the acetal was removed with 33% H_2SO_4/EtOAc giving the aldehyde 16, which gave 17 after treatment with diethylaminosulfur trifluoride (DAST/CH_2CL_2). Reduction of the aldehyde to the terminal alcohol 18 proceeded smoothly and was followed by conversion to the fluoro (DAST) and chloropropyl ($SOCl_2$/py) analogs 19 and 20, respectively.

For the butyl series, 4-chlorophenylacetonitrile was alkylated with 1-chloro-4-acetoxybutane using NaH in DMF, followed by homologation and treatment with potassium triazole (re-acetylating when necessary). Removal of the acetoxy group with NaOH/MeOH gave the 4-butanol intermediate 25. The 4-fluorobutyl

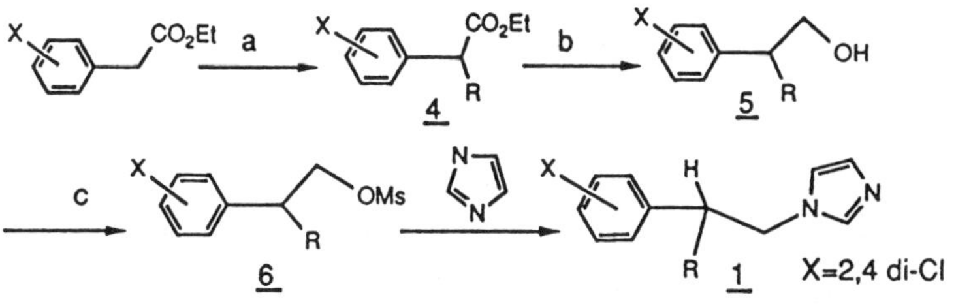

a=base; b=LAH,Et_2O; c=MsCl,TEA;
base=NaH,KH

Figure 1. Synthesis of 2-substituted-2-(2,4-dichlorophenyl) ethylimidazole.

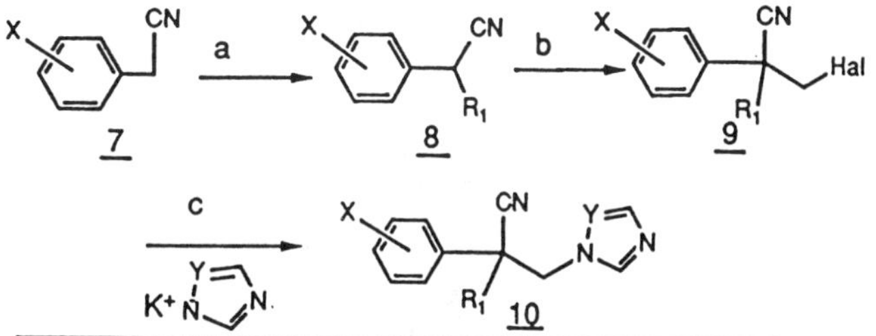

a=base,RCl; b=base,DMSO,CH_2Br_2 or CH_2Cl_2; c=DMSO
base=NaOH;NaH;KH

Figure 2. Three step synthesis of 2-substituted-2-cyano-phenethylazoles.

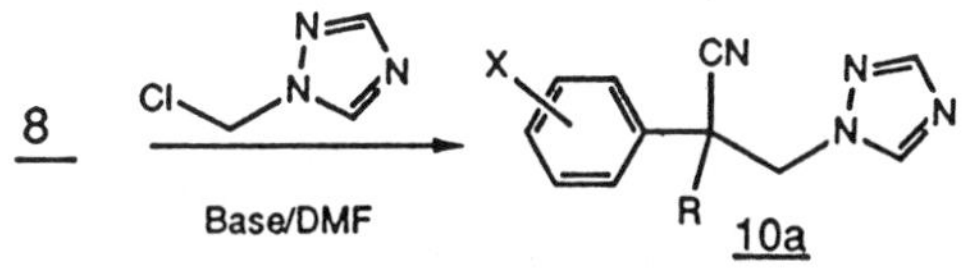

Base = NaOH, NaH, KH

Figure 3. Two step synthesis of 2-substituted-2-cyano-phenethyltriazole.

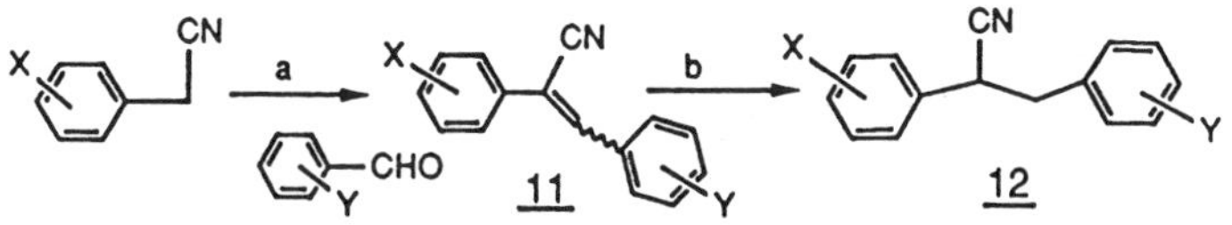

a=NaOH,MeOH; b=$NaBH_4$,THF,EtOH

Figure 4. Preparation of α-benzyl-phenylacetonitriles.

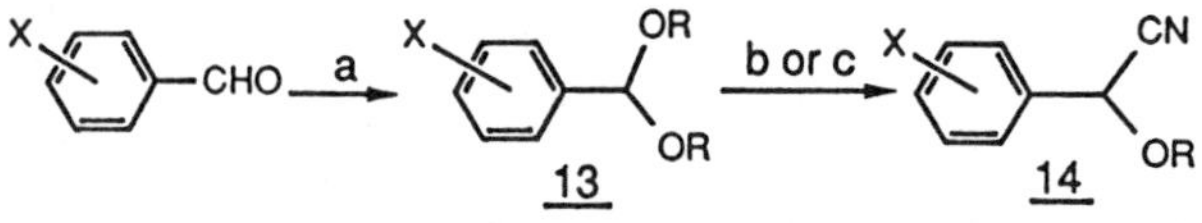

a=ROH,H+; b=TMSCN,SnCl$_4$; c=ClCOCH$_3$,py; NaCN,DMSO

Figure 5. Preparation of α-alkoxy-phenylacetonitriles.

Table I. Halogenated 2-alkyl products and intermediates

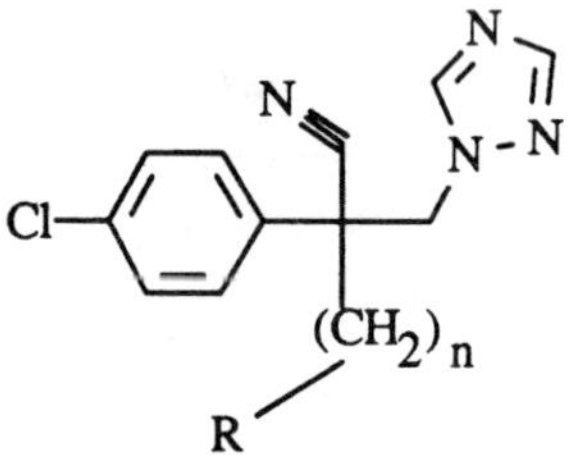

n = 2 compound	R	n = 3 compound	R
15	$C(OEt)_2$	24	CH_2OAc
16	CHO	25	CH_2OH
17	CHF_2	26	CH_2F
18	CH_2OH	27	CH_2Cl
19	CH_2F	28	CHO
20	CH_2Cl	29	CHF_2
21	$C((OCH_2)_2)CH_3$		
22	$COCH_3$		
23	CF_2CH_3		

and 4-chlorobutyl derivatives 26 and 27, respectively, were prepared in the usual manner. The alcohol was oxidized to aldehyde 28 via CrO_3/py, and then fluorinated (DAST/CH_2Cl_2) to give the 4,4-difluorobutyl derivative 29. Internally halogenated, 3-halobutyl derivatives, were prepared by alkylation with the ethylene glycol ketal of 1-chloro-3-butanone, which was converted to the triazole adduct 21. Removal of the ketal provided the 3-oxobutyl analog 22 which gave the difluorobutyl product 23 upon treatment with DAST.

Greenhouse Evaluations

In general, potted plants are treated with technical compound dissolved in 1:1:2, methanol:acetone:water, by spraying the seedling foliage past run-off. Inoculum is applied within 24 hrs. of spraying and the plants incubated 5 to 8 days before disease pressure is evaluated. Detailed test procedures are given in reference 11.

Structure Activity Studies

After extensively surveying major modifications of the structure attached to triazole, a systematic structure-activity study was begun on the phenethyltriazole structure. For this study, the molecule was dissected, as shown below, into 4 quadrants: I) the aryl ring, II) the hydrophobic group, III) the cyano group, and IV) the triazole. The results from investigation of quadrants I, the aryl ring, and II, the

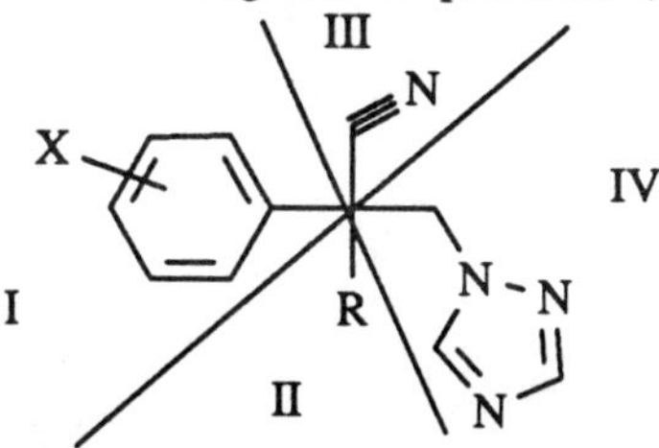

hydrophobic sidechain are presented here. Using unsubstituted phenyl as the base, a series of quadrant II changes were made. A representative compound list is given in Table II. From these compounds, the following structure-activity profile based on *in-vivo* greenhouse testing can be ascertained. There is a large species to species variation on the effect of the substitution on activity, but, in general, the activity peaks at substituents whose chain length is four to five atoms. Non-carbon atoms in the chain, especially oxygen have a negative effect on the activity, and from examining the observed biological activity of n-propyl and butyl vs. i-propyl and i-butyl, and of allyl vs. 2-methallyl, it appears that chain branching has a negative effect on activity. These results are similar to those obtained for miconazole analogues (4) on human fungi, indicating some conservation of the site of action between organisms.

Once the optimum sidechain characteristics had been investigated, aryl substitution (quadrant I) of the cyanophenylethyltriazole was examined. Using butyl as the reference substituent, several mono- and di-substituted phenethyltriazoles were prepared (Table III). Except for the activity of 2-methoxy, 2 and 3 substitution, led to a large loss in activity. Halogen substituents in the 4 position were better than hydrogen, with other substituents whose steric bulk is linear along the attachment bond axis also being active. Though the substitutent effect varies somewhat with the organism, the substituent effect at the three aryl positions can be generally described as follows:

Table II. Control of diseases in greenhouse pot tests of compounds with an unsubstituted phenyl ring

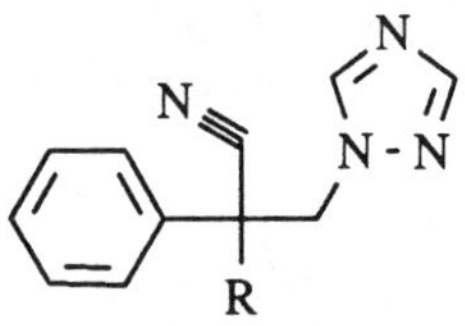

R

rate giving 90% disease control(ug/ml)

substituent	wheat powdery mildew	leaf rust	barley spot blotch
n-propyl	17	220	20
i-propyl	50	>500	>500
n-butyl	25	95	25
i-butyl	29	400	25
n-pentyl	13	76	10
i-pentyl	7	61	25
n-hexyl	1	220	7
cyclohexyl	9	200	300
1-methylbutyl	9	70	>500
methoxy	300	>500	>500
ethoxy	60	>500	75
propoxy	5	400	10
butoxy	10	100	75
$CH_2CH_2OCH_2CH_3$	120	400	19
allyl	19	>500	60
2-methylallyl	82	>500	150
2,3-butenyl	10	120	60
phenyl	25	75	200
benzyl	15	75	150
p-Cl-benzyl	5	5	>500

a) wheat powdery mildew is caused by *Erysiphegraminis f.sp. tritici*, wheat leaf *Puccinia recondita f.sp. tritici* and barley spot blotch by *Cochliobolus sativus*.

Table III. Control of wheat powdery mildew and stem rust in foliar greenhouse tests for phenyl substituted 2-butyl-2-cyano-phenethyltriazoles

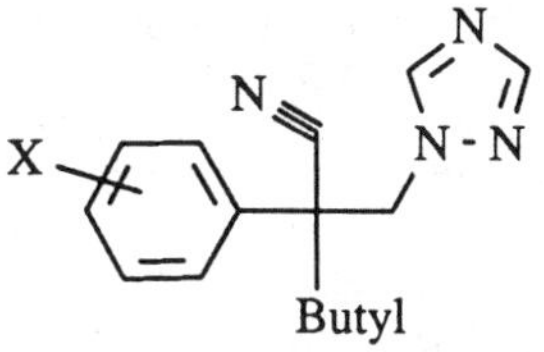

X, N, N, N - N, Butyl

phenyl (X)	rate giving 90% disease control (ug/ml)	
	powdery mildew	stem rust
H	25	60
2-Cl	60	90
2-CN	134	400
2-F	300	300
2-OCH_3	3	500
3-CF_3	150	200
3-Cl	19	150
3-OCH_3	25	450
4-Br	20	33
4-CH_3	150	33
4-Cl(myclobutanil)	2	2
4-CN	10	25
4-F	5	5
4-OC_6H_5	25	500+
4-C_6H_5	7	<5
2,4-Cl	1	19
2-OCH_3,4-Cl	4	19
2,5-OCH_3	2	>500
3,4-Cl	19	15
3,4-OCH_3	300	>500
3,5-CF_3	150	200

a) powdery mildew is caused by *Erysiphe graminis f.sp. tritici* and stem rust by *Puccinia graminis f.sp. tritici.*

ortho H >> Cl > CN > F; OCH_3 varies with organism
meta H >> Cl > OCH_3 > CF_3
para Cl > F > C_6H_5 > CN > Br > H > CH_3 >> OC_6H_5

The direction of activity for disubstituted aryl ring compounds was reasonably predicted by averaging the there is no large interactions between the ring substitutents. With the optimum aryl substituent in hand, the hydrophobic sidechain (quadrant II) was re-investigated. Table IV lists the results which verified that the para-chlorophenyl, butyl substituted compound was one of the best. Some further verification of the substituent scheme was conducted by preparing other mixed quadrant I, quadrant II variants. The best compounds were subjected to additional studies, including systemic and curative tests, and within the scope of alkyl and alkenyl sidechains, myclobutanil, was determined to be the best compound, overall.

Table IV. Control of wheat powdery mildew and leaf rust with para-chloro substitution on the phenyl ring

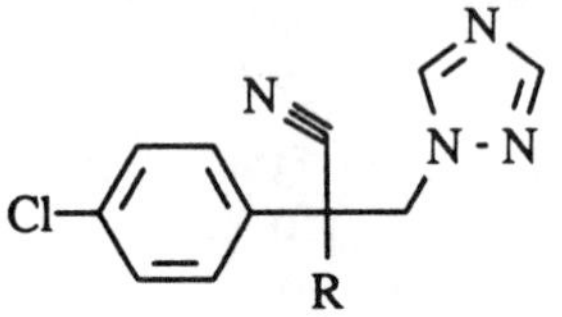

R substituent	rate giving 90% disease control (ug/ml) powdery mildew	leaf rust
n-propyl	1	16
n-butyl(myclobutanil)	2	7
2-methylbutyl	50	75
n-pentyl	2	4
i-pentyl	1	15
n-hexyl	7	100
4,5-pentenyl	25	20
3-flouropropyl	20	50
3-chloropropyl	4	>150
$CH_2CH_2CHF_2$	4	>150
$CH_2CH_2CF_2CH_3$	10	125
4-fluorobutyl	15	75
4-chlorobutyl	2	150
$CH_2CH_2CH_2CHF_2$	0.7	150
$CH_2CH_2CH_2CF_3$	0.4	80
4-methoxybutyl	50	300
$CH_2CH_2CH_2CHO$	300	300
$CH_2CH_2CH(OCH_2CH_3)_2$	10	>150

Literature Cited

1. Janssen Pharmaceutica, Ger Offen. DE 1 940 388, February 26,1970.

2. Heeres, J.; Backx, L.J.J.; Van Cutsem, J.M. J. Med. Chem. 1976, 19, 1148.

3. Ellames, G. J. Modern Synthetic Antifungal Agents; Halsted Press: New York, 1982; pp 49-54

4. Miller, G.A.; Chan Hak Foon. U.S. Patent 4 366 165, December 18, 1982.

5. Weber, W.P.; Gokel G.W. Phase Transfer Catalysis in Organic Synthesis; Reactivity and Structure in Organic Chemistry 4; Springer Verlag: New York, 1977; Chapter 10.

6. Ciba Geigy, European Patent 63 099, April 4, 1982.

7. Makosza, M.; Serafinowa, B. Rocz. Chem. 1965, 39, 1401.

8. Kulp, S.S.; Caldwell, C.B. J. Org. Chem. 1980, 45 171-173.

9. Utimoto, K.; Wakabashyi, Y.; Shishiyama, Y.; Inoue, K.; Nozaki, H. Tett. Lett. 1981, 21 4279-4280.

10. Sterling Drug, U.S. Patent 3 607 942, September 21, 1971.

11. Quinn, J.A.; Fujimoto, T.T.; Egan, A.R.; Shaber, S.H. Pestic. Sci. 1986, 17,357-362.

RECEIVED July 21, 1987

Chapter 29

Prochloraz and Its Analogs

Chemistry, Mode of Action, and Biological Efficacy

Alister C. Baillie

Chesterford Park, United Kingdom Research Station of the Agrochemical Division of Schering AG West Germany, Saffron Walden, Essex, England

Exploration of the area of imidazole-1-carboxamides has led to the discovery of prochloraz, a broad-spectrum fungicide for use on a variety of crops. Prochloraz and its analogues are inhibitors of ergosterol biosynthesis and structure-activity relationships in the area are discussed. In particular, the usefulness of an *in vitro* assay for sterol biosynthesis as a guide to the chemical effort is considered. Finally, the biological activity of prochloraz is briefly described.

In the early 1970s the area of carbamoyl heterocycles had been a fruitful area of synthesis for organic chemists working in the Boots Company in Nottingham, yielding for example, the herbicide epronaz (I) (1) as well as compounds active in other fields.

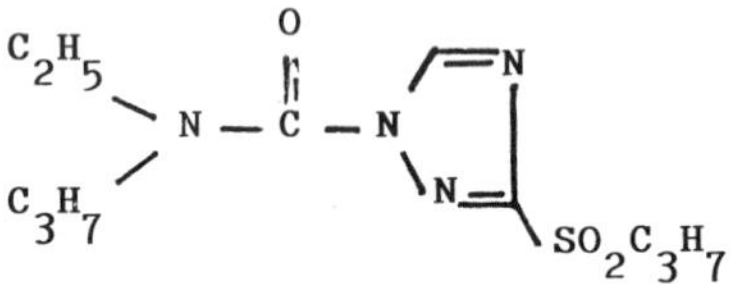

$(C_2H_5)(C_3H_7)N-C(=O)-N$ [triazole ring, $SO_2C_3H_7$]

I

$(C_2H_5)_2N-C(=S)-N$ [imidazole ring]

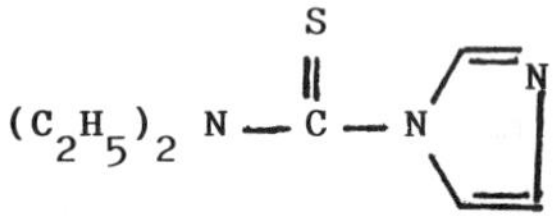

II

Around this time Tolkmith and his colleagues (2) drew attention to the fungicidal activity of the thiocarboxamide (II) and this acted as a spur for workers at the Boots Company to undertake further

0097-6156/87/0355-0328$06.00/0
© 1987 American Chemical Society

synthesis based on this lead. This effort culminated in the discovery of prochloraz (III), a compound that controls important pathogens in cereals and many other crops (3).

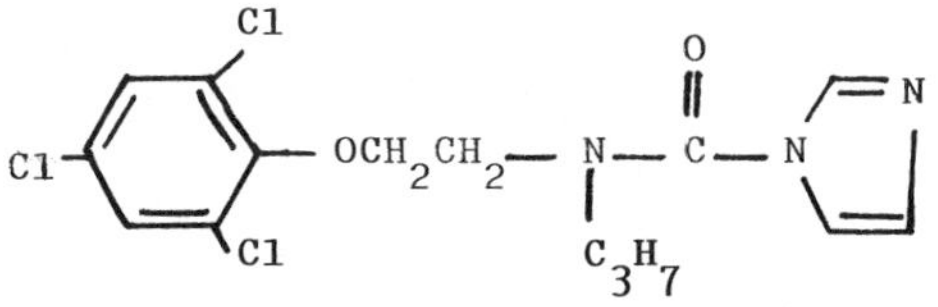

III

The purpose of this paper is to review various aspects of the work done in the prochloraz area in the laboratories of the Boots Company, and latterly (following ownership changes) in the laboratories of FBC Ltd and by the agrochemical division of Schering AG West Germany. The review will describe the synthesis of the various types of compound prepared as the project evolved, and will consider their mode of action and the usefulness of an *in vitro* assay as a guide to synthesis. It will also deal briefly with the biological activity of prochloraz itself. Some of this information has already been published (4).

Initial Synthesis

The effort began with the preparation of simple *N*-alkyl,*N*-aryl-imidazolecarboxamides (e.g.IV) and their *N*-benzyl analogues (e.g.V).

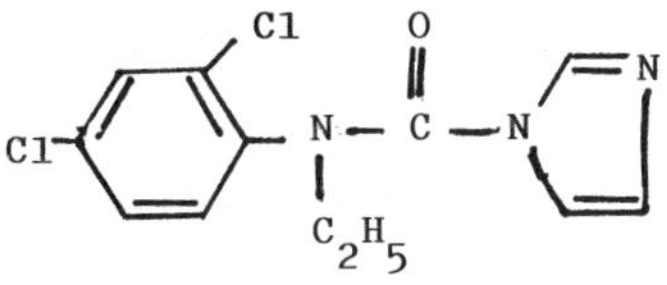

IV

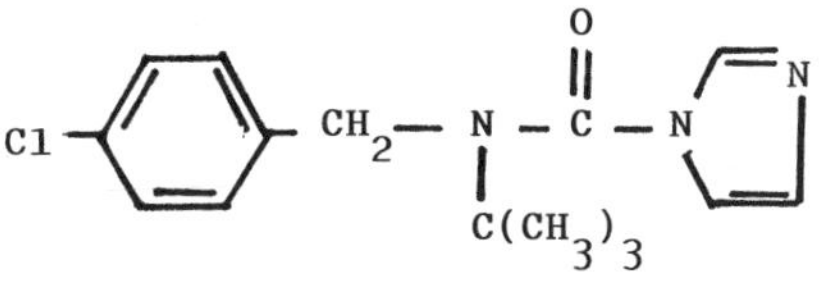

V

These were prepared by the following routes.

(a) $ArNHCOCH_3 \xrightarrow[2.Conc.HCl]{1.NaH/RBr} ArNHR \xrightarrow{COCl_2} Ar\text{-}N(R)\text{-}C(=O)\text{-}Cl$

$\xrightarrow{Imidazole/(C_2H_5)_3N} Ar\text{-}N(R)\text{-}C(=O)\text{-}N$ (imidazole ring)

(b) $ArCH_2Cl \xrightarrow{RNH_2/NaOH} ArCH_2NHR \xrightarrow{as\ (a)} ArCH_2\text{-}N(R)\text{-}C(=O)\text{-}N$ (imidazole ring)

Thus, the appropriately substituted aniline or benzylamine, prepared as shown, was treated with phosgene, and the resulting carbamoyl chloride reacted with imidazole to give the product.

Many of these compounds had good fungicidal activity, which comes as no surprise to us now, but it should be remembered that, when this work was being done, knowledge of the fungitoxic action of azoles and an appreciation of their mode of action (5) were in their infancy. The compounds were particularly active on powdery mildews and some of them (e.g.IV) were systemic by root uptake. Unfortunately they were less active in the field than they had been under glass and they also adversely affected plant growth.

Further synthesis, however, was to prove more fruitful. Thus, using similar procedures, compounds were prepared in which the nitrogen atom carried both an alkyl and an aryloxyalkyl group (cf prochloraz, III).

$ArOH \xrightarrow{BrCH_2CH_2Br/NaOH} ArOCH_2CH_2Br \xrightarrow{as\ before} ArOCH_2CH_2N(R)\text{-}C(=O)\text{-}N$ (imidazole ring)

Compounds containing an alkyl substituent in the chain carrying the aryloxy group were made by a sequence involving reductive amination of the appropriate ketone or aldehyde.

$$\text{(a)}\quad ArOCH_2COCH_3 \xrightarrow{RNH_2/NaBH_4} ArOCH_2CH(CH_3){-}NHR$$

$$\xrightarrow{\text{as before}} ArOCH_2CH(CH_3){-}N(R){-}C(=O){-}N\langle\text{imidazole}\rangle$$

$$\text{(b)}\quad ArOCH(CH_3)CHO \xrightarrow{RNH_2/NaBH_4} ArOCH(CH_3)CH_2NHR$$

$$\xrightarrow{\text{as before}} ArOCH(CH_3)CH_2N(R){-}C(=O){-}N\langle\text{imidazole}\rangle$$

A wide variety of compounds was prepared using these routes (or variations thereon); for example, the length and nature of the N-alkyl chain were varied, as was the length of the alkyl chain carrying the aryloxy group; aryloxyalkyl was replaced by arylthioalkyl; carbamoyl was replaced by thiocarbamoyl, and of course many substituents were introduced in the aryl ring.

The products were generally liquids or relatively low-melting solids and were purified by vacuum distillation or by crystallisation. Experimental details for representative syntheses are available in the patent literature (6, 7), as are procedures for the preparation of complexes of the imidazoles with a number of metals, notably manganese (8).

Several of these compounds were highly active on powdery mildews and had a broader spectrum of activity than their predecessors. In addition, this activity translated well from the glasshouse to the field. The next part of the review will therefore concentrate on these compounds.

Structure - Activity Correlations

In considering these, the first point to note is that substituents on the phenyl ring had the effect one has now come to expect in this field of research. Thus, in a conventional glasshouse test for eradicant activity against *Erisyphe graminis* (powdery mildew of cereals) on barley plants around thirty compounds gave >80% control at 25 ppm and all but one of these contained an aromatic ring bearing two, three or four halogen atoms. The exception was a compound containing *t*-butyl as the aryl substituent, a substituent that is also present in other commercial compounds of this general class. The prochloraz analogue containing an unsubstituted phenyl ring was inactive in this test, while prochloraz was considerably more active than the 2,4-dichloro analogue and, for example, its 2,4,5-trichloro isomer. In polyhalo compounds, one of the halogens could be replaced by a methyl group but, in general, polymethyl compounds were less active than polyhalo analogues.

When the aryl ring was optimally substituted as in prochloraz (III), simple variations of the *N*-alkyl group (for example from propyl to isopropyl, butyl or pentyl), were permissible without much loss in activity as was substitution of either carbon atom of the ethyl portion of the aryloxyethyl group by a methyl group. In some cases the aryloxyethyl chain could be extended to aryloxypropyl without loss of activity, but this was not always true.

Unpredictably, compounds in which the imidazole group was replaced by triazole were very much less active.

In addition to being the most active compound against *E.graminis* in the initial glasshouse screens, prochloraz was the best of a number of analogues in field trials and was the candidate of choice for commercialisation. It is interesting to note that there are a number of important structural differences between prochloraz and other azole fungicides. It is an imidazole, whereas most other important compounds are triazoles, and it can also be regarded as a heterocyclic urea. Although at present it is not clear to what extent this unique type of structure is responsible for the observed spectrum and level of activity of the compound, obviously its chemical properties will influence its uptake, accumulation and metabolism by host plants and pathogens.

Mode of Action Studies

Some information on the mode of action of prochloraz has already been published from these laboratories (4) as has work done elsewhere (e.g. 9). Some additional aspects of our work are described here.

In the light of emerging knowledge on the mode of action of azoles, the effects of prochloraz on the biosynthetic pathway from lanosterol (VI) to ergosterol (VII) (the major sterol in many fungi) were examined as soon as was practicable. This was done using cell-free preparations from yeast and radiolabelled mevalonic acid as the sterol precursor, essentially according to the procedure of Kato and Kawase (10); as a point of experimental detail we now fracture the yeast cells using a bead-beater (which agitates the cells at high speed with glass beads) rather than using the Biox frozen cell press procedure previously described (4).

In our laboratory, the major sterol biosynthesised in untreated extracts was the triene (VIII) (11), rather than ergosterol itself which is, of course, the end product of the pathway in intact cells. It should be noted that VIII arises directly from 14-demethylation of lanosterol. In the presence of 0.1 μM prochloraz (or even 0.01 μM prochloraz in some experiments) the concentration of VIII was significantly reduced, while the level of lanosterol increased (4) indicating clearly that prochloraz inhibited 14-demethylation. At higher fungicide concentrations both the triene and ergosterol were totally absent and only lanosterol was present.

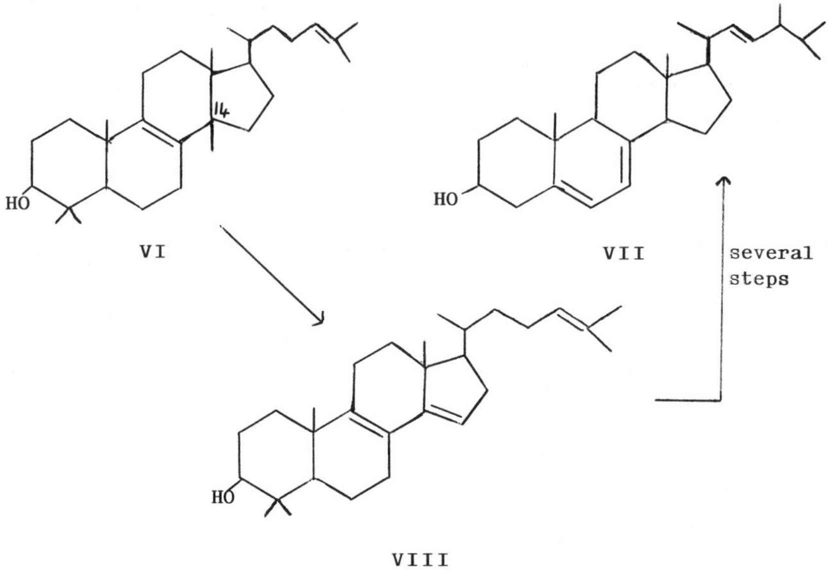

HO 14 VI

HO VII

several steps

HO VIII

In summary, prochloraz, like other azoles, is an ergosterol biosynthesis inhibitor (i.e. it is an EB1) and it does this by blocking 14-demethylation (such compounds are sometimes referred to as demethylation inhibitors, or DMIs). As is now well known, these molecules bind to the sterol binding site of the demethylase enzyme in such a way as to allow the azole to bind to an iron atom in the active site (see below). The normal physiological reaction is therefore prevented.

Reports have appeared, however, indicating some other actions of prochloraz, for example induction of lipid peroxidation (12). Whether these are of practical significance under field conditions is, as yet, unknown.

USE OF THE BIOCHEMICAL ASSAY AS A GUIDE TO SYNTHESIS

As noted previously, much of the synthesis and indeed the preparation of prochloraz itself, preceded the detailed understanding now available on how azoles act. Therefore, when the rapid *in vitro* assay described above became available, its predictive use became an attractive possibility. Experiments were therefore undertaken with the aim of providing a data base of information for potential use in helping to explain structure-activity correlations in compounds already made, and of aiding the continuing synthesis programme. Compounds were tested at concentrations ranging from 0.01 μM to 10 μM and the lowest concentration which perturbed the sterol labelling pattern was noted.

Whereas prochloraz affected sterol biosynthesis at 0.1 μM or less (see above), retrospective testing showed that *N*-alkyl, *N*-substituted benzyl compounds (e.g. V) were active only at 10 μM. Amongst prochloraz analogues, the corresponding triazole was weakly active at 10 μM and compounds in which either oxygen atom had been replaced by a sulphur atom were active at 1.0 μM. The unsubsituted phenoxyethyl analogue (active at 1.0 μM) was also less effective than prochloraz. These results were consistent with the biological data and, although it is difficult to judge such things with hindsight, could have been used to indicate priority areas for further synthesis.

On the other hand, the assay was of limited use in guiding synthesis once the most active area had been established. In the first place, a great many of the compounds prepared were equally active *in vitro* (showing effects on sterol biosynthesis at 0.1 μM) so that no real clues were available to define more detailed priorities. Secondly, a significant number of compounds that showed good *in vitro* activity were poor fungicides *in vivo*. These included, for example, compounds in which the aryl ring carried "unusual" sustituents (in terms of DMIs) such as nitro or ethoxycarbonyl. However, these differences (which presumably reflect adverse transport and/or metabolic factors) are perhaps not unexpected when put in the context of other work on azoles.

Several groups have used molecular graphics techniques to model ways in which ergosterol biosynthesis inhibitors might bind to the active site of their target enzyme (13-14) and we have also looked at prochloraz and its analogues in this way.

Although the exact detail of the pathway from lanosterol to ergosterol probably varies from one pathogenic fungus to another (there are also differences between yeast and other fungi (15)) the results of our mode of action studies (above) led us to model ways in which prochloraz and its analogues could interfere with the demethylase that uses lanosterol as the substrate. In particular, we tried to fit the molecules into the large cage defined by the lanosterol structure, in such a way that the unsubstituted nitrogen atom of the azole could bind to the iron atom in the active site.

Figure 1 shows that prochloraz could fit very well. As expected, many of the analogues could also fit more or less equally well. Since they are hydrophobic molecules one would also expect them to bind well to the lanosterol binding site of the enzyme protein, which would itself be expected to be hydrophobic. However, even the analogue containing the relatively hydrophilic nitro substituent on the aryl ring could bind to the site, as shown by the *in vitro* data. Presumably in this, and related cases, the interactions in the vicinity of the hydrophilic group are not detrimental to binding or, if they are, the hydrophobic binding of the rest of the molecule, and the azole/iron interaction, are dominant. Thus, the modelling studies offered some rationalisation of the experimental finding that many of the prochloraz analogues were equally active *in vitro*.

The discrepancies between *in vitro* and *in vivo* results can also be rationalised. As we have seen, a wide range of analogues inhibited the enzyme. However, it would have been surprising if each of these had been able to reach the target equally well *in vivo*, given the inevitable differences in their transport properties and susceptibility to metabolic breakdown. Absolute agreement between the *in vitro* assay and fungicidal activity could not, therefore, have been expected. In this area of research, as in others, use of the *in vitro* assay has to be allied to a knowledge of existing structure-activity relationships.

In summary then, it is probable that the *in vitro* test could have indicated the most promising areas of research (this is confirmed by our work in other DMI projects) but it was of limited use in fine-tuning such areas.

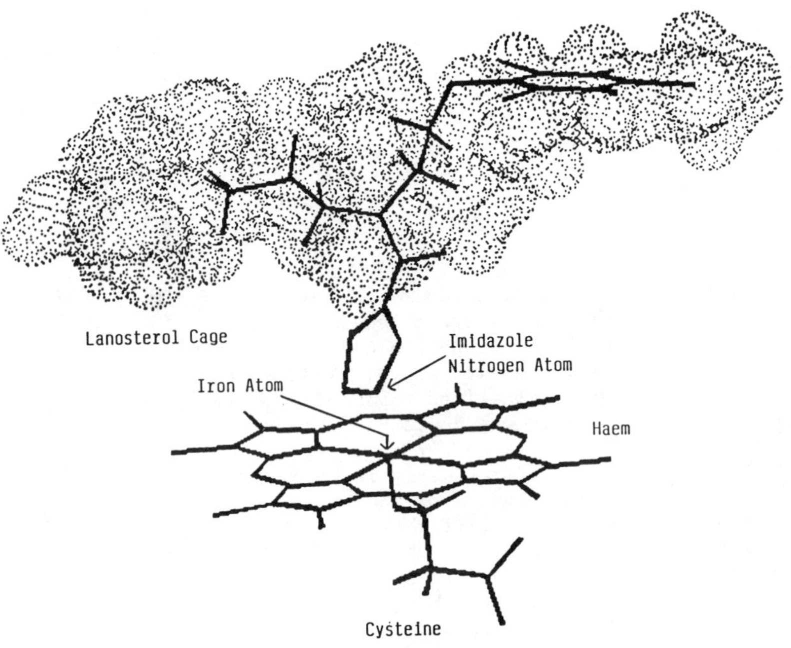

Figure 1. Representation of the interaction of prochloraz with the active site of its target enzyme.

Related Chemistry

As a logical extension to the work on prochloraz, a subsequent examination was made of the related acetamides (IX), which were made using chemistry similar to that already described (16).

$$ArOCH_2CH_2NHR \xrightarrow{ClCH_2COCl/(C_2H_5)_3N} ArOCH_2CH_2N(R)\text{-}C(=O)\text{-}CH_2Cl$$

$$\xrightarrow{\text{Imidazole/NaH}} ArOCH_2CH_2N(R)\text{-}C(=O)\text{-}CH_2\text{-}N(\text{imidazolyl})$$

IX

In general, these compounds were as active in the *in vitro* assay as the corresponding carbamoyl derivatives had been. Structure-activity relationships were roughly similar except that, in this case, the triazoles and imidazoles were equally active *in vitro* and the triazoles were also good fungicides. Some of the compounds prepared in this series showed good biological activity but the best of them did not have any advantages over prochloraz itself. The same was true of the pyridyl analogues (e.g.X) prepared by us and subsequently patented by other workers (17).

$$ArOCH_2CH_2N(R)\text{-}C(=O)\text{-}(\text{pyridyl})$$

X

Biological Activity of Prochloraz

The biological activity of prochloraz has already been reported (4) and will only be summarised here. Although the compound has the same fundamental mode of action as other commercial DMI fungicides, it has a unique spectrum of activity and can be used on a number of crops.

Plant pathogenic fungi controlled include species of *Alternaria*, *Botrytis*, *Botryodiplodia*, *Cercospora*, *Cochliobolus*, *Colletotrichum*, *Fusarium*, *Monilinia*, *Mycogone*, *Penicillium*, *Phoma*, *Pseudocercosporella*, *Pyrenophora*, *Pyricularia*, *Rhynchosporium*, *Sclerotinia*, *Sclerotium*, *Septoria* and *Verticillium* that variously affect the fruits, leaves, roots, seeds, stems or vascular systems of a range of important agricultural and horticultural crop plants. Prochloraz is registered for pre- or, as appropriate, post- harvest control of diseases of cereals, oilseed rape, stone fruit, mushrooms, avocado, citrus, mango, papaya, rice, turf and a number of ornamental plants throughout the world. In Europe it is particularly useful for the control of stem base diseases of cereals, notably eyespot (*Pseudocercosporella*).

Prochloraz, with a log P of around 4.0 and a very low vapour pressure, is not very mobile in plant tissue and it is probable that this contributes, to some extent, to the observed spectrum of activity. In particular, chemical reaching the stem base would not be translocated away from there, whereas less lipophilic azoles would move more readily to the leaves. In addition, the point has already been made that the unique structural features of the compound could also affect the pattern of activity, although there is no direct evidence for this at present.

In any event, it is clear that prochloraz is an extremely effective fungicide which has achieved an important and continuing role in disease control worldwide.

Acknowledgments

I am indebted to many colleagues who have worked on this project over a number of years, and without whose contribution this review could not have been written. In particular, I would like to acknowledge the inventive contributions of R.F.Brookes, D.H.Godson, A.F.Hams, D.M.Weighton and W.H.Wells who were employed at the Boots Company.

Literature Cited

1. Copping, L.G.; Brookes, R.F. *Proc. 12th Brit Weed Control Conf.*, 1974, *2*, p809.
2. Tolkmith, H.; Seiber, J.N.; Buddle, P.B.; Mussell, D.R. *Science* 1967, *158*, 1462.
3. Birchmore, R.J.; Brookes, R.F.; Copping, L.G.; Wells, W.H. *Proc. Brit. Crop Protect. Conf. Pests Dis.*, 1977, *2*, 593.
4. Copping, L.G.; Birchmore, R.J.; Wright, K.; Godson, D.H. *Pestic. Sci*. 1984, *15*, 280.
5. Corbett, J.R.; Wright, K.; Baillie, A.C. *The Biochemical Mode of Action of Pesticides, Second Edition*; Academic: London, 1984; p256.
6. Brookes, R.F.; Godson, D.H.; Hams, A.F.; Weighton, D.M.; Wells, W.H. U.S. Patent 3 991 071, 1976.
7. Birchmore, R.J.; Brookes, R.F.; Copping, L.G.; Wells, W.H. British Patent 1 586 998, 1981; *Chem. Abstr*. 1982, *96*, 35261.

8. Birchmore, R.J.; Brookes, R.F.; Copping, L.G.; Wells, W.H. British Patent 1 567 521, 1980; Chem. Abstr. 1979, 90, 89566. (German equivalent).
9. Gadher, P.; Mercer, E.I.; Baldwin, B.C.; Wiggins, T.E. Pestic. Biochem. Physiol. 1983, 19, 1.
10. Kato, T.; Kawase, Y. Agric. Biol. Chem. 1976, 40, 2379.
11. Aoyama, Y; Yoshida, Y. Biochem. Biophys. Res. Commun. 1978, 85, 28.
12. Lyr, H; Edlich, W. Proc. Brit. Crop Protect. Conf. Pests Dis., 1986, 2, 879.
13. Marchington, A.F. Proc. 10th Int. Congr. Plant Protect., 1983, 1, 201.
14. Nyfeler, R.; Huxley, P. Proc. Brit. Crop Protect. Conf. Pests Dis., 1986, 1, 207.
15. Baloch, R.I.; Mercer, E.I.; Wiggins, T.E.; Baldwin, B.C. Phytochemistry 1984, 23, 2219.
16. Wells, W.H. European Patent 84 236, 1983; Chem.Abstr. 1983, 99, 194971.
17. Spatz, D.M. U.S. Patent 4 504 484, 1985.

RECEIVED May 27, 1987

Chapter 30

Application of Molecular Orbital Calculations To Estimate the Active Conformation of Azole Compounds

Toshiyuki Katagi, Nobuyoshi Mikami, Tadashi Matsuda, and Junshi Miyamoto

Laboratory of Biochemistry and Toxicology, Takarazuka Research Center, Sumitomo Chemical Company, 4-2-1 Takatsukasa, Takarazuka, Hyogo 665, Japan

Molecular orbital calculations were introduced to estimate the active conformations of azole compounds at an enzyme active site. The computed data were discussed referring to the spectroscopic information and utilized for the steric fit evaluation.

The active conformation of a biologically active compound bound to the target site(s) affords a valuable information to discuss its efficacy or toxicity at the molecular level. The three-dimensional structure of enzyme active site(s) or binding site(s) of receptor, usually obtained from X-ray analysis, makes it easier to estimate the active conformation of the chemical. However, such information and even the physico-chemical properties of these macromolecules are not available in many cases.

Under these circumstances, it is inevitable to estimate the active conformation of a chemical by another approach. The quantitative structure-activity relationship (QSAR) (1) is one of the important approaches, particularly when the target site of a biologically active compound is unknown. Although X-ray crystallography is also helpful to estimate the active conformation, it provides the conformational information in a solid phase. More important is the conformation of a chemical in solution, which can be assigned in part by spectroscopic studies. Nuclear magnetic resonance (NMR) spectroscopy has been utilized to estimate the relative orientation of each atom in a molecule (2-5). Infra-red (IR) spectroscopy is sometimes a useful tool, especially when hydrogen bonds are present (6). Recently,

0097-6156/87/0355-0340$06.00/0
© 1987 American Chemical Society

resonance raman spectroscopy has been introduced to the structural study of macromolecules such as porphyrin derivatives (7). Furthermore, fluorescence spectroscopy can be used to determine the conformations of a molecule (8,9) and the polarity of microenvironment (10). However, these spectroscopic methods deal with various low energy conformations of molecules in solution or crystal state and it is difficult to seek the active conformation only from the spectroscopic studies.

Recently, the relative energies of various conformations of a chemical have been estimated by molecular orbital calculations. Semi-empirical methods such as PCILO (11,12), CNDO/2 (13), and MNDO (14) are utilized because of their availability with short computation time. However, since the theoretical computations are usually carried out for the 'isolated' molecule, it is not so significant to discuss the efficacy or toxicity of a chemical by using the calculated configuration. Moreover, it is not easy to decide which conformer(s) are involved in the intermolecular interaction with an active site, since the binding conformer may not be the global energy minimum.

Although each of the methods stated above is already known to study the conformations of molecules, an inherent defect in each method makes it difficult to estimate an active conformer. We combined each method as summarized in Figure 1 and applied this strategy to the azole compounds, diniconazole (ER pure) (I) and uniconazole (ES pure) (II) as examples. We estimated their active conformers by the theoretical calculations combined with the spectroscopic analyses, followed by steric fit evaluation with the aid of computer graphics. Prior to steric fit evaluation, the substrate binding assay using the microsomal enzymes was carried out to clarify the intermolecular interactions between the active site(s) and azole compounds.

Mode of action

Two azole compounds (I) and (II), shown in Figure 2, have been developed by Sumitomo Chemical Co., Ltd. (15). (I) shows a significant fungitoxicity by inhibiting oxidative C14 demethylation of the intermediate lanosterol in the biosynthesis of ergosterol in fungi (16). This reaction is known to be catalyzed by fungal cytochrome P-450 enzymes (17,18). In contrast, (II) possessing a similar chemical structure to (I) is a plant growth regulator and retards a stem elongation in higher plants at a recommended dosage. Izumi *et al*. (19) has reported that (II) inhibits the successive metabolic oxidation of the C19 methyl group of intermediate (-)-kaur-16-ene in the biosynthetic pathways of gibberellin. This reaction is considered to be catalyzed by the mixed function oxidases in plants which are spectrophotometrically analogous to those of mammals (20,21). The sites of inhibition by two azole compounds are shown in Figure 3.

Binding assay

It is not so easy to prepare the fungal microsomal fraction and the mixed function oxidases in higher plants. Therefore, the microsomal fraction of rat liver (22) was used instead for the substrate binding assay to ascertain the interaction of (I) and (II) with cytochrome P-450 enzymes. Both (I), (II), and their racemic mixtures showed the Type II substrate difference spectra (23,24) with stoichiometric binding to cytochrome P-450 enzymes. These results strongly suggest that (I) and (II) co-ordinate to the iron atom of the porphyrin moiety in cytochrome P-450 enzymes via the nitrogen atom at the 4-position (N4) of the 1,2,4-triazolyl moiety. In contrast, the *Z*-isomer of (I) (designated as (III)) shows another type of spectra (Type I) which indicate the loose binding of (III) to the cytochrome P-450 enzymes. The difference between Type I and II spectra is shown in Figure 4.

Estimation of the conformations of azole compounds in solution by spectroscopy

To estimate the conformations of (I) and (II) at the enzyme active site of fungi or plants, IR and H-NMR spectra of the azole compounds in solutions were measured. From the results of mode of action and binding assay, (I) and (II) are considered to locate in the close proximity to the prosthetic porphyrin group of cytochrome P-450 enzymes. The polarity of macromolecules close to the porphyrin moiety of apohemoglobin has been determined by fluorescence study to be similar to that of n-octanol (10). In our study, carbon tetrachloride and deuteriochloroform of which polarities were similar to that of n-octanol were used.

Both compounds showed a broad IR absorption at ca. 3,460 cm-1 at concentrations approaching the solubility limit in carbon tetrachloride. The IR absorption spectra of (I) are shown in Figure 5a. Furthermore, the small temperature dependence of the H-NMR chemical shift owing to the hydroxy proton was observed at the concentration of 0.006 mole/liter in deuteriochloroform at -50 ^{o}C to 25 ^{o}C, as shown in Figure 6. In the case of (I) at 0.06 mole/liter, the hydroxy proton showed broad signals with a significant shift to the low-field at the temperature below 0 ^{o}C. These observations strongly suggest that the intramolecular hydrogen bond is formed at a lower concentration.

Which moiety of (I) formed the intramolecular hydrogen bond with the hydroxy proton was estimated as follows. The racemic derivatives of (I), lacking the

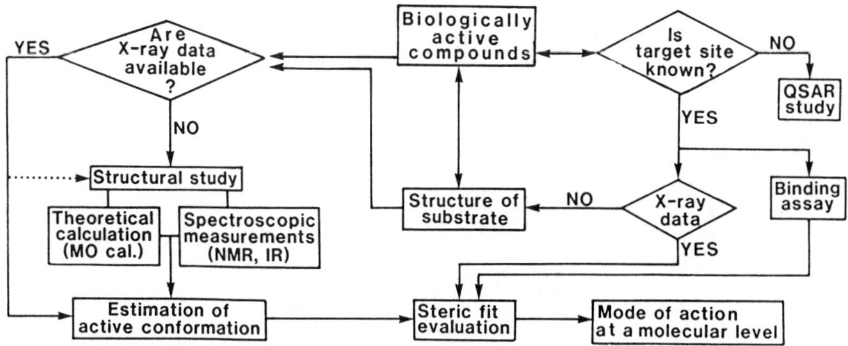

Figure 1 The strategy to estimate the active conformation of biologically active compounds.

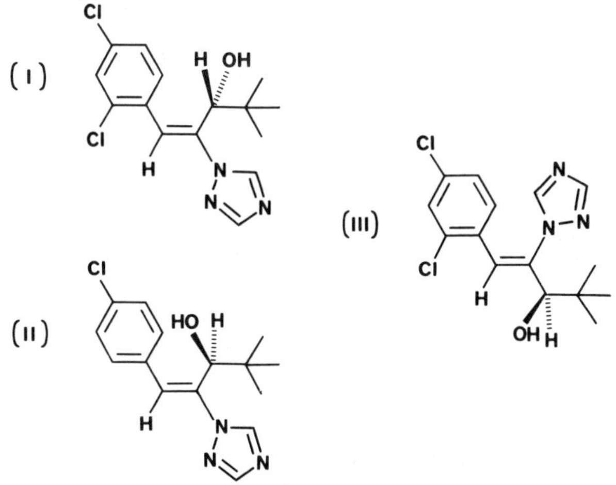

(I) (II) (III)

Figure 2 Chemical structures of azole compounds.

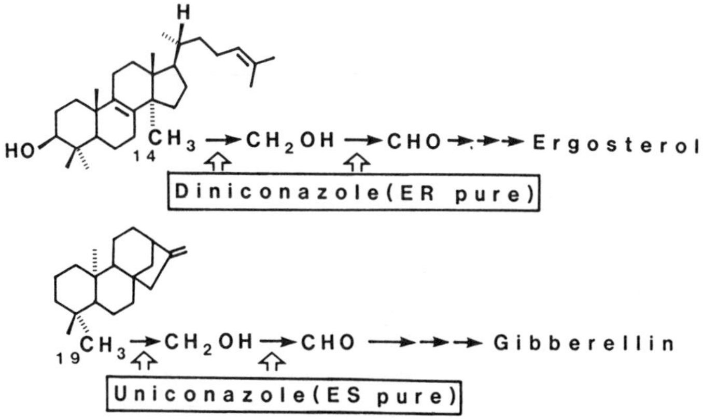

$CH_3 \rightarrow CH_2OH \rightarrow CHO \rightarrow\rightarrow\rightarrow$ Ergosterol

Diniconazole(ER pure)

$CH_3 \rightarrow CH_2OH \rightarrow CHO \rightarrow\rightarrow\rightarrow$ Gibberellin

Uniconazole(ES pure)

Figure 3 The sites of inhibition by azole compounds in the ergosterol and gibberellin biosynthesis.

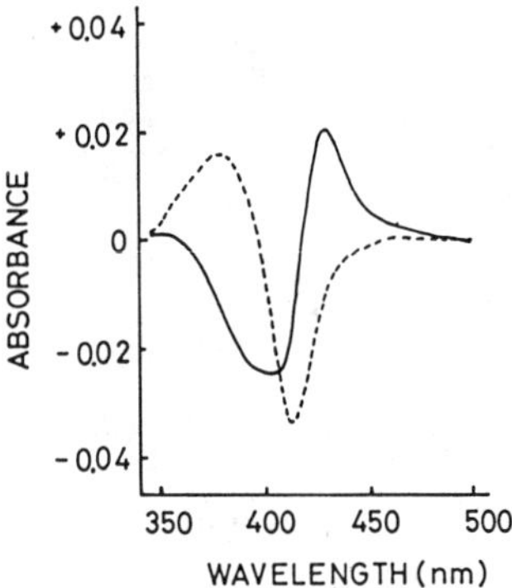

Figure 4 The substrate difference spectra of (I) (——) and (III) (---) with rat liver microsomal enzymes.

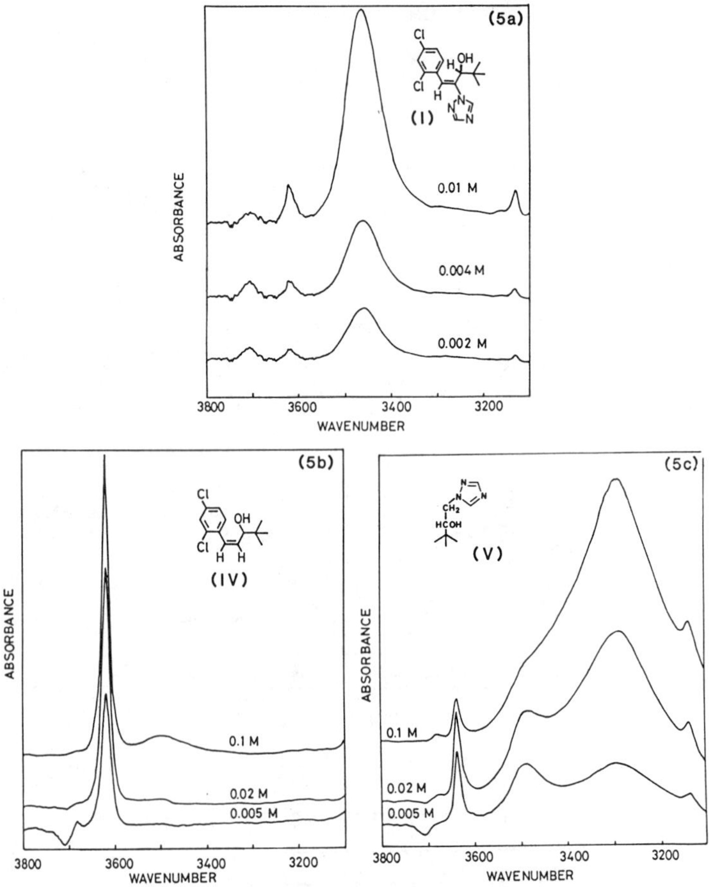

Figure 5 IR absorption spectra of (I), (IV), and (V) in carbon tetrachloride.

1,2,4-triazolyl (IV) or the 2,4-dichlorophenyl moiety (V), were synthesized and subject to IR analysis in carbon tetrachloride. The results are shown in Figure 5b and 5c. (IV) shows a sharp absorption at 3,620 cm-1 owing to a free hydroxy group. In contrast, (V) shows three absorptions at 3,640, 3,490, and 3,240 cm-1 of which intensities varies with the concentration. These absorptions were assigned to be due to a free hydroxy group, intramolecular, and intermolecular hydrogen bonds, respectively. These results indicate that the intramolecular hydrogen bond is formed between the hydroxy proton and the 1,2,4-triazolyl moiety.

To discuss the difference of binding assay between (I) and (III) at the molecular level, the conformation of (III) in solution was estimated as follows. (III) is considered to possess a steric hindrance between the 2,4-dichlorophenyl and 1,2,4-triazolyl moieties. Therefore, the spin-lattice relaxation time (T_1) of the proton at the 6-position of the 2,4-dichlorophenyl moiety was measured by NMR spectroscopy to determine the orientations of the two moieties. Based on the various orientations of two moieties prepared by ACACS system (25), T_1 was calculated and then compared with the observed value. Supposing that the planes defined by the 1,2,4-triazolyl and the 2,4-dichlorophenyl moieties were parallel in the molecule (III), the two dihedral angles θ to define their orientations were incrementally changed. The calculated T_1 values are plotted versus the dihedral angle θ as shown in Figure 7. As the observed T_1 was 3.39 sec, θ was determined to be about 30.0 degrees. The similar orientations of the phenyl rings were reported for *cis*-stilbene and its derivatives (26,27).

Theoretical estimation of the conformations of azole compounds

The MNDO procedure was undertaken for calculations. Most of the theoretical calculations and computer graphics were carried out using ACACS system loaded on a NEC ACOS 430 computer. First, a rough conformational analysis was performed by the PCILO procedure on the initial geometries of (I) and (II) derived from standard values of bond lengths, bond angles, and dihedral angles. Thereafter, the geometries of predominant conformers were optimized by MNDO calculations.

In the case of (III), the MNDO calculations mislead the molecular geometry. Therefore, the two dihedral angles to define the orientations of the 2,4-dichlorophenyl and 1,2,4-triazolyl moieties were fixed to 30.0 degrees which were determined by measurement of T_1. Based upon the optimized molecular geometries of (I) and (II) and their spectroscopic results, we estimated several low energy conformers

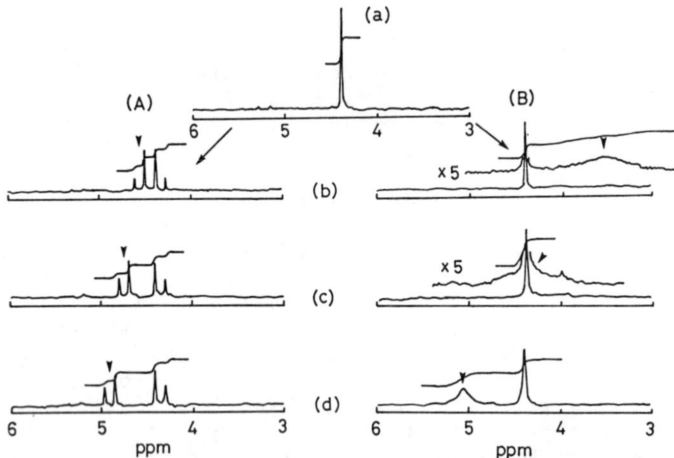

Figure 6 H-NMR spectra of (I) in deuteriochloroform. (A) 0.006, (B) 0.06 mole/liter. (a) 25 °C, (b) 0 °C, (c) -25 °C, (d) -50 °C. The arrows indicate the signal of hydroxy proton.

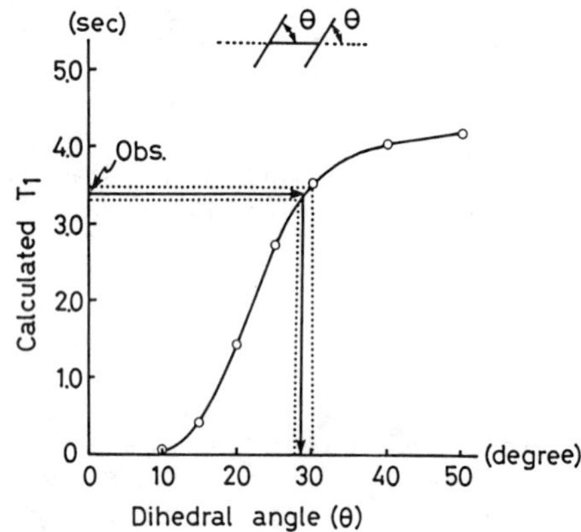

Figure 7 The plot of the calculated T_1 values versus θ.

which possessed an intramolecular hydrogen bond between the hydroxy proton and the nitrogen atom at the 2-position (N2) of the 1,2,4-triazolyl moiety.

The molecular geometries of lanosterol (28) and kaurene (29) were derived from the X-ray crystal structures. In the case of kaurene, the co-ordinates of hydrogen atoms were generated using ACACS system and optimized by the MNDO calculations.

Computer graphics

The steric fit evaluation between the low energy conformers of (I) and that of lanosterol was carried out in such a way that the N4 and C14 methyl carbon atoms locate in close proximity. In the case of (II), the C19 methyl carbon of (-)-kaur-16-ene was used for the evaluation. Based on these results, the conformers of (I) and (II) which well overlapped with the natural substrates were selected.

The results for (I) and (II) are shown in Figure 8. The 1,2,4-triazolyl moiety occupies the space corresponding to the C14 and C19 methyl groups which are susceptible to the enzymatic oxidation, with good overlap of the remaining parts of the molecules. In the case of (II), better overlapping was observed for the conformer which did not possess the intramolecular hydrogen bond (conformer IIb). However, the conformer IIa possessing the intramolecular hydrogen bond seems to be easily converted to the conformer IIb by rotation of the 1,2,4-triazolyl moiety along the C-N axis (Figure 9). The rotational energy barrier was estimated to be ca. 6 kcal/mole by PCILO calculations. It seems that two interconversible conformers of (II) (conformer IIa and IIb) predominate in the vicinity of enzyme active site(s), the latter of which is involved in the inhibition of gibberellin biosynthesis. The observations imply that the polarity of an enzyme active site and its three-dimensional structure are important factors to determine the active conformations of azole compounds.

The above results strongly suggest that the N4 atom of the 1,2,4-triazolyl moiety of (I) and (II) co-ordinates to the active site(s) of oxidase enzymes, which leads to the inhibition of ergosterol and gibberellin biosynthesis, respectively.

The *Z*-isomer (III) is much less fungitoxic than (I) (15). The steric fit evaluation between (I) and (III) by computer graphics indicates the similarity of three-dimensional structure, as shown in Figure 10. The *tert*-butyl moiety of (III) occupies the space where the 1,2,4-triazolyl moiety of (I) locates. It is interesting to compare these results with those of the binding assay. The co-ordination of the *tert*-butyl group to Fe atom of porphyrin moiety of cytochrome

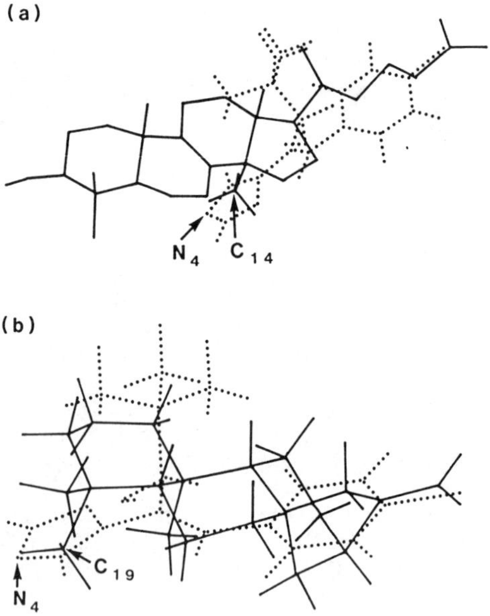

(a)

N_4 C_{14}

(b)

C_{19} N_4

Figure 8 Steric fit evaluation by computer graphics. (a) (I) (---) and lanosterol (——), (b) (II) (---) and (-)-kaur-16-ene (——).

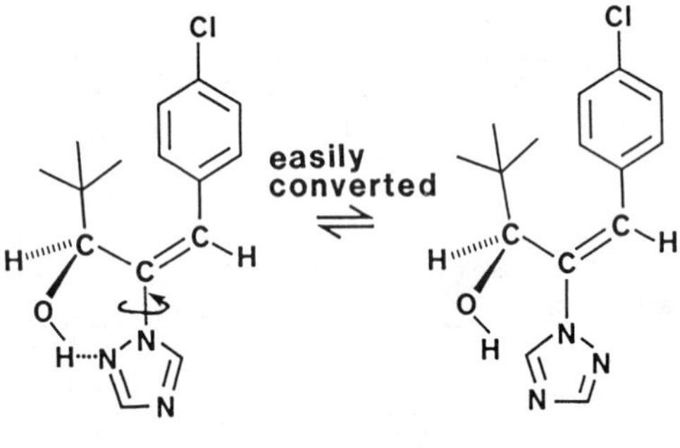

easily converted

Figure 9 The proposed conformational change of uniconazole (ES pure); conformer IIa (left) and IIb (right).

P-450 enzymes is likely to be more loose than that of the N4 atom of the 1,2,4-triazolyl moiety. (III) will be easily replaced by a substrate lanosterol, leading to the less inhibition of ergosterol biosynthesis. Furthermore, the co-ordination profiles of (III) to the active site(s) of cytochrome P-450 enzymes suggest that (III) is susceptible to mammalian metabolism via oxidation of the *tert*-butyl group. Isobe *et al*. reported that oxidation of the *tert*-butyl was a main metabolic pathway in rats for (III) but not for (I) (*30*). These data might support our results regarding the active conformations of the azole compounds at the enzyme active site(s).

Conclusion

We estimated the active conformations of two azole compounds following the strategy proposed above and discussed the interaction between the chemicals and the target sites of macromolecules at the molecular level. The followings are proposed in our study.

1. Diniconazole (ER pure) and uniconazole (ES pure) form the intramolecular hydrogen bond between the hydroxy proton and the N2 atom of the 1,2,4-triazolyl moiety.

2. Theoretical calculations combined with spectroscopic analyses are useful to estimate the low energy conformers of diniconazole (ER pure) and uniconazole (ES pure) in solutions of which polarities are similar to those of the enzyme active sites.

3. The molecular shapes of two azole compounds are similar to those of natural substrates.

4. The N4 atom of the 1,2,4-triazolyl moiety of two azole compounds co-ordinates to the Fe atom of cytochrome P-450 enzymes.

Based on these results, the proposed mode of action of uniconazole (ES pure) is illustrated as an example in Figure 11. Although each of the methods used in this study is already known, the combined application of these methods enables to reduce the number of conceivable active conformations and hence the steric fit evaluation can be performed with high accuracy. The remaining problem is how the azole compounds interact with the non-active sites of enzymes. This is surely related to the difference of biological activity between the optical isomers.

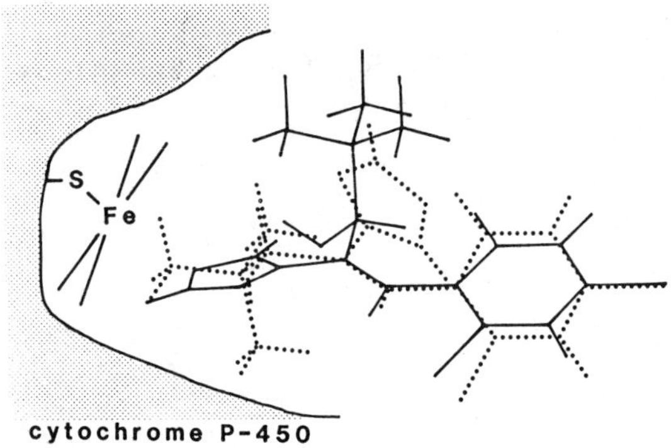

Figure 10 Steric fit evaluation by computer graphics between (I) (——) and its Z-isomer (III) (---).

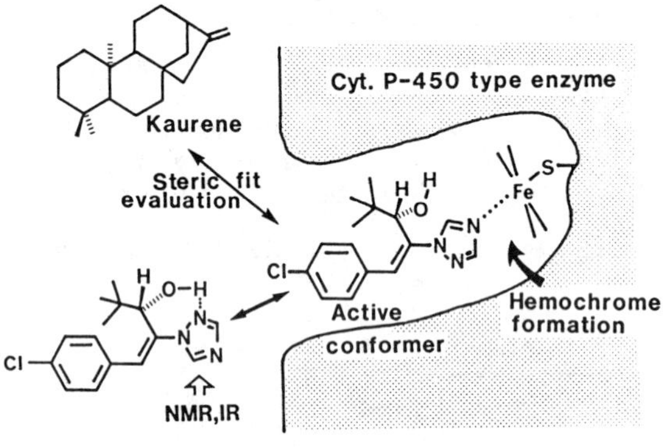

Figure 11 The proposed mode of action of uniconazole (ES pure) at a molecular level.

Literature Cited

1. Hansch, C. In Drug Design; Ariens, E. J., Ed.; Academic: New York, 1971; Vol. I, p 271.
2. Anderson, N. H.; Branch, S. K.; ThomasLoeffler, R. S.; Mann, B. E.; Nowell, I. W.; Walker, P. E. Pestic. Sci. 1984, 15, 310.
3. Houssin, R.; Henichart, J.-P. Org. Magn. Reson. 1981, 16, 202.
4. Elliott, M.; Farnham, A. W.; Janes, N. F.; Johnson, D. M.; Pulman, D. A. Pestic. Sci. 1980, 11, 513.
5. Takasuka, M.; Matsui, Y. J. Chem. Soc. Perkin II 1979, 1743.
6. Novak, A. In Infrared and Raman Spectroscopy of Biological Molecules; Theophanides, T. M., Ed.; NATO Advanced Study Institute Series C, No. 43; D. Dreidel: Boston, 1979.
7. Felton, R. H.; Yu, N.-T. In The Porphyrins; Dolphin, D., Ed.; Academic: New York, 1978; Vol. III, Part A, p 347.
8. Hopfinger, A. J.; Malhotra, D.; Battershell, R. D.; Ho, A. W. J. Pesticide Sci. 1984, 9, 631.
9. Jones, O. T.; Lee, A. G. Pestic. Biochem. Physiol. 1986, 25, 431.
10. Stryer, L. J. Mol. Biol. 1965, 13, 482.
11. Douady, J.; Barone, V.; Ellinger, Y.; Subra, R. Int. J. Quant. Chem. 1980, 17, 211.
12. Boca, R.; Pelikan, P. Int. J. Quant. Chem. 1980, 18, 1361.
13. Pople, J. A.; Beveridge, D. L.; In Approximate Molecular Orbital Theory; McGraw-Hill: New York, 1970.
14. Dewar, M. J. S.; Thiel, W. J. Amer. Chem. Soc. 1977, 99, 4899.
15. Funaki, Y.; Ishiguri, Y.; Kato, T.; Tanaka, S. J. Pesticide Sci. 1984, 9, 229.
16. Takano, H.; Oguri, Y.; Kato, T. J. Pesticide Sci. 1983, 8, 575.
17. Gibbons, G. F.; Pullinger, C. R.; Mitropoulos, K. A. Biochem. J. 1979, 183, 309.
18. Yoshida, Y.; Aoyama, Y.; Takano, H.; Kato, T. Biochem. Biophys. Res. Commun. 1986, 137, 513.
19. Izumi, K.; Kamiya, Y.; Sakurai. A.; Oshio, H.; Takahashi, N. Plant & Cell Physiol. 1985, 26, 821.
20. Dennis, D. T.; West, C. A. J. Biol. Chem. 1967, 242, 3293.
21. Murphy, P. T.; West, C. A. Arch. Biochem. Biophys. 1969, 133, 395.
22. Omura, T.; Sato, R. J. Biol. Chem. 1970, 239, 2370.
23. Schenkman, J. B.; Remmer, H.; Estabrook, R. W. Mol. Pharmacol. 1967, 3, 113.
24. Testa, B.; Jenner, P. Drug Metabolism Rev. 1984, 12, 1.

25. Yoshida, M.; Takayama, C.; Morooka, S.; Yokota, A. 7th Intern. Conf. Compt. Chem. Res. Educ. 1985, No. 32.
26. Suzuki, H. Bull. Chem. Soc. Jpn. 1952, 25, 145.
27. Heatley, F.; Cox, M. K.; Jones, A.; Jacques, B. J. Chem. Soc. Perkin II 1976, 510.
28. Carlisle, C. H.; Timmins, P. A. J. Cryst. Mol. Struct. 1974, 4, 31.
29. Karle, I. L. Acta Crystallgr., Sect B 1972, 28, 585.
30. Isobe, N.; Yanagita, S.; Yoshitake, A.; Matsuo, M.; Miyamoto, J. J. Pesticide Sci. 1985, 10, 475.

RECEIVED May 12, 1987

Chapter 31

Laetisaric Acid

Philip H. Evans, Norbert H. Haunerland, and William S. Bowers

Department of Entomology, University of Arizona, Tucson, AZ 85721

The soil inhabiting basidiomycete fungus *Laetisaria arvalis* secretes an allelochemical which suppresses the growth of several economically important phytopathogenic fungi. We isolated, synthesized and identified this compound as a previously unknown hydroxylated fatty acid (*Z,Z*-9,12-8-hydroxy octadecadienoic acid) and named it laetisaric acid. Our investigation of the chemical structure-biological activity relationships of laetisaric acid analogs has led us to a theory of bioactivation and the design of more potent fungicides. Prospects for the use of laetisaric acid analogs for plant protection are discussed.

Natural products of microbial origin have often led to the development of new agrochemicals, e.g. the streptomycin antibiotics, gibberellins, tetranactin and the avermectins (1,2). The study of microbial allelopathic interactions continues to be a significant source of new chemical information appropriate to the development of biorational pesticides. During a search for allelopathic soil microbes Odvody *et al.* (3) isolated a fungus from sugarbeet residue in the soil of western Nebraska which proved to be a biological control agent for damping off and crown rot diseases of plants. The fungus suppressed *Rhizoctonia* disease in sugarbeets (*Beta vulgaris*), soybeans (*Glycine max*), dry beans (*Phaseolus vulgaris*) and cucumber (*Cucumis sativus*) (4,5). Burdsall *et al.* (6) characterized this basidiomycete fungus as a new organism and named it *Laetisaria arvalis.*

Hoch and Abawi (7) reported the biological control of *Pythium ultimum* root rot of table beets (*Beta vulgaris*) by *L. arvalis,* but also reported that while effectively controlling damping off disease, it was not pathogenic to *P. ultimum.* In dual cultures of *P. ultimum* and *L. arvalis*

0097-6156/87/0355-0353$06.00/0
© 1987 American Chemical Society

growing on potato dextrose agar (PDA) coated microscope slides *L. arvalis* did not parasitize *P. ultimum.* Nevertheless, the hyphae of *P. ultimum* were lysed, resulting in cytoplasmic disorganization and cessation of cytoplasmic streaming (8). When a chloroform extract of *L. arvalis* mycelia was applied to growing *P. ultimum* on a microscope slide it also induced cytoplasmic disorganization and cessation of streaming, followed by the appearance of lipid droplets in the cytoplasm. This suggested the secretion of a diffusable toxin by *L. arvalis.*

Bioassay

While hyphal lysis of *P. ultimum* on PDA microscope slides by *L. arvalis* or mycelial extracts demonstrated the presence of fungicidal activity it was not a quantitative measurement of activity. The growth characteristics of *P. ultimum* on PDA made possible a rapid quantitative bioassay. An inoculum of growing *P. ultimum* mycelia placed in the center of a PDA Petri plate will grow radially until reaching the edge of the plate. The growing mycelial margin is sharply defined and measurable to 1 mm. Thus, radial growth is uniform from the locus of the innoculum and rarely varies more than 2 mm in any direction. Commercial PDA is sufficiently transparent to allow the measurement of the mycelial growth through the agar without opening the Petri plate. The bioassay is simple and rapid and facilitates the isolation of the active fungicidal compound as well as provides the needed quantitative estimation required for structure-activity determination of synthetic analogs. The radial growth assay can be performed on the bench without controlled environmental chambers and is complete within 48 hours. The growth of *P. ultimum* is linear with respect to time until it reaches the edge of the Petri plate (Fig. 1). Bioassay data are therefore obtained over a range of incubation times when growth on experimental plates is compared with the untreated plates. The structural relationship studies have indicated the mode of action and permitted the rational design of more potent analogs.

Growth inhibition of *P. ultimum* is assessed by placing a 5 mm diameter plug from the growth margin of *P. ultimum* growing on PDA into the center of a PDA Petri plate containing the test compound or extract. Chemicals are incorporated into the agar of the test plates at the desired concentration by dispensing the compound, dissolved in 40 µl of methanol, into 40 ml of molten PDA prior to pouring into duplicate 100 x 15 mm Petri plates. The amount of methanol, 1 µl per 1 ml of PDA does not inhibit fungal growth or synergize the growth inhibition of the active compound. The growth of *P. ultimum* on plates containing added chemicals is expressed relative to the growth of *P. ultimum* on untreated plates. When growth of the untreated PDA plate containing *P. ultimum* approaches the edge of the plate the distance from the innoculum plug to the growth margin is measured on four radial lines at 0, 90°, 180°and 270°. The mean of these four measurements is recorded as the radial growth per plate. A duplicate plate is similarly measured and the mean of the eight measurements is the mean growth of the test organism.

Growth of *P. ultimum* is linearly related to the concentration of laetisaric acid (8) and the dose at which growth is inhibited by 50% (ED_{50}) can be calculated by interpolation from a regression curve of growth vs. concentration (Fig. 2). Fine differences of activity may be measured between laetisaric acid and its analogs facilitating a rational approach to the synthetic optimization of activity.

Isolation of Laetisaric Acid

Laetisaria arvalis was grown at 23°C for two weeks on the surface of potato dextrose broth. Mycelial mats from 200 cultures were pooled and blended in a Waring blender for 30 s. This blend was incubated at 23°C for 30 min to allow enzymatic hydrolysis to increase the yield of the fungicidal product. Two volumes of chloroform:methanol (9:1 v/v) were added and the mixture again blended for 30 s. During subsequent work we found that ethyl acetate was a more efficient extracting solvent. We doubt that either of these procedures is optimal and we are examining other extraction techniques. The organic and aqueous phases were separated by centrifugation and the organic phase filtered through silicone treated phase separation paper before concentration under vacuum. Three grams of this crude active extract were loaded on a column of 90 g Florisil (deactivated with 7% water) and eluted sequentially with 300 ml chloroform, 300 ml 50% chloroform in methanol and then with 400 ml of methanol. The activity eluted in the methanol fraction and following concentration *in vacuo* was separated by 0.5 mm preparative silica thin layer chromatography (TLC) by development in benzene:ethyl acetate:formic acid (80:20:1). The active band was scraped from preparative TLC, eluted from the silica by ethyl acetate and rechromatographed two times on preparative silica TLC, eluting with benzene: ethyl acetate: formic acid (80:40:1)(Fig. 3).

The isolation by TLC yielded an active compound which was homogeneous in several normal phase TLC systems. The addition of a small amount of formic acid to the developing solvent resulted in a much sharper TLC spot, indicating an acidic group in the active compound. The active area was not visible under ultraviolet light at 254 nm on indicator TLC plates but was visualized by spraying with 5% phosphomolybdic acid in ethanol and heating to 110°C for 10 min. Infrared spectroscopy indicated hydroxyl and

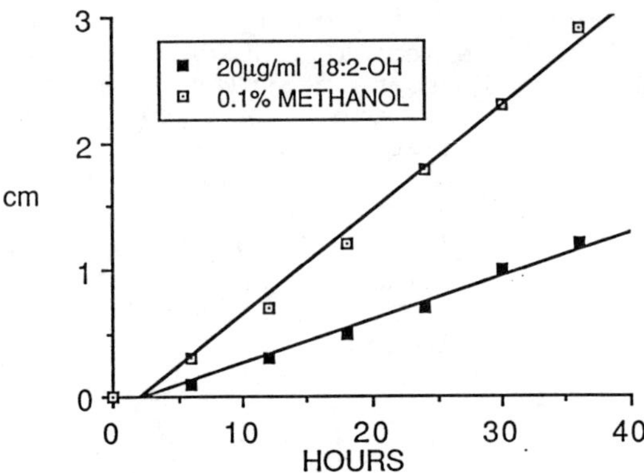

Fig. 1: Radial growth of *P. ultimum* over time with and without 20 µg/ml laetisaric acid in the growth medium.

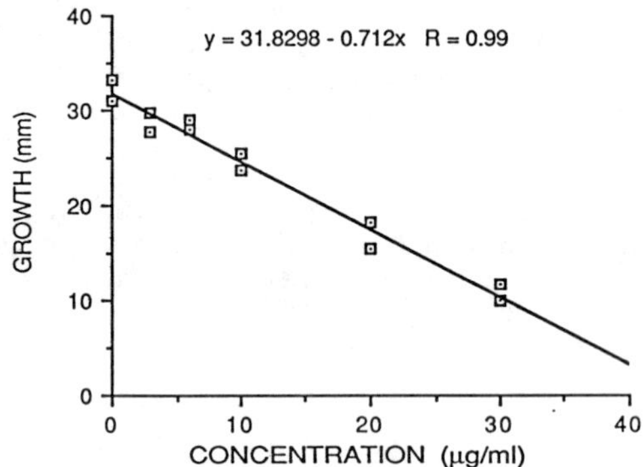

Fig. 2: Radial growth of *P. ultimum* versus concentration of laetisaric acid in the growth medium.

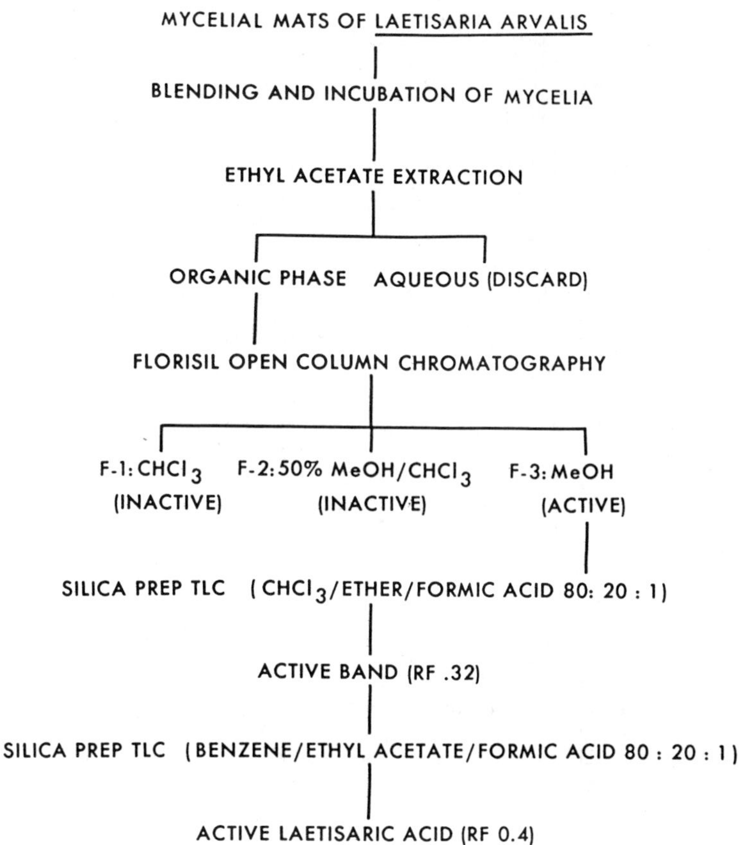

Fig. 3: Isolation of laetisaric acid from *Laetisaria arvalis*.

carboxylic acid groups. Reaction with diazomethane produced a single less polar compound. Capillary gas chromatography of the diazomethane product on a dimethyl silicone and/or Carbowax column gave retention times similar to a twenty carbon fatty acid methyl ester. From its origin and acidic nature we named this bioactive natural product laetisaric acid.

The amount of laetisaric acid in a sample can be readily quantified using the above extraction, thin layer separation, diazomethane derivatization and capillary gas chromatographic procedure. Calculations of the amount of laetisaric acid by bioassay and by the described physical analytical methods are in agreement.

Structure of Laetisaric Acid

The 70 eV electron impact mass spectrum of laetisaric acid methyl ester gives a base peak at m/z 93 and a strong peak at m/z 292 due to a loss of water from the molecular ion at m/z 310. This indicates a molecular formula of $C_{19}H_{34}O_3$. The 400 MHz NMR analysis of laetisaric acid methyl ester in deuterochloroform is characteristic of a fatty acid methyl ester of 34 protons with the presence of a nonconjugated dienol system: 4.45 (1H,dt,J=8.4,6.3Hz), 5.31 (1H,dtt,J=10.7,7.1,1.4 Hz), 5.38 (1H,dtt, J=11.2,8.4, 1.4 Hz), 5.41 (1H,dtt,J=10.7,7.1,1.5 Hz), 5.47 (1H,dt,J=11.2,7.2Hz), 2.87 (1H,dt,J=15.5,7.1Hz), and 2.80 (1H,dt,J=15.5,7.2 Hz). Other signals are 0.89 (3H,t,J=7.7Hz), 1.2 to 1.7 (17H), 2.05 (2H,q,J=7.1Hz), 2.30 (2H,t,J=7.5Hz), and 3.67 (3H,s).

Catalytic hydrogenation of the methyl ester gives methyl stearate (confirmed by GCMS with authentic methyl stearate) as a result of hydrogenolysis and hydrogenation of the dienol system. The geometry of the double bonds as Z (cis) is indicated by the J values of 10.7 and 11.2 in the NMR spectrum. n-Hexanal is an ozonolysis product, indicative of a C-12 unsaturation. These data suggest an eighteen carbon *Z,Z*-9,12 diunsaturated hydroxylated fatty acid. *Z,Z*-9,12 unsaturation is present in the common eighteen carbon fatty acid linoleic acid, a major fatty acid of *Pythium ultimum* (9,10).

Mass spectra of the trimethylsilyl derivative of laetisaric acid gives an ion peak at m/z 239 corresponding to $C_5H_{11}CH{=}CHCH_2{-}CH{=}CH{-}CH{=}OTMS$ and the mass spectra of the oxidized derivative gives a m/z at 165 for $C_5H_{11}CH{=}CHCH_2CH{=}CHC{=}O$. These fragments indicate a hydroxyl at the C-8 position in laetisaric acid.

Synthesis of Laetisaric Acid

We synthesized laetisaric acid to confirm the assigned structure and to produce a sufficient quantity of active material for biological studies. The Grignard coupling of acetylenic intermediates with subsequent catalytic reduction to yield Z double bonds is similar to the method for the total synthesis of arachidonic acid (11,12). An outline of our synthesis of laetisaric acid is shown in Figure 4.

We protect one hydroxyl terminus of the commercially available 1,8-octane diol **1** by reaction with dihydropyran to give the monoalcohol, 8-tetrahydropyranyloxyoctanol **2**. The protected alcohol **2** is oxidized to the aldehyde with pyridinium chlorochromate to give 8-tetrahydropyranyloxyoctanal **3**. 1-Heptyne **4** is coupled with propargyl bromide **5** in a copper catalyzed reaction to produce the diacetylenic 1,4-decadiyne **6**.

Ethyl magnesium bromide is reacted with **6** to produce the diacetylenic Grignard reagent **7**. To this Grignard solution is added **3** to produce 1-tetrahydropyranyloxy-9,12-octadiyn-8-ol **8**. Reduction with a Lindlar catalyst (13) in a methanolic solution of **8** gives 1-THPoxy-9,12,-octadiene-8-ol **9**. Acetylation of **9** with acetic anhydride yields the 8-acetoxy-1-THP oxyoctadec-9,12-diene **10**. The protecting THP group is then removed in ethanol with pyridinium p-toluenesulfonate to give 8-acetoxyoctadec-9,12,-diene-1-ol **11**. Oxidation with Jones reagent in acetone gives 8-acetoxylinoleic acid **12**. Reaction of **12** in methanol with potassium carbonate generates the desired product: *Z,Z*-9,12-8-hydroxyoctadecadienoic acid (laetisaric acid) **13**. Physical and fungicidal properties of our synthetic laetisaric acid are identical with the natural product.

The chain length or carbon number of the starting diol at the first reaction step determines the hydroxyl position with respect to the acid terminus. The position of unsaturation is fixed by selection of acetylenic intermediates which form the Grignard reagent, and the *Z* isomers are developed from the Lindlar reduction. Modifications of these synthetic methods were used to synthesize a variety of analogs (Bowers *et al.*, in manuscript).

Structure Activity Relationships of Synthetic Analogs

The analogs of laetisaric acid were prepared to: 1) determine the structural components of laetisaric acid responsible for fungicidal activity, 2) obtain more active compounds, and 3) gain insight into the biological mode of action of laetisaric acid. The structural determinants of activity of this relatively simple molecule were examined by exploring the contribution of the functional groups (the acid and hydroxyl), the nature of isomerism and the degree of unsaturation, the molecular size or carbon number and the positions of the functional groups on the hydrocarbon chain.

By use of our radial growth bioassay we found that the *Z,Z*-9,12 unsaturation in laetisaric acid is not required for fungicidal activity since synthetic 8-hydroxy stearic

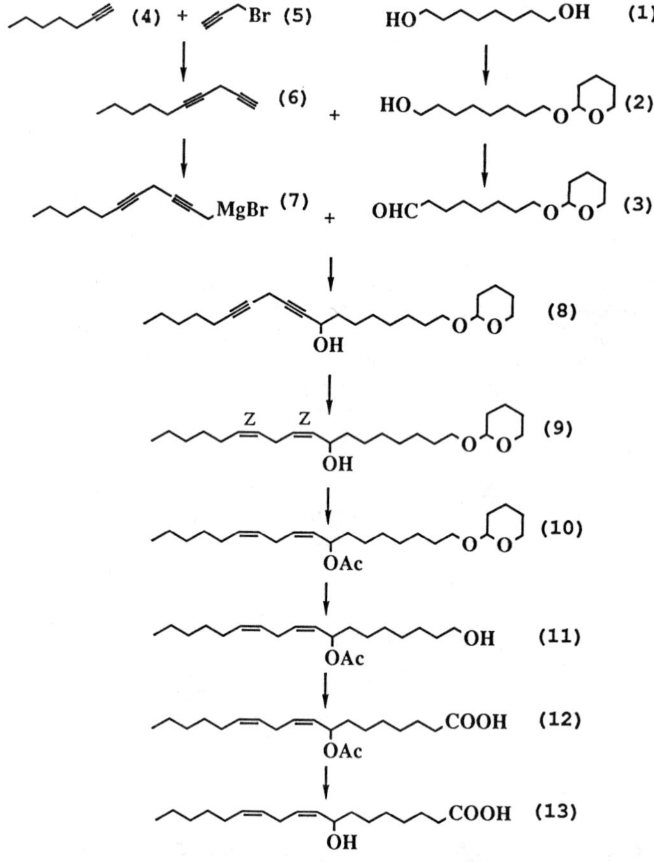

Fig. 4: Chemical synthesis of laetisaric acid.

acid is equally bioactive. We also found stearic acid inactive, demonstrating that hydroxylation of the eighteen carbon acid is required. Replacement of the hydroxyl with a keto function eliminates activity as does the replacement of the C-1 acid with an alcohol.

To determine whether the isomerism and extent of unsaturation of laetisaric acid affects activity, we synthesized and tested a variety of unsaturated analogs. Acetylenic compounds were produced by omitting the catalytic reduction step from the synthesis of laetesaric acid. 8-Hydroxy oleic acid was produced using the appropriate monounsaturated Grignard reagent and the saturated 8-hydroxy stearic acid was synthesized from a decane Grignard reagent. We found no influence on activity by the degree of unsaturation; 8-hydroxy stearic acid is as active as laetisaric acid. Since the saturated analogs are equally active we used the more easily synthesized saturated analogs for the exploration of other structural determinants of activity.

A series of 8-hydroxy saturated fatty acids were synthesized to explore the effect of chain length on activity. The hydroxyl function was maintained on the eight carbon by starting with 1,8-octanediol and the chain length dictated by a reaction with the appropriate carbon number saturated Grignard reagent. The eighteen carbon 8-hydroxy compound demonstrates the most activity in this series (Fig. 5).

A series of compounds were synthesized by the coupling of the appropriate diol and Grignard reagents to determine if the position of hydroxylation is a determinant of activity on C-18 saturated fatty acids. Our bioassay shows a strict requirement of the 8-hydroxy position for activity (Fig. 6).

During the evaluation of a number of synthetic analogs, varying in chain length and position of the hydroxyl, we found that 6-hydroxy hexadecanoic acid, 4-hydroxy tetradecanoic acid and 2-hydroxy dodecanoic acids possess equimolar activity in suppressing growth of *P. ultimum.* The common property of these analogs is not the total carbon number or the position of the hydroxyl from the acid terminus, but the position of the hydroxyl on the C-11 from the lipophilic end of the active molecule.

To explain these data we developed the hypothesis that laetisaric acid and active analogs are metabolized by sensitive fungi, such as *P. ultimum, via* common ß-oxidation to an active 2-hydroxy twelve carbon fatty acid. In the case of laetisaric acid the metabolic product is 2-hydroxydodecadienoic acid. This α-hydroxy compound is apparently not further metabolized by ß-oxidation and accumulates as the ultimate allelopathic agent.

The biorational design of analogous compounds must take into account the asymmetry of 2-hydroxy dodecanoic acid since C-2 is an asymmetric carbon with possible *R* and *S* enantiomers. That the stereochemistry appears to be

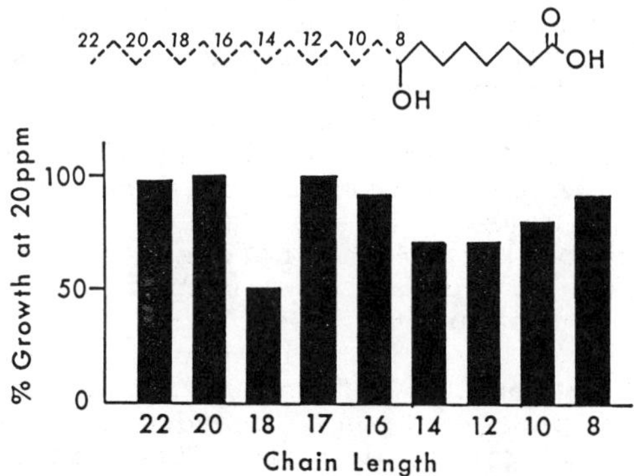

Fig. 5: Radial growth of *P. ultimum* on media containing 20 µg/ml of the indicated chain length 8-hydroxy acids.

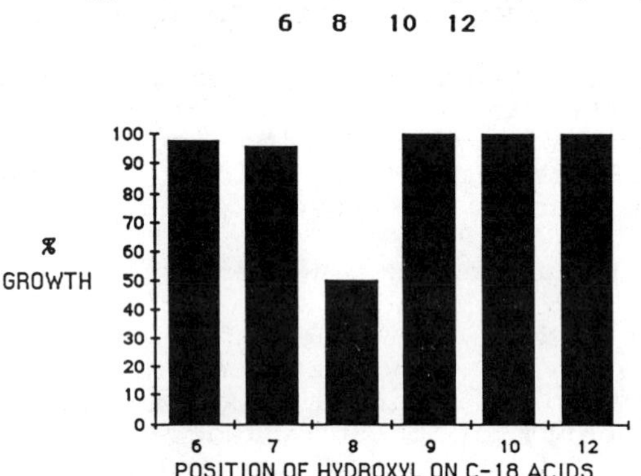

Fig. 6: Radial growth of *P. ultimum* on media containing 20 µg/ml C-18 acids hydroxylated at the position indicated.

irrelevant to biological activity is indicated by the fact that synthetic racemic laetisaric acid, 8-hydroxy stearic acid and 2-hydroxy dodecanoic acid give equimolar fungicidal activity compared to natural laetisaric acid. Nevertheless we separated racemic synthetic 2-hydroxy dodecanoic acid after derivatization with *S*-phenyl ethylamine, resolving the diastereomers by TLC and recovering the *R* and *S* enantiomers (14). Both enantiomers had identical fungicidal activity (Fig. 7).

Discussion

The germicidal properties of fatty acids and their salts are widely recognized (15,16); these compounds are generally regarded as nontoxic to most vertebrate and higher plant species. They are widely used as surfactant adjuvants for the application of herbicides (17). Surfactants are also used for control of apple powdery mildew and apple scab (18,19) and in hydroponic plant culture for the control of *Pythium* and *Olpidium* diseases (20,21). However due to the bipolar nature of many surfactants they are poorly transported through the soil. This physical property prevents their conventional use for control of plant root diseases.

A more promising approach to the use of laetisaric acid in plant protection would be the incorporation of the genetic mechanism for the production of this hydroxylated fatty acid into crop plants, soil or symbiotic bacteria. If a genetic system could be induced to produce laetisaric acid from the ubiquitous linoleic acid in an economically important plant species endogenous resistance to damping off and root rot diseases would result. The production of laetisaric acid by associated bacteria could prevent establishment of root pathogens. Early results of experiments on the biosynthesis of laetisaric acid indicate that the microsomes of *L. arvalis* are capable of producing laetisaric acid from linoleic acid. Evaluation of the feasiblity of transfer of the genes for production of laetisaric acid from linoleic acid will require a more depthful study of the biosynthesis of laetisaric acid.

Another approach to the use of *L. arvalis* for plant protection may be the enhancement of laetisaric acid production either by increasing *L. arvalis* soil population density, selecting for higher yielding strains of *L. arvalis* with increased gene frequency coding for laetisaric acid production or stimulating the production of laetisaric acid in the resident population. We need to know if the production of laetisaric acid is induced by the presence of *P. ultimum* or whether the laetisaric acid secreted is a constituitive secondary fungal metabolite. Preliminary results show that a higher yield of laetisaric acid is obtained after endogenous enzymatic hydrolysis suggesting that *L. arvalis* may be induced to release free laetisaric

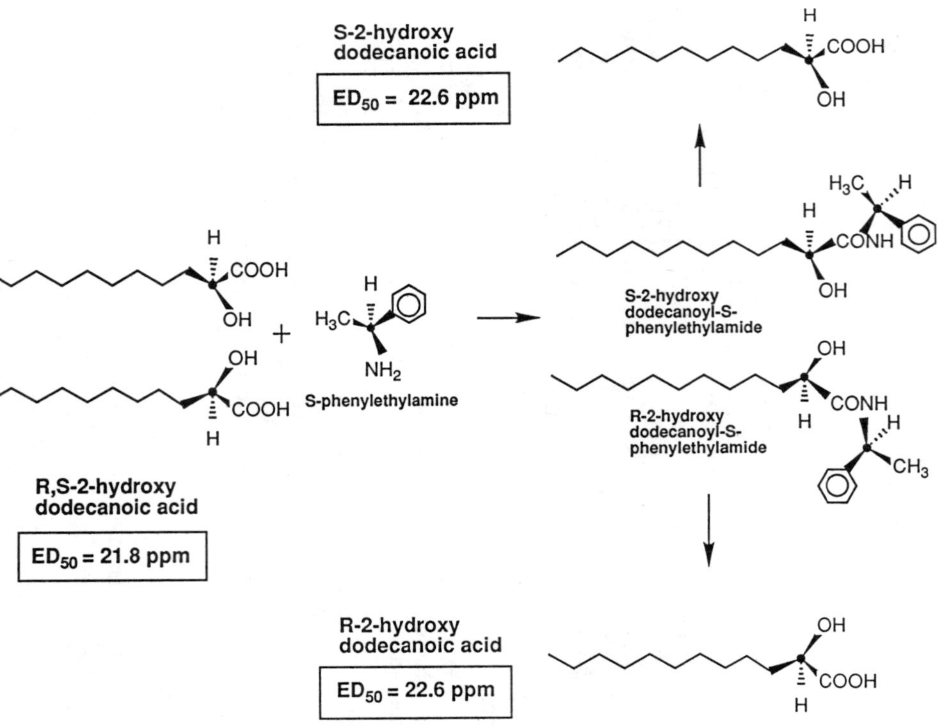

Fig. 7: Separation and activity of *R* and *S* 2-hydroxy dodecanoic acids.

acid. Discovery of an inducer could lead to enhancement of the production of laetisaric acid by the resident population of *L. arvalis* in the soil, thereby suppressing *Pythium*, *Rhizoctonia* and other soilborne plant diseases. Several groups are investigating specific biological interactions involving unusual fatty acids. For example an hydroxylated fatty acid structurally similar to laetisaric acid, (+)-8-hydroxy hexadecanoic acid, is an endogenous spore germination inhibitor of the fern *Lygodium japonicum* (22,23).

We have speculated on but do not understand the mechanism causing the lytic activity of laetisaric acid. The active twelve carbon metabolite of laetisaric acid may poison a key enzyme in lipid metabolism or disrupt the integrity of the fungal cell membrane by insertion or dissolution as has been shown in *Escherichia coli* with sodium dodecyl sulfate and Triton X-100 (24,25). Why the C-12 molecule is most active remains to be determined. Kinetic studies of lipid metabolism and physicochemical and ultrastructural investigations of membranes treated with the putative active metabolite may answer these questions.

The hydroxylated fatty acids hold the promise of being safe, simple and specific plant protectants. Our work on laetisaric acid demonstrates how the investigation of allelochemical interactions may lead to the development of new biorational agrochemicals.

Literature Cited

1. Rice, E.L. Pest Control with Natures Chemicals. University of Oklahoma Press; Norman, 1983.
2. Putnam, A.R.; Tang, C-S. The Science of Allelopathy. John Wiley and Sons; New York, 1986.
3. Odvody, G.N.; Boosalis, M.G.; Kerr, E.D. Phytopathology 1980, 70, 655-658.
4. Lewis, J.A.; Papavizas, G.C. Phytopathology 1980, 70, 85-89.
5. Odvody, G.N.; Boosalis, M.G.; Lewis, J.A.; Papavizas, G.C. Proc. Am. Phytopathol. Soc. 1977, 4, 158.
6. Burdsall, H.H.; Hoch, H.; Boosalis, M.G.; Setliff, E.C. Mycologia 1980, 72, 728-736.
7. Hoch, H.; Abawi G. Phytopathology 1979, 69, 417-419.
8. Bowers, W. S.; Hoch, H.; Evans, P.H.; Katayama, M. Science 1986, 232, 105-106.
9. Weete, J.D. Fungal Lipid Biochemistry: Distribution and Metabolism, Plenum, New York, 1974.
10. Bowman, R.D.; Mumma, R.O. Biochim. Biophys. Acta 1967, 144, 501-510.
11. Ege, S.N.; Wolovsky, R.; Gensler, W.J. J. Am. Chem. Soc., 1961, 83, 3080-3085

12. Rachlin, A.I.; Wasyliw, N.; Goldberg, M.W. J. Org. Chem. 1961, 26, 2688-2693.
13. Fieser, M.; Fieser, L.F. Reagents for Organic Synthesis John Wiley and Sons, New York,1967; p 566.
14. Karlsson, K. A.; Pascher, I. Chem. Phys. Lipids 1974, 12, 65-7416.
15. Wyss, O.; Ludwig, B.J.; Joiner, R.R. Arch. Biochem. 1945, 7, 415-425.
16. Li, C.Y.; Lu, K.C.; Trappe, J.M.; Bollen, W.B. Forensic Sci. 1970, 16, 329.
17. Norris, R.F. In Adjuvants for Herbicides; Weed Science Society of America, 1978.
18. Clifford, D.R.; Hislop, E.C. Pestic. Sci. 1975, 6, 409-418.
19. Burchill, R.T.; Swait, A.A.J. Ann. Appl. Biol. 1977, 87, 229-231.
20. Tomlinson, J.A.; Thomas, B.J. Ann. Appl. Biol. 1986, 108, 71-80.
21. Stenghellini, M.E.; Tomlinson, J.A. Phytopathology 1987, 77, 112-114.
22. Yamane, H.; Sato, Y.; Takahashi, N.; Takeno, K.; Furuya, M. Agric. Biol. Chem. 1980, 44, 1697-1699.
23. Masoka, Y.; Sakakibara, M.; Mori, K. Agric. Biol. Chem. 1982, 46, 2319-2324.
24. Woldringh, C.L.; VanIterson, J. Bacteriol. 1972, 111, 801-813.
25. Camille, P.; Fletcher, G.; Wulff, J.L.; Earhart, C.F. J. Bacteriol. 1973, 115, 717-722.

RECEIVED May 27, 1987

OTHER CONTROL METHODS

Chapter 32

Synthesis of Alkyl *N*-Cyano-*N*-substituted Carbamates, Thiolcarbamates, and *N,N*-Disubstituted Cyanamides

Lydia Suba, Tann Schafer, Peter G. Ruminski, and John J. D'Amico

Monsanto Agricultural Company, 800 North Lindbergh Boulevard, St. Louis, MO 63167

The reaction of S, S' alkyl and benzyl cyanodithioimidocarbonate (1-5) with potassium hydroxide in an acetone medium afforded the O-potassium S-alkyl and benzyl cyanothioimidocarbonates (6-10). The reaction of the potassium salts with alkyl, allyl or benzyl halides furnished the titled thiolcarbamates (11-29).

The reactions of S, S' methyl cyanodithioimidocarbonate with potassium hydroxide in alkyl or benzyl alcohol furnished the O-alkyl and benzyl O-potassium cyanoimidocarbonates (30-34). The reaction of the potassium salts (30, 32 or 33) with a 10% excess of alkyl, allyl or benzyl halides afforded the unknown titled carbamates (35-46). The reaction of 31 with 10% excess benzyl bromide or 34 with 10% excess methyl iodide gave the same product, N-benzyl-N-methyl cyanamide (47). The reactions of 31 with 10% and 55% excess allyl bromide afforded N-allyl-N-methyl cyanamide (48) and N,N-diallyl cyanamide (49), respectively. The reaction of 32 with 28% excess of allyl iodide furnished N-allyl-N-propyl cyanamide (50).

Possible mechanisms, supporting NMR, IR and mass spectra data and biological activity are discussed.

Kazuo Nishio and co-workers (2a,b,c) reported the synthesis of the titled compounds by the following reactions:

$$\begin{matrix} CH_3S \\ C_6H_5CH_2S \end{matrix}\!\!>\!C{=}N{-}C{\equiv}N + KOH \xrightarrow[\text{reflux}]{\text{acetone}} K{-}\underset{\substack{|\\ CN}}{N}{-}\overset{\substack{O\\ \|}}{C}{-}SCH_2C_6H_5 + CH_3SH \qquad (1)$$

$$K{-}\underset{\substack{|\\ CN}}{N}{-}\overset{\substack{O\\ \|}}{C}{-}SR + R'X \xrightarrow[\text{reflux}]{\text{acetone}} R'{-}\underset{\substack{|\\ CN}}{N}{-}\overset{\substack{O\\ \|}}{C}{-}SR + KX \qquad (2)$$

where R=alkyl, alkenyl or benzyl
where R'=alkyl, alkenyl or alkynyl

0097-6156/87/0355-0368$06.00/0
© 1987 American Chemical Society

Upon reviewing the cited patents in the above reference, we would like to make the following comments: (1) in all examples the elemental analysis were not reported, (2) the % yield was reported for only three compounds, (3) the structure assignment for the potassium salt (reaction 1) is incorrect and (4) with the exception of the infrared data (reaction 1) which were misinterpreted, no other spectral data were reported. Furthermore we question the products obtained in reaction 1. In our opinion reaction 1 would yield a mixture containing both the methyl and benzyl mercaptan and two potassium salts as illustrated by the following pathway:

$$CH_3S{-}C(SCH_2C_6H_5){=}N{-}C{\equiv}N \xrightarrow[HOH]{KOH} CH_3S{-}C(OH)(SCH_2C_6H_5){-}N(H){-}C{\equiv}N \longrightarrow (KO)(C_6H_5CH_2S)C{=}N{-}C{\equiv}N + CH_3SH$$

$$CH_3S{-}C(OH)(SCH_2C_6H_5){-}N(H){-}C{\equiv}N \longrightarrow (KO)(CH_3S)C{=}N{-}C{\equiv}N + C_6H_5CH_2SH$$

We have published extensively concerning the synthesis of N,N-disubstituted thiolcarbamates (3) and moderate attention has been focused on the synthesis of compounds derived from potassium cyanodithioimidocarbonate (4-7). Moreover, since we disagree with their proposed structure of the potassium salt in the solid state and Nishio furnished limited proof for their proposed structures, it appeared desirable to report our work in this area of chemistry.

The key intermediates, S, S' alkyl and benzyl cyanodithioimidocarbonates (2-5), were prepared by the reactions of potassium cyanodithioimidocarbonate (4) with the alkyl or benzyl halides (Table I).

$$2RX + (KS)_2C{=}N{-}C{\equiv}N \xrightarrow[H_2O]{25\text{-}30\ ^{\circ}C} (RS)_2C{=}N{-}C{\equiv}N \qquad (3)$$

1 (5), R=$-CH_3$; 2, R=$-C_2H_5$; 3, R=$-C_3H_7$; 4, R=$-C_4H_9$; 5 (8), R=$-CH_2C_6H_5$

The reaction of 1-5 with potassium hydroxide in an acetone medium afforded the O-potassium S-alkyl and benzyl cyanothioimidocarbonates (6-10) and not the structure as shown in reaction 1 (Table II).

$$(RS)_2C{=}N{-}C{\equiv}N + KOH \xrightarrow[reflux]{acetone} (KO)(RS)C{=}N{-}C{\equiv}N + RSH \qquad (4)$$

6, R=$-CH_3$; 7, R=$-C_2H_5$; 8, R=$-C_3H_7$; 9, R=$-C_4H_9$; 10, R=$-CH_2C_6H_5$

Analysis, infrared (neat) and NMR spectra were in agreement for the proposed structures of 6-10. The presence of C≡N and C=N absorption bands at 2170-2180 and 1585-1590 cm^{-1}, respectively, and the absence of the C=O absorption band at 1680-1700 cm^{-1} for 6 and 10 (Table II) furnished conclusive evidence for our structures (6-10) and thus ruled out their proposed structure (reaction 1). Nishio and coworkers (2b) reported the following infrared spectral data and assignment for 10: 2180 (C≡N) and 1580 cm^{-1} (C=O) which is

Table I. S, S' Alkyl and Benzyl Cyanodithioimidocarbonates

$$2\ RX + (KS)_2C{=}N{-}C{\equiv}N \xrightarrow[\substack{25\text{-}30\ ^oC \\ X=Br\ or\ I}]{H_2O} (RS)_2C{=}N{-}C{\equiv}N$$

No.	R	Reaction Time (Days)	Mp ^oC or (N_D^{25})	% Yield[a]	NMR, δ (ppm) $CDCl_3$-Me_4Si
1 (5)	$-CH_3$	7	55-6	84	2.64 (s,6,CH_3)
2	$-C_2H_5$	7	(1.5827)	90	1.40 (t,6,CH_2<u>CH_3</u>) 3.20 (q,4,<u>CH_2</u>CH_3)
3	$-C_3H_7$	8	(1.5623)	94	———
4	$-C_4H_9$	6	(1.5484)	89	———
5 (8)	$-CH_2C_6H_5$	1	83-4	94	4.40 (s,4,CH_2) 7.40 (s,10,C_6H_5)

[a]Satisfactory analytical data (±0.2) for C,H,N and S were reported.
(Reprinted with permission from reference 1(b), p 5. Copyright 1987 Gordon and Breach.)

Table II. O-Potassium S-Alkyl and Benzyl Cyanothioimidocarbonates

$$(RS)_2C{=}N{-}C{\equiv}N + KOH \xrightarrow[\text{Reflux}]{\text{Acetone}} (KO)(RS)C{=}N{-}C{\equiv}N + RSH$$

No.	R	Mp °C (dec.)	Reflux Period Hrs.	% Yield	NMR, δ (ppm) D_2O-Me_4-Si
6[a]	$-CH_3$	225-7[b]	6	95[d]	2.3 (s,3,SCH_3)
7	$-C_2H_5$	220-5	1.5	56[e]	1.2 (t,3,$CH_2\underline{CH_3}$) 2.9 (q,2,$\underline{CH_2}CH_3$)
8	$-C_3H_7$	229-31[c]	22	69[f]	———
9	$-C_4H_9$	220-2	22	62[f]	———
10[g]	$-CH_2C_6H_5$	257-9[c]	72	30[f]	4.1 (s,2,CH_2) 7.4 (s,5,C_6H_5)

[a] IR (CsI): 2935 (aliph C-H), 2170 (C≡N) and 1585 cm^{-1} (C=N).

[b] Recrystallization from ethanol-water. (c) Recrystallization from methanol.

[d] Calcd: C, 23,36; H, 1.96; K, 25.35; N, 18.16; O, 10.37; S, 20.79.
Found: C, 23.57; H, 1.88; K, 25.28; N, 17.88; O, 10.68; S, 20.51

[e] Calcd: N, 14.00; S, 16.10; K, 19.60.
Found: N, 14.10; S, 16.12; K, 19.60.

[f] Satisfactory analytical data (±0.4%) for C, H, N and S were reported.

[g] IR (KBr): 2950 (aliph C-H), 2180 (C≡N) and 1590 cm^{-1} (C=N).

(Reprinted with permission from reference 1(b), p 5. Copyright 1987 Gordon and Breach.)

comparable to our data (Table II). However, their assignment of 1580 cm^{-1} absorption band due to the presence of C=O instead of C=N group is erroneous. Accordingly, this misinterpretation of the infrared spectrum led them to the incorrect structure (reaction 1).

The reactions of the potassium salts (6-9) with alkyl, allyl or benzyl halides in dimethylformamide at 80-90 °C furnished the alkyl-N-cyano-N-substituted thiolcarbamates (11-29).

$$(KO)(RS)C{=}N{-}C{\equiv}N + R'X \xrightarrow[\text{80-90 °C, 48 hrs.}]{\text{DMF}} R'{-}N(CN){-}C({=}O)SR + RX \quad (5)$$

R and R' are shown in Table III

The proposed mechanisms for reactions 4 and 5 are depicted in Scheme I. As noted, we favor addition to the conjugated system followed by elimination of the mercaptan instead of the nucleophilic displacement mechanism.

Analysis, infrared, NMR and mass spectra were in agreement for the proposed structure of 11-29, (Table III and Scheme II). Initially we had anticipated that oxygen alkylation would have occurred to give the intermediate A followed by the Chapman rearrangement to give 11-29.

$$(KO)(CH_3S)C{=}N{-}C{\equiv}N + CH_3I \xrightarrow[\text{50-60 °C}]{\text{DMF}} \left[(CH_3O)(CH_3S)C{=}N{-}C{\equiv}N\right] \text{ A} \quad (6)$$

$$\text{A} \;\not\xrightarrow{\text{Chapman Rearrangement}}\; CH_3{-}N(CN){-}C({=}O)SCH_3 \quad \underline{11} \text{ (formed directly from the reactants)}$$

Even when reaction 6 was conducted at low temperature no evidence was obtained for the formation of intermediate A. This conclusion was based on the examination of the analytical data of a crude sample, heated sample (100-116 °C for 16 hours) and a distilled sample of 11. All three samples furnished comparable index of refraction, infrared and NMR spectra. The presence of C≡N and C=O absorption bands at 2230 and 1700 cm^{-1}, respectively, and the absence of C=N absorption band at 1585 cm^{-1} for all three samples furnished conclusive evidence that no oxygen alkylation occurred but instead nitrogen alkylation resulted to give the thiolcarbamates (11-29).

We now wish to report that replacing the O-potassium S-alkyl cyanothioimidocarbonates with O-alkyl and benzyl O-potassium cyanoimidocarbonate afforded the synthesis of the previously unknown titled carbamates or the N,N-disubstituted cyanamides.

By replacing acetone with methyl, ethyl, propyl, butyl or benzyl alcohol as a solvent, the reaction of S, S' methyl cyanodithioimidocarbonate (5) with potassium hydroxide furnished the unexpected key intermediates, O-alkyl and benzyl O-potassium cyanoimidocarbonates (30-34, Table IV).

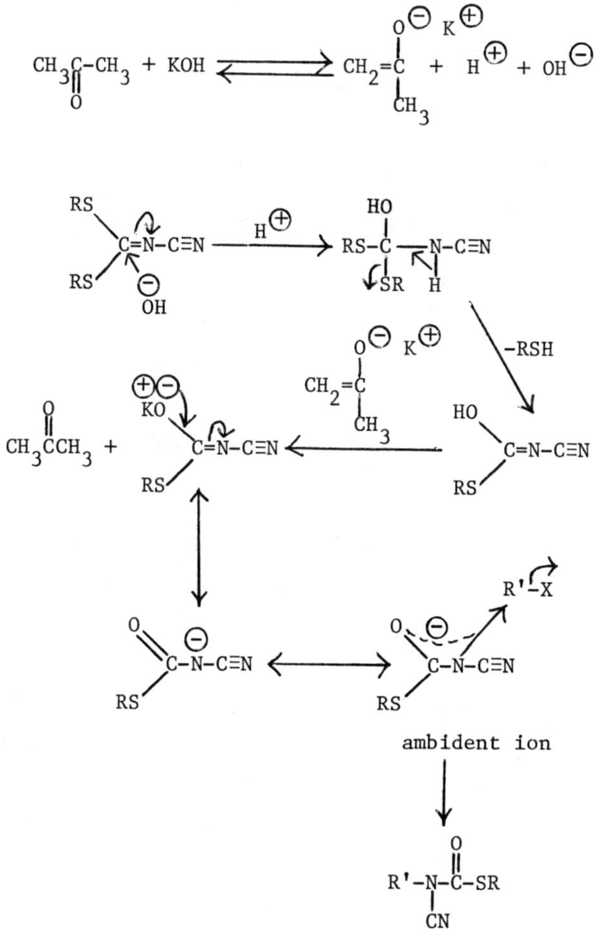

Scheme I. (Reprinted with permission from reference 1(b), p 3. Copyright 1987 Gordon and Breach.)

Table III

Alkyl-N-Cyano-N-Substituted Thiolcarbamates

$$\begin{matrix}KO \\ RS\end{matrix}\!\!>\!C{=}N{-}C{\equiv}N + R'X \xrightarrow{DMF} R'{-}\underset{\underset{CN}{|}}{N}{-}\overset{\overset{O}{\|}}{C}{-}SR$$

X=Cl, Br or I

No.	R	R'	bp °C/mm	% Yield	NMR, δ (ppm) $CDCl_3$-Me_4Si	Ir(cm^{-1}) Neat	$M^{+\cdot}$ Rel. Intensity
11[a]	$-CH_3$	$-CH_3$	66/0.3 N_D^{25}=1.5050	37[c]	2.50(s,3,SCH_3) 3.32(s,3,NCH_3)	2230(C≡N) 1700(C=O)	130 (23)
12[a]	$-CH_3$	$-C_2H_5$	74-5/0.55 N_D^{25}=1.4950	37[b]	1.38(t,3,$\underline{CH_3}CH_2N$) 2.50(s,3,$\underline{CH_3}S$) 3.75(q,2,$CH_3\underline{CH_2}N$)	2230(C≡N) 1700(C=O)	144 (24)
13	$-CH_3$	$-C_3H_7$	83-4/0.3 N_D^{25}=1.4902	44[b]	1.00(t,3,$N(CH_2)_2\underline{CH_3}$) 1.80(sextet,2,$NCH_2\underline{CH_2}CH_3$) 2.50(s,3,$SCH_3$) 3.70(t,2,$N\underline{CH_2}CH_2CH_3$)	2220(C≡N) 1680(C=O)	158 (18)
14	$-CH_3$	$-CH_2C_6H_5$	150-2/0.5 N_D^{25}=1.5645	45[b]	2.40(s,3,SCH_3) 4.70(s,2,$N\underline{CH_2}$) 7.40(s,5,$\underline{C_6H_5}$)	2230(C≡N) 1670(C=O)	206 (12)
15	$-CH_3$	$-C_5H_{11}$	87-9/0.5 N_D^{25}=1.4859	63[b]	0.7-1.1(m,3,$N(CH_2)_4\underline{CH_3}$) 1.1-2.1(m,6,$NCH_2(\underline{CH_2})_3CH_3$) 2.45(s,3,$SCH_3$) 3.67(t,2,$N\underline{CH_2}$)	2235(C≡N) 1690(C=O)	186 (5)

16	$-CH_3$	$-C_4H_9$	64-5/0.2 $N_D^{25}=1.4873$	51[b]	0.8-1.1(m,3,$N(CH_2)_3\underline{CH_3}$) 1.1-2.0(m,4,$NCH_2(\underline{CH_2})_2CH_3$) 2.45(s,3,$SCH_3$) 3.63(t,2,$N-\underline{CH_2}$)	2238(C≡N) 1685(C=O)	172 (15)
17	$-CH_3$	$-CH_2CH=CH_2$	100-7/3.6 $N_D^{25}=1.5113$	45[b]	2.45(s,3,SCH_3) 4.20(d,2,$N\underline{CH_2}$) 5.13-6.30(m,3,$NCH_2\underline{CH=CH_2}$)	2240(C≡N) 1695(C=O)	156 (16)
18	$-C_2H_5$	$-CH_2C_6H_5$	137-40/0.8 $N_D^{25}=1.5537$	43[b]	1.20(t,3,$\underline{CH_3}CH_2$) 2.87(q,2,$\underline{CH_2}CH_3$) 4.60(s,2,$N\underline{CH_2}$) 7.23(s,5,C_6H_5)	2240(C≡N) 1690(C=O)	220 (20)
19	$-C_2H_5$	$-CH_2CH=CH_2$	85-8/1.0 $N_D^{25}=1.5011$	33[b]	1.33(t,3,$\underline{CH_3}CH_2$) 3.03(q,2,$\underline{CH_2}CH_3$) 4.23(d,2,$N\underline{CH_2}$) 5.13-6.33(m,3,$NCH_2\underline{CH}=\underline{CH_2}$)	2240(C≡N) 1690(C=O)	170 (25)
20	$-C_2H_5$	$-C_3H_7$	96/2.0 $N_D^{25}=1.4869$	28[b]	1.0(t,3,$\underline{CH_3}CH_2CH_2$) 1.33(t,3,$SCH_2\underline{CH_3}$) 1.73(sextet,2,$CH_2\underline{CH_2}CH_3$) 3.00(q,2,$S\underline{CH_2}CH_3$) 3.62(t,2,$N\underline{CH_2}CH_2CH_3$)	2240(C≡N) 1690(C=O)	172 (17)
21	$-C_2H_5$	$-C_2H_5$	89-90/2.2 $N_D^{25}=1.4892$	40[b]	1.35(t,6,$SCH_2\underline{CH_3}$ and $NCH_2\underline{CH_3}$) 3.02(q,2,$S\underline{CH_2}CH_3$) 3.70(q,2,$N\underline{CH_2}CH_3$	2240(C≡N) 1690(C=O)	158(7)

Continued on next page

Table III (continued)

No.	R	R'	bp °C/mm	% Yield	NMR, (ppm) $CDCl_3$-Me_4Si	Ir (cm^{-1}) Neat	M⁺· Rel. Intensity
22	$-C_2H_5$	$-CH_3$	55/0.3 N_D^{25}=1.4968	41[b]	1.33(t,3,$SCH_2\underline{CH_3}$) 3.00(q,2,$S\underline{CH_2}CH_3$) 3.27(s,3,$N\underline{CH_3}$)	**2240**(C≡N) 1690(C=O)	144 (10)
23	$-C_3H_7$	$-CH_3$	83-6/0.55 N_D^{25}=1.4928	38[b]	0.92(t,3,$S(CH_2)_2\underline{CH_3}$) 1.63(q,2,$SCH_2\underline{CH_2}CH_3$) 2.95(t,2,$S\underline{CH_2}CH_2CH_3$) 3.23(s,3,$N\underline{CH_3}$)	2240(C≡N) 1690(C=O)	158 (2)
24	$-C_3H_7$	$-C_2H_5$	79-81/0.5 N_D^{25}=1.4881	46[b]	0.8-1.9(m,8,$CH_2\underline{CH_2}\underline{CH_3}$) and $\underline{CH_3}CH_2N$) 2.98(t,2,$S\underline{CH_2}CH_2CH_3$) 3.70(q,2,$N\underline{CH_2}CH_3$)	2230(C≡N) 1685(C=O)	172 (7)
25	$-C_3H_7$	$-C_3H_7$	96-9/0.9 N_D^{25}=1.4855	34[b]	1.0(t,6,$S(CH_2)_2\underline{CH_3}$ and $N(CH_2)_2\underline{CH_3}$) 1.48-2.08(m,4,$SCH_2\underline{CH_2}CH_3$ and $NCH_2\underline{CH_2}CH_3$) 3.0(t,2,$S\underline{CH_2}CH_2CH_3$) 3.63(t,2,$N\underline{CH_2}CH_2CH_3$)	2240(C≡N) 1690(C=O)	186 (14)
26	$-C_3H_7$	$-CH_2CH=CH_2$	78-9/0.2 N_D^{25}=1.4969	51[b]	1.0(t,3,$S(CH_2)_2\underline{CH_3}$) 1.74(q,2,$SCH_2\underline{CH_2}CH_3$) 3.02(t,2,$S\underline{CH_2}CH_2CH_3$) 4.2(d,2,$N-\underline{CH_2}$) 5.2-6.2(m,3,$\underline{CH=CH_2}$)	2240(C≡N) 1690(C=O)	184 (10)

27	$-C_3H_7$	$-CH_2C_6H_5$	155/0.9 N_D^{25}=1.5476	46[b]	0.9(t,3,S$(CH_2)_2CH_3$) 1.53(q,2,$SCH_2CH_2CH_3$) 2.90(t,2,$SCH_2CH_2CH_3$) 4.63(s,2,NCH_2) 7.3(s,5,C_6H_5)	2240(C≡N) 1690(C=O)	234 (5)
28	$-C_4H_9$	$-C_2H_5$	88–90/0.6 N_D^{25}=1.4857	52[b]	0.8–2.15(m,10,NCH_2CH_3) and $SCH_2(CH_2)_2CH_3$) 3.0(t,2,SCH_2) 3.7(q,2,N-CH_2)	2230(C≡N) 1695(C=O)	186 (28)
29	$-C_4H_9$	$-CH_2CH=CH_2$	110–2/1.0 N_D^{25}=1.4970	22[b]	0.9(brt,3,S$(CH_2)_3CH_3$) 1.08–1.9(m,4,$SCH_2(CH_2)_2CH_3$) 3.0(t,2,SCH_2) 4.08(d,2,$NCH_2CH=CH_2$) 5.08–6.1(m,3,$CH_2CH=CH_2$)	2240(C≡N) 1690(C=O)	198 (5)

[a]Mass spectrum m/e (rel. intensity)

11 – 130(23(M^{+}), 84(4), 83(100), 77(3), 76(2), 75(75), 73(3), 58(5), 47(39) and 45(14)
12 – 144(24)(M^{+}), 98(4), 97(80), 75(100), 69(60), 47(26), 46(5) and 45(9)

[b]Satisfactory analytical data (±0.4%) for C, H, N and S were reported

[c]Calcd: C, 36.91; H, 4.65; N, 21.52; O, 12.29; S, 24.64
Found: C, 36.82; H, 4.69; N, 21.46; O, 12.10; S, 24.54

(Reprinted with permission from reference 1(b), p 6–8. Copyright 1987 Gordon and Breach.)

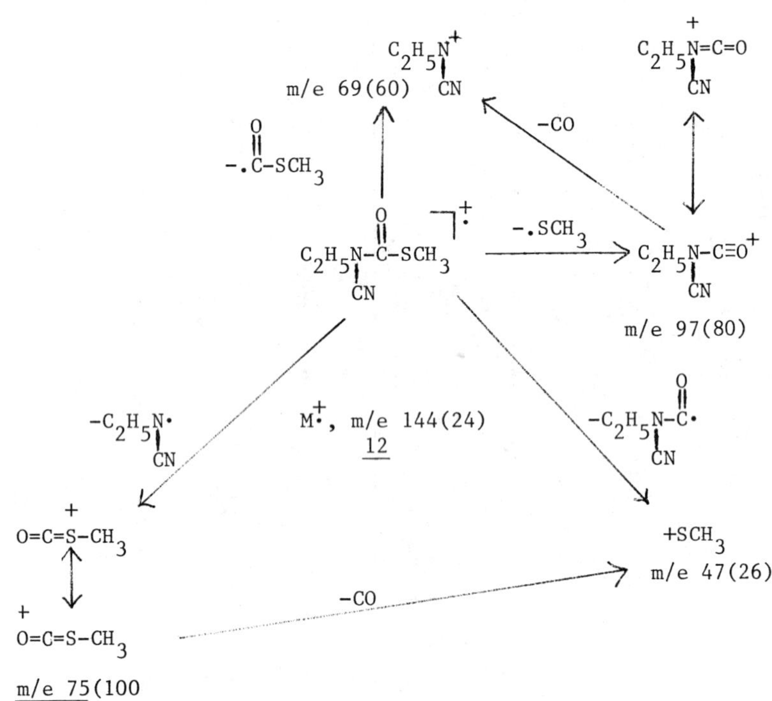

Scheme II. (Reprinted with permission from reference 1(b), p 4. Copyright 1987 Gordon and Breach.)

Table IV. O Alkyl and Benzyl O Potassium Cyanoimidocarbonates

$$(CH_3S)_2C{=}N{-}C{\equiv}N + ROH \xrightarrow{KOH} (KO)(RO)C{=}N{-}C{\equiv}N + 2CH_3SH$$

No.	R	Mp °C (dec.)	Heating Period Hrs.	Heating Period T °C	% Yield	NMR, δ (ppm) Me_2SOd_6-Me_4Si
30[a]	$-C_2H_5$	196-7[b]	6	75-80	87[c]	1.05 (t,3,$CH_2\underline{CH_3}$) 3.80 (q,2,$\underline{CH_2}CH_3$)
31	$-CH_3$	238-9	6	50-60	68[d]	3.40 (s,3,CH_3)
32	$-C_3H_7$	159-61	22	54-58	65[f]	———
33	$-C_4H_9$	153-5[e]	48	78-80	79[f]	———
34	$-CH_2C_6H_5$	229-31[e]	48	80-90	99[f]	5.1 (s,2,CH_2) 7.4 (s,5,C_6H_5)

[a]IR (CsI): 3000 (aliph C-H), 2170 (C≡N) and 1580 cm^{-1} (C=N)

[b]Recrystallization from ethanol.

[c]Calcd: C, 29.80; H, 3.75; K, 24.75; N, 17.38; O, 24.81.
Found: C, 30.17; H, 3.78; K, 24.48; N, 16.98; O, 24.44.

[d]Calcd: C, 26.08; H, 2.19; K, 28.30; N, 20.27.
Found: C, 26.02; H, 2.13; K, 28.19; N, 20.10.

[e]Recrystallization from methanol. [f]Analytical data (±0.4%) for C, H and N were reported.

(Reprinted with permission from reference 1(b), p 223. Copyright 1987 Gordon and Breach.)

$$(CH_3S)_2C{=}N{-}C{\equiv}N + ROH \xrightarrow[50-90\ ^oC]{KOH} (KO)(RO)C{=}N{-}C{\equiv}N + 2CH_3SH \qquad (7)$$

30, R=$-C_2H_5$; 31, R=$-CH_3$; 32, R=$-C_3H_7$; 33, R=$-C_4H_9$; 34, R=$-CH_2C_6H_5$

Analysis, infrared (neat), and NMR spectra were in agreement for the proposed structures of (30-34). Based on elemental analysis and NMR spectra the alternate carbamate structure NCKNC(=O)OR had to be considered in reaction 7. However, the carbamate structure was ruled out on the basis of the infrared spectral data. In 30 the presence of C≡N and C=N absorption bands at 2170 and 1580 cm^{-1}, respectively and the absence of the C=O absorption band at 1700-1755 cm^{-1} furnished conclusive evidence for the proposed structures (30-34).

The reaction of the potassium salts (30, 32 or 33) with a 10% excess of alkyl, allyl or benzyl halides in dimethylformamide at 80-90 °C afforded the titled carbamates (35-46).

$$(KO)(RO)C{=}N{-}C{\equiv}N + \underset{10\%\ excess}{R'X} \xrightarrow[80-90\ ^oC]{DMF} R'{-}N(CN){-}C(=O){-}OR \qquad (8)$$

R and R' as shown in Table V.

Analysis, infrared, NMR and mass spectra were in agreement for the proposed structures of 35-46. The proposed mechanisms for reactions 7 and 8 are depicted in Scheme III.

The reaction of 31 with 10% excess benzyl bromide or 34 with 10% excess methyl iodide gave the same product, N-benzyl-N-methyl cyanamide 47.

$$\underset{31}{(KO)(CH_3O)C{=}N{-}C{\equiv}N} + \underset{10\%\ excess}{C_6H_5CH_2Br} \xrightarrow[80-90\ ^oC,\ 22\ hrs.]{DMF} \underset{47}{C_6H_5CH_2{-}N(CN){-}CH_3} + CO_2 \qquad (9)$$

$$\underset{34}{(KO)(C_6H_5CH_2O)C{=}N{-}C{\equiv}N} + \underset{10\%\ excess}{CH_3I} \xrightarrow[80-90\ ^oC,\ 22\ hrs.]{DMF} 47 + CO_2$$

The reaction of 31 with 10% and 55% excess allyl bromide afforded N-allyl-N-methyl cyanamide (48) and N,N-diallyl cyanamide (49), respectively.

$$\underset{31}{(KO)(CH_3O)C{=}N{-}C{\equiv}N} \xrightarrow[CH_2=CHCH_2Br;\ DMF - 80-90\ ^oC;\ 72\ hrs.]{10\%\ excess} \underset{48}{CH_2{=}CHCH_2{-}N(CN){-}CH_3} + CO_2 \qquad (10)$$

$$31 \xrightarrow[CH_2=CHCH_2Br;\ DMF - 80-90\ ^oC;\ 72\ hrs.]{55\%\ excess} \underset{49}{(CH_2{=}CHCH_2)_2{-}N{-}CN} + CO_2 + CH_3Br$$

Table V

Alkyl N-Substituted Carbamates

$$\begin{matrix} KO \\ RO \end{matrix} \!\!>\! C{=}N{-}C{\equiv}N + \underset{\text{10\% excess}}{R'X} \xrightarrow[\text{80-90 °C}]{\text{DMF}} R'N(CN){-}C({=}O){-}OR$$

X=Br or I

No.	R	R'	Reaction Time-Days	bp °C/mm	% Yield	NMR, δ (ppm) $CDCl_3$-Me_4Si	Ir (cm^{-1}) Neat	M⁺· Rel. Intensity
35	$-C_2H_5$	$-CH_2C_6H_5$	2	122-5/0.7 N_D^{25}=1.5149	30[a]	1.20(t,3,OCH_2CH_3) 4.18(q,2,OCH_2CH_3) 4.55(s,2,NCH_2) 7.33(s,5,C_6H_5)	2250(C≡N) 1750(C=O)	204(15)[b]
36	$-C_2H_5$	$-CH_2CH{=}CH_2$	2	53-5/0.3 N_D^{25}=1.4532	41[a]	1.30(t,3,OCH_2CH_3) 4.07(d,2,$NCH_2CH{=}CH_2$) 4.27(q,2,OCH_2CH_3) 5.03-6.20(m,3,$CH_2CH{=}CH_2$)	2250(C≡N) 1755(C=O)	154(7)[b]
37	$-C_2H_5$	$-C_2H_5$	1	79-81/3.2 N_D^{25}=1.4355	46[a]	1.30(t,6,OCH_2CH_3 and NCH_2CH_3) 3.57(q,2,NCH_2CH_3) 4.27(q,2,OCH_2CH_3)	2245(C≡N) 1750(C=O)	142(12)[b]
38	$-C_2H_5$	$-C_3H_7$	3	66-8/0.8 N_D^{25}=1.4389	41[a]	0.97(t,3,$NCH_2CH_2CH_3$) 1.30(t,3,OCH_2CH_3) 1.70(q,2,$NCH_2CH_2CH_3$) 3.47(t,2,$NCH_2CH_2CH_3$) 4.25(q,2,OCH_2CH_3)	2240(C≡N) 1750(C=O)	156(3)[b]

Continued on next page

Table V (continued)

No.	R	R'	Reaction Time-Days	bp °C/mm	% Yield	NMR, δ (ppm) $CDCl_3$-Me_4Si	Ir (cm^{-1}) Neat	$M^{+\cdot}$ Rel. Intensity
39	$-C_2H_5$	$-CH_3$	1	42/0.4 N_D^{25}=1.4393	27[a]	1.30(t,3,$OCH_2\underline{CH_3}$) 3.17(s,3,NCH_3) 4.25(q,2,$O\underline{CH_2}CH_3$)	2250(C≡N) 1755(C=O)	128(8)[b]
40	$-C_3H_7$	$-CH_3$	1	74-6/1.4 N_D^{25}=1.4332	41[a]	0.92(t,3,$O(CH_2)_2\underline{CH_3}$) 1.70(q,2,$OCH_2\underline{CH_2}CH_3$) 3.18(s,3,$NCH_3$) 4.14(t,2,$O\underline{CH_2}CH_2CH_3$)	2210(C≡N) 1755(C=O)	142(10)[b]
41	$-C_3H_7$	$-C_2H_5$	1	81/1.6 N_D^{25}=1.4375	48[a]	1.0(t,3,$O(CH_2)_2\underline{CH_3}$) 1.32(t,3,$NCH_2\underline{CH_3}$) 1.73(q,2,$OCH_2\underline{CH_2}CH_3$) 3.6(q,2,$N\underline{CH_2}CH_3$) 4.2(t,2,$O\underline{CH_2}CH_2CH_3$)	2210(C≡N) 1755(C=O)	156(10)[b]
42	$-C_3H_7$	$-C_3H_7$	1	90/1.6 N_D^{25}=1.4385	67[a]	0.98(t,6,$O(CH_2)_2\underline{CH_3}$ and $N(CH_2)_2\underline{CH_3}$) 1.73(q,4,$OCH_2\underline{CH_2}CH_3$ and $NCH_2\underline{CH_2}CH_3$) 3.55(t,2,$N\underline{CH_2}CH_2CH_3$) 4.2(t,2,$O\underline{CH_2}CH_2CH_3$)	2210(C≡N) 1755(C=O)	170(7)[b]

43	$-C_3H_7$	$-CH_2C_6H_5$	1	144–6/1.2 N_D^{25}=1.5093	41[a]	0.85(t,3,$O(CH_2)_2\underline{CH_3}$) 1.63(q,2,$OCH_2\underline{CH_2}CH_3$) 4.15(t,2,$O\underline{CH_2}CH_2CH_3$) 4.68(s,2,$N\underline{CH_2}$) 7.3(s,5,$C_6\underline{H_5}$)	2210(C≡N) 1755(C=O)	218(8)[b]
44	$-C_4H_9$	$-C_3H_7$	1	78–9/0.5 N_D^{25}=1.4361	71[a]	0.93(m,6,$N(CH_2)_2\underline{CH_3}$ and $O(CH_2)_3\underline{CH_3}$ 1.1–1.9(m,6,$NCH_2\underline{CH_2}CH_3$) and $OCH_2(\underline{CH_2})_2CH_3$ 3.23(t,2,$N\underline{CH_2}CH_2CH_3$) 4.1(t,2,$O\underline{CH_2}(CH_2)_2CH_3$)	2250(C≡N) 1755(C=O)	185[c]
45	$-C_4H_9$	$-C_2H_5$	1	76–8/0.8 N_D^{25}=1.4348	57[a]	0.85(m,3,$O(CH_2)_3\underline{CH_3}$) 1.05–1.95(m,7,$NCH_2\underline{CH_3}$) and $OCH_2(\underline{CH_2})_2CH_3$) 3.5(q,2,$N\underline{CH_2}CH_3$) 4.15(t,2,$O\underline{CH_2}(CH_2)_2CH_3$)	2250(C≡N) 1750(C=O)	171[c]
46	$-C_4H_9$	$-CH_3$	1	68–71/0.9 N_D^{25}=1.4351	19[a]	0.9(m,3,$O(CH_2)_3\underline{CH_3}$) 1.1–1.8(m,4,$O(\underline{CH_2})_2CH_2CH_3$) 3.2(t,3,$N\underline{CH_3}$) 4.2(t,2,$O\underline{CH_2}(CH_2)_2CH_3$)	2250(C≡N) 1765(C=O)	157[c]

[a]Satisfactory analysis (±0.4%) were reported for C, H and N
[b]Electron impact mass spectra
[c]Chemical ionization mass spectra $(M + 1)^{+\cdot}$

(Reprinted with permission from reference 1(b), p 224–5. Copyright 1987 Gordon and Breach.)

$$ROH + KOH \rightleftharpoons RO^{-}K^{+} + H^{+} + OH^{-}$$

$$(CH_3S)_2C{=}N{-}C{\equiv}N \xrightarrow[\;^{-}OR\;]{H^{+}} CH_3S{-}C(OR)(SCH_3){-}N(H){-}C{\equiv}N$$

$$\xrightarrow{-CH_3SH} (RO)(CH_3S)C{=}N{-}C{\equiv}N \xrightarrow[\;^{-}OH\;]{H^{+}} (RO)(HO)C(SCH_3){-}N(H){-}C{\equiv}N$$

$$\xrightarrow{-CH_3SH} (RO)(HO)C{=}N{-}C{\equiv}N \xrightarrow{K^{+}} (RO)(K^{+}\,^{-}O)C{=}N{-}C{\equiv}N \leftrightarrow (RO)(O{=})C{-}N^{-}{-}C{\equiv}N \leftrightarrow (RO)(^{-}O)C{=}N{-}C{\equiv}N$$

ambident anion

$$\xrightarrow{R'{-}X} R'{-}N(CN){-}C({=}O){-}OR$$

Scheme III. (Reprinted with permission from reference 1(b), p 220. Copyright 1987 Gordon and Breach.)

The reaction of 32 with 28% excess of allyl iodide gave N-allyl-N-propyl cyanamide (50).

$$\underset{\underline{32}}{\begin{matrix} KO \\ C_3H_7O \end{matrix} \!\!>\! C{=}N{-}C{\equiv}N} \xrightarrow[\text{DMF - 80-90 °C, 48 hrs.}]{\text{28\% excess } CH_2{=}CHCH_2I} \underset{\underline{50}}{CH_2{=}CHCH_2{-}\underset{CN}{N}{-}C_3H_7} + CO_2 \quad (11)$$

The proposed mechanisms for the formation of 47, 48, 49 and 50 are shown in Scheme IV.

The determination of the optimum conditions for the synthesis of the unsymmetrical cyanamides similar to 47, 48 and 50 by our novel method (reactions 9, 10 and 11) would be very desirable. The hydrolysis of these mixed cyanamides would provide a useful synthesis of secondary mixed amines (reaction 12) which is not possible by Vliet's method (9) (reaction 13) which affords only secondary symmetrical amines.

$$R{-}\underset{R'}{N}{-}CN \xrightarrow{H_2O} R{-}\underset{R'}{N}H + CO_2 + NH_3 \quad (12)$$

$$2\ RBr \xrightarrow{Na_2NCN} R_2NCN \xrightarrow{H_2O} R_2NH + CO_2 + NH_3 \quad (13)$$

In summary, depending on reaction condition, we have described a novel and versatile direct synthesis of alkyl N-cyano-N-substituted carbamates or N,N-disubstituted cyanamides. The required intermediates can be prepared in good yields from cyanamide, carbon disulfide, potassium hydroxide, alkyl or benzyl alcohols and alkyl or benzyl halides which are readily available and inexpensive.

Nishio and co-workers (2a,b,c) claimed the following biological activity: (1) thiolcarbamate derivatives represented by the general formula NCR'NC(=O)SR, where R and R' are alkyl, alkenyl or alkynyl groups, can be used as a bactericide, fungicide, insecticide, miticide or herbicide, (2) compounds of the general formula NCR'NC(=O)-SR, where R'=alkyl or alkenyl and R=benzyl and its p-chloro derivative are active as miticide, herbicide and antimicrobicide and (3) thiolcarbamate derivatives represented by the general formula (KO)(RS)C=NCN where R=benzyl and M=K (compound 10) are effective in controlling microorganisms such as Piricularia oryzae and Xanthomonas citri.

Concerning our evaluation program the titled thiolcarbamates and carbamates exhibited activity as plant growth regulators for soybean and corn. The most active compounds possessed the general formula NCR'NC(=O)SR, where R'=ethyl or propyl and R=methyl (compounds 12 and 13). However, additional synthesis and testing are needed in order to determine the true merits of the titled compounds for this application.

$$RO-\overset{O}{\overset{\|}{C}}-\underset{CN}{\underset{|}{N}}-R' \xrightarrow{Nu} RO\overset{O}{\overset{\|}{C}}Nu + \underset{CN}{\underset{|}{\overset{\ominus}{N}}}-R'$$

$$R'-\underset{CN}{\underset{|}{\overset{\ominus}{N}}} + R-O-\overset{O}{\overset{\|}{C}}-\underset{CN}{\underset{|}{N}}-R' \longrightarrow R-\underset{CN}{\underset{|}{N}}-R' + CO_2 + \underset{CN}{\underset{|}{\overset{\ominus}{N}}}-R'$$

No.	R	R'	excess Halide
47	$-CH_3$	$-CH_2C_6H_5$	10% Benzyl bromide
	$-CH_2C_6H_5$	$-CH_3$	10% Methyl iodide
48	$-CH_3$	$-CH_2CH=CH_2$	10% Allyl bromide
50	$-C_3H_7$	$-CH_2CH=CH_2$	28% Allyl iodide

$$\underset{\underline{48}}{CH_3\underset{CN}{\underset{|}{N}}-CH_2CH=CH_2} \xrightarrow[\text{allyl bromide}]{\text{55\% excess}} \left[(CH_2=CHCH_2)_2\underset{CH_3}{\underset{|}{N}}-CN\right]^{\oplus} Br^{\ominus} \xrightarrow{-CH_3Br} \underset{\underline{49}}{(CH_2=CHCH_2)_2NCN}$$

Scheme IV. (Reprinted with permission from reference 1(b), p 222. Copyright 1987 Gordon and Breach.)

Literature Cited

1. (a) Presented at the 191st National Meeting of American Chemical Society, Agrochemicals Division, New York City, N.Y.
   (b) The experimental details of the synthesis of these compounds can be found in: Phosphorus and Sulfur, 1987, 29, 1-10, ibid, 1987, 29, 219-226.
2. (a) Nishio, K., Yoshinaga, E. and Takita, K., (Kumiai Chemical Industry Co. Ltd.) Japan, Kokai 73 99,331, 1973. Chem. Abstr., 1974, 81, 10446m.
   (b) Nishio, K., Saito, M., Kawada, S. and Takita, K., (Kumiai Chemical Industry Co. Ltd.) Japan, Kokai 73 96,724, 1973. Chem. Abstr., 1974, 80, 104873e.
   (c) Nishio, K., Kato, T., Kawada, S. and Takita, K., (Kumiai Chemical Industry Co. Ltd.) Japan, Kokai 73 96,725, 1973. Chem. Abstr., 1974, 80, 104872d.
3. D'Amico, J. J. and Schafer, T., Phosphorus and Sulfur, 1980, 8, 301.
4. (a) Hantzsch, A. and Wolveskamp, M., Justus Liebigs Ann. Chem., 1904, 321, 265.
   (b) D'Amico, J. J. and Campbell, R. H., J. Org. Chem., 1967, 32, 2567.
5. D'Amico, J. J., Boustany, K., Sullivan, A. B. and Campbell, R. H., Int. J. Sulfur Chem., 1972, Part A, Volume 2, Number 1, 37-41.
6. D'Amico, J. J., (Monsanto Co.) U.S. Patent 3,299,129, 1967.
7. Ruminski, P. G., Suba, L. A. and D'Amico, J. J., 1984, Phosphorus and Sulfur, 19, 335.
8. Fromm, E. and von Gonez, D., 1907, Ann., 355, 196.
9. (a) Vliet, E. B., 1924, J. Am. Chem. Soc., 46, 1305.
   (b) Vliet, E. B., 1943, Org. Synthesis, Coll. Vol. 1, 203.

RECEIVED July 20, 1987

Chapter 33

Asymmetric Synthesis of Selected Insect Pheromones

P. E. Sonnet [1], P. L. Guss [2], J. H. Tumlinson, T. P. McGovern [3], and R. T. Cunningham [4]

Insect Attractants, Behavior, and Basic Biology Research Laboratory, Agricultural Research Service, U.S. Department of Agriculture, Gainesville, FL 32604

This is a review of synthetic efforts made at these laboratories in recent years. Stereoisomers of sex pheromones of various insect species were synthesized in order to facilitate identification and permit more thorough evaluation of their potential in insect control programs. Syntheses are described for pheromones of the stable fly, tsetse fly, southern and western corn rootworms, and the Mediterranean fruit fly attractant, trimedlure. In each instance centers of asymmetry were generated that made use of diastereomer formation using readily available (R)- and (S)-α-methylbenzylamine. Resolutions were achieved either by preparative HPLC, or fractional crystallization of amides. The latter technique was rendered synthetically useful for the preparation of configurationally pure acids by virtue of transformations wrought upon the amides that made them subject to cleavage under very mild conditions.

[1]Current address: Eastern Regional Research Center, Agricultural Research Service, U.S. Department of Agriculture, Wyndmoor, PA 19118

[2] Deceased

[3]Current address: Organic Chemicals Synthesis Laboratory, Agricultural Research Service, U.S. Department of Agriculture, BARC-West, Beltsville, MD 20705

[4]Current address: Tropical Fruit and Vegetable Research Laboratory, Agricultural Research Service, U.S. Department of Agriculture, Hilo, HI 96720

This chapter is not subject to U.S. copyright.
Published 1987, American Chemical Society

The Agricultural Research Service of the USDA has supported investigations of chemical cues that have led to useful alternative measures in pest control. Some of these are designed as early detection systems; others are being used to reduce infestations directly (1). Because insect behavioral responses are generally keyed to stereochemistry, the investigation of chemical structure must be concluded with syntheses and studies performed on stereoisomers of the identified natural products. We describe here some of our work in this area emphasizing syntheses of rootworm pheromone stereoisomers -- compounds that we expect will have application both in detection and control. We also describe our synthesis of the stereoisomers of a purely "synthetic" attractant, namely trimedlure, a mixture of materials that has been employed as a bait in monitoring for Mediterranean fruit fly for a long time.

Biological Activity vs. Stereostructure

Usually when a male insect is presented with a racemic candidate pheromone, it does respond sexually (2) (Figure 1). Examination of the responses toward stereoisomers generally results in the following: strong response toward one enantiomer; little or no response toward the other enantiomer or other stereoisomers. Occasionally an insect may respond to both enantiomers of a structure; and occasionally one enantiomer actually inhibits the male's response to the "active" isomer. In such cases, the original isolation/identification adventure could unearth the situation as a problem that hinders identification. Since the initial research generally culminates in a synthesis of the assigned structure that is not stereodifferentiated, the inactivity of the candidate synthetic may cause the champagne to be set aside while collaborators eye each other with grave suspicion.

The point has often been made, but seems worth repeating, that there is as yet no substitute for asymmetric synthesis in assigning stereostructure to most insect semiochemicals. The amount of natural product available is usually far less than 1 mg. More important, the centers of asymmetry are often far removed from the chemical functionality that one traditionally employs as leverage for spectral evaluation of configuration. As a rule, stereocontrolled syntheses of a set of stereoisomers follows initial assignment of structure, and a methodical investigation of the activity of these isomers individually and as mixtures is then conducted.

Resolution of Carboxylic Acids

Among simple structures that are suitable as key synthetic intermediates, α-branched carboxylic acids are easily prepared and versatile (Figure 2). One would like to obtain such a material from an available chiral pool and proceed, but few α-branched alkanoic acids are available as natural products. (S)-2-Methylbutyric acid, uniquely, can be obtained in 99% enantiomeric excess (ee) by Jones oxidation of the commercially available alcohol (3).

1. Response to one enantiomer, not the other

   Very common

---

2. Response optimal to a ratio of enantiomers

   OH OH

   S R

   Gnathotricus sulcatus =65:35 ratio *S*:*R*

---

3. Response to one enantiomer, other is inhibitory

   OH

   S

   Gnathotricus retusus. Does not respond to the pheromone of *G. sulcatus*

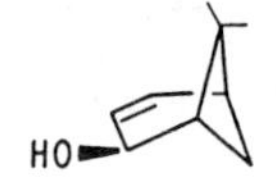

S,*cis*-verbenol

Ips calligraphus and *typographus*

$(C_{10}H_{21})$

7*R*,8*S*

Gypsy moth

(C_8H_{17})

R

Japanese beetle

Figure 1. Relationship of Biological Activity to Enantiomeric Composition

A number of methods for generating such acids in high configurational purity by asymmetric induction are known in which the use of chiral amide enolates may be cited (4, 5). The degree of configurational bias in these reactions is often excellent although they show dependency on the alkylating agent. They are, in fact, least effective for the less hindered halides, e.g., methyl iodide. Nevertheless, faced with the task of developing a useful route to an agricultural chemical, one could indeed opt for such an approach, particularly if a few percent of the unwanted enantiomer can be removed easily, or offers no problem in the product's application.

Resolution of diastereomeric amides by preparative HPLC has been developed for α-branched alkanoic acids, and has been employed to prepare dimethyl branched alkanes implicated in tsetse fly sexual communication (6). In much of our own work we have made use of fractional crystallization whereby racemic acids are converted to amides of either (R)- or (S)-α-methylbenzylamine. These amines are available from Hexcel Corp., Zeeland, MI, and the diastereomeric amides can be analyzed for purity chromatographically.

One such method employs cholesteric liquid crystals, such as cholesterol p-chloro cinnamate, as stationary phases for capillary gas chromatography (7) (Figure 3). The basis of the chromatographic resolutions of these amides is related to the rigidity of a central backbone containing the amide link (8). For the purposes of this comparison, the greater the size difference between the two alkyl groups on the acid residue, the better the separation. As a corollary, the more highly organized the liquid phase, the greater the differentiation between diastereomers also. In the liquid crystal phase, it appears that the high degree of organization optimizes the nonpolar phase's capacity to distinguish the solute's length to breadth ratio (9) and retains the more linear diastereomer.

In order to reap the reward of purification, we had to develop methods to cleave the amides without racemizing the acid (Figure 4). The usual hydrolytic procedures were too severe; and recently developed milder methods generally required base that caused some loss of configurational purity. Deprotonation of the pure amide with a strong, but nonnucleophilic base followed by reaction of the anion with, e.g., methyl chloroformate produces an acyl urethan. For simple α-alkylacyl groups reaction of the acyl urethan with nucleophiles occurs preferentially on the acyl group, so cleavage to the acid can be affected with, e.g., cold aqueous base. An alternative sequence involves reaction of the amide anion with ethylene oxide to give a hydroxyethylated analog. The acyl group migrates from nitrogen to oxygen under acid catalysis. We have found that the crude aminoester intermediate can be conveniently reduced by lithium aluminum hydride to the corresponding carbinol. Since the recovered amides from the fractionations can be converted to free amines and racemic acids, the process can be repeated. It quickly provides quantities of α-substituted acids and carbinols in $\geq$ 99.6% enantiomeric excess (ee).

1. Available natural products
2. Asymmetric induction
3. Resolution

   fractional crystallization of amides
   (R- and S- α-methylbenzylamine)

$$CH_3CH_2COOH \xrightarrow[\text{2) RX}]{\text{1) 2LDA}} CH_3CH(R)COOH \xrightarrow[\text{2) } \alpha\text{-MBA}]{\text{1) } SOCl_2} CH_3CH(R)C(O)NHCHCH_3Ph$$

Figure 2. Synthesis of Enantiomers of α-Branched Carboxylic Acids

$R_1R_2CH(CO)NHCHCH_3Ph$

R_1	R_2	SE-54 α	C-20M α	CpCC α
CH_3	C_2H_5	1.021	1.018	1.036
CH_3	i-C_3H_7	1.040	1.046	1.064
CH_3	n-C_3H_7	1.060	1.056	1.071
CH_3	n-C_4H_9	1.058	1.068	1.100
n-C_5H_{11}	n-C_6H_{13}	1.000	1.000	1.011

CpCC = CHOLESTEROL para-Chlorocinnamate

α = Ratio of Corrected Retention Volumes

Figure 3. Comparison of GLC separations of diastereomeric amides on several liquid phases

Methyl Branched Alkanes (Stable Fly, Tsetse Fly-Type Hydrocarbons)

An example of the application of this sequence is the synthesis of the stereoisomers of 15,19-dimethyltritriacontane (Figure 5) (10). Propionic acid was alkylated with 1-bromotetradecane and the sequence just described followed to obtain (R)- and (S)-2-methylhexadecanols. Using known methods, the alcohols were converted to aldehydes of one greater carbon number and also to phosphonium salts. The aldehydes and salts were condensed in Wittig condensations, and the resulting alkenes reduced to give the three stereoisomers of the target alkane. These structures have been implicated as a sex excitant for the stable fly (11), and one of the tsetse fly species (12).

Southern Corn Rootworm

The southern corn rootworm is a member of the genus Diabrotica, family Chrysomelidae. This genus contains a large number of pest species that feed upon include corn, cucumber, squash and melon. Mint and mesquite grass have also been attacked by an occasional species (13).

The sex pheromone structure, 10-methyl-2-tridecanone, was synthesized using the carboxyl group as the source of the methyl branch (14) (Figure 6). Undecylenic acid was α-propylated and resolved via amides. The procedure followed allowed us to obtain the alcohols,(R)- and (S)-2-propyl-10-undecenol (≥99.6% ee). The corresponding bromide was reduced with lithium triethylborohydride (15); then the double bond was converted to a methyl ketone by a) oxymercuration, b) reduction of the C-Hg bond with sodium borohydride, and c) oxidation with dichromate. The male southern corn rootworm responds only to the (R)-configuration; no biological activity was noted for the (S)-enantiomer. Therefore, in this instance the racemic compound would be predicted to monitor this species adequately.

Western Corn Rootworm

Another important member of this family is the western corn rootworm, *Diabrotica virgifera virgifera* LeConte. Our research with this insect's sex pheromone gave ample indication that much can be learned both by biologists and chemists if a project to identify chemical cues is not focused solely on a designated pest species, but is instead broadened to encompass closely related species.

The structure of the western corn rootworm sex pheromone is 8-methyl-2-decanol propanoate (16) and four stereoisomers are possible (Figure 7). In our synthesis (3), we coupled a chiral 5-carbon unit to a 6-carbon fragment that had the requisite substitution to allow resolution at the oxygenated carbon. As mentioned earlier, (S)-2-methylbutyric acid was available to us from the alcohol. D-Isoleucine served as a source for the (R)-acid. Nitrosation, followed by decarboxylative oxidation of the intermediate hydroxyacid led to the (R)-2-methylbutyric acid in 96% ee. The process of fractional crystallization was

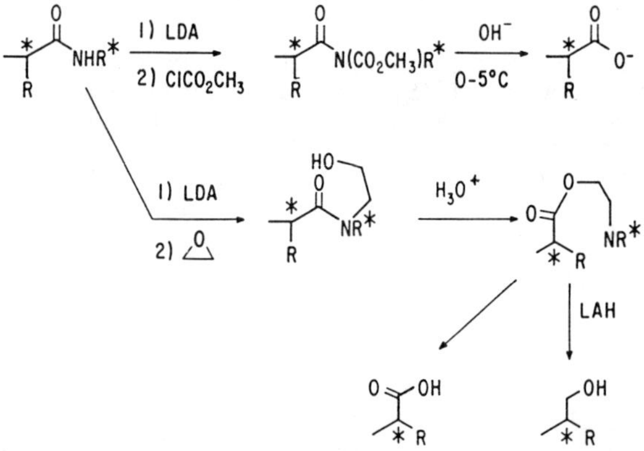

Figure 4. Cleavage of diastereomerically pure amides

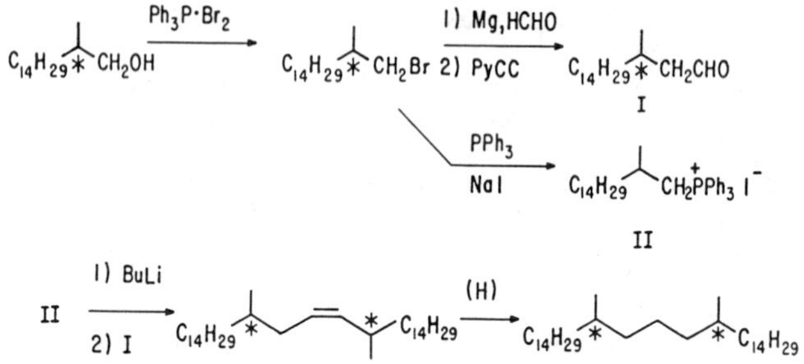

Figure 5. Synthesis of the stereoisomers of 15,19-dimethyltritriacontane

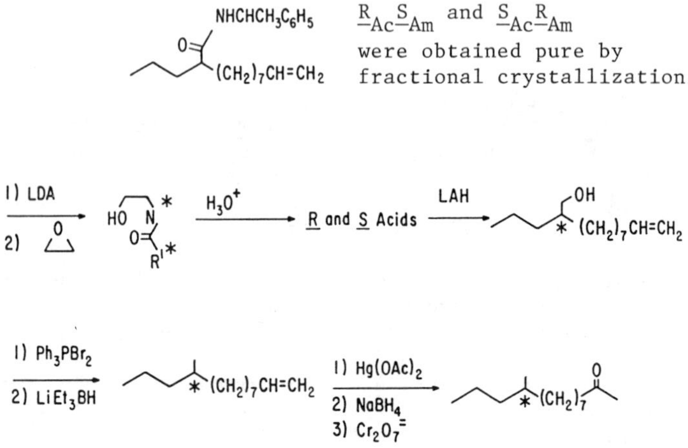

$\underline{R}$Ac$\underline{S}$Am and $\underline{S}$Ac$\underline{R}$Am were obtained pure by fractional crystallization

Figure 6. Synthesis of the southern corn rootworm sex pheromone stereoisomers

unsuccessful for this particular amide, and it was resolved by preparative HPLC (silica gel: THF, EtOAc, hexane; 1:2:7). The purified diastereomers were hydroxyethylated and then hydrolyzed with 1N HCl under reflux. The acids obtained were each 94% ee.

The (R)- and (S)-acids were then reduced to the alcohols and converted to derivatives suitable for organometallic coupling to the ethylene ketal of 6-bromo-2-hexanone (Figure 8). Hydrolytic cleavage of the ketal, and reduction gave 8-methyl-2-decanol that has strong configurational bias at the 8-carbon. The alcohols were converted to carbamates with (R)-α-naphthylethyliosocyanate (synthesized from (R)-α-naphthylethylamine) and resolved by preparative HPLC (silica gel: EtOAc, hexane; 7:93). Separation is also possible though less efficient with the more available α-methylbenzylisocyanate. The pure alcohols are then obtained from the carbamates (LAH) and these were then propionylated.

Examination of the responses of other Diabroticites yielded very interesting results. The western corn rootworm responded most strongly to the 2R,8R-isomer, and less so to 2S,8R. Another species, the Mexican corn rootworm, *D. v. zeae* Krysan & Smith, was found to respond identically. Their ranges differ, though, and reproductive isolation might have occurred by that geographical partitioning. The northern corn rootworm, *D. l. barberi* Smith & Lawrence, was known to be attracted to the western species (northern male to western female), but mating was mechanically deterred. The male was only responsive to the 2R,8R-isomer, however. Although it was attracted to the racemate, high concentrations show lessened response and, in fact, the 2S,8R-isomer was inhibitory.

Diabrotica longicornis (no common name) was only recently accorded species status to separate it from the northern corn rootworm. Its stereobias (2S,8R) offered convincing evidence that this insect indeed possessed its individual communications system (17). Two other nonpests, *D. porracea* and *D. lemniscata*, also responded to the 2S,8R-isomer. Finally, we have discovered that traps containing the acetate ester (2R,8R) caught *D. cristata* (18). So far it appears that the hydrocarbon center must be (R) for rootworm perception. Even that isomer most effective for inhibition had the 8R configuration. The obligatory nature of that asymmetric center allows preparations that are racemic at that site (the [S] is not perceived). The ester site is, however, species differentiating and syntheses must be geared to the biological result desired.

Mediterranean Fruit Fly

As a closing example of the value of asymmetric synthesis in the area of insect chemistry, we describe the synthesis of the stereoisomers of trimedlure, a material discovered by empirical screening and used to monitor for "Medfly" (Figure 9). The commercial preparation of this attractant mixture involves a nonselective addition of HCl to a substituted cyclohexene. The several products are shown in abbreviated form (Figure 9); the *t*-butyl esters of this mixture of acids has been employed for many years as a bait for the medfly (19). Each component,

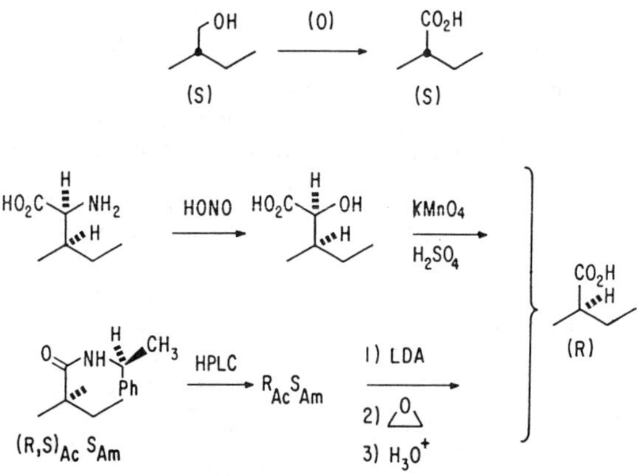

(O)

(S) (S)

HONO

$KMnO_4$

H_2SO_4

HPLC

1) LDA

2)

3) H_3O^+

(R)

$(R,S)_{Ac}\ S_{Am}$

$R_{Ac}S_{Am}$

Figure 7. Syntheses of (R)- and (S)-2-methylbutyric acid

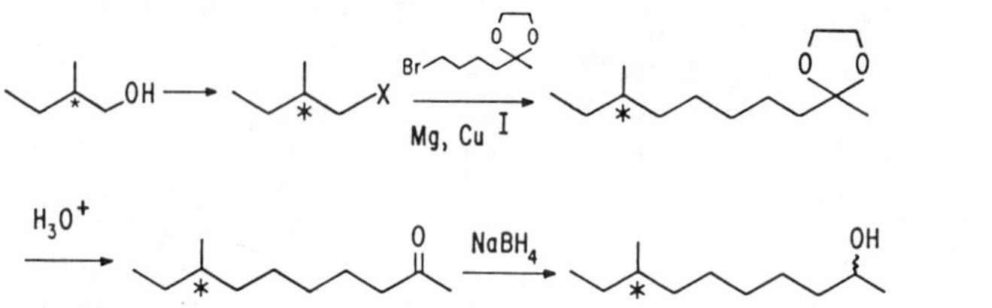

Mg, Cu I

H_3O^+

$NaBH_4$

a) X is halogen/tosylate
b) Alcohol site resolved (HPLC) as α-Naphthylethyl carbamates

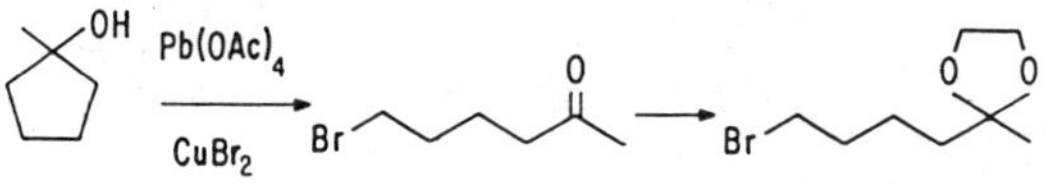

$Pb(OAc)_4$

$CuBr_2$

Figure 8. Synthesis of the western corn rootworm sex pheromone stereoisomers

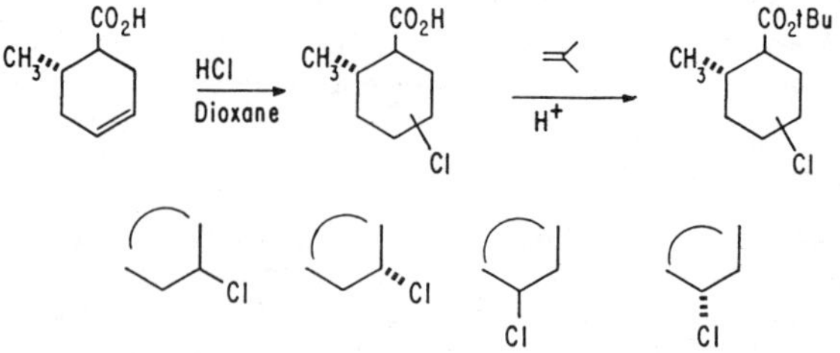

HCl
Dioxane

H^+

Figure 9. Commercial synthesis of "trimedlure", a synthetic attractant for Mediterranean fruit fly. (Reproduced from Reference 21. Copyright 1966, American Chemical Society.)

however, is a racemate, and the racemate labeled "C" (20) has been shown previously to be most active.

The unsaturated acid, a compound that could not be prepared readily by asymmetric induction, seemed a good candidate for resolution. In fact, this acid was resolved by fractional crystallization of diastereomeric amides (Figure 10), and then the pure diastereomers were cleaved by means described above. Other ploys suggested themselves (recrystallization of salts rather than amides, recrystallization of amides of purified HCl adducts, etc.), but these alternative approaches were unsuccessful (21). Additionally, hydrolysis of intermediate aminoesters gave poor yields of the desired unsaturated acids, and the hydrolysis was instead interrupted to reduce the crude aminoester-acid product with LAH. The rotations of the carbinols and acids were the basis for initial assignment of absolute configuration.

Further evidence was obtained from spectral data. Because of the rigidity of the amide link and the consequent solution conformation preferences as mentioned earlier, the ring-methyl group is opposed by either the methyl or phenyl substituents on the amine based asymmetric center (Figure 11 illustrates the likely major solution conformations). The phenyl ring's anisotropy shifts the ring-methyl protons significantly upfield. This observation was made repeatedly with various synthetic intermediates and the subject was described in our original publication (21).

We also felt that the relative solubilities of the diastereomeric amides (or their crystal lattice energies) might be related to the sense of steric bulk disymmetry about that central backbone. If one could perform a chemical reaction, such as addition to the double bond, that could alter the distribution of steric bulk, one could hope to invert diastereomer solubility. Addition of a symmetrical reagent, such as bromine, avoids positional isomerism and the stability of the bromonium ion ensures stereoselectivity. Thus each diastereomeric amide gave only one bromine adduct. The solubilities were indeed dramatically altered and, since bromine is easily removed (Zn, acetic acid) it became possible to use the amide mixture that had been recovered from purification to claim the more soluble diastereomer as its bromine adduct. A process was established to obtain both enantiomeric cyclohexene acids using only one chiral amine.

A derivative based on chiral oxazolidones has been described by Pirkle (22) that can be used to gain information about configuration (Figure 12). Again a strong conformational bias is afforded such compounds in solution both by the nature of the bonding involved and the tendency for the carbonyls to be aligned in opposition. The effects of alignment result in differential shielding of substituents thus permitting NMR to be used as a probe for absolute configuration. The oxazolidone shown (Figure 12) was synthesized from (R)-phenylglycine via the corresponding alcohol. The phenyl substituent of this chiral auxiliary shields the ring methyl protons of the 1S,6S unit by

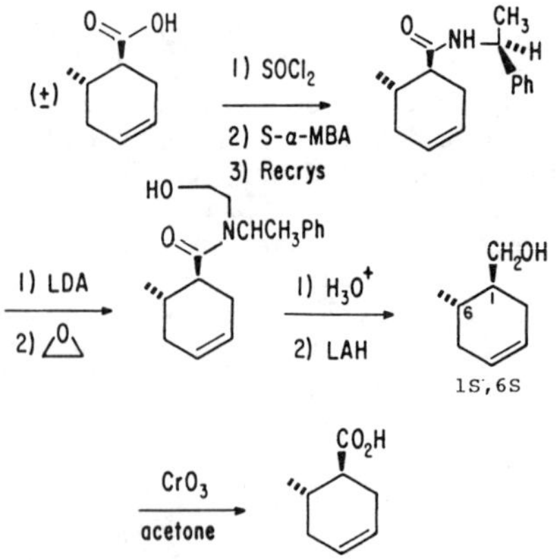

1) $SOCl_2$
2) S-α-MBA
3) Recrys

1) LDA
2) ethylene oxide

1) H_3O^+
2) LAH

1S,6S

CrO_3
acetone

Figure 10. Synthesis of the stereoisomers of trans-6-methyl-3-cyclohexene carboxylic acid

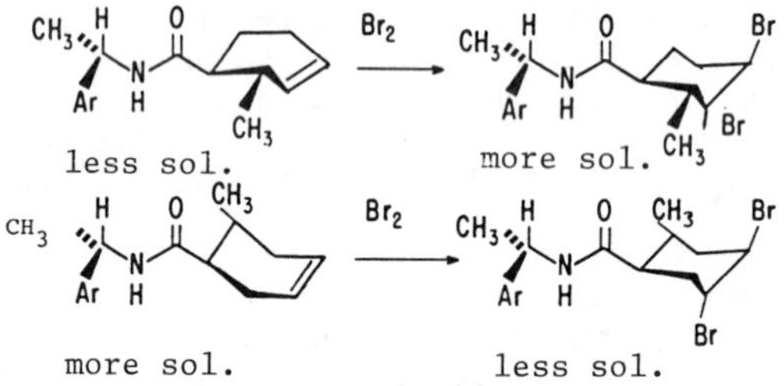

less sol. → (Br_2) → more sol.

more sol. → (Br_2) → less sol.

purified dibromide —Zn→ corresponding unsat. diastereomer

Figure 11. Relationship of stereostructure to solubility of key synthetic intermediates in the synthesis of trimedlure stereoisomers

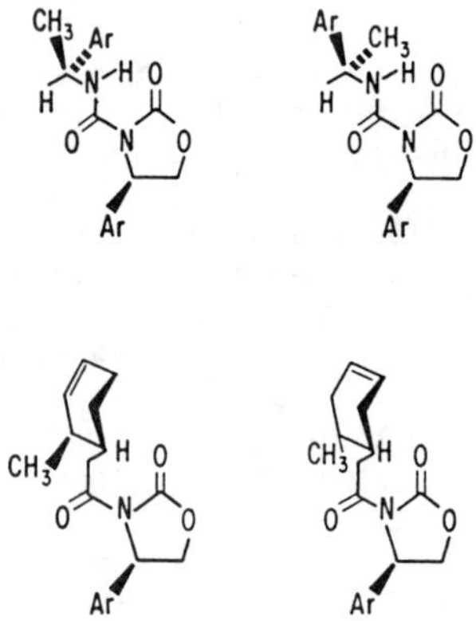

Figure 12. (R)-4-phenyl-1,2,3-oxazolidone derivatives

0.2 ppm, offering additional confirmation of configurational assignments.

The syntheses were completed by following essentially the commercial procedure and adding HCl to enantiomerically pure cyclohexene acids. The esterified mixtures were then subjected to preparative HPLC. Each isolated component would, of course, be configurationally pure. Commercial trimedlure was tested in field traps with wicks that had been baited with 50 mg each (Figure 13). The 1S,2S,4R-enantiomer of "C" was more effective even at 5 mg/wick. Since this enantiomer makes up more than 10% of the commercial lure, and another component (as a racemate) has also shown some activity, there is a hint that isomeric purity may provide a better lure.

Since, the original presentation of this paper, the pheromone of the Mediterranean fruit fly has been identified (23). The compounds, 3,4-dihydro-2H-pyrrole, ethyl-E-3-octenoate, E,E,-α-farnesene, and geranyl acetate, bear no obvious resemblance to the active components of trimedlure. The origin of the biological activity of the synthetic, therefore, remains enigmatic.

Structure	Compound	Configuration	Total Caught (15 reps)
Commercial Trimedlure (50 mg/wick)		-	963
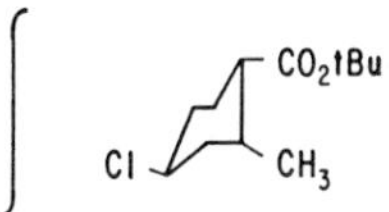 CO_2tBu, Cl, CH_3	"C"	1S,2S,4R	1584
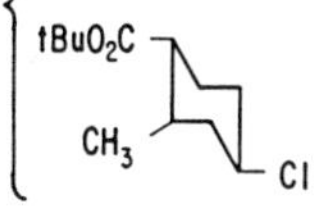 $tBuO_2C$, CH_3, Cl	"C"	1R,2R,4S	273
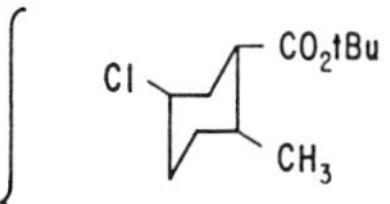 CO_2tBu, Cl, CH_3	"A"	1S,2S,5R	529
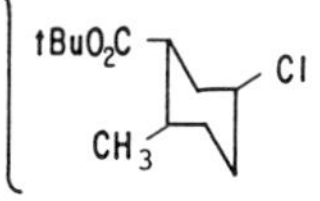 $tBuO_2C$, Cl, CH_3	"A"	1R,2R,5S	402

Figure 13. Stereoisomers tested at 5 mg/wick.

Literature Cited

1. Leonhardt, B. A.; Beroza, M. "Insect Pheromone Technology", ACS Symposium Series 190, Am. Chem. Soc., Washington, D. C., 1982.
2. Silverstein, R. M., "Enantiomeric Composition and Bioactivity of Chiral Semiochemicals in Insects," in "Chemical Ecology: Odour Communication," Ritter, F. J., Ed., Elsevier/North-Holland Biochemical Press, New York, 1979, pp. 133-146.
3. Sonnet, P. E.; Carney, R. L.; Henrick, C. A. J. Chem. Ecol. 1985, 11, 1371-1385.
4. Evans, D. A.; Takacs, J. M.; McGee, L. R.; Ennis, M. D.; Mathre, D. J.; Bartroli, J. Pure and Appl. Chem. 1981, 53, 1109-1127.
5. Evans, D. A. Aldrichimica Acta 1982, 15, 23-32.
6. Ade, E.; Helmchen, G.; Heilegenmann, G. Tetrahedron Lett. 1981, 21, 1137-1140.
7 Sonnet, P. E.; Heath, R. R. J. Chromatogr. 1982, 238, 41-50.
8. Pirkle, W. H.; Hauske, J. R. J. Org. Chem. 1977, 42, 1839-1844.
9. Sakagami, S. J. Chromatogr. 1982, 246, 121-125, and earlier refs. cited.
10. Sonnet, P. E. J. Chem. Ecol. 1984, 10, 771-781.
11. Sonnet, P. E.; Uebel, E. C.; Harris, R. L.; Miller, R. W. J. Chem. Ecol. 1977, 3, 245-249.
12 Carlson, D. A.; Langley, P.A.; Huyten, P. Science 1978, 201, 750-753.
13. Smith, R. F. Bull. Entomol. Soc. Am. 1966, 12, 108-110.
14. Sonnet, P. E. J. Org. Chem. 1982, 47, 3793-3796.
15. $LiEt_3BH$ has a limited shelf life, cf footnote (14) of ref. 14.
16. Guss, P. L.; Tumlinson, J. H.; Sonnet, P. E.; Proveaux, A. J. J. Chem. Ecol. 1982, 8, 545-556.
17. Krysan, J. L.; Wilkin, P. H.; Tumlinson, J. H.; Sonnet, P. E.; Carney, R. L.; Guss, P. L. Ann. Entomol. Soc. Am. 1986, 79, 742-746.
18. Guss, P. L.; Carney, R. L.; Sonnet, P. E.; Tumlinson, J. H. Environ. Entomol. 1983, 12, 1296-1300.
19. Chambers, D. L. "Attractants for fruit fly survey and control," in "Chemical Control of Insect Behavior: Theory and Application," H. H. Shorey & J. J. McKelvey, Jr., Eds., John Wiley & Sons, Inc. New York, 1977, pp. 327-344.
20. Mcgovern, T. P.; Beroza, M. J. Org. Chem. 1966, 31, 1472-1477.
21. Sonnet, P. E.; McGovern, T. P.; Cunningham, R. T. J. Org. Chem. 1984, 49, 4639-4643.
22. Pirkle, W. H.; Simmons, K. A. J. Org. Chem. 1983, 48, 2520-2527.
23. Baker, R.; Herbert, R. H.; Grant, G. G. J. Chem. Soc., Chem. Commun. 1985, 824-825.

RECEIVED May 15, 1987

Chapter 34

Chemical Hybridizing Agents

Synthesis of Racemic *cis*- and *trans*-Methanoproline

Willy D. Kollmeyer [1], S. K. Barrett, and D. H. Flint [1]

Biological Sciences Research Center, Shell Agricultural Chemical Company, P.O. Box 4248, Modesto, CA 95352

Chemicals that affect pollen viability have potential value to plant breeders for production of F_1 hybrids and seed. The non-protein amino acid [1R-(1α,2β,5α)]-3-azabicyclo[3.1.0]-hexane-2-carboxylic acid, otherwise known as cis-3,4-methano-L-proline, is such a material. It was originally isolated from the seeds of Aesculus parviflora, and the sole literature synthesis involved methylenation of a dihydroproline derivative with hazardous diazomethane. In this work, a new and convenient method capable of yielding multigram amounts of both cis- and trans-methanoproline isomers as racemic hydrochloride salts has been devised. This route, which starts from 1,2-cyclopropanedicarboxylic acid and proceeds via 3-azabicyclo[3.1.0]hexane derivatives, is described.

In plant breeding programs the search for improved hybrids involves crossing different parental lines and evaluating the resulting F_1 progeny. Control of male fertility is an important step in this process (1). For example, a corn plant can be emasculated mechanically with ease, because the male flowers are located in the upper part of the plant at a suitable distance above the female flowers. Detasseling prevents any self-pollination, and a plant altered in this way can only function as a female parent. Then, by relying upon natural cross-pollination, the breeder can use an unaltered plant in an adjacent row as the male parent.

[1]Current address: Experimental Station, E. I. du Pont de Nemours & Co., Wilmington, DE 19898

0097–6156/87/0355–0401$06.00/0
© 1987 American Chemical Society

This simple but basic technique has been used to great advantage in the development and production of superior corn hybrids. Even though cytoplasmic male sterility supplanted detasseling for a time, mechanical control of male fertility is currrently the method of choice in hybrid corn seed production (1).

Cytoplasmic Male Sterility. Unfortunately, large-scale mechanical emasculation cannot be applied to all crops of interest. In wheat, for example, the pollen-bearing anthers and female stigmas lay side by side within each floret of a spikelet. Removal of anthers with small, hand-held instruments obviously has utility only for small-scale hybridization experiments. Nevertheless, by crossing a female parent endowed with cytoplasmic male sterility with a male parent that has fertility-restoring genes, one can achieve hybrid wheat seed production. This technology, however, has limitations: compared to detasseling in corn, it is much more time consuming and does not allow all existing lines to be examined as experimental parents (1).

Chemical Hybridizing Agents. For these reasons chemical control of male fertility has been a long sought goal, especially for crops that are normally self-pollinating such as wheat (1-8). An effective chemical hybridizing agent could have potential value not only for plant breeding research studies, but also for commercial production of F_1 hybrids.

Recently, the non-protein amino acid [1R-(1α,2β,5α)]-3-azabicyclo[3.1.0]hexane-2-carboxylic acid, commonly known as *cis*-3,4-methano-L-proline, was patented as a chemical hybridizing agent for small grain cereal crops (9). This compound was originally isolated from the seeds of *Aesculus parviflora* (10), and the sole literature synthesis involved methylenation of a chiral dihydroproline derivative with hazardous diazomethane (11). Unfortunately, neither of these sources was suitable for providing large quantities of methanoproline for plant breeding field studies. To this end, we devised a new synthesis capable of providing multigram amounts of *cis*- and *trans*-methanoproline isomers as racemic, hydrochloride salts. This route, which starts from 1,2-cyclopropanedicarboxylic acid and proceeds via 3-azabicyclo-[3.1.0]hexane derivatives, is reported here. Experimental details are given in the patent literature (12, 13).

Synthesis of Methanoproline

Following the general procedure of McCoy(14), we subjected a mixture of ethyl chloroacetate and ethyl acrylate to base-catalyzed cyclocondensation (see Figure 1). This reaction provided diethyl 1,2-cyclopropanedicarboxylates 1 as a mixture consisting predominently of the *cis*-isomer. Further enhancement of the *cis* product was achieved by saponification of the reaction mixture to the isomeric mixture of 1,2-cyclopropanedicarboxylic acids 2 and subsequent treatment with thionyl chloride. As a consequence vacuum distillation could be used to cleanly separate the resulting mixture of *cis*-1,2-cyclopropanedicarboxylic acid anhydride 3 and *trans*-1,2-cyclopropanedicarboxylic acid chloride 4 (15). In this way the anhydride 3 was obtained readily in 35-40 g batches starting from one mole each of ethyl chloroacetate and ethyl acrylate (ca. 35% yield overall).

The next sequence involved conversion of the anhydride 3 to 3-azabicyclo[3.1.0]hexane 9 as shown in Figure 2. Although the ^{1}H NMR spectrum of this bicyclic amine has been described in the literature (16), details of its preparation have not been given. In this work treatment of the anhydride 3 with benzylamine at elevated temperature gave good yields of the corresponding bicyclic imide 5. By altering the reaction conditions, we isolated the intermediate acid amide 7 and its benzylammonium salt 6. Reduction of the bicyclic imide 5 to the N-benzyl bicyclic amine 8 with the soluble reagent sodium bis(2-methoxyethoxy)aluminum hydride (Redal) was essentially quantitative. Although amine 8 could be distilled, crude product was sufficiently pure for the next step. Thus, palladium-catalyzed hydrogenolysis of either material afforded the desired bicyclic amine 9. Even though this conversion was essentially quantitative, a lower isolated yield resulted from carryover of amine 9 with the ethanolic forerun in the workup by distillation. This inconvenience was circumvented by adding to the solution one equivalent of hydrochloric acid before removal of ethanol. Then the well-behaved hydrochloride 10 was obtained in quantitative yield as a crystalline mass by removing solvent at reduced pressure. When prepared according to Figure 2, the bicyclic amine 9 afforded a ^{1}H NMR spectrum that compared favorably with the literature spectrum (16).

Another route to amine 10 used the isomerically-mixed 1,2-cyclopropanedicarboxylic acid 2 directly without recourse to the anhydride 3. Thus, ca. one mole of crude acid 2 was treated with benzylamine at 180°C to afford a crystalline sample of impure imide 5 (72%). Nevertheless, when this impure material was reduced with lithium aluminum hydride, the amine 8 (68%) was isolated by distillation in a high state of purity. As before, catalytic hydrogenolysis of the N-benzyl group led to a quantitative yield of the bicyclic amine hydrochloride 10. In this

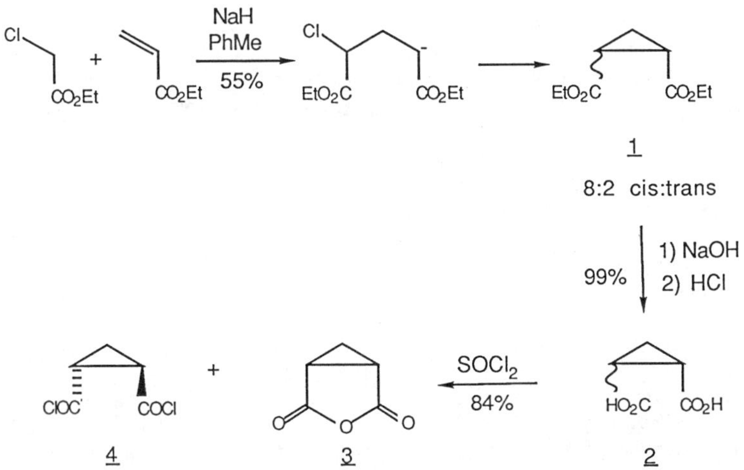

Figure 1. Synthesis of 1,2-Cyclopropanedicarboxylic Acid and Derivatives

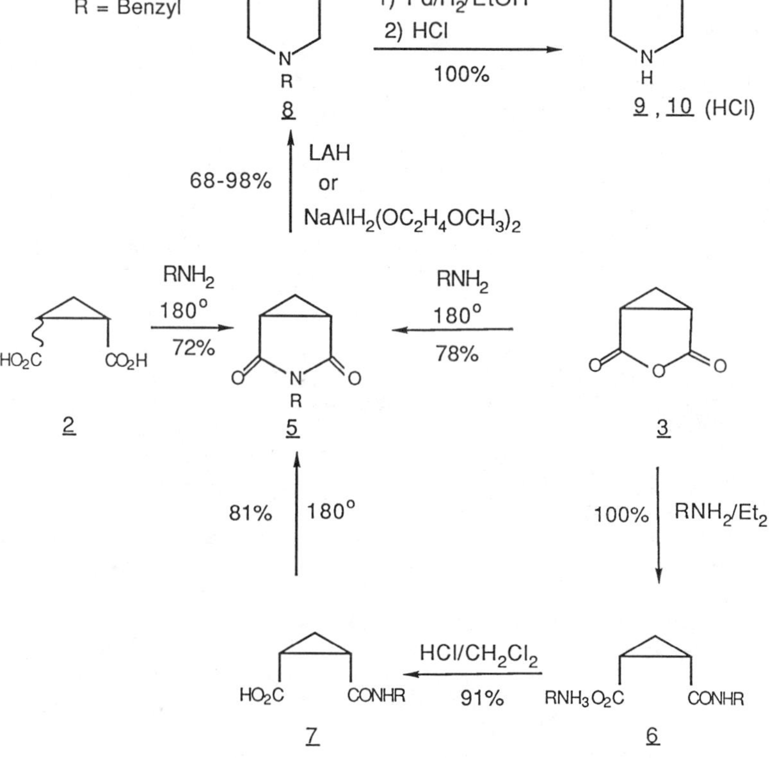

Figure 2. Synthesis of 3-Azabicyclo[3.10]hexane

way, amine 10 was obtained in 27% overall yield starting from ethyl chloroacetate and ethyl acrylate. By comparison, the preparation of amine 10 via anhydride 3 afforded an overall yield of 30%.

The next stage of the methanoproline synthesis made use of the chemistry of piperidine and pyrrolidine to which the chemistry of bicyclic amine 9 is clearly related. The literature teaches the N-chlorination and dehydrochlorination of piperidine or pyrrolidine to afford solutions of the reactive cyclic imines 1-piperideine (17, 18) and 1-pyrroline (19). These electrophlic imines readily add hydrogen cyanide (20-22); and hydrolyses of the resulting α-cyano amines constitute straightforward routes to pipecolic acid (21) and proline (22), respectively. Therefore, the model reactions shown in Figure 3 were carried out for application to the chemical conversion of bicyclic amine 9. (At the time of this work, Reference 22 had not yet appeared.) Of special note was the two stage use of sodium bisulfite followed by sodium cyanide: in this way, handling hydrogen cyanide *per se* was avoided.

With this experience in hand, the amine hydrochloride 10 was transformed into the aminonitrile 14 as shown in Figure 4. This entire sequence was carried out on an approximate 0.5 mole scale via five separate reactions without isolation of intermediates to give a 67% overall yield of aminonitrile 14 based on amine 10. Thus, the amine hydrochloride 10 was neutralized with concentrated potassium hydroxide, and the liberated free amine 9 was taken up in ether. Treatment of this solution with N-chlorosuccinimide (NCS) gave a solution of the N-chloroamine 11. Further addition of ethanolic potassium hydroxide effected dehydrochlorination. The resultant bicyclic imine 12 in ethanolic ether was sequentially treated with aqueous sodium bisulfite and then solid sodium cyanide. The desired aminonitrile 14 was isolated as a distillable liquid.

A further modification (not shown in Figure 4) eliminated the need for a separate neutralization of amine salt 10 and replaced the previous chlorinating agent N-chlorosuccinimide with ordinary household bleach. Thus, salt 10 was added directly to an aqueous mixture of sodium bicarbonate and sodium hypochlorite. The resulting N-chloroamine 11 was taken up in ether and processed as before to give nitrile 14 in an overall yield of 64%. This compared favorably with the previous yield of 67% for the conversion of amine hydrochloride 10 to nitrile 14.

The last step, barium hydroxide-catalyzed hydrolysis of the aminonitrile 14 followed by sulfuric acid neutralization, gave a racemic mixture of *cis*- and *trans*-methanoproline. After removal of barium sulfate and solvent, trituration of the residue with ethanol afforded

$(CH_2)n$ NCS Et_2O → $(CH_2)n$ N–Cl → KOH EtOH → $(CH_2)n$ N

n=o, pyrrolidine
n=1, piperidine

$NaHSO_3$ H_2O

$(CH_2)n$ CO_2H ← 1)$Ba(OH)_2$ 2) H_2SO_4 ← $(CH_2)n$ CN ← NaCN H_2O ← $(CH_2)n$ SO_3Na

n=0, proline, 79% n=0, 33%
n=1, pipecolic acid, 65% n=1, 63%

Figure 3. α-Carboxylation of Pyrrolidine and Piperidine

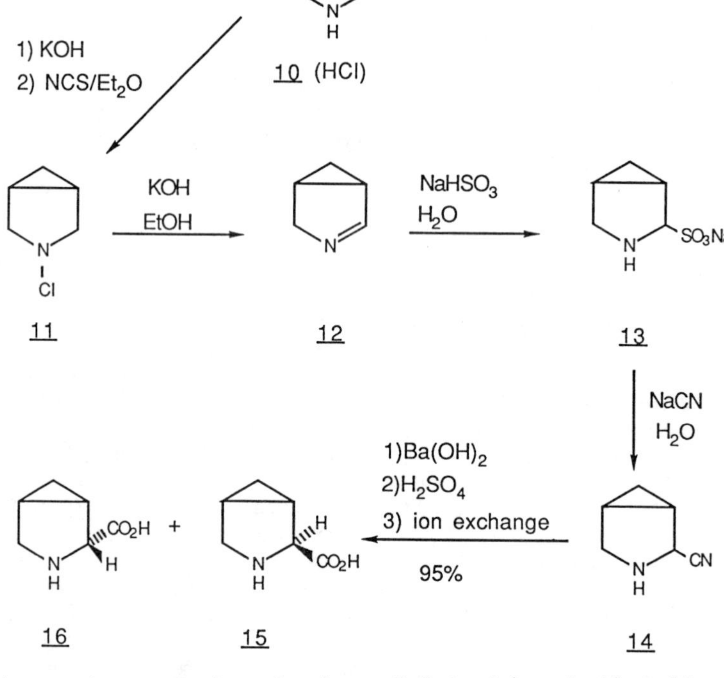

Figure 4. α-Carboxylation of 3-Azabicyclo[3.1.0]-hexane

a trans-enriched crystalline material (ca. 1.5:1 trans:cis by ^{1}H NMR). Concentration of the mother liquor gave a tacky solid enriched in the cis-isomer (ca. 2.2:1). The combined crude product (95%) had an overall trans:cis isomer ratio of 55:45.

The cis-enriched fraction was purified in 5 g batches by ion exchange chromatography on Dowex 50-X8 resin with 1.5 N hydrochloric acid as eluent. Under these conditions, the cis-isomer eluted first (11). Both amino acids 15 and 16 were obtained as analytically pure, crystalline hydrochlorides upon evaporation of the acid eluates. No evidence (^{1}H NMR) of any cyclopropyl ring opening was noted.

The cis and trans isomers of methanoproline, either individually (11) or as a mixture, are easily recognized and distinguished from one another by ^{1}H NMR. The methine proton of the $NCHCO_2$ group occurs as a doublet at δ 4.3 (D_2O) in the cis isomer, whereas the trans isomer has a singlet at δ 4.1. The hydrochloride salts 15 and 16 show a similar splitting pattern, but the signals occur at slightly lower fields: cis, δ 4.4, doublet; trans, δ 4.2, singlet. These splitting patterns, which arise from coupling with the adjacent cyclopropyl proton, are in qualitative agreement with the Karplus rule (23). On this basis the precursor aminonitrile 14 appeared to be a trans isomer, because the NCHCN proton resonance was a singlet at δ 3.9. However, GCMS analysis revealed two components, each having an appropriate parent ion with m/z 108. The isomeric composition of nitrile 14 was, therefore, unclear.

Further improvements to this route to methanoproline and the syntheses of related amino acids have been reported elsewhere (24). In this way, chemical manipulation of 3-azabicyclo[3.1.0]hexane has allowed the preparation of multi-kilogram quantities of both cis- and trans-methanoprolines (24).

LITERATURE CITED

1. Poehlman, J. M. "Breeding Field Crops", 2nd ed.; Avi Publishing Company, Inc.: Westport, Connecticut, 1979; Chapters 6 and 11.
2. Hoaglund, A. R.; Elliot, F. C.; Rasmussen, L. W. Agron. J. 1953, 45, 468-472.
3. Chopra, V. L.; Jain, S. K.; Swaminathan, M. S. Indian J. Genet. Plant Breed. 1960, 20, 188-199.
4. Porter, K. B.; Wiese, A. F. Crop Science 1961, 1, 381-382.
5. Kaul, C. L.; Singh, S. P. Indian J. Plant Physiol. 1967, 10, 112-118.
6. Rowell, P. L.; Miller, D. G. Crop Science 1971, 11, 629-631.
7. Fairey, D. T.; Stoskopf, N. C. ibid 1975, 15, 29-32.

8. Berhe, T.; Miller, D. G. ibid 1978, 18, 35-38.
9. Kerr, M. W. U.S. Patent 4,047,930, 1977.
10. Fowden, L.; Smith A. Phytochem. 1969, 8, 437-443.
11. Fujimoto, Y.; Irreverre, F.; Karle, J. M.; Karle, I. L.; Witkop, B. J. Am. Chem. Soc. 1971, 93, 3471-3477.
12. Kollmeyer, W. D. U.S. Patent 4,183,857, 1980.
13. Kollmeyer, W. D. U. S. Patent 4,225,499, 1980.
14. McCoy, L. L. J. Am. Chem. Soc., 1958, 80, 6568-6572.
15. Oda, R.; Shono, T.; Oku, A.; Takao, H. Makromolekulare Chemie 1963, 67, 124-131.
16. Wendisch, D.; Naegele, W. Org. Magn. Resonance 1970, 2, 619-624.
17. Schopf, C.; Komzak, A.; Braun, F.; Jacobi, E.; Bormuth, M. L.; Bullnheimer, M.; Hagel, I. Justus Liebigs Ann. Chem. 1948, 559, 1-42 .
18. Bender, D. R.; Bjeldanes, L. F.; Knapp, D. R.; Rapoport, H. J. Org. Chem. 1975, 40, 1264-1269.
19. Fuhlhage, D. W.; VanderWerf, C. A. J. Am. Chem. Soc. 1958, 80, 6249-6254.
20. Grob, C. A.; Fischer, H. P.; Link, H.; Renk, E. Helv. Chim Acta 1963, 46, 1190-1206.
21. Bohme, H.; Ellenberg, H.; Herboth, O. E.; Lehners, W. Chem. Ber. 1959, 92, 1608-1613.
22. Schmidt, U.; Poisel, H. Angew. Chem. Int. Ed. Engl. 1977, 16, 777.
23. Jackman, L. M.; Sternhell, S. "Applications of Nuclear Magnetic Resonance Spectroscopy in Organic Chemistry", 2nd ed.; Pergamon Press: New York, 1969; pp. 281-283.
24. Day, J. A.; Kollmeyer, W. D.; Mason, R. F.; Searle, R. J. G.; Wood, D. A. "Pesticide Chemistry: Human Welfare and the Environment"; Miyamoto, J.; Kearney, P. C., Eds.; Vol. 1, Pergamon Press: Oxford, 1983; pp. 159-164.

RECEIVED May 15, 1987

Chapter 35

Overview of Synthetic Approaches to Strigol and Its Analogs

O. D. Dailey, Jr., Armand B. Pepperman, Jr., and S. L. Vail

Southern Regional Research Center, Agricultural Research Service, U.S. Department of Agriculture, New Orleans, LA 70179

Strigol is a very effective germination stimulant for parasitic weeds in the genus Striga (witchweed). This compound is available only in minute quantities from natural sources. An attractive method of control of witchweed and other parasitic weeds such as Orobanche (broomrape) would involve treatment of an infected field with a biosynthetic product (such as strigol) or synthetic analog to induce suicidal germination of the weed seed in the absence of a host plant. The need exists to prepare sufficient quantities of strigol and its analogs to permit extensive laboratory testing and to determine their utility as control agents when applied to infested fields. The total syntheses of strigol developed by Sih, Raphael, and Brooks are discussed. In addition, a number of partial syntheses, representing alternative approaches to intermediates in Sih's preparation, are presented. A new synthetic route to strigol, utilizing the inexpensive starting materials mesityl oxide and ethyl acetoacetate, has been developed. Finally, a number of simplified two-, three-, and four-ring analogs of strigol have been prepared, several of which have shown activity as Striga and Orobanche germination stimulants.

(+)-Strigol is a very effective germination stimulant for the parasitic weeds in the genus Striga (witchweed) (1). Recently the absolute structure of natural (+)-strigol has been established as shown in 1 (2). Natural (+)-strigol induces greater than 50% germination of witchweed [Striga asiatica (L.) Kuntze] seeds at a concentration of 10^{-11} M (1). Synthetic (±)-strigol effects comparable germination in the concentration range of 10^{-10} to 10^{-12} M (3,4). In one study (5), synthetic (±)-strigol showed activity at 10^{-16} M, but these results have not been reproduced.

This chapter is not subject to U.S. copyright.
Published 1987, American Chemical Society

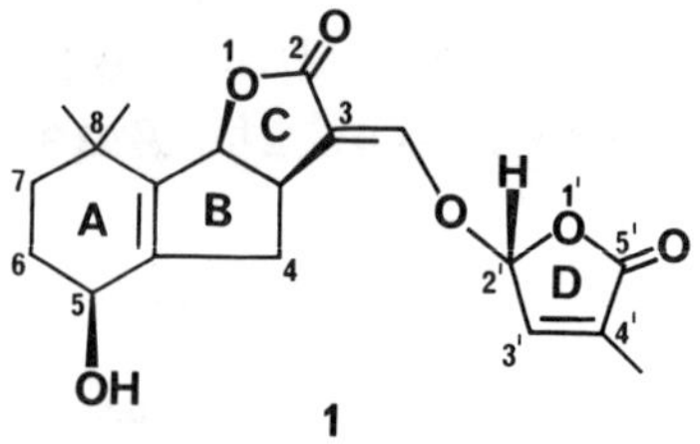

The parasitic weeds of *Striga* species are thought to germinate primarily in response to a *chemical* signal of the host plant. Corn, rice, sugarcane, and *Sorghum* are the major crop plants affected by *Striga*. Recently, *the first* characterization of a germination stimulant for *Striga* derived from a natural host (*Sorghum*) was reported (6). The compound, a hydroquinone derivative, is highly unstable and consequently would have no practical utility. Strigol was originally isolated in small quantities from the root exudates of cotton (a nonhost plant) (1). It has not been identified in exudates of any host plant nor does it appear to be available from any natural source in the quantities required for field testing.

Striga asiatica (L.) Kuntze, one of several species of *Striga* found commonly in the Eastern Hemisphere, was found in North and South Carolina in 1956 (7). The seed has the capability to remain dormant and viable in the ground for fifteen to twenty years until stimulated by a chemical or chemicals released by the young roots of certain plants. The germinated seed rapidly develops a radicle, which receives a second chemical signal from the host (the haustorial initiation factor) upon contact with the host root. Thereupon, the tip of the radicle is transformed into a haustorium which attaches itself to the host root. The *Striga* derives carbohydrates, water, minerals, and some photosynthates from the infected parasitized plant which generally appears drought-stricken and often dies if the parasitic plant is not removed. Crop losses approaching 100% occur in heavily infested fields (7-9). In 1957, federal and state quarantines were invoked to prevent the spread of witchweed. Although the quarantine program has been effective, and the control and eradication program has permitted considerable acreage to be removed from quarantine, the problem still exists and further research is needed (10).

Because of the lengthy periods of viability of the seeds of *Striga* and *Orobanche* (broomrape) in the soil, effective control of these parasitic weeds is extremely difficult. An attractive method of control would involve treatment of an infected field with a biosynthetic product (such as strigol) or synthetic analog to induce suicidal germination of the weed seed in the absence of a host plant. The results of field tests with ethylene (11) and synthetic strigol analogs (12) offer evidence of the utility of this method of control.

To date, probably less than ten grams of (±)-strigol has been synthesized. For extensive field studies and basic biological studies a large quantity (in excess of 100 g) is required. Although several syntheses of strigol have been reported, the need for an economic synthesis adaptable to large scale preparation still exists.

Syntheses of Strigol

Four total syntheses of strigol have been reported in the literature (13-15). In each case, (±)-strigol was prepared by a convergent synthesis in which the final step was the alkylation of the tricyclic hydroxymethylene lactone **2** with the bromobutenolide **3**.

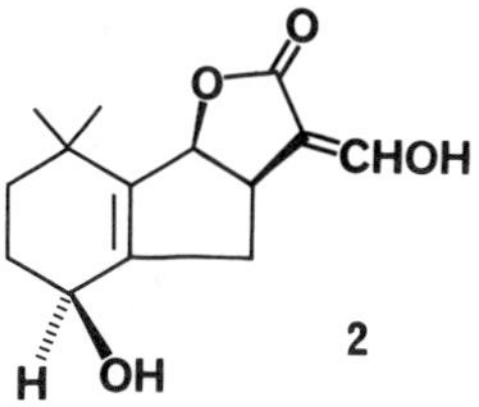

2

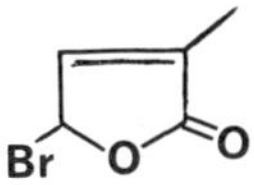

3

Shortly after the structure of strigol was established, its total synthesis was reported by Sih and co-workers (13) and by Raphael *et al.* (14). Sih's synthetic approach will be presented in its entirety as it provides a useful framework for discussion of other total and partial syntheses of strigol.

Sih's Synthesis of Strigol. Sih and co-workers utilized citral as starting material for the preparation of **2**, representing the A, B, and C rings of strigol. The anil of citral was converted to a mixture of α-cyclocitral **(4)**, and β-cyclocitral **(5)** (Equation 1).

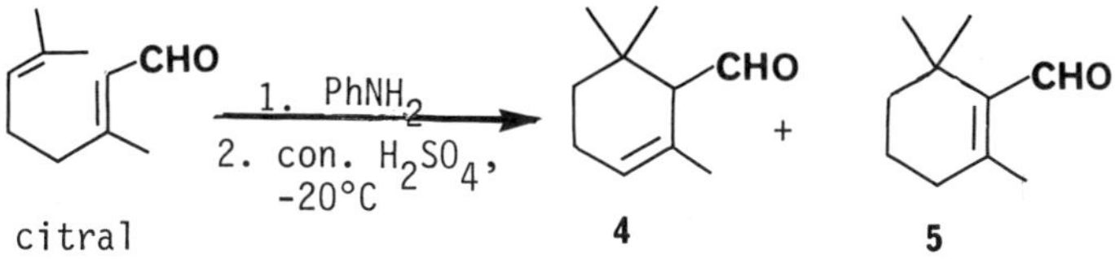

citral —(1. $PhNH_2$; 2. con. H_2SO_4, -20°C)→ **4** + **5** (1)

Depending upon the conditions employed, either **4** or **5** could be obtained in good yield, and both were converted to the enone **9** by separate routes. As shown in Scheme I, **9** could be prepared from α-cyclocitral (4) in four steps in 34% overall yield. The best route developed for the transformation of β-cyclocitral (5) to **9** is outlined in Scheme II. Enone **9** could be obtained in five steps in 47% overall yield as follows: reaction of **5** with oxygen in heptane at 0-5°C in the presence of 5% platinum on carbon furnished the crude acid **10** in 70% yield; methylation afforded the pure ester **11** in 84% yield; treatment with bromine at 0-10°C provided the crude bromo ester **12** in quantitative yield; hydrolysis of **12** gave the hydroxy ester **13** in 81% yield following column chromatography; finally, Jones oxidation furnished **9** in 98% yield.

The elaboration of the tricyclic hydroxymethylene lactone **2** is summarized in Scheme III. Treatment of enone **9** with a 20% excess of N-bromosuccinimide (NBS) in refluxing carbon tetrachloride under the

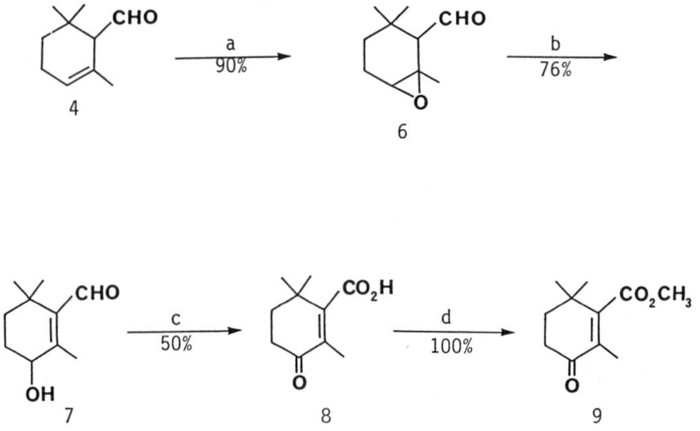

CHO

a 90%

CHO

b 76%

4

6

CHO

c 50%

CO_2H

d 100%

CO_2CH_3

OH 7

8

9

[a]MCPBA. [b]Pyrrolidine, ether. [c]CrO_3/H_2SO_4. [d]CH_3I, K_2CO_3.

Scheme I. Sih's conversion of α-cyclocitral to enone 9.

CHO

a 70%

CO_2H

b 84%

5

10

CO_2CH_3

c 100%

CO_2CH_3

d 81%

11

Br 12

CO_2CH_3

e 98%

CO_2CH_3

OH 13

9

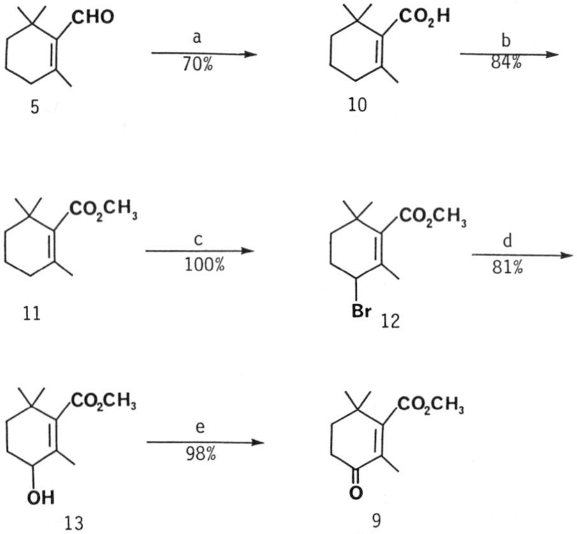

[a]O_2, 5%Pt/C, heptane. [b]CH_3I, K_2CO_3, acetone. [c]Br_2, $CHCl_3$, $h\nu$, N_2, 0-10 °C. [d]H_2O,Δ. [e]CrO_3/H_2SO_4.

Scheme II. Sih's conversion of β-cyclocitral to enone 9.

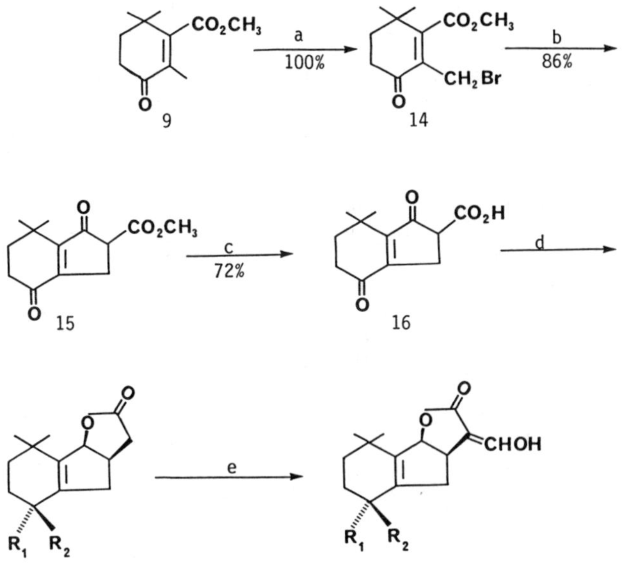

CO_2CH_3 a 100% CO_2CH_3 CH_2Br b 86%

9 14

CO_2CH_3 c 72% CO_2H d

15 16

e CHOH

R_1 R_2 R_1 R_2

17, R_1 = H; R_2 = OH 26%

18, R_1 = OH; R_2 = H

2, R_1 = H; R_2 = OH 78%

[a] NBS, CCl_4, hν, Δ. [b] (1) $NaCH(CO_2CH_3)_2$; (2) HOAc.
[c] (1) $BrCH_2CO_2CH_3$, K_2CO_3, acetone; (2) HOAc, 6 N HCl, Δ.
[d] (1) DIBAH, CH_2Cl_2, -70 °C; (2) 20% H_2SO_4. [e] HCO_2CH_3, NaH, ether.

Scheme III. Synthesis of the tricyclic hydroxymethylene lactone 2.

illumination of an incandescent lamp afforded a quantitative yield of crude bromo ester **14**. Reaction of **14** with the sodium salt of dimethyl malonate and subsequent neutralization with acetic acid furnished the bicyclic diketone **15** in 86% yield. Alkylation with methyl bromoacetate and subsequent acid hydrolysis gave the diketo acid **16** in 72% yield. Treatment of **16** with 3.5 equivalents of diisobutylaluminum hydride (DIBAH) afforded a mixture of hydroxy lactones **17** and **18**. Column chromatography and crystallization of the purified mixture afforded the desired isomer **17** in 26% yield. Formylation of **17** provided the hydroxymethylene lactone **2** in 78% yield.

The synthetic route followed for the preparation of the bromobutenolide **3** is presented in Scheme IV. 3-Methyl-2-furoic acid **19** was prepared in three steps by the literature method (16). Three additional steps produced **3**: photooxygenation of **19** in ethanol with subsequent stannous chloride reduction of epoxides to give the alkoxybutenolide **20** (17); hydrolysis in boiling water to the hydroxybutenolide **21** (18); treatment of **21** with carbon tetrabromide and triphenylphosphine (19).

Finally, alkylation of **2** with excess **3** in the presence of anhydrous K_2CO_3 in hexamethylphosphoric triamide (HMPA) afforded a diastereomeric mixture of (±)-strigol **1** and (±) -2'-epistrigol (**22**, Equation 2). Column chromatography and crystallization of the isolated components furnished **1** in 27% yield and **22** in 18% yield. Using citral as starting material, the overall yield of **1** was 0.6% _via_ α-cyclocitral **(4)** or 0.9% _via_ β-cyclocitral **(5)**.

Raphael's Syntheses of Strigol. In 1974, Raphael and co-workers presented two synthetic routes to (±)-strigol (14). These two approaches differ in the steps in the preparation of the hydroxy lactone **17**. The first approach utilizes 2,2-dimethylcyclohexanone **23** as starting material (Scheme V). Treatment of the condensation product **24** with phosphorus pentoxide in methanesulfonic acid at room temperature for 5 minutes produced the bicyclic enone **25** (representing the A and B rings of strigol) in 53% yield. Reaction of **25** with sodium hydride and diethyl oxalate followed by methyl bromoacetate and subsequent removal of the oxalyl grouping by treatment with sodium methoxide in refluxing methanol afforded the methyl ester **26** in 52% yield. In order to introduce the 5-hydroxy group of strigol, **26** was converted to the mixture of acetoxy-esters **27** in 64% yield by sequential treatment with NBS and silver acetate in acetic acid. The hydrolysis products **28** were reduced with DIBAH to afford a mixture of **17** and **18**. Separation by preparative layer chromatography provided the desired alcohol **17** in 22% yield and crude **18** in 23% yield. The overall yield of **17** from **23** was 3.5%; in Sih's synthesis **17** was prepared from citral in 4.2% yield.

The remaining steps of Raphael's synthesis of strigol were the same as Sih's with the exception that bromobutenolide **3** was prepared in a different manner (Equation 3). 2-Methyl-3-butenoic acid was converted to 3-methyl-2(5H)-furanone (**29**) by the method of Frank-Neumann and Berger (reported yield: 75%) (20). Reaction of **29** with NBS in the presence of benzoyl peroxide afforded **3** in 82% yield.

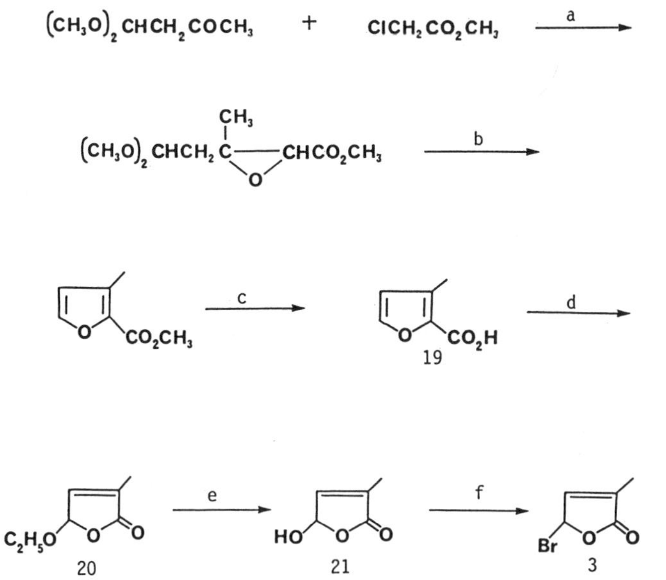

$(CH_3O)_2CHCH_2COCH_3$ + $ClCH_2CO_2CH_3$ $\xrightarrow{a}$

$(CH_3O)_2CHCH_2C(CH_3)$—$CHCO_2CH_3$ (epoxide, O) $\xrightarrow{b}$

CO_2CH_3 $\xrightarrow{c}$ CO_2H 19 $\xrightarrow{d}$

C_2H_5O 20 $\xrightarrow{e}$ HO 21 $\xrightarrow{f}$ Br 3

[a] $NaOCH_3$, ether. [b] 150-160 °C. [c] OH^-. [d] O_2, C_2H_5OH, V_2O_5, hν/Sens. [e] H_2O, Δ. [f] CBr_4, Ph_3P.

Scheme IV. Sih's preparation of the bromobutenolide 3.

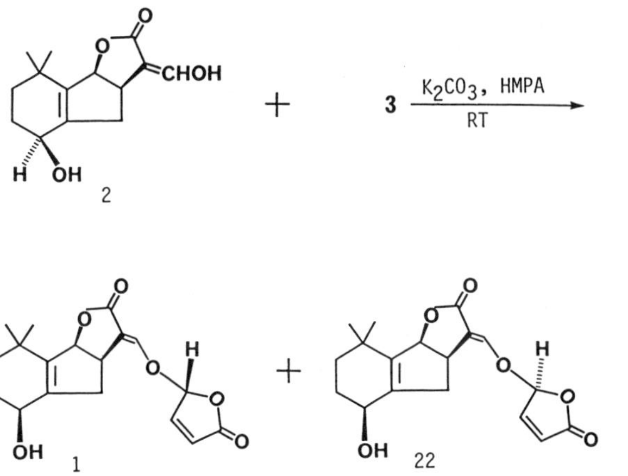

CHOH, H OH 2 + 3 $\xrightarrow[RT]{K_2CO_3,\ HMPA}$

OH 1 + OH 22

Equation 2. Synthesis of strigol and epistrigol (22).

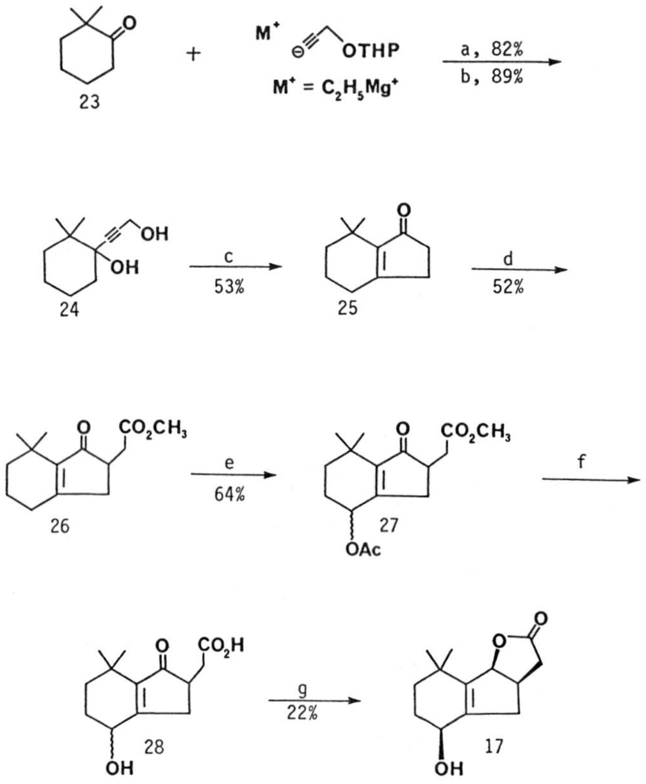

23 + M^+ OTHP $M^+ = C_2H_5Mg^+$ a, 82% b, 89%

24 c 53% 25 d 52%

26 e 64% 27 f

28 g 22% 17

[a] (1) THF, Δ; (2) NH_4Cl. [b] H_2SO_4, CH_3OH, RT. [c] P_2O_5, CH_3SO_3H, RT, 5 min. [d] (1) NaH, $(CO_2Et)_2$, PhH, RT; (2) $BrCH_2CO_2CH_3$, Δ, acetone; (3) $NaOCH_3$, CH_3OH, Δ; (4) 2 N HCl. [e] NBS, αα'-azobis-isobutyronitrile, CCl_4, Δ; (2) HOAc, AgOAc, Δ. [f] (1) CH_3OH, 6 N NaOH, 0 °C; (2) 10 N HCl. [g] (1) DIBAH, CH_2Cl_2, -70 °C; (2) CH_3OH; (3) H_3O^+; (4) chromatography.

Scheme V. Raphael's first route to strigol. Conversion of 2,2-dimethylcyclohexanone to hydroxy lactone 17.

$$\text{CH}_2{=}\text{CH}{-}\text{CH}(\text{CH}_3)\text{CO}_2\text{H} \xrightarrow[\text{CH}_2\text{Cl}_2]{\text{Br}_2} \text{BrCH}_2{-}\text{CHBr}{-}\text{CH}(\text{CH}_3)\text{CO}_2\text{H} \xrightarrow[\text{CHCl}_3]{\text{Et}_3\text{N}} \tag{3}$$

$$\mathbf{29} \xrightarrow[\text{CCl}_4\ \Delta]{\text{NBS, } (\phi\text{CO})_2} \mathbf{3}\ (\text{Br})$$

Raphael's second synthetic route is shown in Scheme VI. In this approach, the bicyclic nitro enone **31**, possessing the proper functionality for elaboration of the A-ring hydroxy of **1**, was prepared by the acid-catalyzed cyclization of nitrodiketone **30**. Attempts to introduce the second A-ring methyl group by treatment of **31** with lithium dimethylcuprate failed. Reaction of **31** with titanium tetrachloride afforded the diketone **32** which was selectively monoketalized to **33**. Reaction with lithium dimethylcuprate furnished the gem-dimethyl compound **34**, which was converted to the diester **35**. Treatment of **35** with acid in an atmosphere of oxygen yielded the unsaturated diketo acid **16** directly, which can be elaborated to strigol as described by Sih. According to Raphael's data, the second route to strigol afforded **16** in 2.4% overall yield.

Brooks' Synthesis of Strigol. In 1982, through a cooperative agreement with the Southern Regional Research Center, D. W. Brooks undertook an improved synthesis of strigol which would be suitable for multigram preparation. The preliminary results of this effort were reported in 1983 with the synthesis of methyl 3-oxo-2,6,6-trimethylcyclohex-1-ene-1-carboxylate **9** in 48% yield from α-ionone **36** (Scheme VII) (21). Sih's procedure (Scheme II) afforded **9** in 26% yield from citral.

In 1985, Brooks reported an improved total synthesis of (±)-strigol utilizing α-ionone as starting material (Scheme VIII) (15,22). The synthesis is patterned after that of Sih and co-workers (Schemes I and III, Equation 2). There are many common intermediates (**6**,**7**,**14**,**41**,**16**,**17**) but all except **7** are prepared by new or modified methods. The conversion of **17** to strigol was in accordance with Sih's procedure except that N-methylpyrrolidone was used instead of HMPA in the reaction of **2** with **3**. Details of the synthesis are discussed by Brooks et al. in the following chapter.

In summary, Brooks' synthesis provided (±)-strigol in 10 steps and 4.4% overall yield from α-ionone or 12 steps and 6.8% overall yield with the recycling of **18**. The preparation is suitable for scale-up and requires only one chromatographic separation.

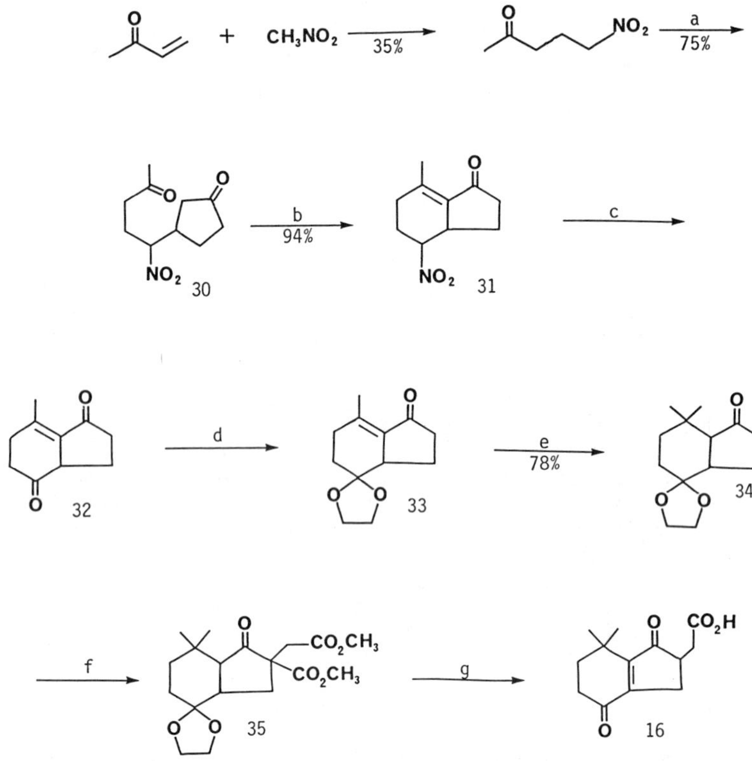

$+ CH_3NO_2$ → 35% ; NO_2 →[a] 75%

NO_2 30 →[b] 94% → NO_2 31 →[c]

32 →[d] 33 →[e] 78% → 34

→[f] CO_2CH_3 CO_2CH_3 35 →[g] CO_2H 16

[a] Cyclopentenone, diisopropylamine, $CHCl_3$, 60 °C. [b] TsOH, PhH, Δ. [c] (1) CH_3OH, $NaOCH_3$; (2) $TiCl_4$, NH_4OAc (aq.). [d] $HOCH_2CH_2OH$, TsOH, PhH, Δ. [e] (1) $LiCuMe_2$, ether, -5 °C, 2 h; (2) satd. NH_4Cl (aq.). [f] (1) Methoxymethylmagnesium carbonate, DMF, 150 °C, N_2, 6 h; (2) 1 N HCl; (3) CH_2N_2; (4) $BrCH_2CO_2CH_3$, acetone, K_2CO_3, Δ. [g] 5% H_2SO_4, O_2, $CH_3OCH_2CH_2OCH_3$, Δ.

Scheme VI. Raphael's second route to strigol. Elaboration of the diketo acid 16.

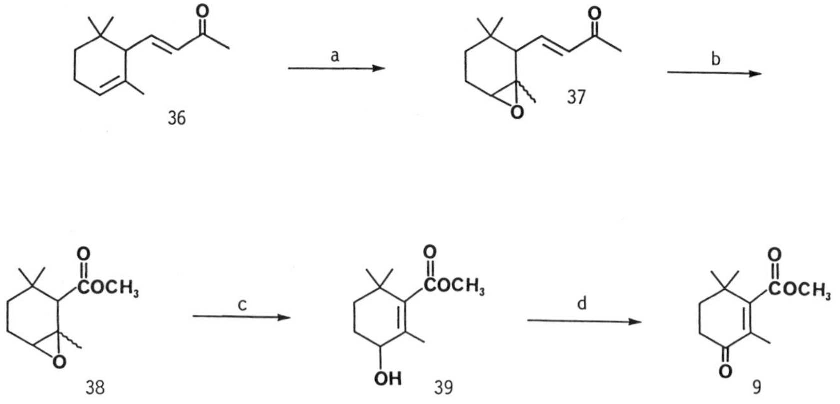

[a] MCPBA, CH_2Cl_2. [b] (1) $NaIO_4$, $KMnO_4$ (cat.), t-BuOH; (2) CH_3I, K_2CO_3, $(CH_3)_2CO$. [c] $NaOCH_3$, CH_3OH. [d] PCC, CH_2Cl_2.

Scheme VII. Brooks' conversion of α-ionone to enone 9.

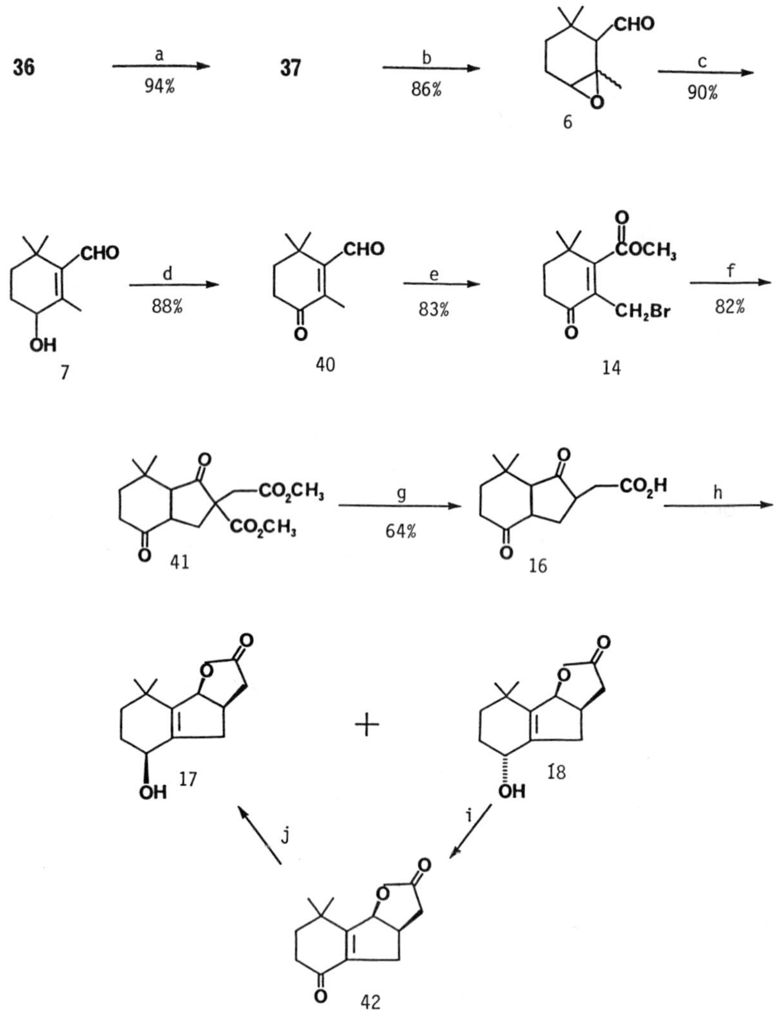

[a] 30% CH_3CO_3H, HOAc, NaOAc, 0 °C. [b] (1) O_3, CH_3OH, -78 °C; (2) Zn, HOAc. [c] Pyrrolidine, ether, 25 °C. [d] Jones reagent. [e] (1) NBS, CCl_4, $h\nu$, 70 °C; (2) CH_3OH, 0 °C. [f] (1) NaH, $CH_2(CO_2CH_3)_2$; (2) $BrCH_2CO_2CH_3$. [g] 6 N HCl, HOAc, 100 °C. [h] $CeCl_3(H_2O)_7$, $NaBH_4$, 0 °C. [i] PCC, CH_2Cl_2, 25 °C. [j] $NaBH_4$.

Scheme VIII. Brooks' improved route to strigol. Conversion of α-ionone to hydroxy lactone 17.

Partial Syntheses of Strigol

A number of partial syntheses of strigol have been reported in the literature (23-27). These syntheses represent alternative approaches to intermediates in Sih's synthesis.

In 1976, Dolby reported the preparation of the hydrindan **15** (Scheme IX) (23). Dimethylpyruvic acid **45** was prepared according to the procedure of Ramage and Simonsen (28). The condensation of hippuric acid (**43**) and acetone yields the oxazolone **44**, which affords **45** upon treatment with concentrated hydrochloric acid. The Friedel-Crafts acylation of ethylene with glutaric anhydride afforded 5-oxo-6-heptenoic acid **46** in low yield (14-45%). Base-catalyzed condensation of **45** with **46** gave the crude dibasic acid **47** in 79% yield. Treatment of **47** with excess diazomethane provided the diester **48** in quantitative yield. The esterification also can be accomplished in 90% yield with DBU and iodomethane (L. J. Dolby, University of Oregon, personal communication, 1979). Base-catalyzed cyclization of **48** afforded **15** in 98% yield.

In 1979, Cooper and Dolby (24) reported a new synthesis of 3-methyl-5-hydroxy-2(5H)-furanone, **21**, precursor to bromobutenolide **3**. Compound **21** was prepared in five steps in 34% overall yield from 3-(p-toluenesulfonyl)butanal.

In 1983, a one-step synthesis of the acid **8** from a mixture of α- and β-cyclocitrals **4** and **5** (Equation 4) was reported (26). A mixture of 45% **4** and 55% **5** in dioxane - water (9:1) was treated with calcium carbonate and freshly crystallized NBS (5.1 equivalents total) to

CHO 4 + CHO 5 —[NBS, $CaCO_3$, 9:1 dioxane-H_2O, hν, Δ]→ CO_2H O 8 (4)

afford **8** in 40% yield (72% yield from **5**). This represents a significant improvement over Sih's process (Scheme I). However, subsequent attempts to reproduce the procedure were unsuccessful (D. W. Brooks, Purdue University, personal communication, 1984).

Synthetic Studies at the Southern Regional Research Center

In 1978, a project was undertaken at the Southern Regional Research Center with the goal of preparing sufficient quantities of strigol and its analogs to permit the broad spectrum of tests necessary to understand the role of these compounds in the germination, growth, and reproduction of witchweed and others parasitic weeds, and to determine their utility as control agents when applied to infested fields. We decided to initiate our investigations in the large-scale preparation of strigol through the modification and improvement of one of the existing synthetic sequences. We selected Sih's synthesis of strigol through α-cyclocitral because it appeared to present fewer experimental problems (29). In several cases the literature yields

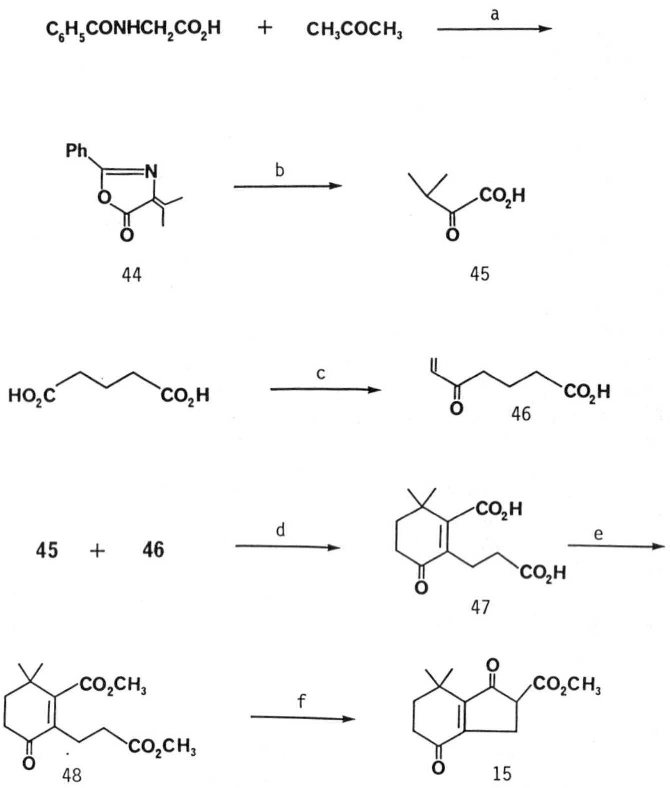

$C_6H_5CONHCH_2CO_2H$ + CH_3COCH_3 $\xrightarrow{a}$

44 $\xrightarrow{b}$ 45

$HO_2C(CH_2)_3CO_2H$ $\xrightarrow{c}$ 46

45 + 46 $\xrightarrow{d}$ 47 $\xrightarrow{e}$

48 $\xrightarrow{f}$ 15

[a] Ac_2O, NaOAc, 110 °C. [b] con. HCl. [c] $AlCl_3$, $CH_2{=}CH_2$, CH_2Cl_2.
[d] (1) 1.5 N KOH (aq.), Δ, 2 h; (2) con. HCl. [e] CH_2N_2 or CH_3I, DBU.
[f] (1) 0.78 N $NaOCH_3$, CH_3OH, Δ, N_2, 2 h; (2) HOAc, 1% HCl.

Scheme IX. Dolby's partial strigol synthesis. Preparation of the hydrindan 15.

could not be duplicated; preparations of **7**, **8**, **15**, **16**, and **17** gave considerably lower yields. Whereas Sih reported that oxidation of **7**

CHO, OH 7 —Jones reagent→ CHO, O 49 —Ag_2O→ CO_2H, O 8 (5)

with excess Jones reagent provided keto acid **8** in 45-55% yield, yields of only 30% were obtainable in our laboratory. We developed a two-step procedure (25) that provided for a substantial improvement in the yield of **8** (Equation 5). In this procedure **7** was treated with Jones reagent over a shorter reaction time to afford the keto aldehyde **49** which was oxidized with alkaline silver(I) oxide to **8** in 70-85% overall yield.

Recently, we developed a new synthetic route to strigol (27; Dailey, Jr., O. D. *J. Org. Chem.*, in press). This approach utilizes ethyl 4-oxo-2,6,6-trimethylcyclohex-2-ene-1-carboxylate **50** as starting material (Scheme X). The primary synthetic target was the diketo acid **16**, an intermediate in the latter stages of both the Sih and Brooks strigol syntheses (Schemes III and VIII).

Enone **50** was prepared in molar quantities by the zinc chloride catalyzed condensation of mesityl oxide with ethyl acetoacetate using a modification of the procedure of Surmatis, *et al.* (30). Distillation of the crude product mixture afforded material consisting of **50** and the isomeric **51** in ratios ranging from 7:1 to better than 10:1 (NMR analysis) in yields in the 27-37% range. The distilled material was sufficiently pure for use in the subsequent reaction.

Enone **50** could be converted to olefin **53** by two different procedures. Treatment of a 8:1 mixture of **50** and **51** with 1,2-ethanedithiol and boron trifluoride etherate (31) and subsequent distillation of the crude product afforded pure dithioketal **54** in 81% yield. Compound **51** did not react under the conditions employed. Raney nickel desulfurization of the dithioketal **52** to **53** was accomplished in high yield (>80%) on a 10-30 g scale; however, the yields decreased substantially (24-29%) when the reaction was done on a larger scale (>100 g).

In the event, a new method was developed for the direct conversion of **50** to **53**. Compound **50** is cleanly reduced to **53** in one to two hours upon treatment with a 2.5-4.0 molar excess of triethylsilane and boron trifluoride etherate at 80-95°C. Compound **51** does not react under these conditions. The reaction proceeded in good yield over a wide range of substrate quantity. Olefin **53** was obtained in 72% yield from 100 g of a 9:1 mixture of **50** and **51**. There are examples in the literature of the reduction of simple aliphatic ketones to the corresponding hydrocarbons using gaseous boron trifluoride and triethylsilane in dichloromethane (32). However, we know of no report of the reduction of a ketone to a methylene compound using boron trifluoride etherate and triethylsilane.

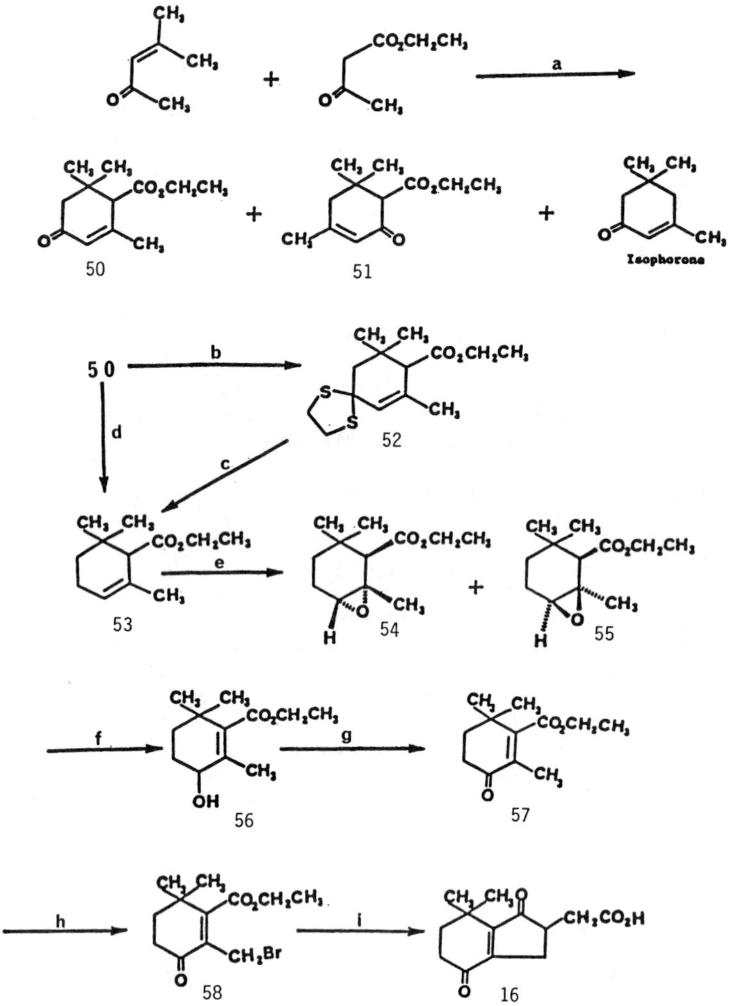

[a] $ZnCl_2$, toluene, heptane, Δ. [b] $HSCH_2CH_2SH$, $BF_3 \cdot Et_2O$, 0 °C→RT. [c] W-2 Raney nickel, EtOH, RT. [d] $BF_3 \cdot Et_2O$, Et_3SiH, 80-95 °C. [e] CH_3CO_3H, NaOAc, CH_2Cl_2, RT. [f] NaOEt, EtOH. [g] Jones reagent. [h] NBS, CCl_4, hν. [i] (1) $CH_2(CO_2CH_3)_2$, NaH, THF, 0 °C; (2) $BrCH_2CO_2Et$, 0 °C→RT; (3) HOAc, 6 N HCl, 66-100 °C.

Scheme X. Dailey's synthesis of the diketo acid 16.

Large scale epoxidation of **53** (50-100 g) with peracetic acid (33) consistently furnished the epoxides **54** and **55** in essentially quantitative yield. Treatment of the epoxides (40-100 g) with sodium ethoxide in refluxing ethanol provided allylic alcohol **56**. Oxidation of **56** (0.50 mmol-0.50 mol) with the Jones reagent (13,34) consistently afforded enone **57** in yields of 95% or better. In large scale conversions of **53** to **57**, the crude intermediate compounds **54**, **55**, and **56** were used directly in the subsequent reaction without further purification. Typically, for the three-step process, **57** is obtained in 95% yield, sufficiently pure for the next reaction.

The conversion of **57** to bromoketone **58** was not as straightforward as expected. The literature procedure (13) for the bromination of the methyl ester **9** (light initiation, 20% excess NBS, refluxing carbon tetrachloride) gave highly variable results. In all instances, a significant amount of bromoketone **59** was formed as

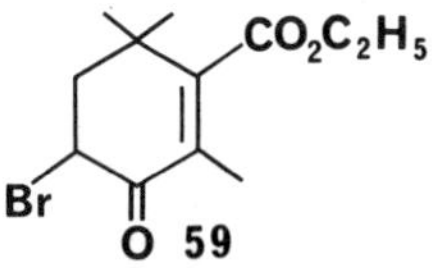

59

side-product. When less than one gram of **57** was brominated, the product mixture consisted of 85-90% **58** and 10-15% **59**. On a larger scale (using 15 to 45 g of **57**) the percentage of **59** increased to 25-42%. It was established that heating the reaction mixture at reflux increased the amount of **59** formed. The amount of **59** formed could be kept at an acceptably low level (0-15%) by using the light as the sole source of heat and maintaining the temperature of the reaction mixture at or below 50°C. In a modification of Brooks' procedure (15, Scheme VIII), bromoketone **58** could be converted directly to diketo acid **16** in 60% yield. The two literature methods for conversion of **16** to the hydroxy lactone **17** were investigated: reduction with diisobutylaluminum hydride (13) and treatment with ceric chloride followed by excess sodium borohydride (15). The latter method was found to give superior results. The synthesis of strigol may be completed as described in the literature (13,15).

Sih's synthesis (13) using citral as starting material affords diketo acid **16** in 16% yield in eight steps. Brooks' procedure (15) using α-ionone as starting material provides **16** in 28% yield in seven steps. With ethyl 4-oxo-2,6,6-trimethylcyclohex-2-ene-1-carboxylate **50** as starting material, **16** can be produced in 38% yield in six steps. The relative low cost of mesityl oxide and ethyl acetoacetate more than offsets the low yield of the condensation reaction producing **50**. Each step of the new synthetic route to **16** is suitable for large-scale production, being based upon inexpensive starting materials and reagents and requiring no chromatographic purification.

Syntheses of Strigol Analogs

Since 1974, the syntheses of a large number of simplified analogs of strigol have been reported. The vast majority of these analogs retain the structure of the C and D rings of strigol.

In 1974, Cassady and Howie reported (35) the preparation of the dilactones **62** and **63** (Equation 6). Compound **63** showed antitumor activity. Results of testing for seed germination activity have not been reported.

CH_3CN, RT, 24 h

60, R = H
61, R = CH_3

(6)

62, R = H
63, R = CH_3

Johnson's Syntheses of Strigol Analogs. The greatest volume of work in the preparation of synthetically simpler analogs of strigol has been performed by Johnson and coworkers (12,36-39) who have prepared two-, three-, and four-ring analogs.

Whereas the bromobutenolide **3** was invariably utilized in the syntheses of strigol, Johnson employed the chloride **64** (38) or the sulfonate **65** (37). Compound **64** could be prepared as shown in Equation 7.

$CH_3CO_2-CH{=}CH_2$ + $CH_3COCO_2C_2H_5$ $\xrightarrow{TiCl_4}$ $CH_3CO_2-CH(Cl)-CH_2-C(OH)(CH_3)CO_2C_2H_5$

(7)

$\xrightarrow[H_2O]{EtOH\text{-}HCl,}$ $\xrightarrow{SOCl_2}$

64

CH_3SO_3

65

Johnson's syntheses of two- and three-ring analogs of strigol were first reported in the form of patents (37,38). Of the two-ring analogs prepared, compound **66** (Equation 8), labeled GR5 (36), showed low-level activity in promoting the germination of both Striga and Orobanche spp. The methyl derivative **67** showed increased activity, especially for Striga spp.

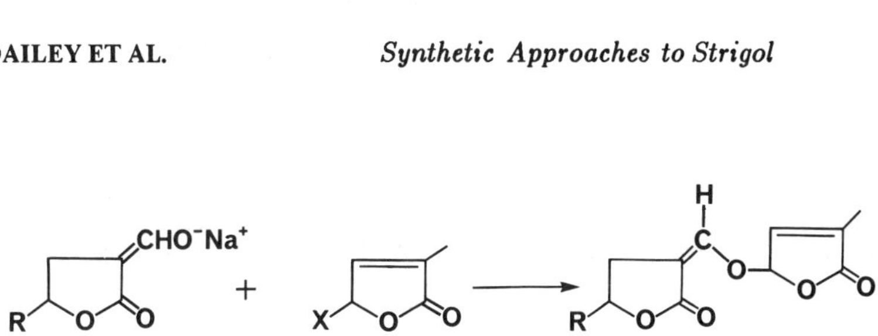

64, X = Cl
65, X = CH_3SO_3

66, R = H
67, R = CH_3

(8)

The three-ring analogs of strigol were prepared from **64** or **65** and the sodium salt of the appropriate bicyclic oxymethylenelactone (36,39). Of the compounds prepared, the isomeric GR-7 (**68**) and GR-28 (**69**), were highly effective in promoting germination of the seeds

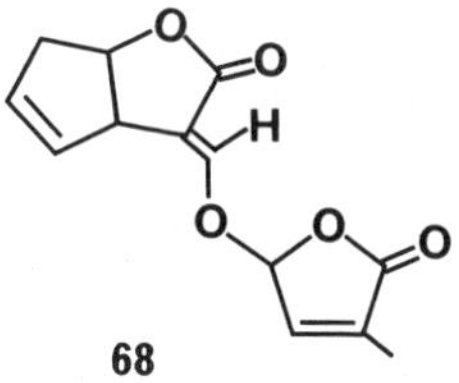

68

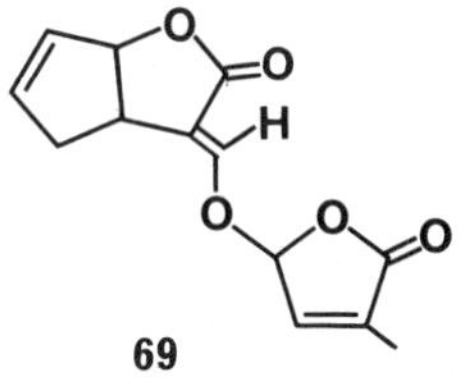

69

of Striga and Orobanche spp. Both **68** and **69** incorporate the B, C, and D rings of strigol and **69** contains the double bond in the same relative position as in strigol. Unfortunately, extensive field studies established that GR-7 exhibited low soil stability, particularly in alkaline media (36). Compound **69** proved to be considerably less stable than **68** towards light, heat, and alkali (39). Of the four-ring analogs of strigol, GR-18 (**70**) and GR-24 (**71**) (36, 39) have received the most attention. Compound **71**, which possesses the greatest structural similarity to strigol, proved to be the most active and most stable of all three- and four-ring analogs in both the laboratory and limited field trials.

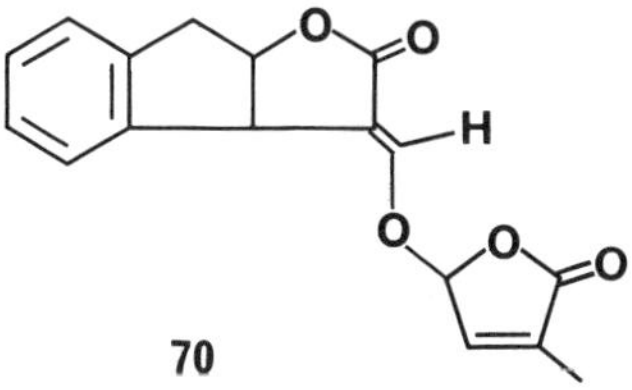

70

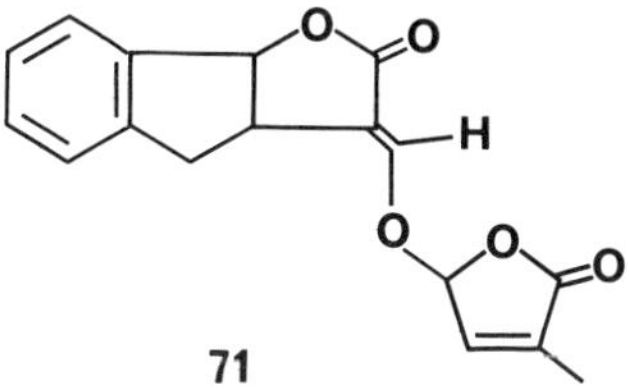

71

The synthesis of the ABC-ring portion of **71** is shown in Scheme XI (39). Indan-1-one was converted to 1-oxo-indan-2-ylacetic acid **72** by the method of Groves and Swan (40). Reduction of **72** with sodium borohydride produced the alcohol **73** which was treated with p-toluenesulfonic acid to provide the tricyclic lactone **74** (41). Subsequent formylation and condensation with either butenolide **3** or **65** affords **71**. Larger quantities of **71** are required for adequate evaluation, and optimization of its synthesis is required for its manufacture to be economically feasible (36).

The strigol analogs prepared by Johnson and co-workers are normally obtained almost exclusively as the natural E-isomers. Each geometric isomer can exist as two diastereomers (39). Compounds **68** and **70** have been separated into their diastereoisomeric forms. In each case, the two diastereomers were almost equally active as germination stimulants (36).

Other Syntheses of Strigol Analogs. In 1979, Cook and Co-workers reported the synthesis of the aromatic analog **75** (42), which contains all but one of the carbon atoms of strigol. It was about 2% as active as strigol as a seed germination stimulant. The diastereomeric compound **76** exhibited one-hundredth of the activity of **75**.

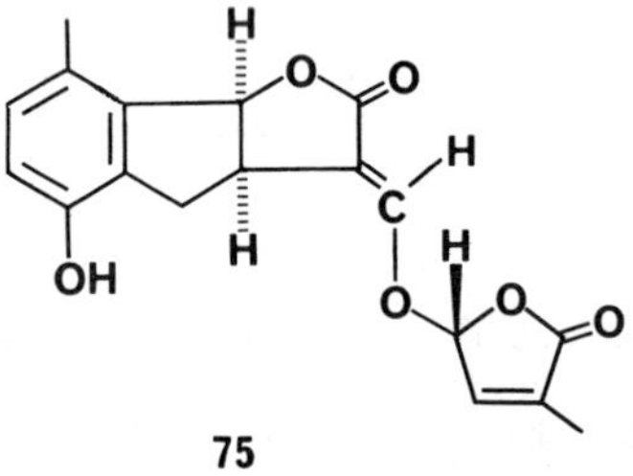

75 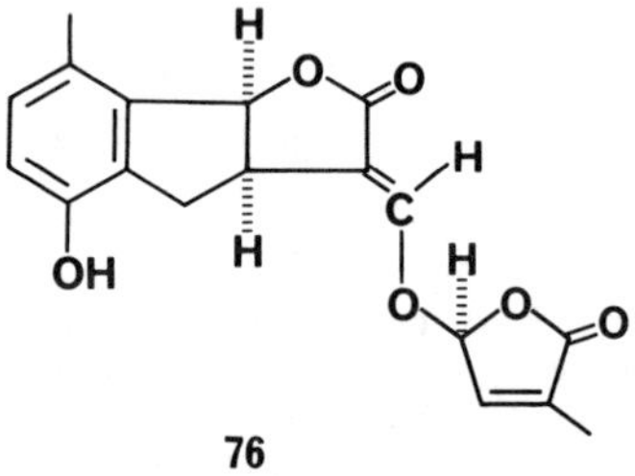 **76**

Finally, Brooks (22) has reported the syntheses of the AD-ring analog **77** and the ABD-ring analog **78**. His syntheses of additional analogs are reported in the following chapter of this volume.

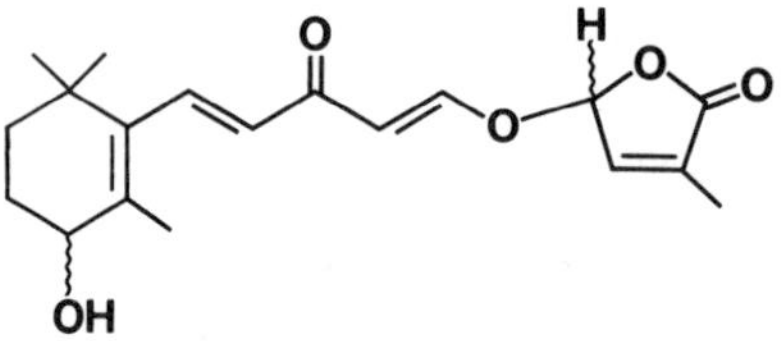

77 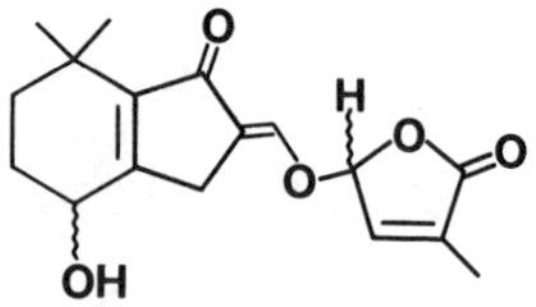 **78**

Strigol has been evaluated as a germination stimulant for several parasitic weeds in addition to witchweed. It has also been tested as a germination regulator for non-parasitic weed species. A large number of precursors and analogs of strigol have been evaluated as germination stimulants, germination inhibitors, growth inhibitors,

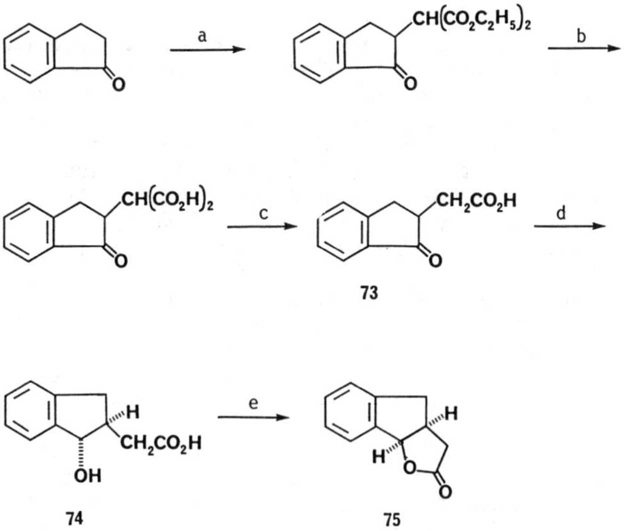

$CH(CO_2C_2H_5)_2$

a

b

$CH(CO_2H)_2$

c

CH_2CO_2H

d

73

H

CH_2CO_2H

OH

74

e

H

H

O

O

75

[a] (1) Br_2; (2) $NaCH(CO_2Et)_2$, benzene,Δ. [b] KOH, EtOH,Δ.
[c] 170 °C. [d] $NaBH_4$. [e] TsOH, benzene,Δ.

Scheme XI. Preparation of the ABC-ring portion of GR-24.

fungicides, insecticides, and herbicides. These topics, as well as structure-activity correlations, are discussed in detail in our companion paper "Biological Activity of Strigol, its Precursors, and Analogs" found elsewhere in this book.

Conclusion

Strigol, a potent weed seed germination stimulant, is available only in minute quantities from natural sources. This compound is a potential control agent for parasitic weeds of the genera *Striga* and *Orobanche*. Multigram quantities are required for extensive laboratory testing and field studies. In response to this need, a number of synthetic studies have been undertaken. Total syntheses of strigol have been reported by Sih, Raphael (two routes), and Brooks. A practical economically feasible synthesis, suitable for large-scale production, would utilize inexpensive starting materials and require a minimum of chromatographic purification. The final step of all the reported total syntheses of strigol is the alkylation of the tricyclic hydroxymethylene lactone **2** with the bromobutenolide **3**. Sih's synthetic approach provides **2** in slightly higher yield than either of Raphael's routes and appears to be more adaptable to large-scale preparation. Compound **3** can be prepared from 2-methyl-3-butenoic acid in high yield in three steps as reported by Raphael. Sih's synthesis of **3**, although lengthier, requires considerably less expensive starting materials. In 1985, Brooks reported the conversion of α-ionone to (±)-strigol in ten steps in 4.4% overall yield. The preparation is suitable for scale-up and requires only one chromatographic separation. Sih's synthesis afforded strigol in less than 1% yield. Recently, Dailey reported the conversion of ethyl 4-oxo-2,6,6-trimethylcyclohex-2-ene-1-carboxylate **50** to the diketo acid **16**, an intermediate in the latter stages of both the Sih and Brooks syntheses, in six steps in 38% yield. This process is quite suitable for large-scale production, being based upon inexpensive starting materials and reagents and requiring no chromatographic purification.

A large number of simplified analogs of strigol have been prepared. Such compounds, requiring shorter and less expensive syntheses, may have utility even if their activities are less than that of strigol. Upon consideration of such factors as stability, ease of synthesis, and expense of synthesis, none of the analogs prepared to date are superior or equivalent to strigol. The four-ring analog GR-24, **(71)**, appears to be the most promising analog presently available. However, larger quantities are required for evaluation, and optimization of its synthesis is required for its manufacture to be economically feasible.

Interest in utilizing strigol as a germination stimulant for *Striga* continues, particularly in Africa and Asia. The strigol syntheses of Sih and Raphael and the improvements and modifications introduced by Brooks and Dailey should serve as the foundation of any practical preparation.

Literature Cited

1. Cook, C. E.; Whichard, L. P.; Wall, M. E.; Egley, G. H.; Coggon, P.; Luhan, P. A.; McPhail, A. T. J. Am. Chem Soc. 1972, 94, 6198.
2. Brooks, D. W., Bevinakatti, H. S.; Powell, D. R. J. Org. Chem. 1985, 50, 3779.
3. Hsiao, A. I.; Worsham, A. D.; Moreland, D. E. Weed Sci. 1981, 29, 101.
4. Pepperman, A. B.; Connick, Jr., W. J.; Vail, S. L.; Worsham, A. D.; Pavlista, A. D; Moreland, D. E. Weed Sci. 1982, 30, 561.
5. Eplee, R. E.; English, T. J.; White, W. B. Proc. So. Weed Sci. Soc. 1976, 29, 409.
6. Chang, M.; Netzly, D. H.; Butler, L. G.; Lynn, D. G. J. Am. Chem. Soc. 1986, 108, 7858.
7. Shaw, W. C., Shepherd, D. R.; Robinson, E. C.; Sand, P. F. Weeds 1962, 10, 182.
8. Riopel, J. L. In "Vegetative Compatibility Responses in Plants"; Moore, R., Ed.; Academic Press: New York, 1983; pp. 13-34.
9. Ramaiah, K. V.; Parker, C.; Vasudeva Rao, M. J.; Musselman, L. J. "Striga Identification and Control Handbook; Information Bulletin No. 15; International Crops Research Institute for the Semi-Arid Tropics: Patancheru, A. P., India, 1983.
10. Pavlista, A. D. Weeds Today, 1980, 11 (2), 19.
11. (a) Egley, G. H.; Dale, J. E. Weed Sci. 1970, 18, 586 (b) Eplee, R. E. Ibid. 1975, 23, 433.
12. Johnson, A. W.; Rosebery, G.; Parker, C. Weed Res. 1976, 16, 223.
13. Heather, J. B.; Mittal, R. S. D.; Sih, C. J. J. Am. Chem. Soc. 1974, 96, 1976; 1976, 98, 3661.
14. MacAlpine, G. A.; Raphael, R. A.; Shaw, A.; Taylor, A. W.; Wild, H. J. J. Chem. Soc., Chem. Commun. 1974, 834; J. Chem. Soc., Perkin Trans. 1, 1976, 410.
15. Brooks, D. W.; Bevinakatti, H. S.; Kennedy, E.; Hathaway, J. J. Org. Chem. 1985, 50, 628.
16. Burgess, D. M. J. Org. Chem. 1956, 21, 102; "Organic Syntheses"; Rabjohn, N., Ed.; Wiley: New York, 1963, Collect. Vol. 4, p. 649, p. 428.
17. Farina, F.; Martin, M. V. An. Quim. 1971, 67, 315.
18. Van der Merwe, J. P.; Farbers, C. F. J. S. Afr. Chem. Inst. 1964, 17, 149.
19. Weiss, R. G.; Snyder, E. I. J. Org. Chem. 1971, 36, 403.
20. Franck-Neumann, M.; Berger, C. Bull. Soc. chim. France 1968, 4067.
21. Brooks, D. W.; Kennedy, E. J. Org. Chem. 1983, 48, 277.
22. Brooks, D. W.; Kennedy, E.; Bevinakatti, H. S. ACS Symp. Ser. 1985, 268, 437.
23. Dolby, L. J.; Hanson, G. J. J. Org. Chem. 1976, 41, 563.
24. Cooper, G. K.; Dolby, L. J. J. Org. Chem. 1979, 44, 3414.
25. Pepperman, A. B. J. Org. Chem. 1981, 46, 5039.
26. Sierra, M. G.; Spanevello, R. A.; Ruveda, E. A. J. Org. Chem. 1983, 48, 5111.
27. Dailey, Jr., O. D.; Vail, S. L. ACS Symp. Ser. 1985, 268, 427.

28. Ramage, G. R.; Simonsen, J. L. J. Chem. Soc. 1935, 532.
29. Pepperman, Jr., A. B.; Blanchard, E. J. ACS Symp. Ser. 1985, 268, 415.
30. Surmatis, J. D.; Walser, A.; Gibas, J.; Thommen, R. J. Org. Chem. 1970, 35, 1053.
31. Liu, H. J.; Hung, H. K.; Mhehe, G. L.; Weinberg, M. L. D. Can. J. Chem. 1978, 56, 1368.
32. Fry, J. L.; Orfanopulos, M.; Adlington, M. G.; Dittman, Jr., W. R.; Silverman, S. B. J. Org. Chem. 1978, 43, 374.
33. Reif, D. J.; House, H. O. "Organic synthesis"; Wiley: New York, 1963, Collect. Vol. 4, p. 860.
34. Bowden, K.; Heilbron, I. M.; Jones, E. R. H.; Weedon, B. C. L. J. Chem. Soc. 1946, 39.
35. Cassady, J. M.; Howie, G. A. J. Chem. Soc., Chem. Commun. 1974, 512.
36. Hassanali, A. In "Striga: Biology and Control"; Ayensu, E. S.; Doggett, H.; Keynes, R. D.; Marton-Lefeore, J.; Musselman, L. J.; Parker, C.; Pickery, A.; Eds.; ICSU Press: Paris, 1984; pp. 125-132.
37. Johnson, A. W.; Rosebery, G. U. S. Patent 4,002,457, 1977.
38. Johnson, A. W.; Hassanali, A. Ger. Offen. 2,240,801, 1978; Chem. Abstr. 1978, 88, 190,581.
39. Johnson, A. W.; Gowda, G.; Hassanali, A.; Knox, J.; Monaco, S.; Razavi, Z.; Rosebery, G. J. Chem. Soc., Perkin Trans. 1 1981, 1734.
40. Groves, L. H.; Swan, C. A. J. Chem. Soc. 1951, 867.
41. House, H. O.; Babad, H.; Toothill, R. B.; Noltes, A. W. J. Org. Chem. 1962, 27, 4141.
42. Kendall, P. M.; Johnson, J. V.; Cook, E. E. J. Org. Chem. 1979, 44, 1421.

RECEIVED May 12, 1987

Chapter 36

Synthetic Studies of Strigol and Its Analogs

Dee W. Brooks[1], Eileen Kennedy[2,4], H. S. Bevinakatti[2,5], Armand B. Pepperman, Jr.[3], and Judith M. Bradow[3]

[1]Abbott Laboratories, Abbott Park, IL 60064
[2]Department of Chemistry, Purdue University, West Lafayette, IN 47907
[3]Southern Regional Research Center, Agricultural Research Service, U.S. Department of Agriculture, New Orleans, LA 70179

An improved total synthesis of (±)-strigol (**1**), a potent seed germination stimulant for *Striga* and other related parasitic plants, is described along with the determination of the absolute configuration of natural (+)-strigol. Several new analogs of strigol with seed germination activity have been prepared and some initial testing results are provided.

Strigol (**1**) was isolated from root exudates of cotton (*Gossypium hirsutum* L.) and the relative structure was established by Cook and co-workers.(1) Considerable interest in strigol arose due to its potent germination stimulant activity for seeds of witchweed (*Striga asiatica*), a parasitic plant which causes considerable damage to crops of the *Gramineae* family such as corn, sorghum and sugarcane.(2,3) Witchweed seeds can remain dormant in the soil for several years until favorable conditions prevail including exposure to some type of chemical germination stimulant.(4-6) The concept of using a chemical signal to break dormancy and induce germination of weed seeds is relevant to designing new approaches for weed control. For parasitic weeds such as witchweed, inducing germination in the absence of a host plant would result in starvation of the seedling and hence offers an alternative to herbicide treatment. Prior to the isolation of strigol many compounds were surveyed for germination activity for witchweed and related root parasites.(3) Strigol was found to be more potent than other stimulants examined (50% germination at 10^{-11} M).(2)

[4]Current address: Dow Chemical Company, Building 768, Midland, MI 48667
[5]Current address: Alchemie Research Center, P.O. Box 155, Thane Belapur Road, Thane 400 601, Maharashtra, India

0097-6156/87/0355-0433$06.00/0
© 1987 American Chemical Society

In 1956, *Striga asiatica*, was discovered in both North and South Carolina.(3) The species found in the United States, renamed *Striga lutea*, (1) has a wide geographical distribution and attacks numerous members of the *Gramineae* family. In 1957 a Federal quarantine was invoked to minimize the spread of *Striga lutea* , and eradication directed research programs were instituted by the United States Department of Agriculture. Evaluation of herbicides(7), methods of cultivation (3), and the development of resistant crop species (8-11) were studied. Research was also directed toward the isolation and identification of natural, plant-produced germination stimulants and the development of effective synthetic stimulants.

The fact that strigol is not readily available from natural sources motivated efforts to develop efficient total synthetic schemes. Several partial (12-17) and three total syntheses (18-20) have been reported. Interest in potential field testing of strigol as a control agent in witchweed infested areas provided further impetus to develop improved synthetic routes applicable on a multigram scale. Another aspect involved the elucidation of structure-activity relationships for strigol with the objective of designing more potent and/or simpler analogs with appropriate properties and activity.

The biological mechanism of strigol mediated seed germination is not completely understood. However, some results indicate that *Striga* and *Orobanche* germination stimulants are produced in the extending root zones of a large variety of plants.(21,22) Recently, Lynn and coworkers have identified a hydroquinone derivative as the first example of a natural host-derived (*Sorghum bicolor*) germination stimulant for witchweed.(23) When the donor stimulant is presented to the seed of a parasitic plant rapid cell expansion leads to the emergence of a radicle. In the presence of a host plant, the root apex swells at the point of contact forming a bell shaped tissue known as the haustorium, which attaches to the host root. Growth proceeds from the haustorium by penetration of a compatible host cortex to provide vascular continuity between host and parasite. The parasitic seedling grows underground for several weeks depending entirely upon the host for nourishment and during this time causes extensive injury to the host plant. After some time a flowering shoot emerges above the soil. The weed then produces chlorophyll and becomes semi-parasitic. Within about one month flowers appear which produce very small seeds.(3) In cases where the seed is stimulated to germinate in the absence of a host plant, the haustorium of the parasite either does not develop or cannot successfully attach to the roots of the non-host plants. Most parasitic weeds of this type are native to the Eastern Hemisphere and cause significant crop destruction in Africa, Asia and the Middle East.

Total Synthesis of (±)-Strigol (**1**)

The total synthesis of (±)-strigol developed by Sih and co-workers (18), formed the basis for our efforts to devise an improved practical synthesis. The general plan involved consecutive A+B+C+D ring formation and the connection of four key bonds as shown in Scheme 1.

Scheme 1. Synthetic Strategy

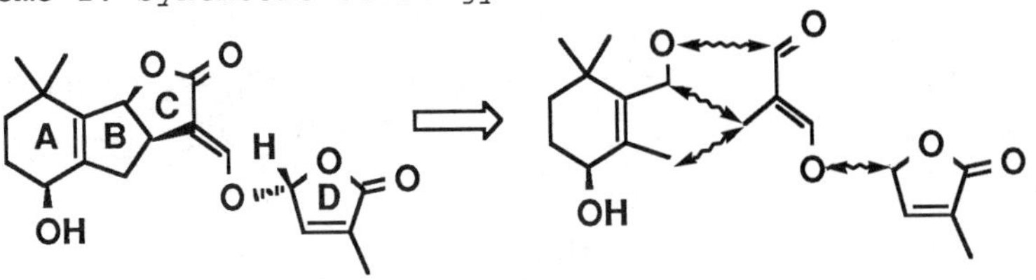

Our total synthesis of (±)-strigol is outlined in Scheme 2. Commercially available α-ionone (**2**) was chosen as the starting material, as it contained the required carbon framework and functionality appropriate for elaboration to an A-ring intermediate. Epoxidation with 30% peracetic acid followed by ozonolysis of the enone functionality gave the aldehydes **4a,b**. Epoxide opening with pyrrolidine gave the hydroxy aldehyde **5** and selective oxidation of the hydroxy group with chromic acid in acetone (Jones' method) provided the keto aldehyde **6**. This product was converted to the methyl ester bromide **8** by a one-pot reaction involving treatment of **6** with N-bromosuccinimide in carbon tetrachloride followed by the addition of methanol. This step circumvented a troublesome oxidation step of previous synthetic studies.(14,18) Optimization of this reaction provided a reproducible one-pot procedure for the preparation of the diester **9** from **8**. Acid catalyzed hydrolysis and decarboxylation of crude **9** gave the acid **10**. Reduction of an aqueous solution of the sodium salt of acid **10** with $NaBH_4$ in the presence of $CeCl_3$ followed by acidification, gave an equal mixture of isomeric hydroxy lactones **11** and **12**. The desired isomer **11** crystallized from an ether solution of the isomeric mixture. The undesired isomer was salvaged by oxidation to the keto lactone **13** followed by stereoselective reduction with $NaBH_4$ to give **11** (76%) and **12** (14%). The hydroxymethylene lactone **14** was then prepared and subjected to O-alkylation with the bromobutenolide **15** using excess K_2CO_3 in N-methyl-pyrrolidinone. This provided a mixture of (±)-strigol (**1**)(35%) and (±)-epistrigol (**16**)(39%), which were separated by chromatography. The total synthesis of (±)-strigol was accomplished in ten steps and 4.4% overall yield from α-ionone or twelve steps and 6.8% overall yield if recycling of **12** is considered.(20)

Scheme 2. Total Synthesis of (±)-Strigol

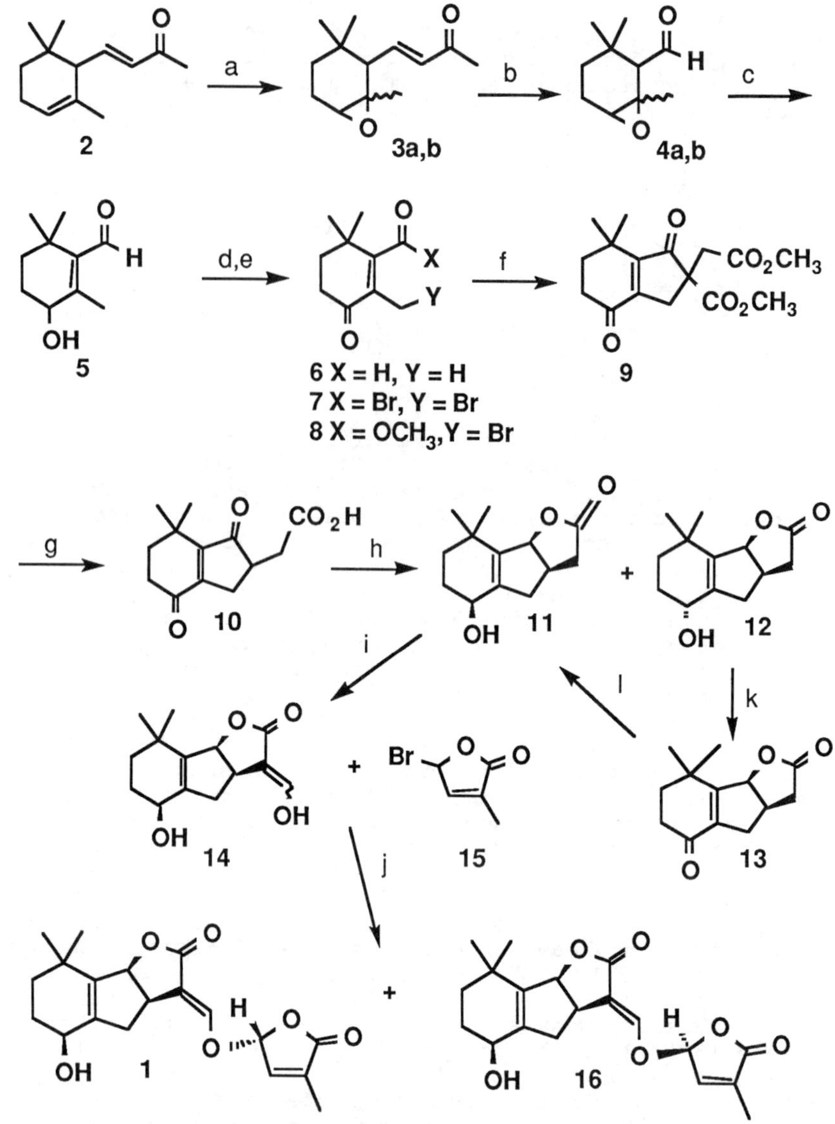

2 —a→ 3a,b —b→ 4a,b —c→

5 —d,e→ 6 X = H, Y = H; 7 X = Br, Y = Br; 8 X = OCH_3, Y = Br —f→ 9

—g→ 10 —h→ 11 + 12

11 —i→ 14 + 15 —j→ 1 + 16

12 —k→ 13 —l→ 11

Reagents: (a) CH_3CO_3H, CH_3CO_2H, 0°C, 94%; (b) 1. O_3, CH_3OH, -78°C, 2. Zn, CH_3CO_2H, -30 to 25°C, 86%; (c) pyrrolidine, ether, 25°C, 90%; (d) H_2CrO_4, acetone, 0°C; (e) 1. NBS, CCl_4, 70°C, 2. CH_3OH, 0°C, 83%; (f) 1. NaH, $CH_2(CO_2CH_3)_2$, THF, -10 to 25°C, 2. $BrCH_2CO_2CH_3$, 25°C. 82%; (g) 6N HCl, CH_3CO_2H, 100°C, 64%; (h) 1N NaOH, $CeCl_3(H_2O)_7$, $NaBH_4$, 0°C, 75%; (i) NaH, EtOCHO, ether, 25°C, 93%; (j) K_2CO_3, NMP, 25°C, 39%; (k) PCC, CH_2Cl_2, 25°C, 74%; (l) $CeCl_3(H_2O)_7$, $NaBH_4$, EtOH, 0°C, 76% **11**.

Absolute Configuration of (+)-Strigol

Our approach to solve the absolute configuration of natural (+)-strigol was to identify an appropriate optically pure derivatizing agent of known absolute configuration that would convert (±)-strigol into a separable diastereomeric mixture. X-Ray crystallographic analysis of one pure diastereomer would establish the configuration of chiral centers in strigol relative to the known chiral center in the derivatizing agent. Finally, removal of the derivatizing group to regenerate one enantiomer of strigol and comparison of the optical rotation with that reported for the natural product would complete the determination of absolute configuration.

We found that (R)-(-)-1-(1-naphthyl)ethyl isocyanate (25) proved effective in this case to provide equal amounts of two diastereomeric carbamates **17** and **18**, which were separated by chromatography on silica gel (30-50% THF in hexane). The carbamate **17** with the larger R_f on silica gel was readily crystallized by slow evaporation of an ethyl acetate and tetrahydrofuran mixture to provide suitable crystals for X-ray analysis. The carbamate **17** was then subjected to the method developed by Pirkle and Hauske (26) for the mild cleavage of carbamates. Thus, treatment with triethylamine and trichlorosilane provided the corresponding enantiomer of strigol with observed $[a]_D$ +270° (c 0.2, $CHCl_3$) compared to the literature value(18) for natural (+)-strigol, $[a]_D$ +293° (c 0.15, $CHCl_3$). Therefore, the absolute configuration of (+)-strigol was established as that depicted by **1**. It is noteworthy to mention that the absolute structure shown for (+)-strigol in the earlier literature which was arbitrarily chosen by Cook and co-workers (2) and thereafter depicted by others (18,20) was, fortunately, the correct enantiomer. The full experimental details of this investigation and the details of the X-ray crystallographic analysis are available.(24)

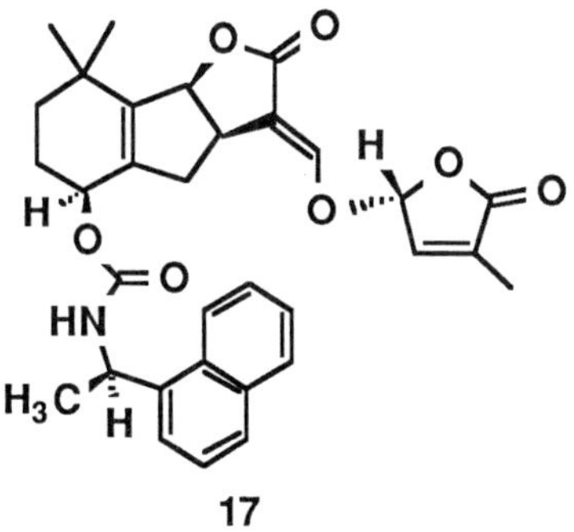

17

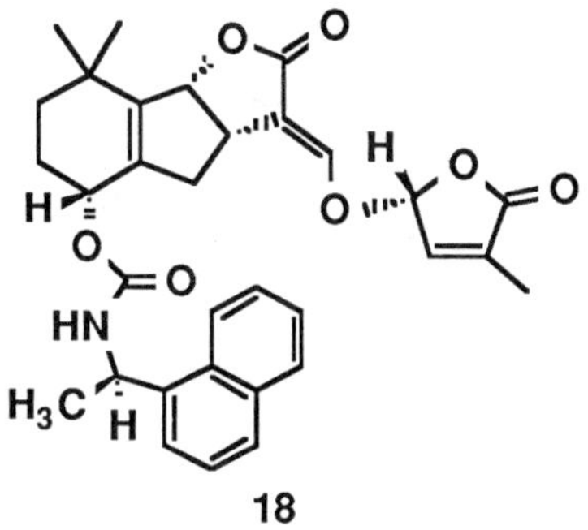

18

Analogs of Strigol

A variety of strigol analogs have been synthesized and tested as germination stimulants with seeds of *Striga* and *Orobanche* (27-30). To provide a general overview, the structures and *in vitro* activity of some of the many compounds that have been evaluated are summarized in Scheme 3. The compounds 20-23 are early synthetic intermediates from the total synthesis of strigol and the hydroxy aldehyde **22** exhibits activity similar to strigol. Compound **26** is a simple C-D ring analog and compound **27** is a B-C-D analog. The A-B-C-D analog **29** containing an aromatic A-ring was substantially less active than strigol. From the studies reported thus far strigol remains as one of the consistently most potent germination stimulants for *Striga* seeds, but amazingly, the simple synthetic A-ring analog **22** and butenolide **25** are approximately equally active.

Our interest in preparing strigol analogs was centered on both early and advanced synthetic intermediates from the total synthetic studies. From the previous description of known analogs a trend of observing activity in compounds containing A and/or D ring units of strigol led us to design other A-D analogs. The A-D ring analog **32** was readily prepared in three steps. Treatment of the epoxide **3a,b** with sodium methoxide in methanol gave the isomeric alcohol **30** which was converted to the hydroxymethylene derivative **31** in a standard fashion. Condensation of **31** with bromobutenolide **15** using excess K_2CO_3 in N-methylpyrrolidinone completed the preparation of **32** in 30% overall yield from **3a,b**. This analog is very closely related to strigol in that it has the same number of carbons and relative positioning of the A and D rings. The analog **32** is more conformationally flexible than strigol and evaluation of its biological activity is in progress.

Reagents: (a) Na, CH_3OH, 25°C, 75%; (b) NaH, EtOCHO, ether, 25°C, 84%; (c) K_2CO_3, N-methylpyrrolidinone, 25°C, 46%.

Scheme 3. Some Synthetic *Striga* Seed Germination Stimulants

(% germination, concentration, reference)

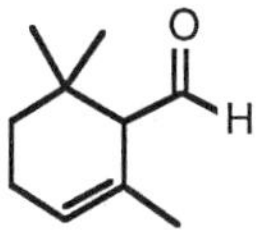

O H OH OH CO$_2$H EtO

20 (55%, 10^{-7}M, 27)

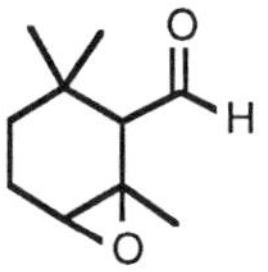

21 (60%, 10^{-9}M, 27)

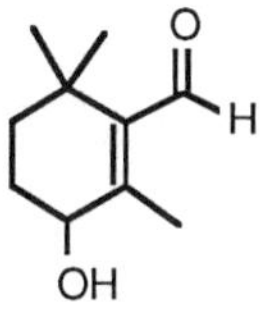

22 (60%, 10^{-11}M, 27)

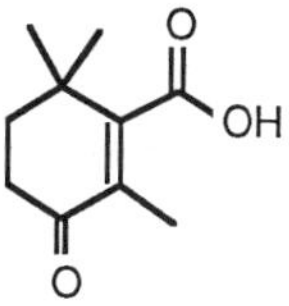

23 (50%, 10^{-4}M, 27)

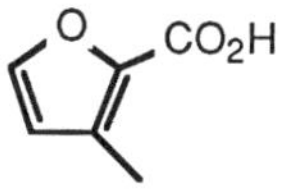

24 (40%, 10^{-9}M, 27)

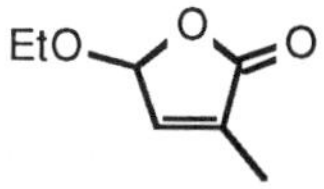

25 (72%, 10^{-10}M, 27)

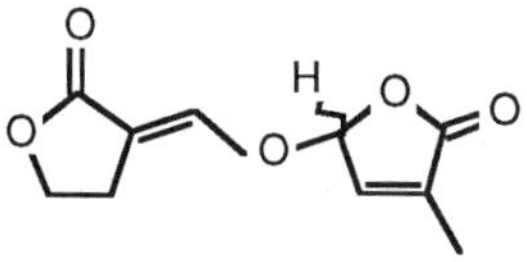

26 (61%, 10^{-7}M, 28)

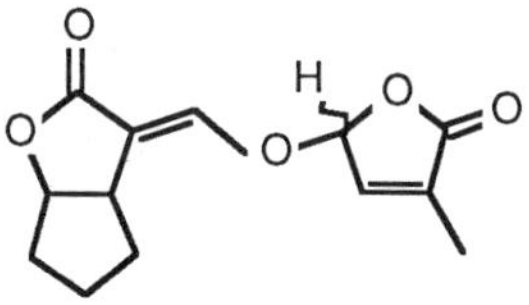

27 (68%, 10^{-8}M, 27)

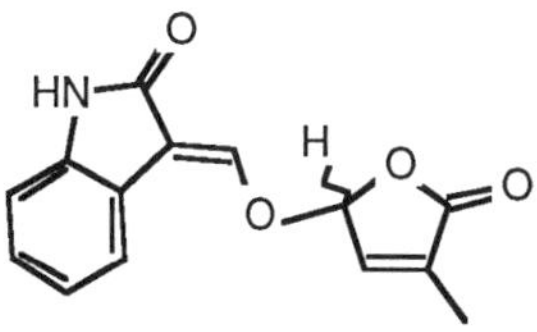

HN

28 (>50%, 10^{-7}M, 28)

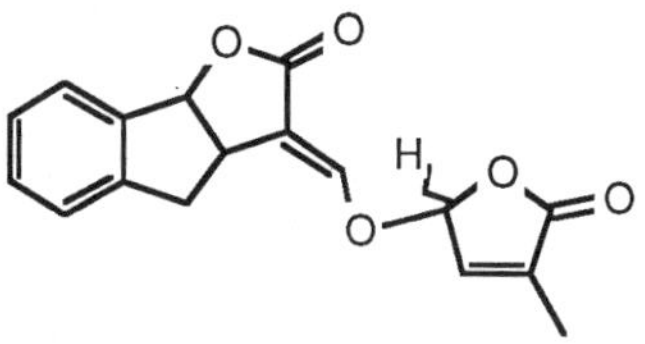

29 (>50%, 10^{-7}M, 28)

We were also interested in forming A-D ring analogs in which the two rings were directly attached. The potassium salt of **23** was condensed with bromobutenolide **15** and the bromophthalide **34** to give the analogs **33** and **35** respectively.

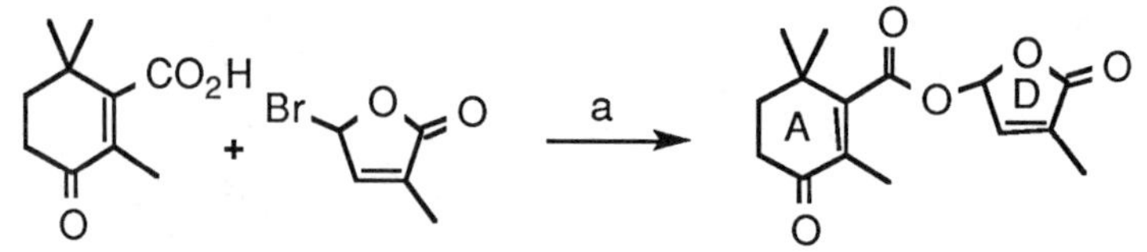

Reagents: (a) K_2CO_3, N-methylpyrrolidinone, 25°C.

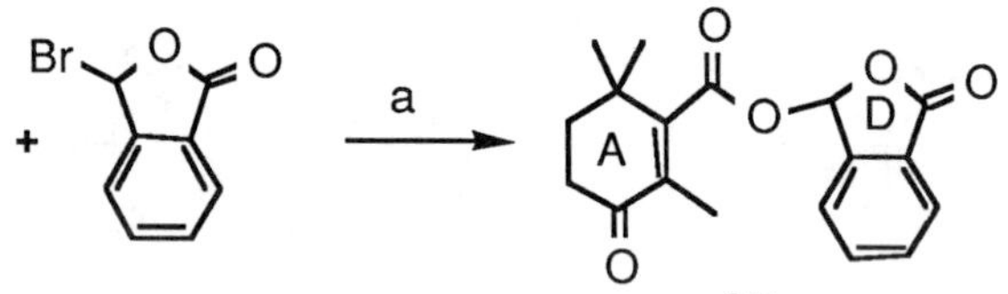

Access to analogs where the A ring is fused to a butenolide unit was provided from the bromoacid **36** by treatment with aqueous base yielding the ketolactone **37** which was smoothly reduced to the hydroxy analog **38**.

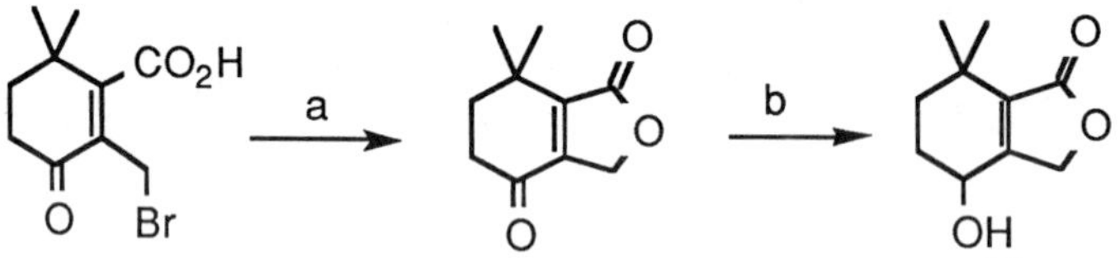

Reagents: (a) 1. KOH, n-C_4H_9OH, reflux, 2. 6N HCl; (b) $CeCl_3(H_2O)_7$, $NaBH_4$, CH_3OH, 25°C, 83%.

The availability of diketoacid **10** from our strigol synthesis prompted us to examine synthetic entry to A-B-D ring analogs. Following the esterification process used for **23**, we found that the acid **10** could be similarly esterified with bromobutenolide **15** and bromophthalide **34** to provide the analogs **39** (41%) and **40** (70%) respectively.

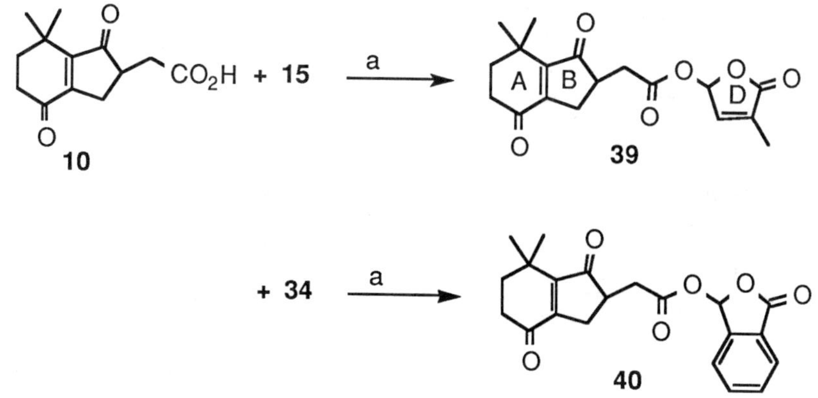

Reagents: (a) K_2CO_3, acetone.

In an effort to further delineate the structure activity features of the D ring in strigol, we prepared the phthalide analog **41** which stimulated 78% germination at 10^{-6}M in the witchweed bioassay.

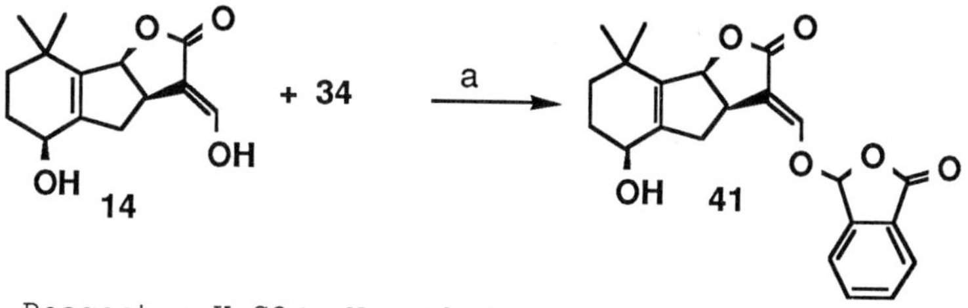

Reagents: K_2CO_3, N-methylpyrrolidinone, 25°C.

We were also interested in examining the results of replacing the D ring with an open chain analog. The closest analog would be methyl angelate (**42**) but attempts to brominate it led to the formation of methyl bromotiglate (**43**). Therefore we used **43** to condense with **44** to provide the acyclic D ring analog **45** which caused 78% germination at 10^{-6} M. This compound might be compared to the analog **26** which caused 61% germination at 10^{-7}M.

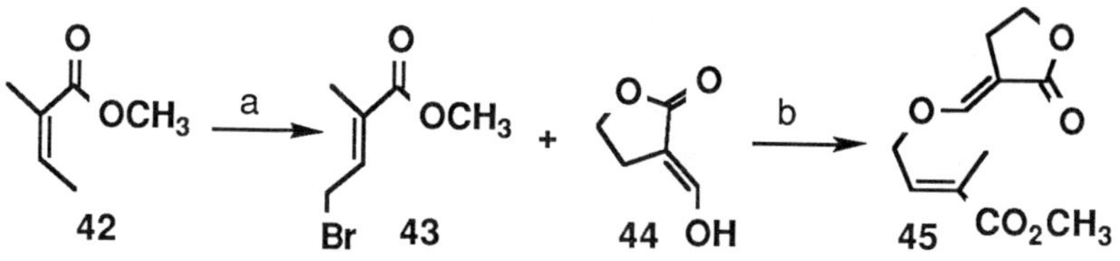

Reagents: (a) N-bromosuccinimide, CCl_4, 70°C; (b) 1. Na, CH_3OH, ether, 25°C, 2. N-methypyrrolidinone.

Another very simple analog **46** was designed which incorporated mainly the C -D ring unit. Reduction of the sodium salt of 3-benzoyl propionic acid (**47**) and subsequent acidic workup provided the lactone **48**. This lactone was converted to the hydroxymethylene derivative **49** and the sodium salt of **49** was condensed with bromobutenolide **15** to give the C-D analog **46** as a mixture of diastereomers. This mixture was tested in the witchweed assay and found to cause 54% germination at 10^{-9} M. It remains to be established if there is a significant difference in activity for each diastereomeric isomer as seen for strigol and epi-strigol.

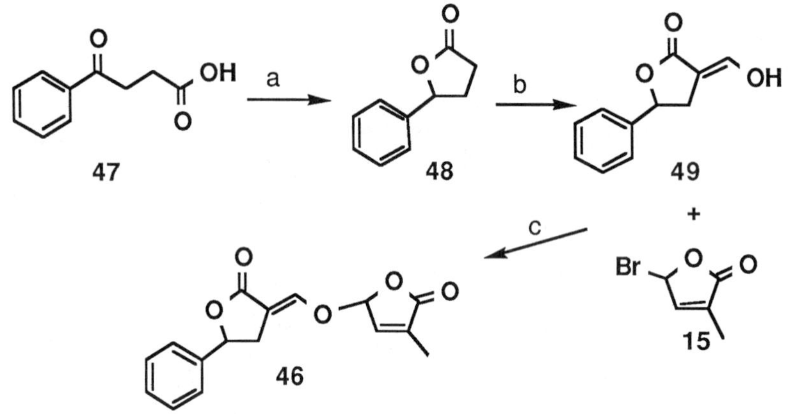

Reagents: (a) NaOH, $NaBH_4$, 25°C; (b) NaH, EtOCHO, ether, 25°C; (c) NaH, N-methylpyrrolidinone.

Striga Germination Bioassay

Striga seeds were initially surface sterilized with 1% aqueous NaOCl, followed by two deionized water rinses and then were pre-incubated in 10mL of deionized water in the dark at 28°C for 10 days. Samples of pre-incubated seeds were collected on 5 μm Metricel filters (Gelman Type GA-1) and floated in 10mL test solution or control solution (either 0.1% dimethyl sulfoxide or deionized water). For the germination incubations, seeds and test solution were transferred to 96 well plastic culture dishes (0.4 mL/well and 4 replicates of 8 wells each for a given assay). The *Striga* seeds were then incubated in the dark for 3 days at 28°C before evaluation of germination (radicle protrusion) under 40X magnification. Each experiment was repeated at least twice. Where necessary, test solution pH was adjusted to 6.8 with 0.1N KOH.

Conclusion

An improved total synthesis of strigol has been accomplished which is amenable to scale up. The absolute structure of strigol has been established. Several simple analogs have shown significant activity as witchweed seed germination stimulants, and some features of the structure-activity relationships have been elucidated. Access to additional analogs which await testing has been achieved . These results and further investigations will hopefully lead to effective synthetic compounds for the control of witchweed and related parasitic plants.

Acknowledgments

We express our appreciation to the United States Department of Agriculture and Purdue University for support of this research and Dr. S. Vail for helpful discussions during the course of this work.

Literature Cited

1. Cook, C. E.; Whichard, L. P.; Turner, B.; Wall, M. E.; Egley, G. E. Science (Washington, D.C.) 1966, 154, 1189.
2. Cook, C. E.; Whichard, L. P.; Wall, M. E.; Egley, G. E.; Croggon, P.; Luhan, P. A.; McPhail, A. T. J. Am. Chem. Soc. 1972, 94, 6198.
3. Shaw, W. C.; Shepherd, D. R.; Robinson, E. L.; Sand, P. F. Weeds 1962, 31, 552.
4. Egley, G. H.; Dale, J. E. Weed Sci. 1970, 18, 586.
5. Worsham, A. D.; Moreland, D. E.; Klingman, G. C. J. Exp. Botany 1964, 15, 556.
6. Okonkwo, S. N. C. Am. J. Botany 1966, 53, 142.
7. Langston, M. A.; English, T. J.; Eplee, R. E. Proc. Second Intl. Symposium on Parasitic Weeds 1979, 273.
8. Parker, C.; Reid, D. C. *ibid.* 1979, 79.
9. Tidiane Ba, A. *ibid*., 1979, 128.
10. Basler, F.; Haddad, A. *ibid*., 1979, 254.
11. Williams, C. N. Nature 1959, 184, 1511.
12. Dolby, L. J.; Hanson, G. J. J. Org. Chem. 1976, 41, 563.
13. Cooper, G. K.; Dolby, L. J. J. Org. Chem. 1979, 44, 3414.
14. a. Pepperman, A. B. J. Org. Chem. 1981, 46, 5039, b. Pepperman, A. B.; Blanchard, E. J. In "The Chemistry of Allelopathy" Thompson, A. C., Ed.; ACS Symposium Series; 1985, 268, Chapter 28.
15. Brooks, D. W.; Kennedy, E. J. Org. Chem. 1983, 48, 277.
16. Sierra, M. G.; Spanevello, R. A.; Ruveda, E. A. J. Org. Chem. 1983, 48, 5111.
17. Daily, O. D.; Vail, S. L. In "The Chemistry of Allelopathy" Thompson, A. C., Ed.; ACS Symposium Series; 1985, 268, Chapter 29.
18. Heather, J. B.; Mittal, R. S. D.; Sih, C. J. J. Am. Chem. Soc. 1974, 96, 1976; 1976, 98, 3661.

19. MacAlpine, G. A.; Raphael, R. A.; Shaw, A.; Taylor, A. W.; Wild, H. J. J. Chem. Soc. Chem. Commun. 1974, 834; J. Chem. Soc., Perkin Trans. 1976, 1, 410.
20. a. Brooks, D. W.; Bevinakatti, H. S.; Kennedy, E.; Hathaway, J. J. Org. Chem. 1985, 50, 628; b. Brooks, D. W.; Kennedy, E.; Bevinakatti, H. S. In "The Chemistry of Allelopathy" Thompson, A. C., Ed.; ACS Symposium Series; 1985, 268, Chapter 30.
21. Brown, R. In "Handbuch der Pflanzenphysiologie"; Springer-Verlag; Berlin, 1965: Vol XVIz; pp925-932.
22. Egley, G. H.; Dale, J. E. Weed Sci. 1971, 19, 678.
23. Chang, M.; Netzly, D. H.; Butler, L. G.; Lynn, D. G. J. Am.Chem. Soc. 1986, 108, 7858.
24. Brooks, D. W.; Bevinakatti, H. S.; Powell, D. R. J. Org. Chem. 1985, 50, 3779.
25. Pirkle, W. H.; Simmons, K. A.; Boeder, C. W. J. Org. Chem. 1979, 44, 4891.
26. Pirkle, W. H.; Hauske, J. R. J. Org. Chem. 1977, 42, 2781.
27. Vail, S. L.; Dailey, O. D.; Connick. W. J.; Pepperman, A. B. In "The Chemistry of Allelopathy" Thompson, A. C., Ed.; ACS Symposium Series; 1985, 268, Chapter 31.
28. Johnson, A. W.; Gowda, G.; Hassanaldi, A.; Knox, J.; Monaco, S.; Razavi, Z.; Rosebery, G. J. Chem. Soc., Perkin 1 1981, 1734.
29. Pepperman, A. B.; Connick, W. J.; Vail, S. L.; Worsham, A. D.; Pavlista, A. D.; Moreland, D. E. Weed Science 1982, 30, 561.
30. Johnson, A. W.; Rosebery, G.; Parker, C. Weed Research 1976, 16, 223.

RECEIVED May 12, 1987

Chapter 37

Biological Activity of Strigol, Its Precursors, and Its Analogs

Armand B. Pepperman, Jr., O. D. Dailey, Jr., and S. L. Vail

Southern Regional Research Center, Agricultural Research Service, U.S. Department of Agriculture, New Orleans, LA 70179

Strigol, a natural product isolated from root exudates of cotton (*Gossypium hirsutum* L.) was found to be an extremely potent seed germination stimulant for the parasitic plant, witchweed (*Striga asiatica*). Elucidation of the structure of strigol led to the synthesis of many analogs. The results of these synthetic efforts, and the evaluation of these compounds as germination stimulants, germination inhibitors, growth inhibitors, fungicides, insecticides, and herbicides are discussed.

A chemical isolated from the root exudates of cotton (*Gossypium hirsutum* L.) was shown to be an extremely potent seed-germination stimulant for witchweed [*Striga asiatica* (L.) Kuntz] (1). The structure of the compound was elucidated by Cook *et al* (2), and given the trivial name, strigol, **1**, (Insert Figure 1). The compound contains three rings (A, B, and C) joined to a fourth (D) by a methyleneoxy bridge. The first total synthesis of (±)-strigol was reported in 1974 by Heather *et al* (3). The details of the synthesis and the resolution of (±)-strigol into its enantiomers was reported by the same group in 1976 (4). At about the same time, MacAlpine and coworkers reported another method for the total synthesis of (±)-strigol (5,6). In subsequent discussion, the use of the term strigol implies the (±)-enantiomeric mixture. The same convention will be used for the analogs and for epistrigol.

Witchweed is an economically important root-parasite that affects many warm-season grasses, including such important crop members of the Gramineae family as corn (*Zea mays* L.), grain sorghum [*Sorghum bicolor* (L.) Moench], and sugarcane (*Saccharum officinarum* (L.) (7). The ability of viable witchweed seed to remain dormant in the soil for many years, only to germinate when favorable conditions prevail, makes eradication difficult (8). Usually, seed will not germinate unless pretreated in a warm, moist environment for several days prior to exposure to a chemical stimulant released from the roots of both host and non-host species (9). After germination, the

This chapter is not subject to U.S. copyright.
Published 1987, American Chemical Society

seedling attaches itself to the host plant through an organ called the haustorium and draws all its nutrients and water from the host, causing severe damage.

Application of a chemical to break dormancy and/or to stimulate germination of weed seeds is a recent development in weed management and may be used increasingly in the future. The principle has been used with witchweed to induce germination in the absence of its obligate host plants, causing the seedling to die of starvation. This "suicidal germination" has been shown to be an effective control and/or eradication procedure, as field tests with ethylene (10) and synthetic analogs of strigol (11) have significantly reduced viable seed populations. The isolation and characterization of the natural witchweed seed germination stimulant of sorghum has recently been reported (12). The compound is an hydroquinone with a fifteen-carbon aliphatic substituent on the ring. This natural stimulant is much less active than strigol and is readily oxidized to the benzoquinone which is inactive as a germination stimulant for witchweed, precluding its use as a control agent.

The synthesis of strigol and its derivatives and the possibility of using these compounds for weed control and eradication has stimulated interest for their use in other parasitic and dormant weed seeds. A number of strigol analogs and precursors have been prepared and evaluated, permitting the proposal of structure-activity correlations. In this paper, we review these results and discuss the implications of these investigations.

Discussion and Results

Witchweed bioassays were generally conducted on seed that has been conditioned in water for 7-14 days, the conditioning solution removed, and the seed washed before being treated with the terminal solution which contained the suspected seed germination stimulant (13, 14). After 1 to 2 days, germination was determined by microscopic examination for radicle protrusion through the seed coat. *Orobanche* species and other *Striga* species seeds were handled in generally the same manner. Other weed and crop seeds were pretreated and terminated in the appropriate manner as described in the reference.

Strigol and Epistrigol

Strigol is the standard for this class of compounds, because it is a natural isolate that has been characterized and synthesized, and it is the most potent witchweed seed germination stimulant yet discovered. At concentrations of 10^{-14} to 10^{-6} M, strigol induced 35-100% of properly conditioned seed (1, 13), normally requiring 10^{-12} to 10^{-11} M for maximum germination (>80%). Hsiao *et al* (13) found that conditioning witchweed seeds in strigol solutions, rather than water, had an adverse effect on the responsiveness of the seeds to strigol stimulation. The higher the concentration of strigol in the pretreatment solution, the higher the concentration of strigol that is required in the terminal solution to achieve maximum germination. Pepperman *et al* (14) found that 10^{-10}M strigol and 10^{-6} M epistrigol, **2**, (Insert Figure 2) were the lowest concentrations

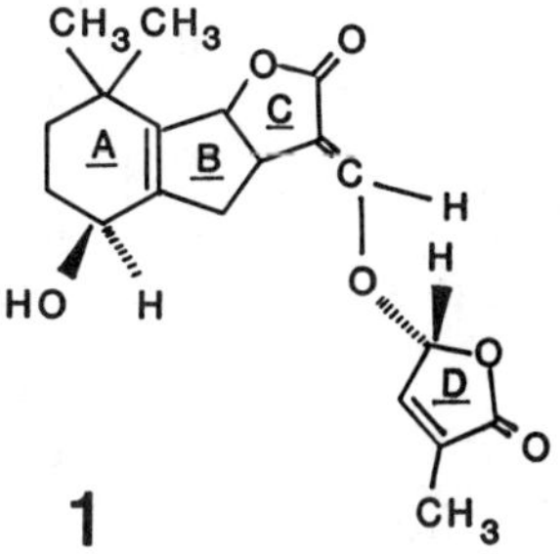

1

Figure 1 -- Structure of strigol (**1**) with A-B-C-D-rings designated.

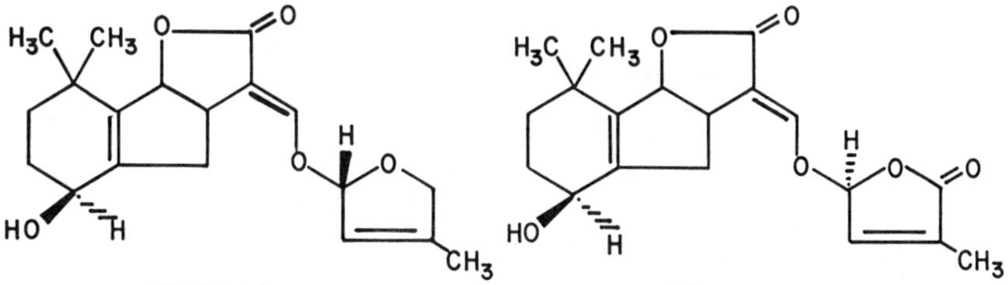

STRIGOL

EPISTRIGOL

1

2

Figure 2 -- Structures of strigol (**1**) and epistrigol (**2**).

capable of inducing greater than 80% germination of witchweed seeds. These authors also noted the very poor water solubility of both strigol and epistrigol and observed that activity was enhanced if DMSO was used as the solvent carrier.

Strigol appears to be relatively stable in soil, but because of its limited solubility, it is only fractionally leached past the top layer of soil. After 21 days of leaching daily with 1.27 cm. of simulated rainfall, about 86% of the applied strigol remained in the top 2.5 cm. of soil. Even with the small amounts present in the soil profile from 7.5-30 cm., significant numbers of witchweed seed did germinate (15). These results suggest that strigol has a potential for effective use in a witchweed control or eradication program.

In several field studies conducted at Whiteville, N.C., strigol consistently stimulated 10-20% more witchweed seed germination than some of the analogs which had comparable activity in *in vitro* studies. Seed germination was about 75% even at a soil depth of 10 cm (16,17). Strigol and corn root exudates both cause germination of witchweed seed without any evidence of haustorial formation (18). Addition of gum tragacanth extract to the germinated seedlings effected formation of the haustoria. The active compounds of the gum tragacanth extract responsible for haustorial formation have been isolated and several derivatives synthesized (19-21). The compounds bear little structural similarity to strigol.

Strigol is also effective as a germination stimulant for clover broomrape (*Orobanche minor*), a related parasitic weed (22). Visser and Johnson (23) tested strigol and some of its analogs as germination stimulants for *Alectra vogelii* and *Alectra orobanchoides*, which belong to another genus of root parasitic weeds of the same family as *Striga* (*Scrophulariaceae*). *A. vogelii* parasitizes legumes and *A. orobanchoides* parasitizes sunflower. Strigol was active at the relatively high concentrations of 10^{+2} to 10^{+3} ppm (10^{-4} to 10^{-3} M) and 10^{+1} to 10^{+3} ppm (10^{-5} to 10^{-3} M) respectively. In the same study, several analogs were found to be more effective than strigol as *Alectra* seed germination stimulants. Due to the low solubility of strigol it is possible that this reflects solubility differences rather than structural requirements.

The first example in which strigol was tested as a germination regulator for non-parasitic weed species was reported by Bradow (24), who showed that strigol and epistrigol were essentially inactive as germination stimulants for chilled and unchilled shepherdspurse seed (*Capsella bursa-pastoris*), although several analogs were quite active. A study on strigol dormancy regulation over a broad concentration range for temperature stressed lettuce seed (25), indicated that strigol was inhibitory of germination at 10^{-16} M for Grand Rapids lettuce seed and at 10^{-6} and 10^{-12} M for Great Lakes lettuce seed. As will be discussed in detail later, some of the strigol analogs stimulated germination. Some increase in the rate of germination in non-dormant Grand Rapids lettuce seed with strigol was observed. Neither strigol nor epistrigol was active in regulating germination of 26 weed and crop seeds (Bradow, J. M., Connick, W. J. Jr.; Pepperman, A. B. Manuscript in review).

Four Ring Analogs of Strigol

In this paper the use of four-ring, three-ring, or two-ring designates the number of rings the analog possesses of the original strigol nucleus, not necessarily the total number of rings the compound possesses. Thus the four-ring analogs (4-RAS) contain the A, B, C, and D rings. There have been fewer four-ring analogs prepared, since the main advantage in synthesizing analogs is reduced steps, time, complexity, and expense. With all four rings present, there is a small reduction in the difficulty of the synthesis since the 4-RAS reported thusfar have an aromatic A-ring, eliminating the problem of the stereochemistry of the hydroxyl group on the A-ring.

Johnson and coworkers (26) prepared a few 4-RAS compounds, two of which are shown in Figure 3 (Insert Figure 3) GR-24, **3**, is the most active synthetic compound made by this group, having activity of the same magnitude as strigol for Striga species, and is the most active known compound for inducing germination of Orobanche species. GR-24 has the same general ring geometry, with respect to the A- and C-rings, and contains the double bond in the B-ring in the same relative position as in strigol. It was found to be more stable to alkali, heat, and light than most of the other analogs. GR-18, **4**, was also prepared by Johnson's group and has the aromatic A-ring and double bond one carbon further away from the C-ring lactone or isomeric to **3**. Because of its structural similarity to strigol one would predict greater activity for **3** than **4**. Johnson claims (26) that this is the case but the data have not appeared in the scientific literature. Menetrez, however, has evaluated GR-24 against Striga asiatica and found it to have activity comparable to strigol, inducing 89-97% germination over the concentration range of 10^{-5} to 10^{-12} M (27). Kendall and coworkers (28) prepared compound **5** which is similar to GR-24, in having an aromatic A-ring with the double bond and C-ring in the same relative position as in strigol. In addition, **5** has the -OH at the 4-position and a methyl group at the 1-position of the A-ring. Kendall's compound has more structural similarity to strigol than **3**, yet its activity is only about 2% that of strigol for witchweed germination.

GR-24 has also been tested against Alectra spp. (23) and induced greater than 50% germination of A. vogelii at 10^{-3} to 10^{-7} M. Against A. orobanchoides it gave greater than 50% germination at 10^{-3} to 10^{-6} M. This activity is comparable to strigol for A. orobanchoides and superior for A. vogelii. Promotion of germination of dormant unchilled shepherdspurse seeds by GR-24 occurred at 10^{-3} and 10^{-4} M wherein 60-80% of the seeds germinated compared to 10% in the untreated control (24). This was the first evidence that strigol analogs have bioregulatory activity in non-parasitic weed seeds. Strigol was essentially ineffective against these seeds. In a broad screen bioassay versus 26 different weed and crop seeds stimulation of germination of Amarathus retroflexus, Eragrostis curvula, and Lactuca sativa (cv. Grand Rapids, Light sensitive and Light insensitive), all occurred with GR-24 (Bradow, J. M.; Connick, Jr., W. J., Pepperman, A. B. manuscript in preparation).

Although the 4-RAS have not been tested as extensively as the three-ring and two-ring analogs of strigol, GR-24 is particularly attractive from the standpoint of activity and stability and appears to be a prime candidate for field evaluation and further study toward optimizing and simplifying the synthetic procedure.

Three-ring Analogs of Strigol

The three-ring analogs of strigol (3-RAS) are the most widely studied of the analogs, primarily due to their relative ease of synthesis compared to strigol and the 4-RAS, and because of generally greater stability and often greater activity than the 2-RAS. The 3-RAS are comprised of the B, C, and D rings of strigol (Insert Figure 4). In particular, a large amount of work has been done with **6,** which was first prepared by Johnson and coworkers who called it GR-7 (11). The germination data for parasitic weeds in the presence of 3-RAS are shown in Table 1 (Insert Table 1). In the U.S. Patent describing the preparation and testing of several analogs, Johnson and Rosebery (29) found GR-7 to stimulate germination of *S. asiatica* and *S. hermonthica* as well as *O. ramosa* and *O. crenata*. Only non-dormant *O. aegyptica* was unaffected. The lowest effective concentration of GR-7 was reported as 10^{-10} M for *S. asiatica*. Other workers in the field found the lowest concentration of GR-7 to give significant germination was 10^{-8} M (14, 30). Pepperman *et al* (14) tested strigol and 3-RAS under the same set of conditions and found strigol to be 100 times more active than GR-7.

Both *A. vogelii* and *A. orobanchoides* were significantly stimulated to germinate by GR-7. over a wide concentration range. GR-28, **7**, was also evaluated against these parasites and found to be somewhat less active at the lower concentrations for both species (23). The semi-parasite *Cistanche phelypea* germinated to a moderate degree (about 42%) over a wide concentration range of 10^{-4} to 10^{-8} M (31).

Germination stimulation of dormant shepherdspurse seed by **6** occurred at 10^{-3} to 10^{-4} M (Insert Table 2) and was comparable to that observed for GR-24. Bioassays of 26 weed and crop seeds showed significant stimulatory activity by **6** with two lettuce cultivars and non-dormant *Amaranthus palmeri* (25 and Bradow, J. M.; Pepperman, A. B.; and Connick, W. J., Jr. manuscript in preparation). The observed effects, while significant, were smaller than the dramatic effects observed in the parasitic weeds. For these studies, the preparation of **6** was carried out in a variation of Johnson's synthesis, and the product was separated into two isomers, **6a** and **6b,** which were assigned the structures shown, based on the melting point and TLC mobility similarities to strigol and epistrigol (32). In Grand Rapids lettuce the higher-melting isomer (HMI) was more active than the lower-melting isomer (LMI), whereas in Great Lakes the LMI was stimulatory over a wide concentration range. In Great Lakes, the HMI was stimulatory only at 10^{-4} M and inhibitory at the lower concentrations of 10^{-8}, 10^{-10}, and 10^{-14} M. The lettuce seed germination is sensitive to the stereochemistry of **6,** as is *Amaranthus palmeri*, where only the HMI had significant effects on the germination of this non-dormant seed (Bradow, J. M., Connick, W. J., Jr., and Pepperman, A. B., Manuscript in review).

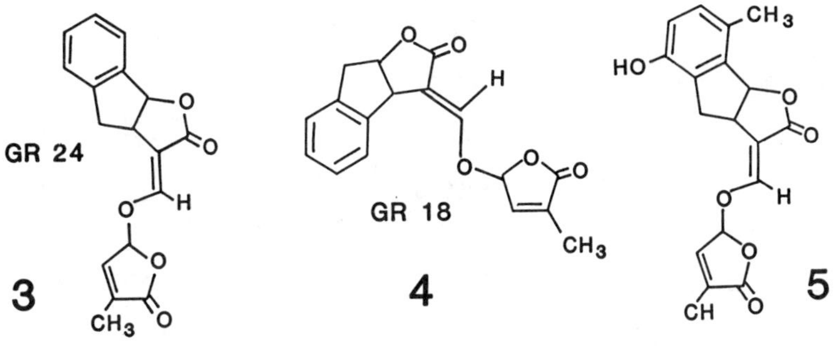

GR 24
3
GR 18
4
5

Figure 3 -- Structures of 4-ring analogs of strigol (4-RAS).

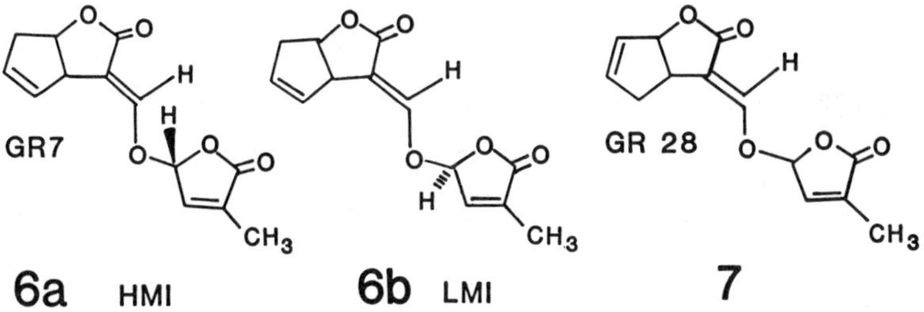

GR7
6a HMI
6b LMI
GR 28
7

Figure 4 -- Structures of 3-ring analogs of strigol (3-RAS); high-melting isomer (HMI = **6a**), low-melting isomer (LMI = **6b**).

TABLE 1
GERMINATION STIMULATION ACTIVITY OF A THREE-RING ANALOG OF STRIGOL, GR-7 (**6**) ON PARASITIC WEEDS

SPECIES	ACTIVITY % germination at concentration	REFERENCE
Striga asiatica	55% at 10^{-10} M	(29)
	60% at 10^{-8} M	(29)
	58% at 10^{-7} M	(14) a)
	68% at 10^{-8} M	(14) a)
	>85% at 10^{-8} M	(30)
	>80% at 10^{-5} and 10^{-6} M	(27)
Striga hermonthica	53% at 10^{-8} M	(29)
	58% at 10^{-7} M	(29)
Orobanche aegyptica	no significant effects on non-dormant seed	(29)
Orobanche ramosa	ca. 50% at 10^{-6} to 10^{-8} M	(29)
Orobanche crenata	64% at 10^{-6} M	(29)
	49% at 10^{-7} M	(29)
Orobanche minor	No significant difference from water control	(22)
Alectra vogelii	53-98% from 10^{-9} to 10^{-3} M	(23)
Alectra orobanchoides	47-91% from 10^{-9} to 10^{-3} M	(23)
Cistanche phelypaea	ca. 42% at 10^{-4} to 10^{-8} M	(31)

a) Mixture of two isomers[Two isomers of GR-7 exist and have been separated (31)]. The higher melting isomer was only 10% as active as the lower melting isomer.

TABLE 2
GERMINATION STIMULATION ACTIVITY OF A THREE RING ANALOG OF STRIGOL, GR-7 (6) ON NON-PARASITIC WEEDS

SPECIES	ACTIVITY % germination at concentration	REFERENCE
Capella bursa-pastoris	60-80% at 10^{-4} to 10^{-3} M	(24)a)
Lactuca sativa Grand rapids cv.	20-30% greater than control for temperature stressed lettuce seed at 10^{-4} or 10^{-6} M b)	(25)
Great Lakes cv.	10-25% stimulatory at 10^{-4} to 10^{-10} and 10^{-16} M c)	(25)
Amaranthus palmeri	13.5% stimulatory for non-dormant seed at 10^{-4} M. d)	e)

a) The isomer mixture was not tested but there was no significant difference between the higher melting isomer (HMI) and the lower melting isomer (LMI).

b) HMI. (LMI gave +13% at 10^{-4} M).

c) LMI. (HMI gave +32% at 10^{-4} M but inhibitory from -20% to -36% at 10^{-8}, 10^{-10}, and 10^{-14} M).

d) HMI. (LMI had no significant effect).

e) Bradow, J. M. et al, manuscript in review.

Although GR-28, **7**, was active against Alectra species, and was claimed (26) to be particularly effective for germination of Orobanche and Striga spp. (possibly better than GR-7 although data is not provided), it has not been widely studied because it proved to be considerably less stable towards light, heat, and alkali than GR-7. Derivatization of **6**, such as epoxidation of the C-ring double bond, hydrogenation of the C-ring double bond, or replacement of the double bond between C-3 and C-4 of the D-ring with a benzene ring, all caused decreased germination activity (33). Testing of a number of derivatives having different alkyl or aryl groups at the 3, 4, or 5 positions of the D-ring [2(5H)-furanones] showed that only the analogs possessing 4-methyl and 3-t-butyl substituents were as effective as **6** (33). These derivatives possess improved alkaline stability and would be good candidates for future field studies.

Two-Ring Analogs of Strigol.

The 2-RAS are the easiest and least expensive to prepare of the analogs but are often less active than the 3-RAS, 4-RAS, and strigol. These differences are clearly shown in the study by Pepperman et al (14), wherein the lowest concentrations of 2-RAS (**8** in Figure 5, Insert Figure 5) which were active as witchweed seed germination stimulants were 10^{-7} M (61% germination) and 10^{-6} M (86% germination). The 3-RAS (GR-7) was active at the lowest concentration of 10^{-8} M (68% germination). The 3-RAS was about 10 times as active as the 2-RAS and only 1% as active as strigol both against S. asiatica and S.hermonthica (29). The available data for **8** (called GR-5 by Johnson), is summarized in Table 3, (Insert Table 3). It was inactive against A. vogelii whereas the 3-RAS is highly active, but **8** was active at levels of about 10^{-6} M versus the other parasitic weeds, which is comparable to the 3-RAS. In the non-parasitic weed seeds, the 2-RAS and 3-RAS have approximately the same activity versus Capsella bursa-pastoris (24), and both Lactuca sativa cultivars(25).

Johnson (26) claimed an increase in activity, particularly for Striga spp., when a 4-methyl group is introduced into the butyrolactone fragment, structure **9**. The introduction of the extra carbon in the lactone ring (structure **10**) reduced activity. While the 2-RAS are not as active as strigol or the 4-RAS, they are sometimes as active as the 3-RAS, and easier to prepare, making them very attractive for large-scale use. A disadvantage of the 2-RAS is their poorer stability to alkali, heat, and light (Pepperman, unpublished results) which may require application of more chemical to achieve the same level of control. Despite this drawback, the economics still might be favorable and further field-testing appears to be warranted.

Strigol Precursors and Fragments

Pepperman et al (14) prepared and tested 30 strigol precursors, analogs, and fragments for germination stimulation activity in witchweed. Seven of these compounds were A-ring precursors, of which four were active. The data for the active compounds are summarized in Table 4 (Insert Table 4), and the structures are given in Figure 6

TABLE 3
GERMINATION STIMULATION ACTIVITY OF A TWO-RING ANALOG OF STRIGOL, GR-5 (**8**)

SPECIES	ACTIVITY % germination at concentration	REFERENCE
Striga asiatica	56% at 10^{-8} M 61% at 10^{-7} M 86% at 10^{-6} M 86% at 10^{-6} or 10^{-5} M	(29) (14) (14) (27)
Striga hermonthica	56-70% at 10^{-7} to 10^{-5} M	(29)
Orobanche aegyptica	70-80% over a range of 10^{-9} to 10^{-6} M	(29)
Orobanche crenata	52% at 10^{-6} M	(29)
Alectra vogelii	Inactive	(23)
Alectra orobanchoides	>50% over a range of 10^{-8} to 10^{-3} M	(23)
Capsella bursa-pastoris	60-80% at 10^{-4} to 10^{-3} M	(24)
Lactuca sativa Grand Rapids cv.	temperature stressed (28°C) 17% higher than control at 10^{-6} M	(25)
Great Lakes cv.	10-25% at 10^{-10} to 10^{-6} M	(25)

TABLE 4
WITCHWEED GERMINATION STIMULANT ACTIVITY OF STRIGOL PRECURSORS AND FRAGMENTS

COMPOUND #	% GERMINATION
11	55 at 10^{-7} M
12	60 at 10^{-9} M
13a	70 at 10^{-10} M 60 at 10^{-11} M
13b	50 at 10^{-4} M
14	40 at 10^{-9} M
15c	72-76 at 10^{-10} and 10^{-9} M a)
15f	60 at 10^{-5} M

a) Johnson et al. reported 25-50% germination at 10^{-6} to 10^{-3} M against O. ramosa for **15a** and **15c** (11).

(Insert Figure 6). The activity of **13a** was comparable to the activity of strigol. Alpha-cyclocitral, **12**, was only slightly less active than **13a**. Unfortunately, **13a** is unstable, readily oxidizing in air to the acid, **13b**, which is only moderately active. Oxidation of **12** also occurs readily. The facile oxidation of **12** and **13a** precludes any practical application in the field. Some of the A-ring and AB-ring precursors have also been found to be active in germination studies with Orobanche ramosa (34). Earlier observations by Johnson et al indicated that the bis-lactone structure (2-RAS) was the minimum structural requirement for activity against Striga species (11), but the work on strigol precursors (14), indicates the importance of the A-ring as a factor in strigol's activity. Brooks has prepared some analogs containing the A- and D-rings connected by open-chain bridges and the results are reported elsewhere in this volume.

Of seven D-ring precursors tested with witchweed (Insert Figure 7), the ethyl derivative, **15c**, showed significant germination activity at 10^{-10} and 10^{-9} M concentration. Two others, 3-methyl-2-furoic acid, **14**, and the dimeric compound, **15**, showed moderate levels of germination activity (see Table 4); 40% at 10^{-9} M and 60% at 10^{-5} M respectively (14). Johnson et al (29) observed no significant effect on S. hermonthica with **15a c**, and **e** but moderate activity on O. aegyptica for **15a** and **15c**. Johnson et al (11) also reported moderate activity for the same two compounds against O. ramosa. Vail et al (35) found that both **15c** and the oxybisfuranone, **15f**, were active as germination stimulants in Striga asiatica and Orobanche ramosa.

Evaluation of twelve butenolides (Pepperman, A. B. and Bradow, J. M., manuscript in preparation) as germination regulators for 26 weed and crop seeds, showed a small amount of activity. Eleven monocots tested against all 12 compounds showed only 16 significant responses, most of which were inhibitory. Stimulation of non-dormant Lolium perenne and Sorghum bicolor and of dormant Bromus secalinus was observed with **15a**. Seventeen dicots (three varieties of lettuce) tested with the same 12 compounds gave about 50 significant responses, of which the majority were inhibitory. Dormant Lactuca sativa (both light-sensitive and light insensitive), Amaranthus palmeri, and Amaranthus retroflexus were particularly sensitive to the butenolides, being inhibited or stimulated by the majority of the test compounds. In this same study, some of the butenolides were assayed against S. asiatica, and shown to be effective. In particular, the allyloxy derivative (**15h**) gave 40-60% germination over the range of 10^{-7} 10^{-10} M. The sec-butoxy derivative (**15g**) was moderately active (20-40% germination) at 10^{-5} to 10^{-9} M. Menetrez, however, obtained greater than 80% germination at 10^{-5} to 10^{-6} M for **15g** (27). The dimer (**15f**), the 3-RAS (**6**), and the 2-RAS (**8**) all gave >80% germination at 10^{-5} and 10^{-6} M in Menetrez's work. The 3-RAS and 2-RAS both gave about 50% germination at 10^{-8} M (27). Menetrez also noted significant interaction between the pregermination incubation period and pregermination temperature; with 14 days incubation and temperatures above 28°C affording the highest germination percentages. A more complex but significant interaction was observed between the analog used and the length of the germination period. Other researchers have recognized and pointed

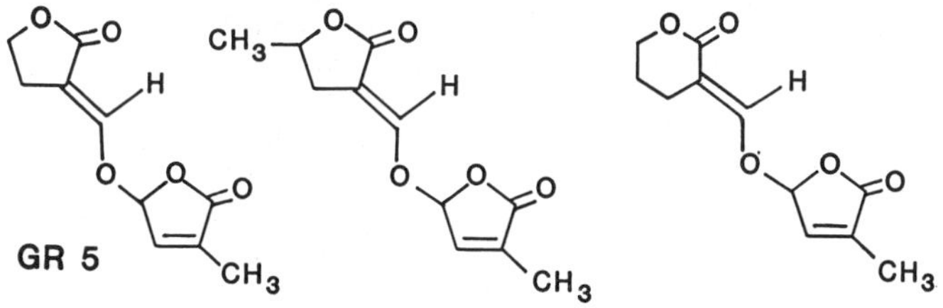

8 9 10

Figure 5 -- Structures of two-ring analogs of strigol (2-RAS).

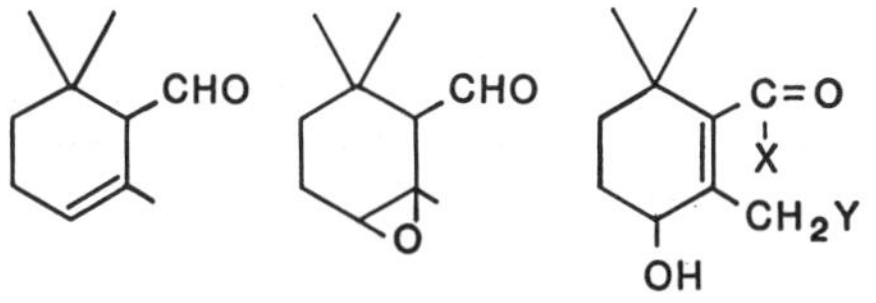

11 12 13

a, X=Y=H
b, X=OH, Y=H
c, $X=OCH_3$, Y=H
d, $X=OCH_3$, Y=Br

Figure 6 -- Structures of A-ring precursors of strigol.

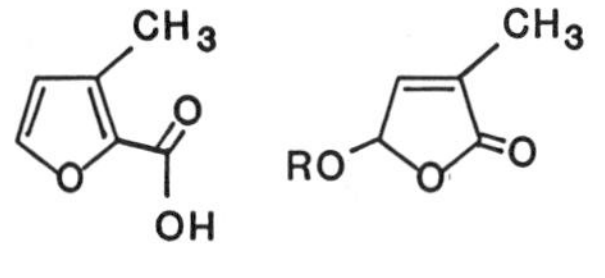

14 15

a, R=H
b, $R=CH_3$
c, $R=CH_3CH_2$
d, $R=CH_3CH_2CH_2$
e, $R=(CH_3)_3\,CH$
f, R = 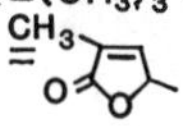
g, $R=CH_3CH_2CH(CH_3)$
h, $R=CH_2=CHCH_2$
i, $R=CH_3(CH_2)_{10}CH_2$
j, $R=CH_3CH(CH_3)CH_2$
k, R =
l, R = -CH_2

Figure 7 -- Structures of D-ring precursors of strigol.

out the variables and difficulties involved with witchweed seed germination bioassays; citing effects of length of the incubation period, temperature during the incubation period, method of pretreatment of seed, fungal contamination, and exposure to the stimulant before completion of the preconditioning period (13,14,27,36). The differences in activity observed by different groups may be attributed to variations in one or more of these parameters. Similar problems have been documented in *Striga hermonthica* bioassays (37).

Field Tests of Analogs

A limited amount of data on field-testing of strigol analogs has been reported, primarily involving GR-7 and GR-24. GR-7 was reported to be stable when incorporated in dry soil and to decompose slowly in wet soil (38). It was concluded that GR-7 was satisfactory for controlled stimulation of *S. hermonthica* in the African savanna.

Eplee and coworkers (16) found that both GR-7 and GR-24 gave approximately 50% witchweed seed germination as far down as 22.5 cm in the soil, when surface applied. Surface application was more effective than pre-plant incorporation, probably due to microbial breakdown. The same group also studied residual activity of GR-7, GR-24, and strigol, finding moderate to high activity after 7 days, (about 70% for GR-7 and strigol, 43% for GR-24). After 14 days, activity dropped off dramatically to 20% for GR-7, and about 38% for strigol and GR-24. After 28 days, none of the compounds caused any significant germination (17). Under the conditions required for conditioning of witchweed seed, the soil life of GR-7, GR-24, and strigol appears to be about 7-10 days.

Ogborn observed that the analogs are most effective when applied at the start of the rains since they diffuse slowly downwards behind the wetting front. Lateral diffusion is minimal so the analogs must be broadcast over the whole soil surface. Significantly profitable crop increases resulted when the analogs were properly applied. In this same study, there was no evidence that GR-7 was active as a germination stimulant for *Striga gesneroides* (39).

Field results indicate a diminished activity when strigol and its analogs are applied to soil, especially alkaline soils, due to soil bonding and/or degradation or microbial attack (16, 17, 37-39). Factors affecting the activity of strigol and its analogs in soil are pH, moisture at the time of application, soil type, physiological status of seeds at the time of application, and amount of rainfall in the first 7-10 days after application. Since witchweed seeds must undergo an after-ripening period and preconditioning period before responding to the germination stimulant, timing is a critical factor in any evaluation of germination stimulants (36). The presence of the stimulant during the preconditioning period has a deleterious effect on the number of seeds germinated (13), further emphasizing the importance of the time of application.

Other Biological Activity

Several of the butenolides (**15b, c, d, e, h, i, j, k, l**) were tested in a broad screen bioassay for fungicidal, herbicidal, and insecticidal activity. Only one compound, the lauryl butenolide (**15i**) showed any herbicidal activity, giving complete control of barnyardgrass. Other weeds in the test were morningglory, cocklebur, velvetleaf, nutsedge, crabgrass, cheatgrass, and wild oats (Pepperman, A. B. unpublished data). Insecticidal activity was demonstrated by all of the butenolides tested, at low to moderate levels, against one or more insects including fall armyworm, tobacco budworm, boll weevil, two-spotted spidermite, and aster leafhopper. Fungicidal activity of the butenolides was also at a low to moderate level but all of the butenolides showed some activity against one or more plant diseases such as broad-bean botrytis, peanut late leaf spot, apple scab, wheat powdery mildew, rice blast, and grape downy mildew. Further work will be required to assess the insecticidal and fungicidal potential of the butenolides.

In some ongoing work, several of the butenolides (**15f, i, j, k, l,**) were shown to be growth inhibitory in a wheat coleoptile bioassay (Cutler, H. G., and Pepperman, A. B. unpublished results). The activity was greatest at 10^{-3} M but some of the compounds retained part of their activity at 10^{-4} M. The simple alkyl butenolides, **15c, e,** and **g,** were inactive. Strigol was inactive but its epimer, epistrigol, had growth inhibitory activity at both 10^{-3} and 10^{-4} M concentrations indicating the stereochemical sensitivity of the growth regulator bioassay. Cassady and Howie (40) prepared a 2-RAS derivative with a 5-methyl group instead of a 3-methyl group and found it had cytotoxic activity against *Hela* cells.

Conclusions

Cook predicted that strigol and related compounds might be representative of a new class of plant hormones (2). While this prediction may not have been borne out, strigol and its analogs have demonstrated biological activity in a variety of systems. Activity at hormonal concentrations has been demonstrated in the germination of parasitic weeds of the *Striga*, *Orobanche*, and *Alectra* species. In addition, some of the analogs show either germination stimulation or inhibition at millimolar concentrations in various weed and/or crop seeds. Growth inhibition of wheat coleoptiles was observed for some D-ring strigol precursors and a moderate level of fungicidal and insecticidal activity was found for the same type of compounds. Sufficiently large quantities of the analogs must be prepared for proper field evaluation and identification of the most active and stable compounds for use in eradication of parasitic weeds. Evaluation of strigol and related compounds for other types of biological activity appears to be a promising area for future research.

Literature Cited

1. Cook, C. E.; Whichard, L. P.; Turner, B.; Wall, M. E.; Egley, G. H. Science 1966, 154, 1189-90.
2. Cook, C. E.; Whichard, L. P.; Wall, M. E.; Egley, G. H.; Coggon, P.; Luhan, P. A.; McPhail, A. T. J. Am. Chem. Soc. 1972, 94, 6198-99.
3. Heather, J. B.; Mittal, R. S. D.; Sih, C. J. J. Am. Chem. Soc. 1974, 96, 1976-77.
4. Heather, J. B.; Mittal, R. S. D.; Sih, C. J. J. Am. Chem. Soc. 1976, 98, 3661-69.
5. MacAlpine, G. A.; Raphael, R. A.; Shaw, A.; Taylor, A. W.; Wild, H. J. J. Chem. Soc., Chem. Commun. 1974, 834-35.
6. MacAlpine, G. A.; Raphael, R. A.; Shaw, A.; Taylor, A. W.; Wild, H. J. J. Chem. Soc., Perkin Trans. I, 1976, 410-16.
7. Shaw, W. C.; Shepherd, D. R.; Robinson, E. L.; Sand, P. F. Weeds 1962, 10, 182-92.
8. Saunders, A. R. Union of South Africa Dep. Agric. Sci. Bull. 1933, No. 128, 56 pp.
9. Brown, R. Nature 1945, 155, 455-56.
10. Eplee, R. E. Weed Science 1975, 23, 433-36.
11. Johnson, A. W.; Rosebery, G.; Parker, C. Weed Res. 1976, 16, 223-27.
12. Chang, M.; Netzly, D.H.; Butler, L.G.; Lynn, D.G. J. Am. Chem. Soc. 1986, 108, 7858-60.
13. Hsiao, A. I.; Worsham, A. D.; Moreland, D. E. Weed Science 1981, 29, 101-4.
14. Pepperman, A. B.; Connick, W. J. Jr.; Vail, S. L.; Worsham, A. D.; Pavlista, A. D.; Moreland, D. E. Weed Science 1982, 30, 561-66.
15. Hsiao, A. I.; Worsham, A. D.; Moreland, D. E. Weed Science 1983, 31, 763-65.
16. Eplee, R. E.; Harris, C. E.; Norris, R. S.; Nance, J. G. Ann. Rep. Witchweed Lab., U. S. Dept. of Agric., Animal and Plant Health Insp. Service, Plant Protection and Quarantine Program, 1981, pp. 22-27.
17. Eplee, R. E.; Harris, C. E.; Norris, R. S.; Nance, J. G. Ibid, 1982, p. 41.
18. Nickrent, D. L.; Musselman, L. J.; Riopel, J. L.; Eplee, R. E. Ann. Bot. 1979, 43, 233-36.
19. Lynn, D. G.; Steffens, J. C.; Kamat, V. S.; Graden, D. W.; Shabanowitz, J.; Riopel, J. L. J. Am. Chem. Soc. 1981, 103, 1868.
20. Kamat, V. S.; Graden, D. W.; Lynn, D. G.; Steffens, J. C.; Riopel, J. L. Tetrahedron Lett., 1982, 23, 1541.
21. Steffens, J. C.; Lynn, D. G.; Kamat, V. S.; Riopel, J. L. Ann. Bot. 1982, 50, 1.
22. Spelce, D. L.; Musselman, L. J., Z. Pflanzenphysiol., 1981, BD104, 281-83.
23. Visser, J. H.; Johnson, A. W. S. Afr. J. Bot. 1982, 1, 75-6.
24. Bradow, J. M. Weed Science 1985, 34, 1-7.
25. Pepperman, A. B.; Connick, W. J.; Bradow, J. M. 1983, Abstract 208, 23rd Annual Mtg. of Weed Science Society of America, St. Louis, Mo.

26. Johnson, A. W.; Gowda, G.; Hassanali, A.; Knox, J.; Monaco, S.; Razavi, Z.; Rosebery, G. J. Chem. Soc., Perkin I, 1981, 1734-43.
27. Menetrez, M. E. PhD. Thesis, North Carolina State University, Raleigh, North Carolina, 1985.
28. Kendall, P. M.; Johnson, J. V.; Cook, C. E. J. Org. Chem., 1979, 44, 1421-24.
29. Johnson, A. W.; Rosebery, G. U. S. Patent 4,002,459. 1977.
30. Stevens, R. A.; Eplee, R. E. Proc. 2nd Symp. On Parasitic Weeds, 1979, p. 211.
31. Ismail, A. M. A. Phytomorphology 1982, 32, 241-45.
32. Connick, W. J., Jr.; Pepperman, A. B. J. Agric. Food Chem. 1981, 29, 984-86.
33. Hassanali, A. In Striga: Biology and Control; Ayensu, E. S.; Doggett, H.; Keynes, K. D.; Marton-Lefevre, J.; Musselman, L. J.; Parker, C.; Peckering, A. Ed. ICSU Press, Paris, 1984; pp. 125-132.
34. Vail, S. L.; Blanchard, E. J.; Dailey, O. D.; Riopel, J. L. 1986, Abstract 185, 26th Annual Mtg. of Weed Science Society of America, Houston, Texas
35 Vail, S. L.; Pepperman, A. B.; Connick, W. J.; Riopel, J. L. 1985, Abstract 223, 25th Annual Mtg. of Weed Science Society of America, Seattle, Wash.
36. Musselman, L. J. Ann. Rev. Phytopathol. 1980, 18, 463-89.
37. Babiker, A. G. T.; Hamdoun, A. M. Weed Research, 1982, 22, 111-115.
38. Ogborn, J. E. A.; Mansfield, R. A. Proc. 2nd Symp. on Parasitic Weeds, 1979, p. 298, Raleigh, N. C.
39. Ogborn, J. E. A. Ibid. p. 308.
40. Cassady, J. M.; Howie, G. A. J. Chem. Soc., Chem. Commun. 1974, 512-13.

RECEIVED May 12, 1987

Author Index

Affiliation Index

Subject Index

A

B

C

G

H

I

Production and indexing by Colleen P. Stamm
Jacket design by Carla L. Clemens

Elements typeset by Hot Type Ltd., Washington, DC
Printed and bound by Maple Press Co., York, PA

Recent Books

Personal Computers for Scientists: A Byte at a Time
By Glenn I. Ouchi
276 pp; clothbound; ISBN 0–8412–1000–4

The ACS Style Guide: A Manual for Authors and Editors
Edited by Janet S. Dodd
264 pp; clothbound; ISBN 0–8412–0917–0

Silent Spring Revisited
Edited by Gino J. Marco, Robert M. Hollingworth, and William Durham
214 pp; clothbound; ISBN 0–8412–0980–4

Chemical Demonstrations: A Sourcebook for Teachers
By Lee R. Summerlin and James L. Ealy, Jr.
192 pp; spiral bound; ISBN 0–8412–0923–5

Phosphorus Chemistry in Everyday Living, Second Edition
By Arthur D. F. Toy and Edward N. Walsh
362 pp; clothbound; ISBN 0–8412–1002–0

Pharmacokinetics: Processes and Mathematics
By Peter G. Welling
ACS Monograph 185; 290 pp; ISBN 0–8412–0967–7

Chemistry of High-Temperature Superconductors
Edited by David L. Nelson, M. Stanley Whittingham, and Thomas F. George
ACS Symposium Series 351; 329 pp; 0–8412–1431–X

Reversible Polymeric Gels and Related Systems
Edited by Paul S. Russo
ACS Symposium Series 350; 292 pp; 0–8412–1415–8

The Chemistry of Acid Rain
Edited by Russell W. Johnson and Glen E. Gordon
ACS Symposium Series 349; 337 pp; 0–8412–1414–X

Sources and Fates of Aquatic Pollutants
Edited by Ronald A. Hites and S. J. Eisenreich
Advances in Chemistry Series 216; 558 pp; ISBN 0–8412–0983–9

Nucleophilicity
Edited by J. Milton Harris and Samuel P. McManus
Advances in Chemistry Series 215; 494 pp; ISBN 0–8412–0952–9

For further information and a free catalog of ACS books, contact:
American Chemical Society
Distribution Office, Department 225
1155 16th Street, NW, Washington, DC 20036
Telephone 800-227-5558